Liver Imaging
CURRENT TRENDS AND
NEW TECHNIQUES

Contents

Preface and Acknowledgments xi

Contributing Authors xiii

I. OVERVIEW

1. Liver Tumor Imaging: Issues for the 1990s	J. T. Ferrucci	1
2. Principles of Hepatic Lesion Detection by MRI and CT	D. D. Stark	19

II. LESION DETECTION BY MRI AND CT: TECHNIQUES AND RESULTS

3. Hepatic CT: Techniques, Applications, and Results	P. C. Freeny	28
4. Hepatic Imaging Using High-Field MRI	W. D. Foley	39
5. Midfield MRI of the Liver	D. D. Stark	49
6. Ultralow-Field MRI of the Liver	R. F. Thoeni	58

III. LESION DETECTION BY MRI AND CT: COMPARATIVE STUDIES

7. Hepatic Lesions Detected by MRI and CT Comparative Studies: The National Institutes of Health Experience	J. A. Frank, A. J. Dwyer, D. L. Miller, and J. W. Reinig	64

8. Emory Experience With Both CT and MRI in the Detection of Focal Liver Disease	M. E. Bernardino	73

IV. SPECIAL MRI TECHNIQUES FOR LIVER LESION IMAGING

9. STIR MRI of the Liver	W. P. Shuman, A. A. Moss, and R. L. Baron	82
10. Chemical-Shift Imaging of the Liver	J. K. T. Lee	91
11. Steady-State MRI of the Liver	S. E. Harms, D. P. Flamig, and K. A. Glastad	96

V. FAST IMAGING

12. Fast-Scan MRI of the Abdomen	J. Frahm	105
13. Ultrafast MRI of the Liver	S. Saini and M. S. Cohen	114
14. MRI Fluoroscopy: Applications of Ultrashort TR Real-Time MRI	S. J. Riederer	119
15. Magnetization-Prepared Rapid Gradient-Echo (MP-RAGE) MRI	E. E. de Lange, J. P. Mugler III, and J. R. Brookeman	128

VI. TISSUE CHARACTERIZATION: PRIMARY AND SECONDARY MALIGNANCY

16. Radiologic-Pathologic Correlation in Liver Tumors	P. R. Ros	137
17. MRI of Hepatic Metastatic Disease	J. Wittenberg	153
18. Hepatocellular Carcinoma: CT and MRI	K. Ohtomo, Y. Itai, and Y. Sasaki	162
19. Differentiation of Malignant Liver Tumors by Subsecond Dynamic CT	R. Langer, M. Langer, C. Zwicker, F. Astinet, and R. Felix	170

VII. TISSUE CHARACTERIZATION: BENIGN TUMORS

20. Benign Tumors of the Liver	D. Mathieu and E. S. Zafrani	177
21. CT and MRI of Hepatic Cavernous Hemangiomas	S. Saini	190
22. Hepatic Hemangiomas: A Comparison of 99^mTc-Labeled Red Blood Cell SPECT and MRI for Definitive Diagnosis	B. A. Birnbaum and J. C. Weinreb	201

23. *Color Doppler Flow Mapping of Liver Tumors*	L. Bolondi, S. Gaiani, S. Li Bassi, G. Benzi, G. Zironi, V. Santi, A. Rigamonti, and L. Barbara	209
24. *Hepatic Cavernous Hemangioma: Diagnosis by Means of Rapid Dynamic Nonincremental CT*	J. Gaa and S. Saini	212

VIII. STAGING LIVER TUMORS FOR THERAPEUTIC INTERVENTION

25. *Principles of Hepatic Surgery*	R. A. Malt	217
26. *Hepatic and Portal Venous Anatomy in Cross-Sectional Imaging for Hepatic Resections*	D. A. Turner, T. A. S. Matalon, A. Doolas, and B. Silver	223
27. *Staging Liver Tumors for Therapeutic Intervention: Determination of Resectability by CT-Angiography*	R. C. Nelson	237
28. *Intraoperative Ultrasonography of Liver*	J. F. Simeone	247
29. *Application of a Three-Dimensional Workstation to Liver Tumor Volumetrics*	M. A. Goldberg, P. F. Hahn, D. D. Stark, and J. T. Ferrucci	256

IX. HEPATIC VASCULAR DISEASES

30. *Imaging of the Budd-Chiari Syndrome*	P. F. Hahn and E. K. Yucel	260
31. *Portal Hypertension: Doppler US Flow Imaging*	L. Barbara, L. Bolondi, S. Gaiani, S. Li Bassi, G. Zironi, and G. Benzi	269
32. *Magnetic Resonance Angiography (MRA) of the Hepatic Vein and Portal System*	Y. Yuasa and K. Hiramatsu	277
33. *Radiology of Liver Transplantation: Complications and Interventions*	M. P. Federle and W. L. Campbell	283

X. SPECTROSCOPY

34. *Magnetic Resonance Spectroscopy of the Liver: A Review*	D. J. Meyerhoff and M. W. Weiner	289
35. *Metabolic Liver Disease Observed Through MRS: Hepatic Encephalopathy*	B. D. Ross	298

XI. DIFFUSE LIVER DISEASES

36. Hepatitis, Fatty Liver, and Cirrhosis	Y. Itai and K. Ohtomo	306
37. Iron Storage Diseases	J. P. Kaltwasser, U. Straube, and R. Gottschalk	313

XII. PHARMACEUTICAL DEVELOPMENT

38. Principles for Design of Liver Contrast Agents	D. D. Stark	326

XIII. NONSPECIFIC AGENTS

39. Gadolinium-DTPA: Lesion Detection and Differential Diagnosis	M. Laniado, M. Skalej, H. Bongers, and G. Kölbel	340
40. Gd-DOTA: Chemistry, Toxicity, and Clinical Results	B. Bonnemain, A. C. Neiss, D. Doucet, S. Beauté, and D. Meyer	349
41. Dynamic Gadolinium-DTPA–Enhanced MRI of the Liver Using the RASE Technique	S. A. Mirowitz and J. K. T. Lee	358

XIV. BILIARY AGENTS

42. Hepatobiliary Agents for MRI: Rationale and Preliminary Evaluation	R. B. Lauffer	365
43. Hepatobiliary Contrast Agents: An Overview of the Development of Manganese Dipyridoxyl Diphosphate (Mn-DPDP)	S. M. Rocklage and M. VanWagoner	374
44. Hepatobiliary Contrast Agents for MRI	F. Cavagna, P. Tirone, E. Felder, and C. de Haën	384

XV. PARTICULATES

45. Particulate Biodegradable Contrast Medium for CT of the Liver	T. Gjøen, E. Holtz, P. Strande, J. Klaveness, P. Leander, and A. Berg	394
46. Ferrite Particles: Rationale and Clinical Results (Midfield)	J. T. Ferrucci	403
47. Iron Oxide: High-Field MRI Clinical Results	G. Marchal, P. Van Hecke, P. Demaerel, E. Decrop, and A. L. Baert	415

48. *Superparamagnetic Starch Microspheres: A Reticuloendothelial MRI Contrast Agent* A. K. Fahlvik, E. Holtz, and J. Klaveness *425*

Index *431*

Preface

Few physicians would dispute the dramatic impact ultrasonography, computed tomography (CT), and magnetic resonance imaging (MRI) have had on the clinical diagnosis and therapy of liver diseases over the last several years. It is now taken for granted that in modern, well-equipped radiologic facilities these noninvasive "body imaging" methods can routinely disclose difficult-to-diagnose entities such as subcentimeter metastases, Budd-Chiari syndrome, regenerating nodules, traumatic lacerations, and hemosiderosis, to name a few.

Most physicians would agree that there will be even more and better technological advances in the field of imaging. Fast and ultrafast CT and MRI scanning, color flow Doppler ultrasonography, three-dimensional computer-aided imaging, liver-specific CT and MRI contrast agents, and MRI spectroscopy are among the newer techniques to be applied to the liver. These all promise anatomic, physiologic, and metabolic data that will greatly extend accuracy and safety in clinical diagnosis. Moreover, quantitative measurements of the liver's various cellular and biochemical functions should become almost commonplace.

This volume summarizes the recent past and probes the immediate future of the technologically and clinically demanding field of liver imaging. It has been assembled from presentations at an International Symposium on Liver Imaging held in late June 1990 in Boston, under the auspices of the Department of Radiology and the Liver-Biliary-Pancreas Center of the Massachusetts General Hospital and the Division of Continuing Medical Education of the Harvard Medical School. During the three-day meeting, over 200 registrants received presentations from some 50 invited speakers, heard 25 original proffered scientific papers, and viewed technical exhibits by commercial firms. Twelve different countries were represented by the various speakers.

A principal scientific focus of this volume and the symposium is the interface between technologic innovations and their application to clinical imaging. Thus, contributions by engineers, physicists, and biochemists are intermingled with those of diagnostic radiologists. We believe that we have identified the key issues and outlined the agenda for liver imaging research and clinical development in the decade of the 1990s.

In a more practical vein, we also recognize that the goal of optimal current clinical performance remains foremost. For the practitioner of body, abdominal, or gastrointestinal imaging there are descriptions of current optimized liver scanning techniques, evolving interpretive criteria, and new pathologic-radiologic insights by experts from all over the world.

In modern medical centers, disorders of the liver increasingly are managed by effective new medical and surgical techniques. Patients with seemingly advanced neoplastic and nonneoplastic conditions are now candidates for a variety of lifesaving interventions. Tomorrow's abdominal radiologists will have an increasingly important role in the evaluation and care of such patients. We hope that this volume will facilitate their contributions.

Joseph T. Ferrucci, M.D.
David D. Stark, M.D.

Acknowledgments

The editors gratefully acknowledge the many collaborating faculty and authors whose pioneering scientific work constitutes the important substance of this volume. We hope they gained knowledge by participating in the symposium just as we did in organizing their contributions for publication.

Further, we especially thank our secretaries, Lynda Bessette, Andrea Kallas, Mary de Alderete, and Paula De Long, whose energy and dedication proved so essential to a timely conclusion of the work.

Special Acknowledgment

Although the content of this volume is derived directly from the symposium presentations, it cannot convey the value of the contributions made by our special Guest Moderators. We therefore particularly thank these individuals, all distinguished professors, for lending their presence and radiologic expertise to ensure a productive scientific exchange.

They are listed, in alphabetical order, with our sincerest gratitude.

Prof. R. Felix, M.D.
Berlin, Germany

Prof. M. Lüning, M.D.
Berlin, Germany

Prof. R. Passariello, M.D.
L'Aquila, Italy

Prof. C. S. Pedrosa, M.D.
Madrid, Spain

Prof. P. Sheedy, M.D.
Rochester, Minnesota

Prof. N. Vasile, M.D.
Paris, France

Prof. K. J. Wolf, M.D.
Berlin, Germany

Contributing Authors

Luigi Barbara, M.D.
First Medical Clinic
University of Bologna
Bologna, Italy

Arne Berg, Ph.D.
Hafslund Nycomed A.S.
Oslo, Norway

Michael E. Bernardino, M.D.
Department of Radiology
Emory University
School of Medicine
Atlanta, Georga

Bernard A. Birnbaum, M.D.
Department of Radiology
New York University Medical Center
New York, New York

Luigi Bolondi, M.D.
First Medical Clinic
University of Bologna
Bologna, Italy

Bruno Bonnemain, Ph.D.
Laboratoire Guerbet
Aulnay-sous-Bois, France

William L. Campbell, M.D.
Department of Radiology
University of Pittsburgh
Pittsburgh, Pennsylvania

Friedrich Cavagna, Ph.D.
Bracco Industria Chimica
Milan, Italy

Eduard E. de Lange, M.D.
Department of Radiology
University of Virginia
Charlottesville, Virginia

Michael P. Federle, M.D.
Department of Radiology
University of Pittsburgh
Pittsburgh, Pennsylvania

Joseph T. Ferrucci, M.D.
Department of Radiology
Massachusetts General Hospital
Boston, Massachusetts

W. Dennis Foley, M.D.
Department of Radiology
Medical College of Wisconsin
Milwaukee, Wisconsin

Jens Frahm, Ph.D.
Max Planck Institute
Göttingen, West Germany

Joseph A. Frank, M.D.
National Institutes of Health
Bethesda, Maryland

Patrick C. Freeny, M.D.
Department of Radiology
Virginia Mason Clinic
Seattle, Washington

Jochen Gaa, M.D.
Department of Radiology
Municipal Hospital
Darmstadt, West Germany

Mark A. Goldberg, M.D.
Department of Radiology
Massachusetts General Hospital
Boston, Massachusetts

Peter F. Hahn, M.D., Ph.D.
Department of Radiology
Massachusetts General Hospital
Boston, Massachusetts

Steven E. Harms, M.D.
Department of Radiology
Baylor University Medical Center
Dallas, Texas

Eckart Holtz, Ph.D.
Hafslund Nycomed A.S.
Oslo, Norway

Yuji Itai, M.D.
Department of Radiology
University of Tokyo
Tokyo, Japan

J. P. Kaltwasser, M.D.
Department of Internal Medicine
J. W. Goethe University
Frankfurt am Main, West Germany

Jo Klaveness, Ph.D.
Hafslund Nycomed A.S.
Oslo, Norway

Ruth Langer, M.D.
Department of Radiology
Free University of Berlin
West Berlin, West Germany

Michael Laniado, M.D.
Department of Radiology
Eberhard Karls University
Tübingen, West Germany

Randall B. Lauffer, M.D.
Department of Radiology
Massachusetts General Hospital
Boston, Massachusetts

Joseph K. T. Lee, M.D.
Mallinckrodt Institute of Radiology
Washington University Medical Center
St. Louis, Missouri

Ronald A. Malt, M.D.
Department of Surgery
Massachusetts General Hospital
Boston, Massachusetts

Guy Marchal, M.D.
Department of Radiology
University Hospitals
Leuven, Belgium

Terence A. S. Matalon, M.D.
Department of Radiology
Rush-Presbyterian St. Luke's Medical Center
Chicago, Illinois

Didier Mathieu, M.D.
Department of Radiology
Hopital Henri Mondor
Paris, France

Dieter J. Meyerhoff, Ph.D.
Department of Medicine
University of California
San Francisco, California

Scott A. Mirowitz, M.D.
Mallinckrodt Institute of Radiology
Washington University Medical Center
St. Louis, Missouri

Albert A. Moss, M.D.
Department of Radiology
University of Washington Medical Center
Seattle, Washington

Rendon C. Nelson, M.D.
Department of Radiology
Emory University
School of Medicine
Atlanta, Georgia

Kuni Ohtomo, M.D.
Department of Radiology
University of Tokyo
Tokyo, Japan

John F. Palmer, M.D.
Division of Oncology and
Radiopharmaceutical Drug Products
Food and Drug Administration
Rockville, Maryland

Stephen J. Riederer, Ph.D.
Department of Radiology
Mayo Clinic
Rochester, Minnesota

Scott M. Rocklage, Ph.D.
Salutar, Inc.
Sunnyvale, California

Pablo R. Ros, M.D.
Department of Radiology
University of Florida College of Medicine
Gainesville, Florida

Brian D. Ross, M.D., Ph.D.
Huntington Medical Research Institutes
Pasadena, California

Sanjay Saini, M.D.
Department of Radiology
Massachusetts General Hospital
Boston, Massachusetts

Joseph F. Simeone, M.D.
Department of Radiology
Massachusetts General Hospital
Boston, Massachusetts

David D. Stark, M.D.
Department of Radiology
Massachusetts General Hospital
Boston, Massachusetts

Ruedi F. Thoeni, M.D.
Department of Radiology
University of California
San Francisco, California

Michael W. Weiner, M.D.
Department of Radiology
University of California
San Francisco, California

Jeffrey C. Weinreb, M.D.
Department of Radiology
New York University Medical Center
New York, New York

Jack Wittenberg, M.D.
Department of Radiology
Massachusetts General Hospital
Boston, Massachusetts

Gerald L. Wolf, M.D., Ph.D.
Department of Radiology
Massachusetts General Hospital
Boston, Massachusetts

Yuji Yuasa, M.D.
Department of Radiology
Keio University
Tokyo, Japan

E. Kent Yucel, M.D.
Department of Radiology
Massachusetts General Hospital
Boston, Massachusetts

Liver Imaging
CURRENT TRENDS AND
NEW TECHNIQUES

I. OVERVIEW

1

Liver Tumor Imaging: Issues for the 1990s

JOSEPH T. FERRUCCI

What issues will interest radiologists dealing with suspected liver tumor patients during the next decade? How will emerging new imaging technologies affect overall accuracy of radiologic diagnosis? Which techniques will flourish? Which will fade? What pathologic-radiologic insights will evolve? The answer will come, at least in part, from ongoing developments in several different areas.

First, recent advances in computed tomography (CT), sonography, and magnetic resonance imaging (MRI) have vastly improved assessment of liver neoplasms just as they have benefited detection of abnormalities in other organs. Liver tumor nodules are now routinely discovered at small size thresholds (millimeters), and in most cases, mass lesions can be characterized with high reliability.

Second, hepatic surgeons now view the patient with primary liver cancer or metastases from colorectal carcinoma as a possible long-term survivor not an end-stage victim. In such cases, precise anatomic descriptions of the number and segmental location of neoplastic deposits are required. Hence radiologic staging of malignant hepatic tumors has become a common clinical task.

Third, commercial manufacturers from the United States, Europe, and Asia are introducing prototype imaging techniques and contrast agents with exceptional potential for liver applications.

New CT and MRI systems can gather data in subsecond intervals, display regional organ perfusion, and provide images formatted in multiple planes. Novel pharmaceuticals specifically targeted both to the hepatic reticuloendothelial system (RES) and to biliary excretion functions provide order of magnitude increases in tissue-tumor contrast.

The power and commitment of resources exemplified by these technical and clinical developments ensures major further advances in clinical imaging of patients with suspected liver cancer. This chapter offers an overview and personal reflections on some of these trends. It was written well before the date of the symposium to preserve whatever originality is possible, and an effort has been made not to preempt the contributions of others.

CLINICAL CONSIDERATIONS
Surgical Advances
In 1989, it was estimated that nearly 150,000 new cases of colorectal carcinoma would be diagnosed in the United States (1). Of these, some 40 percent, or 60,000 patients, will ultimately prove to have liver metastases. Worldwide, primary hepatocellular carcinoma (HCC) is an endemic disorder in many underdeveloped countries; in southeast Asia and sub-Saharan Africa, HCC accounts for

one-third of all malignant neoplasms. Considered globally, primary and secondary liver cancers affect literally millions of persons each year.

Among the most significant therapeutic advances in the management of HCC and colorectal liver metastases is the continued evolution of aggressive surgical techniques (2–7). Techniques for bloodless dissection through the hepatic parenchyma have diminished operative morbidity and mortality, while serial carcinoembryonic antigen assays can lead to the discovery of silent deposits before they grow too large to resect (4,5). It is now estimated that as many as one-fourth of all primary and secondary liver cancers are potentially resectable for cure. In the United States alone, approximately 7000 patients a year with colorectal liver metastases are estimated to be potential candidates for hepatic resection (4,5). When resections have been carried out in patients with three or fewer colon deposits, 20 to 40 percent 5-year survival rates have been obtained in both single-institution and cooperative studies (2,4). Similar favorable results also have been recorded with metastases from visceral sarcomas and endocrine tumors. Moreover, innovative nonoperative techniques for local tumor ablation such as intraoperative cryosurgery, transarterial chemoembolotherapy, and fine-needle intralesion alcohol sclerosis may improve these results further (6).

The Hepatic Substrate

Radiologic assessment of liver tumor suspects is commonly complicated by the coexistence of other abnormalities in the substrate of the liver parenchyma. These may be focal or diffuse, neoplastic or metabolic, and related or unrelated to the neoplasm being evaluated.

Cavernous hemangiomas are so often displayed on T2-weighted MRI images as 5 to 10-mm bright dots as to become a serious confounding nuisance to clinical interpretation (Fig. 1-1). Their prevalence has been traditionally estimated at 5 to 7 percent. However, a recent Finnish study of medicolegal autopsies in 95 men found cavernous hemangiomas in 20 percent of subjects, although the mean size was less than 1.0 cm (8). They are often multiple and may, of course, coexist with metastatic deposits. Thus, when multiple, discrete masses occur, each must be characterized individually. Moreover, hemangiomas have been demonstrated to enlarge with time, and they often develop a central fibrocollagenous scar when over 5.0 cm in diameter, which may give atypical hypovascular filling patterns on CT, radionuclide blood pool scans, and angiography (9–11).

Fatty metamorphosis of the liver appears commonly during the course of malignant disease and may occur as diffuse change or focal deposits. Both patterns cause diagnostic problems and often require correlation of several imaging techniques to resolve. A diffusely fatty liver lowers the attenuation of normal hepatic parenchyma on CT and may cause metastatic deposits to appear isodense and thus obscured. Alternatively, focal areas of normal liver may be spared of fat and retain their normal higher CT density and thus simulate metastatic deposits. In both cases, normal or hyperechoic texture on sonography and normal photon distribution on sulfur colloid scintigraphy are usually diagnostic. Focal deposits of fat also may appear as sharply defined low-density areas simulating metastases on CT (Fig. 1-2). These can enlarge on serial scans simulating disease progression. Focal fatty deposits usually display geographic wedge or pyramidal shapes on CT and leave vessels intact, but again, typical echogenic areas on sonograms and normal scintigraphic findings are confirmatory (12).

Liver fat has not been a major interpretative problem on MRI because conventional spin echo sequences are relatively insensitive to intrahepatic fat content. However, chemical-shift proton spectroscopic imaging sequences are highly sensitive to fat-water proton differences, and so-called phase-contrast techniques show both high contrast between tumor (bright) and fatty liver (dark), giving high cancer detection rates (13). Moreover, in occasional cases where focal fat deposits are suggested by short T1 bright signal areas, the presence of fat can be confirmed as the area becomes dark on a chemical-shift sequence (13).

Regenerating nodules occurring in hepatic cirrhosis may be difficult to differentiate from early or "minimal" hepatocellular carcinoma. They are usually small, 1 to 2 cm in diameter, multiple, and appear hypoechoic on sonography and of high density on CT. Itai et al. (14) found regenerating nodules particularly often shown by MRI as numerous low-intensity areas on T2-weighted images

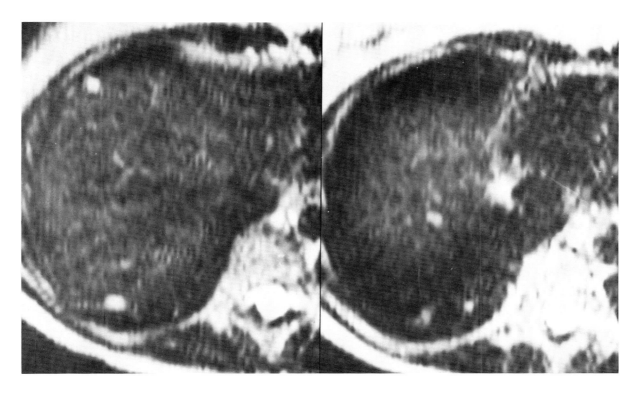

FIGURE 1-1

Incidental hemangiomas? Heavily T2-weighted MRI images of the liver at adjacent levels show five subcentimeter nodules in an adult patient undergoing pretreatment evaluation for lung cancer. Signal brightness is suggestive of hemangiomas (or benign cysts), but lesions are too small to characterize further by other imaging techniques or percutaneous needle biopsy. Management of these millimeter-size "nuisance nodules" is effectively limited to interval follow-up scans.

even when both sonographic and CT findings were normal. They were readily differentiated from hepatomas, which consistently appeared of high signal intensity. Recent pathologic studies of resected specimens have shown hemosiderin deposits in these nodules believed to account for the low MRI signal owing to magnetic susceptibility effects (15).

Tasks of Liver Imaging

Imaging evaluation of liver cancer should be recognized as having several clinically distinct tasks Table 1-1. These are (1) global patient detection, i.e., Does the patient's liver contain tumor deposits? (2) individual lesion detection, i.e., How many lesions are there? (3) individual lesion characterization, i.e., What is the nature of the masses seen? and (4) staging for question of resectability, i.e., If cancerous, is the patient's disease treatable by local measures?

In clinical practice, these functions are rarely confused, although they may not be necessarily performed in every case. In certain instances, a decision as to global status of the patient (cancerous liver or not) suffices; in others, more detailed lesion-by-lesion analysis is sought. Seltzer and Holman (16) have thoughtfully discussed the increasingly important distinctions between global patient diagnosis and lesion-by-lesion diagnosis when comparing techniques. For example, hepatic imaging for staging breast cancer is quickly concluded when a typical positive scan is obtained, whereas patients with colorectal carcinoma often

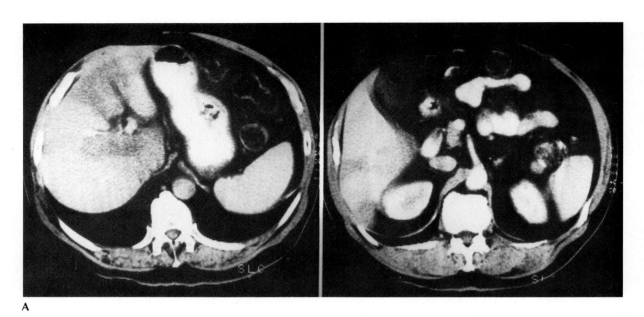

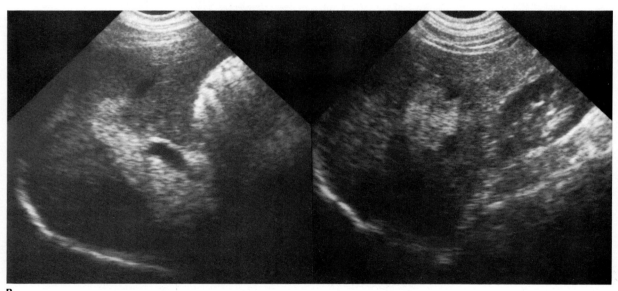

FIGURE 1-2
Focal fat in a patient undergoing chemotherapy for breast cancer. (A) CT scans show multiple discrete low attenuation areas. Occasionally these can simulate metastastic deposits. In this case, geometric wedge shape and peripheral location are strongly suggestive of fat. (B) Sonograms show hyperechoic zones confirmatory of focal fat.

TABLE 1-1. *Tasks of Imaging*

Patient detection
Lesion detection
Lesion characterization
Staging

require more thorough assessment and differential diagnosis of individual lesions because of the possibility of curative surgical extirpation.

However, research publications on liver imaging sometimes blur these sequential tasks. Emphasis has often been directed toward the performance of a technique in terms of sensitivity for lesion detection, with all lesions displayed assumed to be cancerous. The magnitude and significance of the overlap error with incidental benign cysts and hemangiomas are rarely addressed. This will become a more widely recognized issue in the future.

SCREENING AND STAGING

In a 1982 review of hepatic metastasectomy for colon cancer, Marvin Adson, the pioneering liver surgeon from the Mayo Clinic, noted that among the major factors limiting success of surgical approaches was inadequate staging by radiologic imaging techniques (7). Failures occurred both because small lesions went undetected and because operative excision sometimes removed more tissue than was necessary. In the ensuing decade, fundamental advances in imaging technology have greatly improved the diagnosis of liver cancer, largely answering Adson's lament. In addition, even for patients with unresectable disease, more accurate assessments of tumor burden have improved efforts to monitor response to treatment.

Anatomy
Radiologic staging of liver cancer, either primary or metastatic, defines (1) the extent and location of intrahepatic disease, (2) the involvement of surgically critical areas (porta hepatis, inferior vena cava, major bile ducts), and (3) the presence of extrahepatic disease. In institutions where curative hepatic resections or other percutaneous locoregional cancer therapy is available, staging assessments tend to become an automatic feature of most routine CT scan and MRI interpretations.

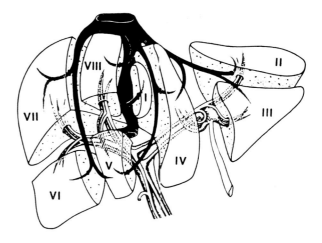

FIGURE 1-3
Segmental surgical anatomy of liver according to French anatomists Couinaud and Bismuth. Eight segments are conceptualized in relation to three major hepatic veins and are numbered in counterclockwise fashion with roman numerals. (From H. Bismuth, Surgical anatomy and anatomical surgery of the liver, World Surg. 6:3, 1982. Reprinted with permission of Springer-Verlag.)

The critical surgical anatomy of the liver is based not on external attachments or lobar landmarks, but on the internal vascular skeleton of the liver (3-5). The French surgical anatomists Couinaud (17) and Bismuth (18) popularized an eight-segment partition based principally on the position of the three major hepatic veins (right, middle, left) (Fig. 1-3). From these somewhat imaginary boundaries, simple and extended multisegmental resections can be fashioned to remove up to 80 percent of liver parenchyma (2-7). Thus, in colorectal metastases, curative resections are feasible for up to four deposits, provided they can be encompassed in a contiguous (multisegmental) en bloc excision (Fig. 1-4). Whenever possible, subsegmental or wedge excisions are employed even though liver parenchyma possesses considerable regenerative potential. By the same token, tumors located centrally with involvement of the portal vein or inferior vena cava are less likely to be resectable (Fig. 1-5).

Further, there is the concept of "surgical" versus "medical" categories for therapy of liver metastases (3). This refers to the likelihood that hepatic secondary deposits from certain primary tumors such as adenocarcinoma of the colon and

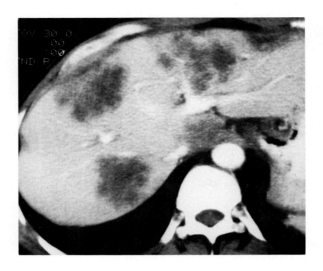

FIGURE 1-4
Dynamic bolus-enhanced CT scan shows metastases from colonic carcinoma considered unresectable because of number (five) and distribution in noncontiguous segments.

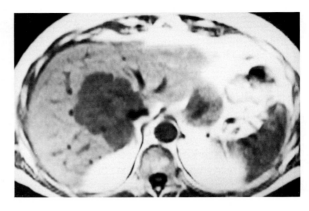

FIGURE 1-5
T1-weighted MRI image shows solitary metastasis from colonic carcinoma considered unresectable because of central location relative to middle and right hepatic veins and inferior vena cava. Central necrosis is also evident.

visceral sarcomas are often few in number, discretely marginated, and might be amenable to local surgical resection or other extirpative procedures, whereas metastases from primary sites such as the breast and pancreas are more often widespread throughout the liver and therefore are generally only amenable to medical management (Fig. 1-6). In the latter group of patients, the only requirement of imaging in order to make treatment decisions is often a simple binary "liver positive" or "liver normal" choice.

Imaging Techniques
At present, some of the historical controversy about which of the many available techniques to use in what circumstance is abating. Table 1-2 shows the various techniques grouped according to their current roles in liver tumor imaging, i.e., screening, staging, and special situations.

Imaging techniques for screening must be generally noninvasive, quickly performed, show high sensitivity for lesion detection at low size thresholds, and have high accuracy in differentiating incidental benign masses from malignant neoplasms. Both CT and MRI fulfill these criteria, provided optimal examination techniques are used. Although CT has been the acknowledged gold standard for liver tumor imaging, it must be performed with dynamic incremental bolus techniques to achieve superior results (19,20). For MRI techniques, both heavily T1- and T2-weighted sequences are required to ensure high detection rates and accurate tissue characterization (21,22). Motion-suppression techniques are generally required as well.

Conventional sonography often discloses hepatic tumor nodules during upper abdominal scanning for abdominal pain, palpable mass, or jaundice. However, its overall false-negative rate for liver metastases exceeds 50 percent, images are not easily reproducible for comparative purposes, and differential diagnosis between benign and malignant nodules is often impossible. Thus sonography is rarely used as a primary screening or surveillance technique in centers where CT and MRI are available.

Imaging the liver for purposes of tumor staging involves more detailed delineation of the anatomic relation of neoplastic deposits to segmental anatomy and to critical anatomic structures such as portal and hepatic veins, inferior vena cava, and major bile ducts. Obtaining this degree of anatomic information frequently requires the greater detail of CT during arterial portography (CTAP) or intraoperative sonography (IOS). The likelihood of obtaining tumor-free margins and

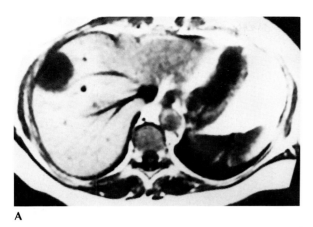 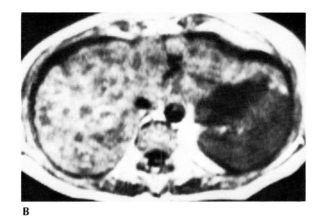

FIGURE 1-6
"Surgical" versus "medical" metastatic disease. (A) "Surgical" deposit. T1-weighted MRI image shows a solitary discrete secondary deposit in area of segment VIII. Lesion was excised. (B) "Medical" deposits. T1-weighted MRI image shows innumerable foci of metastatic disease from primary tumor in breast. Hormonal therapy was used.

TABLE 1-2. *Role of Imaging Techniques for Liver Tumor Assessment*

Screening	Staging	Special Situations
Computed tomography (CT)	Computed tomography with arterial portography (CTAP)	Radionuclide scintigraphy (RN)
and/or	or	
Magnetic resonance imaging (MRI)	Intraoperative ultrasound (IOUS)	Hepatic angiography (HA)

the relative risks of anatomic right and left lobe resection, segmental resection, or multisegmentectomy can thus be weighed. On occasion, good-quality MRI results may provide sufficient information to make specific management decisions concerning surgical approaches. The principal question, however, is whether an apparently free segment of the right and left lobe is in fact uninvolved, permitting the obviously involved segments to be excised.

Scintigraphy and hepatic angiography now play only limited specialized roles. Scintigraphy is occasionally used to facilitate the differential diagnosis of problematic suspected primary liver tumors. Hepatic angiography is generally reserved for problem cases where the differential diagnosis remains in doubt or in patients in whom documentation of arterial anatomy is required for preoperative mapping of the vascular supply.

Invasiveness versus Sensitivity
Clinical comparisons of imaging techniques must consider the degree of invasiveness. Intuitively, the most sensitive tests for detecting liver lesions are often the most invasive. A screening test applied to large numbers of people, many of whom will have no disease, must be a less hazardous study than might be used for detailed anatomic tumor mapping before open hepatic resection. The two principal techniques used for staging, CTAP and IOS, give high lesion detection rates but do involve some risk.

CTAP requires superior mesenteric artery catheterization for administration of contrast material immediately before CT scanning (23–24). Intense hepatic staining resulting from the high dose of iodine directly delivered to the liver and the recording of the highly sensitive CT attenuation values during the portal phase is an extremely accurate method for detecting small liver deposits. Using CTAP, Matsui et al. (23) found 10 of 18 individual colon metastases of less than 15 mm that were not shown by CT, sonography, or angiography (Fig. 1-7). Heiken et al. (24) showed

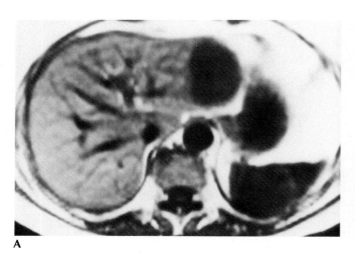
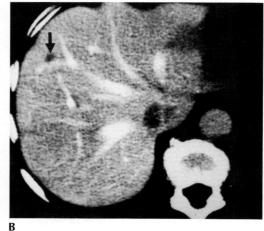

FIGURE 1-7
High sensitivity of CT during arterial portography (CTAP) for lesion detection. (A) Screening MRI image (T1-weighted) shows apparently solitary metastatic deposit replacing lateral portion of left lobe. No other lesions are apparent. (B) CTAP shows a single additional 0.6-cm deposit in peripheral portion of right lobe (arrow). *Surgical excision showed a malignant focus (micrometastasis).*

more than twice as many metastatic deposits with CTAP (81 percent detected) than with standard CT (38 percent detected). Similar results were recorded by Nelson et al. (25). The technique is therefore particularly useful to clear apparently "uninvolved" segments of the liver on screening CT scans or MRI before surgical resection of obvious disease. Unfortunately, CTAP is marred by a high false-positive rate due to laminar flow perfusion defects in up to 30 to 40 percent of cases (26–28). However, such defects can usually be recognized by a typical wedgelike shape and peripheral location. Moreover, the ability of CTAP to provide differential diagnostic information on newly discovered small nodules is uncertain.

IOS is an alternative method for staging that gives superb high-resolution images of subcentimeter liver nodules that may not be palpable to the operating surgeon's fingers (Fig. 1-8). The technique requires excellent cooperation between the surgeon and the sonographer but prolongs the intraoperative manipulation. Estimates of the utility of the procedure vary greatly among operators in different institutions (29,30). I agree with the general assessment of Sugarbaker (5) that when there is high-quality preoperative imaging, the results of IOS tend to be less critical.

Lesion Threshold: The Subcentimeter Nodule
An integral related issue is the question of the threshold size for the ability to both detect and discriminate the nature of liver mass lesions. Until recently, demonstration of metastatic lesions of 1.0 cm in diameter was the best that could be expected with conventional CT, and 30 to 50 percent of individual lesions went undetected (23–25). On the contrary, high-quality MRI techniques frequently display subcentimeter nodules, both benign and malignant, accounting for the greater sensitivity in lesion detection reported from several centers (21,36–38). Moreover, in several series, CTAP has outperformed conventional CT and MRI by an order of magnitude for detection of lesions less than 1.0 cm (23–25,30).

This higher sensitivity for detection of subcentimeter nodules has created the new and daunting problem of characterizing lesions that are usually too small to exhibit distinctive morphologic features. In fact, few authors have addressed the performance of any technique at distinguishing the nature of these tiny subcentimeter nodules (Fig. 1-9). In the only specific study of this problem to date, Brick et al. (31), using conventional CT, were not able to differentiate benign hepatic cysts from solid metastases accurately at

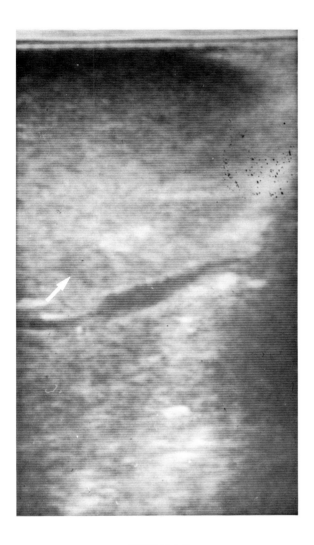

FIGURE 1-8
Intraoperative sonography. Image of left hepatic lobe shows a 1.0-cm metastatic nodule (arrow) above left hepatic vein. Lesion was not evident on preoperative imaging and was not palpable to surgeon. However, in this case, identification of this specific nodule did not alter extent of planned excision.

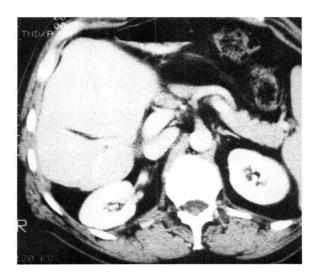

FIGURE 1-9
Conundrum of subcentimeter nodule. Bolus-enhanced CT scan of residual left hepatic lobe after trisegmental resection of right lobe for metastatic colonic cancer. Left lobe has migrated and hypertrophied. A 0.5-cm nodule is clearly displayed in medial segment of left lobe (arrow), but its nature cannot be ascertained because of its small size.

the 1.0-cm level because of partial volume effects. The ultimate solution to assessing the nature of the millimeter-size "dot" now so commonly seen on CT or MRI liver scan remains to be found. For the present, only interval follow-up serial scanning is practical.

CT VERSUS MRI

Several general comments on the CT versus MRI issue are warranted at the outset. Opinions of the comparative merits of CT and MRI for liver tumor imaging have spanned the full spectrum. Thus various reports have concluded that CT remains the gold standard (32), that the results of the two methods are comparable (33–35), and that MRI supercedes CT already (21,36–38). Experienced observers also recognize that the type of CT and MRI equipment available, scanning methods used, and special expertise of the professionals involved greatly influence outcomes and undoubtedly account for the divergent results (39). Moreover, multicenter clinical trials are often disappointing because grouped results often dilute the best efforts and the usual long duration of such studies tends to lag technologic and interpretive refinements. It is also useful to acknowledge that a single liver imaging study may not yield a correct or complete diagnosis under the best of circumstances and it is often critical to integrate the results of multiple imaging studies.

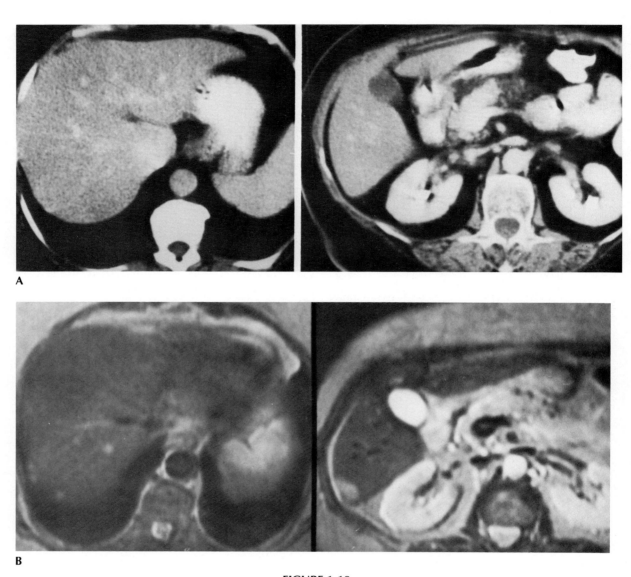

FIGURE 1-10
Superiority of MRI for lesion detection. (A) Two images from a contrast-enhanced CT scan. No lesions are seen. (B) Same sections on T2-weighted MRI scan showing four subcentimeter lesions on cephalad image and a single 2.5-cm lesion on caudad slice.

Notwithstanding these factors, certain elements of current clinical experience with MRI disclose real limitations of CT in terms of sensitivity for lesion detection, differential diagnosis, and invasiveness. As previously noted, several groups have recorded greater sensitivity for lesion detection by MRI (21,36–38) (Fig. 1-10). This may be explained by the inherently greater image contrast in MRI as well as the slice-gap errors of CT when small nodules are present. Spin echo signal-averaged MRI techniques effectively cover the entire liver with high contrast even for subcentimeter nodules (21). Moreover, in two studies the specificity (false-positive rate) also was more favorable with MRI (21,38). This too is an important concern when imaging studies are used for screening. In the best reported CT series, Freeny et al. (40) reported an 85 percent sensitivity for

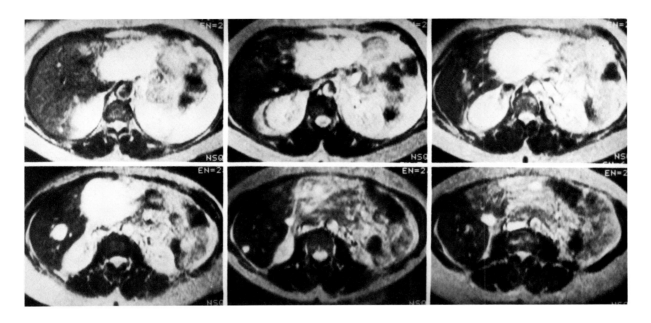

FIGURE 1-11
T2-weighted MRI images show multiple cavernous hemangiomas, with a dominant lesion in left lobe and six to seven smaller nodules scattered throughout right lobe. In patients with suspected metastatic disease and multiple lesions, each nodule must be analyzed individually for optimal patient care. This patient had a palpable liver and normal liver function tests. Based on results of imaging studies, which were considered typical for hemangioma, no further intervention was carried out.

detecting the presence of liver metastases and a 60 percent sensitivity when individual lesion detection was considered. However, the CT technique required to achieve these results is quite demanding, requiring dynamic bolus contrast media injection with power injectors and rapid table incrementation during infusion of contrast material. This allows images to be made during the first 2 minutes after contrast administration (perfusion phase of contrast distribution), during which there is high contrast differential between tumor tissue and normal liver. If images are obtained after equilibrium distribution of contrast material into the interstitial compartment of the liver (2 to 5 minutes), lesions may become isointense with hepatic parenchyma and obscured (41). Moreover, in patients whose primary tumor tends to produce hypervascular liver metastases (islet cell, renal, melanoma), an unenhanced scan should be obtained because 25 percent of cases will be hypervascular and thus isointense, giving false-negative results (42).

Hemangioma is a particularly difficult problem for CT, and no discussion of the two techniques can have clinical relevance unless assessments of metastases and hemangiomas are considered concurrently. Unfortunately, both metastases and hemangiomas may be multiple, may coexist independently, and may be clinically occult (Figs. 1-11 and 1-12). For proper treatment of patients, it is often necessary to analyze each detected liver nodule individually.

In this context, there are three problems with CT in the evaluation of cavernous hemangioma. First, the criteria for differentiation from metastases are typical in no more than 55 percent of cases (44). Even when a typical pattern is present in a patient with a known primary neoplasm, the probability that it represents hemangioma is only 86 percent (43). Second, in many cases, delayed scanning up to 30 minutes after administration of contrast material is required to confirm the typical peripheral centripetal filling sequence. This can represent a throughput problem. Third, because

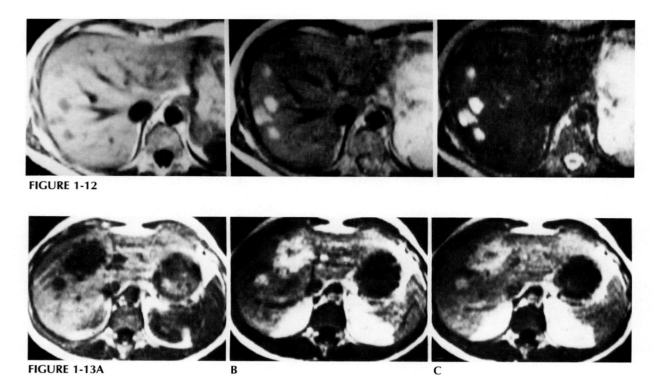

FIGURE 1-12
Another case of multiple hemangiomas in a patient with known retroperitoneal metastases from seminoma. These lesions were stable over a 3-year period. T1-weighted (left), mildly (center), and heavily (right) T2-weighted MRI images.

FIGURE 1-13
Dynamic Gd-DTPA perfusion study for cavernous hemangiomas. Two adjacent hemangiomas in right hepatic lobe surgically proven. Fast SE (225/13, two excitations) spin echo MRI images with IV injection of Gd-DTPA (0.1 μmol/kg of body weight). Before (A), 3 minutes after (B), and 5 minutes after (C) injection. Both lesions show marked and persistent signal enhancement. Dominant lesion shows an area of central scar formation.

of the temporal nature of the diagnostic filling pattern, it is often difficult to assess multiple lesions at different CT slice levels. Hence other studies such as radionuclide blood pool scanning, percutaneous needle biopsy, or MRI are often required. MRI, obviously, shows multiple lesions at multiple slice levels with no need for additional or delayed imaging.

Conversely MRI has shown better than 85 percent accuracy in differentiating hemangiomas and metastases at various field strengths (38,44–46). Heavily T2-weighted spin echo images with TEs greater than 100 ms effectively display the long T2 bright signal typical of slowly flowing blood. A homogeneous "lightbulb" pattern is seen morphologically, while quantitatively the resulting high contrast-to-noise ratio accurately differentiates hemangiomas from metastases (44–46).

More recently, fast MRI with gadolinium has effectively displayed the slow perfusion patterns of hemangioma analogous to contrast-enhanced CT scans (47–52). (Fig. 1-13). Several different dynamic MRI techniques have been used, including fast spin echo and gradient echo methods. All have succeeded in furthering the distinction between hemangiomas and primary and secondary malignant tumors and add a further criterion to the differential diagnosis for problem cases. There is a final advantage of MRI over CT. The inherent dependence of CT on iodinated contrast material for lesion detection and characterization is an additional argument in favor of MRI. It is increasingly difficult to dismiss the risk (high osmolar) or cost (low osmolar) of iodinated contrast media when making judgments about the overall relative desirability of CT versus MRI (53).

An important contrary balancing argument for CT has been its undisputed greater accuracy for displaying extrahepatic diseases such as pancreatic, adrenal, or retroperitoneal pathology (21). The prospect that MRI bowel contrast agents might address this concern has yet to be fulfilled. However, no study has ever compared the clinical impact of trading off accuracy in diagnosing intrahepatic versus extrahepatic disease with either MRI or CT. In the patient with colorectal carcinoma, it may be justifiable to use MRI and forego detail in the retroperitoneum to ensure accuracy within the liver, where there is greater risk of disease as well as a greater risk to the patient's welfare if a diagnostic error occurs. Given the new ultrafast CT and MRI scanning methods and liver-specific contrast agents under development for both, the debate as to which technique is better for liver tumor imaging will no doubt continue for years.

HEPATOCELLULAR CARCINOMA (HCC)

Radiologic evaluation of HCC involves several further specific issues in addition to the general discussion of screening/staging liver cancer given earlier. HCC usually arises as a complication of liver cirrhosis, making initial recognition and differentiation from a regenerative nodule more difficult and limiting the number of patients who can tolerate surgical resection. Only patients with small (3 to 4 cm) encapsulated tumors and well-compensated liver function become candidates for tumor excision (54). However, actuarial survival rates among such patients approach 90 percent at 3 years. Thus recognition of the so-called minimal HCC is an important imaging challenge.

HCC also tends to be a highly aggressive tumor in terms of its local extension; invasion of veins and bile ducts, tendency for arteriovenous shunting, and formation of daughter nodules are common occurrences. Most can be demonstrated radiologically and have obvious implications for setting boundaries of contemplated surgical resection.

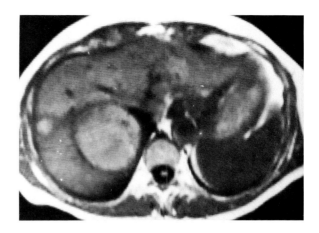

FIGURE 1-14
Hepatocellular carcinoma of right lobe. Typical features are often shown on T1-weighted MRI, as in this case. These include high central signal due to steatosis, low signal capsule, and a 1.5-cm daughter nodule.

Diagnostically, CT scanning following Lipiodol (an iodinated oil, Laboratoire Guerbet, France) injected by means of a catheter placed in the hepatic artery can show subcentimeter HCC lesions, both primary and daughter nodules. However, this technique is presently used only in the Far East. Lipiodol gelatin sponge particles loaded with antitumor drugs also have proved an effective chemotherapeutic method for unresectable lesions (6).

MRI also has proven highly sensitive in the detection, differential diagnosis, and staging of HCC. It is able to recognize the frequent low-signal-intensity capsule, central fatty degeneration, vascular invasion, and daughter nodules that characterize this tumor (Figs. 1-14 and 1-15). Unlike MRI techniques for differentiating metastases from hemangiomas, which rely on T2-weighted sequences, HCC is best characterized by T1-weighted sequences because they provide clear depiction of fat, capsule, and venous involvement (55). More recently, dynamic MRI with gadolinium has been able to confirm the faster flow in HCC as opposed to the stagnant flow in hemangiomas, adding another useful criterion for differential diagnosis (47–52). As in the instance of metastatic liver disease, the powerful diagnostic capabilities of MRI now allow it to rival or exceed CT as a primary liver imaging technique for hepatocellular carcinoma.

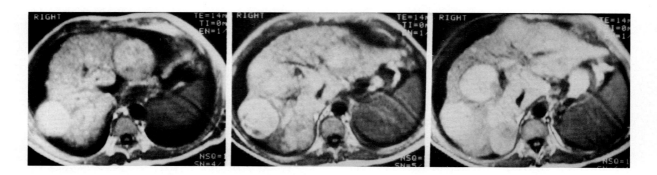

FIGURE 1-15
Multifocal nodular hepatocellular carcinoma with typical features on T1-weighted MRI image. Three adjacent sections. Discrete encapsulated nodules with central high signal due to intralesional fat are highly suggestive morphologic MRI features of hepatoma.

TISSUE CHARACTERIZATION

As is evident from the foregoing, improved accuracy in differential diagnosis (tissue characterization) has been a dominant theme in the development of clinical liver tumor imaging in recent years. As is well known, metastases, hemangiomas, and hepatomas constitute the "big three" categories of liver masses. Whether CT or MRI is used, the parameters for clinical differentiation are (1) signal intensity (contrast-to-noise) values, (2) morphologic architecture features, and (3) hemodynamic perfusion patterns. Although contrast enhanced CT has had an indisputable role, MRI has contributed more by virtue of its inherently richer image contrast. Moreover, scintigraphy adds a unique special dimension for identification and characterization of primary liver tumors. Notwithstanding, tissue characterization of liver masses remains a complex challenge, and tissue sampling by needle or open surgical biopsy is frequently required.

MRI signal intensity ratios have been widely utilized to differentiate hemangiomas from metastases. As initially described by Stark et al. (22), a high signal on late T2-weighted spin echo images typifies hemangiomas as opposed to metastases. For purposes of clinical interpretation, visual comparisons between lesion signal intensity and CSF are substituted for more onerous quantitative measurements.

The abundant morphologic architectural information displayed on both T1- and T2-weighted MRI images also affords reliable differential diagnostic features. In addition to the typical bright "lightbulb" appearance of hemangiomas, Wittenberg et al. (56) also described bright peritumoral edema halo effects and central liquefaction necrosis associated with metastatic deposits. Rummeny et al. (57) documented a high prevalence and diagnostic value of central scar formation as a specific sign of primary liver neoplasms (Fig. 1-16). Ebara et al. (58) described typical MRI morphologic features of hepatocellular carcinoma to include a central high signal area due to steatosis, a low signal peripheral capsule, and daughter nodules. Hahn et al. (59) drew attention to MRI ring phenomena surrounding liver masses usually due to edema, hemorrhage, or fibrosis.

Scintigraphy also plays a unique, albeit limited, role in liver tumor characterization, namely, identification of specific primary liver neoplasms, i.e., hemangioma, focal nodular hyperplasia and hepatic adenoma/hepatoma. The condition suspected is confirmed by the scintigram scan specific for the entity, as shown in Table 1-3. For each condition, a positive photon uptake confirms the suspected diagnosis, although false-negative results occur in all entities. However, use of scintigraphy for liver tumor characterization has declined as the superb capabilities of MRI for liver tumor characterization have been defined.

An interesting new development involves the potential of a variety of different techniques to exploit hemokinetic data for differential diagnosis

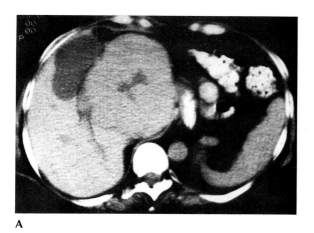 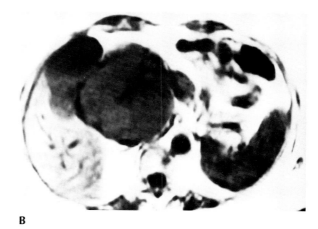

FIGURE 1-16
CT scan (A) and T1-weighted MRI image (B) show central tumor scar. This is a reliable sign that a liver tumor is a primary hepatic neoplasm. However, scars are not specific for any one type of tumor because they occur in adenoma, focal nodular hyperplasia, cavernous hemangioma, and hepatoma. Surgical excision disclosed a hepatic adenoma with foci of hepatocellular carcinoma.

TABLE 1-3. *Scintigraphic Techniques for Characterizing Primary Liver Tumors*

Condition	Radionuclide	Imaging Technique
Cavernous hemangioma	^{99m}Tc	RBC-labeled blood pool scan
Focal nodular hyperplasia	^{99m}Tc	Sulfur colloid and/or HIDA scan
Hepatic adenoma/ hepatoma	^{67}Ga	Citrate scan

TABLE 1-4. *Techniques Using Perfusion Data for Differential Diagnosis*

Computed tomography with iodinated contrast medium
RBC-labeled blood pool scintigraphy
MRI with gadolinium
MRI with iron oxide
Color Doppler flow mapping

(Table 1-4). RBC-labeled scintigraphy displays the slowly flowing blood pool of hemangiomas and accurately distinguishes them from hepatomas and metastases (60). Color Doppler sonographic flow mapping has been found by Tanaka et al. (61) to give a typical network vascular pattern in hepatomas as opposed to metastases (detour pattern) and hemangiomas (dot pattern). MRI contrast enhancement using fast scanning gadolinium was described earlier (47–52). More recently, Hahn et al. (62) found superparamagnetic iron oxide particles to show greater uptake and consequent greater signal loss in hemangiomas than in malignant tumors. Nearly all these methods will most likely undergo further refinement before their ultimate clinical role is clear, but useful information is already being provided.

FUTURE DIRECTIONS

What are likely developments in the next decade? The immediate future will be dominated by exploration of liver applications for fast and ultrafast CT (cine) as well as breathhold and millisecond

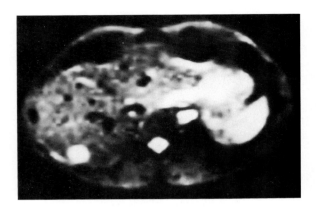

FIGURE 1-17
"Snapshot" ultrafast T2-weighted MRI image showing a hemangioma of the right hepatic lobe. This image was obtained with a modified echo-planar technique in 1/25 s on a 2.0-Tesla advanced NMR system.

"snapshot" MRI techniques (63,64). Saini et al. (64) obtained high-resolution T2-weighted MRI images of the liver and abdomen in 1/25 s working with a modified echo-planar technique at 2.0 Tesla (Fig. 1-17). In addition to the obvious potential for increased patient throughput and analysis of cardiac motion with such techniques, studies of organ and tumor perfusion kinetics will continue and command much attention (47–52). Many of these studies will involve novel MRI contrast agents.

Certainly the entire field of tissue-specific liver contrast agent development will absorb vast amounts of research resources. The richness of the hepatic metabolic milieu will allow molecules to be specifically targeted to the reticuloendothelial system, biliary excretory pathways, and hepatocyte enzyme systems. Particulate superparamagnetic iron oxide (ferrite) particles have already been shown to give a threefold increase in MRI lesion conspicuity and detection sensitivity in early clinical trials (65). Reduction in lesion detection size thresholds from 10 to 2 mm also has been shown after ferrite in implanted rat tumor nodules (66,67). Particulate agents for CT such as perfluorooctylbromide (PFOB) also have increased lesion detection rates in phase I and II clinical trials (68,69).

New relationships between contrast agents and imaging system hardware are also emerging in which the special physical effects of each are exploited and synchronized to optimize results. Thus magnetic susceptibility effects of ferrite particles are exaggerated by gradient echo techniques and may ultimately allow lower doses to be used (70). Other imaging hardware and software developments with liver applications already in clear view are ultralow-field MRI systems (0.02 Tesla), MRI spectroscopy, multiplanar CT and MRI (three-dimensional) imaging, and color flow Doppler ultrasonography. Much has been accomplished, but there is much to be done.

REFERENCES

1. American Cancer Society: Cancer Facts and Figures. Washington, DC, American Cancer Society, 1989.
2. Adson MA, Van Heerden JA, Adson MH, et al: Resection of hepatic metastases from colorectal cancer. Arch Surg 119:647, 1984.
3. Malt RA: Current concepts: Surgery for hepatic neoplasms. N Engl J Med 313:1591, 1985.
4. Sugarbaker PH, Kemeny N: Management of metastatic liver cancer. Adv Surg 22:1, 1988.
5. Sugarbaker PH: Surgical decision making for large bowel cancer metastatic to the liver. Radiology 174:621, 1990.
6. Ferrucci JT, Mathieu DG: Advances in Hepato-Biliary Radiology. St. Louis, Mosby, 1990.
7. Adson MA: Walter B. Cannon lecture: Hepatic metastases in perspective. AJR 140:695, 1983.
8. Karhunen PJ: Benign hepatic tumours and tumour-like conditions in men. J Clin Pathol 39:183, 1986.
9. Freeny PC, Marks WM: Hepatic hemangioma: Dynamic bolus CT. AJR 147:711, 1986.
10. Scatarige JC, Kenny JM, Fishman EK, et al: CT of giant cavernous hemangioma. AJR 149:83, 1987.
11. Choi BI, Han MC, Park JH, et al: Giant cavernous hemangioma of the liver: CT and MR imaging in 10 cases. AJR 152:1221, 1989.
12. Alpern MB, Lawson TL, Foley DW, et al: Focal hepatic masses and fatty infiltration detected by enhanced dynamic CT. Radiology 158:45, 1986.
13. Schertz LD, Lee JKT, Heiken JP, et al: Proton spectroscopic imaging (Dixon method) of the liver: Clinical utility. Radiology 173:401, 1989.
14. Itai Y, Ohnishi S, Ohtomo K, et al: Regenerating nodules of liver cirrhosis: MR imaging. Radiology 165:419, 1987.
15. Ohtomo K, Itai Y, Ohtomo Y, et al: Regenerating nodules of liver cirrhosis: MR imaging with pathologic correlation. AJR 154:505, 1990.

16. Seltzer SE, Holman BL: Imaging hepatic metastases from colorectal carcinoma: Identification of candidates for partial hepatectomy. AJR 152:917, 1989.
17. Couinaud C: Le foie: Études anatomiques et chirurgicales. Paris, Masson, 1957, pp 9–12.
18. Bismuth H: Surgical anatomy and anatomical surgery of the liver. World J Surg 6:3, 1982.
19. Foley WD: Dynamic hepatic CT. Radiology 170:617, 1989.
20. Foley WD, Berland LL, Lawson TL: Contrast enhancement technique for dynamic hepatic computed tomographic scanning. Radiology 147:797, 1983.
21. Stark DD, Wittenberg J, Butch RJ, Ferrucci JT: Hepatic metastases: Randomized controlled comparison of detection with MR imaging and CT. Radiology 165:399, 1987.
22. Stark DD, Felder RC, Wittenberg J, et al: Magnetic resonance imaging of cavernous hemangioma of the liver. AJR 145:213, 1985.
23. Matsui O, Takashima T, Kadoya M, et al: Liver metastases from colorectal cancers: Detection with CT during arterial portography. Radiology 165:65, 1987.
24. Heiken JP, Weyman PJ, Lee JKT, et al: Detection of focal hepatic masses: Prospective evaluation with CT, delayed CT, CT during arterial portography, and MR imaging. Radiology 171:47, 1989.
25. Nelson RC, Chezmar JL, Sugarbaker PH, Bernardino ME: Hepatic tumors: Comparison of CT during arterial portography, delayed CT, and MR imaging for preoperative evaluation. Radiology 172:27, 1989.
26. Freeny PC, Marks WM: Hepatic perfusion abnormalities during CT angiography. Radiology 159:685, 1986.
27. Miller DL, Simmons JT, Chang R, et al: Hepatic metastases detection: Comparison of three CT contrast enhancement methods. Radiology 165:785, 1987.
28. van Beers B, Pringot J, Gigot JF, et al: Nontumorous attenuation differences on computed tomographic portography. Gastrointest Radiol 15:107, 1990.
29. Rifkin ND, Rosato FE, Brauck M, et al: Intraoperative ultrasound of the liver: An important adjunctive tool for decision making in the operating room. Ann Surg 205:466, 1987.
30. Hayashi N, Yamamoto K, Tamaki N, et al: Metastatic nodules of hepatocellular carcinoma: Detection with angiography, CT, and US. Radiology 165:61, 1987.
31. Brick SH, Hill MC, Lande IM: The mistaken or indeterminate CT diagnosis of hepatic metastases: The value of sonography. AJR 148:723, 1987.
32. Glazer GM, Aisen AM, Francis IR, et al: Evaluation of focal hepatic masses: A comparative study of MRI and CT. Gastrointest Radiol 10:263, 1986.
33. Heiken JP, Lee JKT, Glazer HS, Ling D: Hepatic metastases studied with MR and CT. Radiology 156:423, 1985.
34. Chezmar JL, Rumancik WM, Megibow AJ, et al: Liver and abdominal screening in patients with cancer: CT vs. MR imaging. Radiology 168:43, 1988.
35. Barakos JA, Goldberg HI, Brown JJ, Gilbert TJ: Comparison of computed tomography and magnetic resonance imaging in the evaluation of focal hepatic lesions. Gastrointest Radiol 15:93, 1990.
36. Reinig JW, Dwyer AJ, Miller DL, et al: Liver metastasis detection: comparative sensitivities of MR imaging and CT scanning. Radiology 162:43, 1987.
37. Ward BA, Miller DL, Frank JA, et al: Prospective evaluation of hepatic imaging studies in the detection of colorectal metastases: Correlation with surgical findings. Surgery 105:180, 1989.
38. Vlachos L, Trakadas S, Gouliamos A, et al: Comparative study between ultrasound, computed tomography, intra-arterial digital subtraction angiography, and magnetic resonance imaging in the differentiation of tumors of the liver. Gastrointest Radiol 15:102, 1990.
39. Bernardino ME: Focal hepatic mass screening. MR imaging or CT scanning? (Editorial). Radiology 162:282, 1987.
40. Freeny PC, Marks WM, Ryan JA, Bolen WJ: Colorectal carcinoma evaluation with CT: Preoperative staging and detection of postoperative recurrence. Radiology 158:347, 1986.
41. Paushter DM, Zeman RK, Scheibler ML, et al: CT evaluation of suspected hepatic metastases: Comparison of techniques for IV contrast enhancement. AJR 152:267, 1989.
42. Bressler EL, Alpern MB, Glazer GM, et al: Hypervascular hepatic metastases: CT evaluation. Radiology 162:49, 1987.
43. Freeny PC, Marks WM: Patterns of contrast enhancement of benign and malignant hepatic neoplasms during bolus dynamic and delayed CT. Radiology 160:613, 1986.
44. Stark DD, Felder RC, Wittenberg J, et al: Magnetic resonance imaging of cavernous hemangioma of the liver: Tissue specific characterization. AJR 145:213, 1985.
45. Glazer GM, Aisen AM, Francis IR, et al: Hepatic cavernous hemangioma: Magnetic resonance imaging. Radiology 155:417, 1985.
46. Itai Y, Ohtomo K, Furui S, et al: Non-invasive diagnosis of small cavernous hemangioma of the liver: Advantage of MRI. AJR 145:1195, 1985.
47. Hamm B, Wolf KJ, Felix R: Conventional and rapid MR imaging of the liver with Gd-DTPA. Radiology 164:313, 1987.

48. Mano I, Yoshida H, Nakabayashi K, et al: Fast spin echo imaging with suspended respiration: Gadolinium enhanced MR imaging of liver tumors. J Comput Assist Tomogr 11:73, 1987.
49. Yoshida H, Itai Y, Ohtomo K, et al: Small hepatocellular carcinoma and cavernous hemangioma: Differentiation with dynamic flash MR imaging with Gd-DTPA. Radiology 171:339, 1989.
50. Laurent F, Drouillard J, Barat JL, et al: Gadolinium-Dota in hepatic tumors: Assessment in dynamic MRI at 0.5 T. Diag Interv Radiol 1:53, 1989.
51. van Beers B, Demeure R, Pringot J, et al: Dynamic spin-echo imaging with Gd-DTPA: Value in the differentiation of hepatic tumors. AJR 154:515, 1990.
52. Edelman RR, Siegel JB, Singer A, et al: Dynamic MR imaging of the liver with Gd-DTPA: Initial clinical results. AJR 153:1213, 1989.
53. Palmer FJ: The RACR survey of intravenous contrast media reactions: Final report. Australas Radiol 32:426, 1988.
54. Okuda K, Ohtsuki T, Obata H, et al: Natural history of hepatocellular carcinoma and prognosis in relation to treatment: Study of 850 patients. Cancer 56:918, 1985.
55. Rummeny E, Weissleder R, Stark DD, et al: Primary liver tumors: Diagnosis by MR imaging. AJR 152:63, 1989.
56. Wittenberg J, Stark DD, Forman BH, et al: Differentiation of hepatic metastases from hemangioma and cysts by MR. AJR 151:79, 1988.
57. Rummeny E, Weissleder R, Sironi S, et al: Central scars in primary liver tumors: MR features, specificity, and pathologic correlation. Radiology 171:323, 1989.
58. Ehara M, Ohto M, Watauabe Y, et al: Diagnosis of small hepatocellular carcinoma: Correlation of MR imaging and tumor histologic studies. Radiology 159:371, 1986.
59. Hahn PF, Stark DD, Saini S, et al: The differential diagnosis of ringed hepatic lesions in MR imaging. AJR 154:287, 1990.
60. Kudo M, Ikekubo K, Yamamoto K, et al: Distinction between hemangioma of the liver and hepatocellular carcinoma: Value of labeled RBC-SPECT scanning. AJR 152:977, 1989.
61. Tanaka S, Kitamura T, Fujita M, et al: Color Doppler flow imaging of liver tumors. AJR 154:509, 1990.
62. Hahn PF, Stark DD, Weissleder R, et al: Clinical application of superparamagnetic iron oxide to MR imaging of tissue perfusion vascular liver tumors. Radiology 1974:361, 1990.
63. Winkler ML, Thoeni RF, Luh N, et al: Hepatic neoplasia: Breath-hold MR imaging. Radiology 170:801, 1989.
64. Saini S, Stark DD, Rzedzian RR, et al: Forty-millisecond MR imaging of the abdomen at 2.0 T. Radiology 173:111, 1989.
65. Stark DD, Weissleder R, Elizondo G, et al: Superparamagnetic iron oxide: Clinical application as a contrast agent for MR imaging of the liver. Radiology 168:297, 1988.
66. Tsang YM, Stark DD, Chen MC, et al: Hepatic micrometases in the rat with ferrite enhanced MR imaging. Radiology 167:21, 1988.
67. Kawamura Y, Endo K, Watanabe Y, et al: Use of magnetite particles as a contrast agent for MR imaging of the liver. Radiology 174:357, 1990.
68. Mattrey RF, Long DM, Mutter F, et al: Perfluorooctylbromide: A reticuloendothelial specific and a tumor imaging agent for computed tomography. Radiology 145:755, 1982.
69. Bruneton JN, Falewée MN, François E, et al: Liver, spleen, and vessels: Preliminary clinical results of CT with perfluorooctylbromide. Radiology 170:179, 1989.
70. Fretz CJ, Elizondo G, Weissleder R, et al: Superparamagnetic iron-oxide enhanced MR imaging: Pulse sequence optimization for detection of liver cancer. Radiology 172:393, 1989.

2

Principles of Hepatic Lesion Detection by MRI and CT

DAVID D. STARK

The detection of focal hepatic lesions is a paradigm for general principles of image analysis by CT and MRI. The normal liver is a large homogeneous organ with simple morphology and relatively predictable vascular anatomy. Cancer nearly always appears and enlarges as a sphere, with few metabolic or morphologic consequences to complicate detection by imaging. Therefore, liver cancer detection by imaging can be modeled and tested more readily than disease processes in other organ systems.

The diagnostic performance of imaging methods is, of course, dependent on the "quality" of the images themselves. While diagnostic performance can be measured using standard statistical methods, such as receiver-operating-characteristics (ROC) analysis (14), "image quality" cannot be reduced to a simple numerical parameter. Although a group of observers can choose to decide which image is "best," subjective judgments are subject to bias, and qualitative information is less useful than quantitative measurements in scientific investigations of technical performance.

SPATIAL RESOLUTION

Early in the development of cross-sectional imaging, CT scans were assessed mainly in terms of spatial resolution and quantum mottle. During the transition from projective radiography to cross-sectional imaging, the common measure of spatial resolution has evolved from line pairs per millimeter to voxel dimensions (slice thickness and pixel area). Spatial resolution is determined by the operator, who selects a matrix (e.g., 128 × 256) and a field of view. For example, using a 40-cm field of view and a 128 × 256 matrix, pixel dimensions will be 3.125 × 1.56 mm.

SIGNAL-TO-NOISE RATIO

Were it possible to produce infinitesimally small voxels, this would, of course, be ideal. However, there is a direct tradeoff between voxel volume and quantum mottle for CT or signal-to-noise ratio (SNR) for magnetic resonance imaging (MRI). Quantum mottle or low SNR is manifested as the *graininess* of an image (Fig. 2-1). For each MRI examination, the radiologist must choose an appropriate field of view and matrix size and utilize acquisition parameters (pulse sequence and imaging time) that yield sufficient SNR for the specific anatomy under study. The relationship between imaging time and SNR is exponential: SNR increases as the square root of imaging time (SNR $\alpha\ t^{-1/2}$). SNR is also a complex function of field strength and system design fixed by choice at the time of equipment purchase (5,11,13,15,21,25).

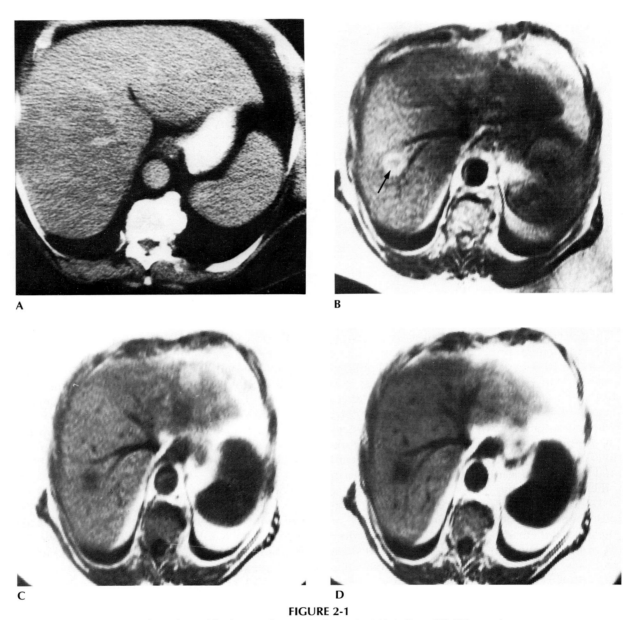

FIGURE 2-1

Imaging in patient with adenocarcinoma of colon metastatic to liver. (A) CT scan shows no lesion. (B) SE 2000/60, four-acquisition (18-min) image shows a single high-intensity metastasis (black arrow) in right hepatic lobe. Because of blurring from respiratory motion, only major hepatic veins are seen. Left lobe of liver is obscured entirely by motion related to cardiac pulsation and overlying ghost artifacts from aortic pulsation. Note ghost artifacts from subcutaneous fat projected outside the patient. Metastasis has increased signal intensity because of long T2 relaxation time relative to surrounding liver tissue (T2-weighted image). (C) Inversion-recovery 1500/15/450 (TR ms/TE ms/TI ms) three-acquisition (10-min) image shows metastasis as a low-signal-intensity region. Because of the use of short TE on this T1-weighted image, smaller hepatic vessels are visible and left hepatic lobe can be seen. Because only three data acquisitions are averaged,

CONTRAST

The subjective terms *image quality* and *anatomic resolution* usually correlate with the product of spatial resolution (1/voxel volume) and the signal-to-noise ratio (SNR). However, anatomic resolution also involves the recognition of boundaries between different tissues, and there are many situations where SNR and spatial resolution are excellent but normal or abnormal anatomy is obscured by the lack of a signal difference. For example, long TR, short TE (so-called proton-density-weighted) images of the brain maximize SNR but minimize signal differences between tissues, and neither normal anatomy nor pathology is well seen. Therefore, *image contrast* is the third parameter fundamental to achieving "quality" CT or MRI images (10,12,26,28).

Image contrast, the relative signal intensity of different tissues, is determined by the physical interaction of tissues with the imaging method. Tissues such as fat and bone differ greatly in electron density (x-ray attenuation) and show high contrast on CT scans. For MRI, the fundamental tissue characteristics are *proton density, relaxation times, motion,* and *resonance frequency*. All four parameters can be exploited as sources of image contrast. However, with four tissue variables interacting with multiple variables of the MRI pulse sequence, image contrast becomes a very complex function. Pitfalls occur because contrast that exists in the physical tissue characteristics might not influence image signal intensity using a particular MRI pulse sequence. In other words, it is the modulation of tissue characteristics by the selected imaging technique (pulse sequence and timing parameters) that determines image contrast.

ARTIFACTS

In addition to spatial resolution, SNR, and contrast, image artifacts must be considered (1–4,6–9, 16,17,27–29). *Noise* is broadly defined as any variation that represents a deviation from the truth. Noise can be random, as in white noise or hiss caused by electronic components. In addition, all imaging techniques occasionally show systematic noise, also known as structured noise or "artifacts" (Figs. 2-1 and 2-2).

CT scan artifacts due to beam hardening or subject motion are examples of structured noise familiar to radiologists. However, CT artifacts are beyond the control of practitioners, since hardware and software remedies are provided as a fixed package by manufacturers. Radiologists have been more directly involved in guiding the development of artifact-suppression methods for MRI.

Unlike the common CT artifacts, MRI artifacts are often projected outside the body and appear on "background" areas of the image as spurious signal intensities or "ghosts" mimicking the real structure that generated the mismapped signal (Figs. 2-3 to 2-5). Mismapping of signal on MRI images can be caused by a variety of defects in instrumentation software or hardware but are most commonly caused by the motion of a signal source (tissue) that interacts adversely with the pulse sequence used to map (create an image) the signals.

TECHNOLOGY ASSESSMENT

A major goal of technology development and assessment is to efficiently obtain quantitative data predictive of the level of clinical performance a given technique will achieve (22,24). Clinical performance, expressed as accuracy, receiver operating characteristics (ROC), or "efficacy," is dependent on numerous clinical variables such as the nature of the patient population selected, therapeutic interventions, and the quality of pathologic proof (23).

Observer performance tested by ROC is essentially a clinical outcome analysis for the technology itself. Observer performance includes innumerable variables that either cannot be isolated

FIGURE 2-1 *(continued)*
ghost artifacts from aorta still overlie left hepatic lobe. Note that ghost artifacts may add to tissue signal constructively, producing a white artifact, or destructively, producing a dark artifact. (D) On SE 260/15, 18-acquisition (10-min) image, ghost artifacts are absent, detailed hepatic vascular structures are sharply defined, and normal left hepatic lobe is well seen because of reduced cardiac-motion-induced artifacts and elimination of ghosts from aorta.

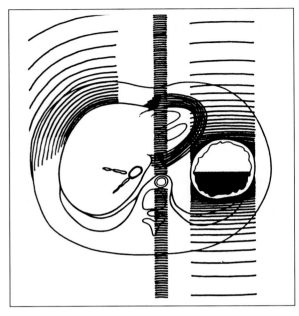

FIGURE 2-2
Schematic transverse image through upper abdomen showing ghost artifacts induced by respiratory motion of subcutaneous fat, aortic and cardiac pulsations, and peristalsis of fluid-containing bowel. For motion in all directions, ghost artifacts are selectively propagated along phase-encoding (vertical) dimension of MRI images reconstructed with two-dimensional Fourier transform.

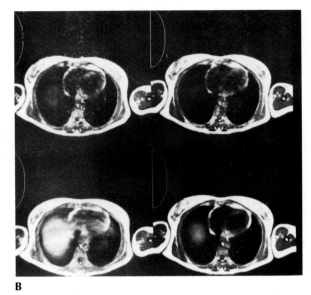

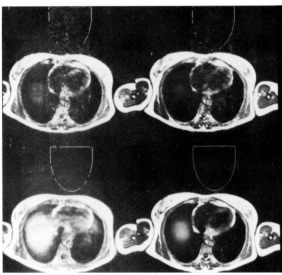

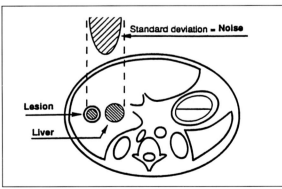

FIGURE 2-3
(A) Schematic diagram of MRI image analysis. Noise has been measured either as the standard deviation or mean signal intensity of background pixels. Region-of-interest measurements in healthy volunteer. In both (B) and (C), the pulse sequence is SE 260/15; top left: 2 acquisitions; top right: 4 acquisitions; bottom left: 8 acquisitions; bottom right: 16 acquisitions. (B) Sampling of statistical (random) noise in laterally placed region of interest avoids ghosts. (C) Sampling of cardiac ghosts (systematic noise) in elliptical region of interest includes aliased ghosts.

for independent study or are inherently nonparametric. For example, performance for the detection of hepatic metastases requires minimizing false-negative and false-positive results. If the diagnostic data (the images) cause interpretive error, stress, or uncertainty in the mind of the observer (the interpreting radiologist), the ROC will reflect this in lower confidence scores.

The interpretation of liver images is complicated by *distractors*, which are real (anatomic) or unreal (noise, artifacts) regions on the image that mask or mimic lesions (18,19). For example, near the hilum of the liver, converging blood vessels can mask or mimic lesions on CT and MRI images. Partial volume averaging of portal structures or structures abutting the liver create similar problems. Artifacts (Fig. 2-1) are the most common problem. All these subjective distractors are most troublesome when image CNR and SNR are reduced. Therefore, CNR and SNR generally reflect overall image quality (22). However, in advanced stages of clinical development, these simple quantitative parameters (SNR and CNR) must be supplemented by ROC analysis to establish diagnostic performance in a clinical setting (23).

Unfortunately, in a clinical setting, the care of an individual is often inconsistent with the design of studies to measure the performance of diagnostic tests in a population of patients. Therefore, clinical trials require large numbers of subjects to average out variations in the study group. It is naive, impractical, and ultimately destructive to medical progress to require randomized, controlled trials (RCTs) at each step in the development of technology. Misunderstandings occur when administrators and scientists from different backgrounds do not clearly define terminology and standards (20). Nevertheless, given the cost and controversy surrounding implementation of expensive methods such as CT and MRI, radiologists must justify their services.

At each step in developing new imaging methods, it is essential to employ parameters that are predictive of diagnostic accuracy. In most circumstances, the product of the SNR and image contrast can be used as a quantitative measure of the information on the image (13,22). Contrast itself is usually expressed as a signal-intensity ratio, e.g., (lesion SI − liver SI)/liver SI, which reduces to the lesion/liver SI ratio − 1. If SNR is taken to be liver SI/noise, the product of contrast × SNR = (lesion SI − liver SI)/noise. To quantitate the conspicuity of a lesion, this signal-difference-to-noise (SD/N) ratio is the appropriate parameter for image analysis. SD/N is loosely known as the contrast-to-noise ratio (CNR), although, strictly speaking, contrast, defined as a ratio, is not directly scaled to image noise.

In evaluating phantoms, animal studies or clinical images, SD/N (CNR) offers a reproducible, quantitative measure of diagnostic performance for purposes of data reduction and statistical analysis. For example, measurements of CNR can be obtained for a particular pathology such as hemangioma to determine which (machine, pulse sequence, contrast agent) technique is best and by what margin of statistical confidence.

Several studies have established a close correlation between CNR and the performance of radiologists in correctly interpreting an image. For example, the threshold size at which a lesison can be detected, the percentage of lesions that are detected, and the confidence in reaching a diagnosis of normal versus abnormal show a close correlation with quantitative image measurements of CNR (24). Therefore, while CNR itself has no role in the management of individual patients, it is an accepted parameter for clinical researchers seeking to define an optimal imaging technique.

COST

Time is the "currency" of imaging, since it determines the cost of the procedure and/or radiation dose to the patient. Since we seek to maximize CNR (benefit) and minimize time (cost), CNR/time is a figure of merit that describes the clinical performance of an imaging technique.

Scan time itself is a complex variable, since the time required for acquisition of a single image is usually much less than the time required to obtain all the images necessary for anatomic coverage of an organ. It is the total examination time that determines throughput and the number of correct diagnoses per day, which, in turn, determines the value of a machine.

SUMMARY

The detection of liver cancer is a challenge to diagnostic medicine of enormous significance worldwide. In addition to being important clinically,

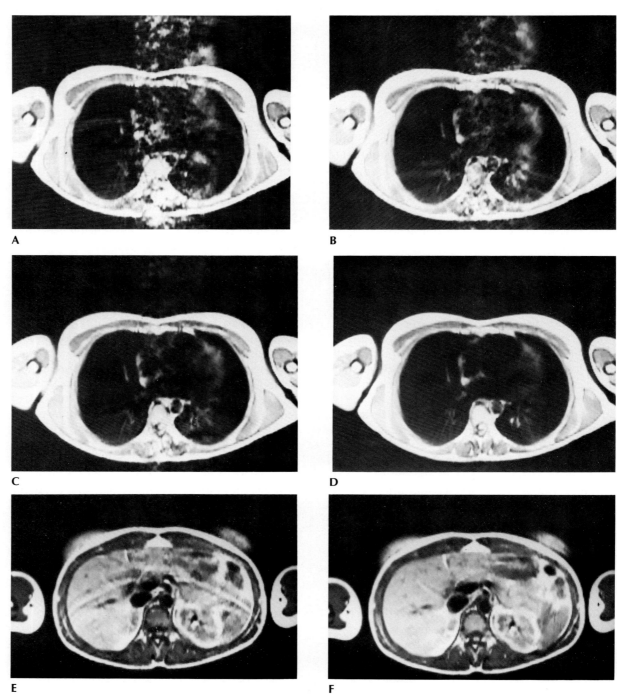

FIGURE 2-4
Results of signal averaging are shown in transverse SE 500/32 images obtained at level of heart (A–D) and pancreas (E–F) in normal volunteer. (A) In image obtained with one data acquisition, 1.1-min scanning time, ghosts of subcutaneous fat and cardiac signal intensity are propagated along phase-encoding axis. (B) In image obtained with two data acquisitions, 2.2-min scanning time, displacement of subcutaneous fat ghost artifacts is

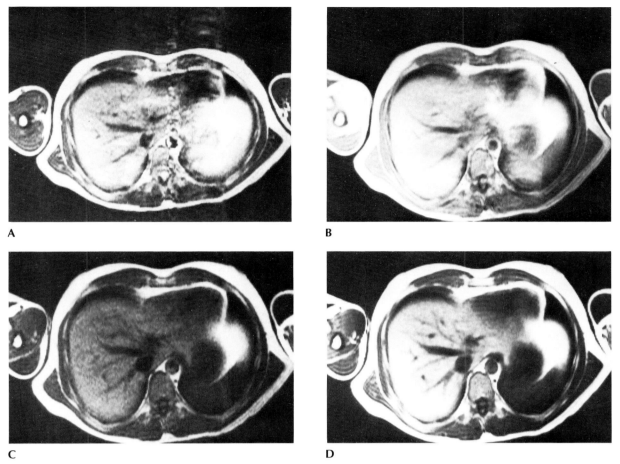

FIGURE 2-5
Transverse images at level of cardiac apex in a healthy, breathing volunteer show effects of changing TE and TR. (A) On SE 2000/60, two-acquisition (9-min) image, left hepatic lobe is blurred because of cardiac motion and obscured by ghost artifacts from heart, inferior vena cava, and aorta. (B) On SE 2000/15, two-acquisition (9-min) image, use of a short TE decreases all types of ghost artifacts and has reduced blurring of left hepatic lobe and pericardial fat. (C) On SE 260/15, two-acquisition (1-min) image, reduction in TR has decreased time of each phase-encoding step and shortened overall imaging time. As a result, blurring is further reduced and edge definition is improved. Hepatic veins are now well seen. However, use of short TR decreases tissue signal intensity and gives image a grainy appearance. (D) On SE 260/15, 16-acquisition (9-min) image, averaging of multiple data acquisitions improves S/N levels. Although time between phase-encoding steps is the same as in part B, ghost artifacts are reduced by signal averaging. Furthermore, more even object sampling during each phase-encoding step has resulted in sharper anatomic delineation of hepatic veins and other structures.

FIGURE 2-4 *(continued)*
doubled. Cardiac ghost artifacts are reduced because two data sets were averaged to form final image. (C) Image was obtained with four data acquisitions, 4.5-min scan time. (D) In image obtained with eight data acquisitions, 9.0-min scan time, ghost artifacts are negligible and cardiac anatomy is resolved. (E) In image obtained with one data acquisition on transverse plane at level of pancreas, prominent ghosts from subcutaneous fat interfere with examination of liver and pancreas. Prominent vascular ghost artifacts are due to inferior vena caval and aortic pulsation. (F) In image obtained with two data acquisitions, subcutaneous fat ghosts are displaced to greater distance because of longer phase-step time; all ghost artifacts show decreased intensity because of signal averaging.

from the perspective of physics, liver cancer imaging is a straightforward problem. However, due to the complexity and continuing evolution of diagnostic imaging technology, important issues are not yet resolved. A major goal of this symposium is to improve interdisciplinary cooperation, which begins with definition of a shared scientific terminology.

The terminology used to describe and analyze cross-sectional images includes both qualitative and quantitative parameters. Quantitation is preferred because it leads to efficient scientific methods for technology development and assessment. Different standards of performance are appropriate for individual scientific disciplines and various stages of technology development.

By selecting appropriate standards of comparison, researchers can identify those techniques which are most promising for development, clinicians can appropriately manage their daily practice, and administrators can establish a rational basis for choosing the technologies that are most deserving of reimbursement. Radiologists have led the development of medical decision analysis for 20 years, and these skills will be especially valuable in the development of hepatic and abdominal MRI.

REFERENCES

1. Bailes DR, Gilderdale DJ, Bydder GM, et al: Respiratory ordered phase encoding (ROPE): A method for reducing respiratory motion artefacts in MR imaging. J Comput Assist Tomog 9:835, 1985.
2. Bellon EM, Haacke EM, Coleman PE, et al: MR artifacts: A review. AJR 147:1271, 1986.
3. Bydder GM, Pernnock JM, Phil M, et al: The short T1 inversion recovery sequence—An approach to MR imaging of the abdomen. Magn Reson Imaging 3:221, 1985.
4. Bydder GM, Young IR: MR imaging: Clinical use of the inversion recovery sequence. J Comput Assist Tomog 9:659, 1984.
5. Edelstein WA, Bottomley PA, Hart HR, Smith LS: Signal, noise, and contrast in nuclear magnetic resonance (NMR) imaging. J Comput Assist Tomog 7:391, 1983.
6. Ehman RL, McNamara MT, Brasch RC, et al: Influence of physiologic motion on the appearance of tissue in MR images. Radiology 159:777, 1986.
7. Felmlee JP, Ehman RL: Spatial presaturation: A method for suppressing flow artifacts and improving depiction of vascular anatomy in MR imaging. Radiology 164:559, 1987.
8. Haacke EM, Lenz GW: Improving MR image quality in the presence of motion by using rephasing gradients. AJR 148:1251, 1987.
9. Haacke EM, Lenz GW, Nelson AD: Pseudo-gating: Elimination of periodic motion artifacts in magnetic resonance imaging without gating. Magn Reson Med 4:162, 1987.
10. Hendrick RE, Nelson TR, Hendee WR: Optimizing tissue contrast in magnetic resonance imaging. Magn Reson Imaging 2:193, 1984.
11. Hendrick RE, Newman FD, Hendee WR: MR imaging technology: Maximizing the signal-to-noise ratio from a single tissue. Radiology 156:749, 1985.
12. Henkelman RM, Hardy P, Poon PY, Bronskill MJ: Optimal pulse sequence for imaging hepatic metastases. Radiology 161:727, 1986.
13. Kaufman L, Kramer DM, Crooks LE, Ortendahl DA: Measuring signal-to-noise ratios in MR imaging. Radiology 173:265, 1989.
14. Metz CE: Basic principles of ROC analysis. Semin Nucl Med V 8:283, 1978.
15. Mugler JP, Brookeman JR: The optimum data sampling period for maximum signal-to-noise ratio in MR imaging. Rev Magn Reson Med 3:1, 1988.
16. Paling MR, Brookeman JR: Respiration artifacts in MR imaging: Reduction by breath holding. J Comput Assist Tomog 10:1080, 1986.
17. Pattany PM, Phillips JJ, Chiu LC, et al: Motion artifact suppression technique (MAST) for MR imaging. J Comput Assist Tomog 11:369, 1987.
18. Seltzer SE, Judy PF: Gaining insight: Improved images enhance understanding. Radiographics 7:1221, 1987.
19. Seltzer SE, Swensson RG, Lentini JF, et al: Detection of liver lesions on medical images: Lessons from psychophysics. Radiology 169:300, 1988.
20. Stark DD: Standards of quality in medical research: Who decides? AJR 151:863, 1988.
21. Stark DD, Hendrick RE, Hahn PF, Ferrucci JT Jr: Motion artifact reduction with fast spin-echo imaging. Radiology 164:183, 1987.
22. Stark DD, Wittenberg J, Edelman RR, et al: Detection of hepatic metastasis by magnetic resonance imaging: Analysis of pulse sequence performance. Radiology 159:365, 1986.
23. Stark DD, Wittenberg J, Butch RJ, Ferrucci JT: Hepatic metastases: Randomized, controlled comparison of detection with MR imaging and CT. Radiology 165:399, 1987.

24. Tsang YM, Stark DD, Chen M, et al: Hepatic micrometastases in the rat: Ferrite enhanced MR imaging. Radiology 167:21, 1988.
25. Wehrli FW, MacFall JR, Glover GH, et al: The dependence of nuclear magnetic resonance (NMR) imaging contrast on intrinsic and pulse sequence timing parameters. Magn Reson Imaging 2:3, 1984.
26. Wehrli FW, MacFall JR, Shutts D, et al: Mechanisms of contrast in NMR imaging. J Comput Assist Tomog 8:369, 1984.
27. Wood ML, Henkelman RM: MR image artifacts from periodic motion. Med Phys 12:143, 1985.
28. Wood ML, Henkelman RM: Suppression of respiratory motion artifacts in magnetic resonance imaging. Med Phys 13:794, 1986.
29. Wood ML, Henkelman RM: The magnetic field dependence of the breathing artifact. Magn Reson Imaging 4:387, 1986.

II. LESION DETECTION BY MRI AND CT: TECHNIQUES AND RESULTS

3

Hepatic CT: Techniques, Applications, and Results

PATRICK C. FREENY

Computed tomography (CT) is a well-established modality for detection of hepatic neoplasms. However, the techniques for performing CT of the liver continue to evolve. This chapter will address the different techniques for contrast administration for hepatic CT, the specific applications of these techniques, and their results.

TECHNIQUES OF HEPATIC CT
Bolus Dynamic CT (BDCT)
Bolus dynamic CT consists of rapid acquisition of axial images of the liver using automatic table incrementation during *simultaneous* intravenous injection of a bolus of 150 to 180 ml of 60 percent contrast agent (Fig. 3-1A). It is generally accepted that BDCT implies that the entire liver is scanned within 2 to 3 min of the onset of the bolus injection of contrast. Current-generation CT scanners are capable of performing scans of 2 s or less at a rate of six to nine scans per minute. Different dynamic scan sequences are used to achieve these results, depending on the performance of the individual scanner. I use a General Electric 9800 Quick CT/T scanner (General Electric, Milwaukee, Wisc.) with a standard sequence consisting of a cluster of three 2-s scans at a speed of 2 s per scan, a 3.5-second interscan delay for table incrementation, and a 10-second intergroup delay for patient breathing. This gives an image repetition rate of nine scans per minute. The average time for a hepatic scan is about 130 to 135 seconds.

Techniques of contrast administration and types of contrast media used for BDCT continue to show considerable variation across the United States. A survey of the members of the Society of Computed Body Tomography from 22 different institutions performed by Zeman and colleagues (1) in 1988 showed that while 17 (77 percent) obtained scans *during* the injection of contrast, only 59 percent of these used a rapid (1 to 2-min) bolus and 41 percent continued to use the older drip-infusion technique. However, subsequent to the survey, many institutions have converted to the bolus technique.

The controversy regarding the accuracy of CT detection of hepatic lesions using a bolus versus a drip infusion of contrast media has, for all practical scientific purposes, finally come to an end. It has now been shown and accepted that *maximal contrast enhancement*, and hence maximal *relative contrast attenuation* of focal hepatic lesions (attenuation of the liver minus attenuation of the lesion) is achieved with a 1 to 2-min injection of 150 to 180 ml of a 60% contrast agent (2–6) (Fig. 3-1B). The most reproducible results are obtained with the use of a programmable power injector that is operated by the CT technologist from the scanning console.

The scan sequence should be initiated following a delay of 20 to 45 s from the onset of the injection. Fifty to 85 ml of contrast material is injected during this delay, allowing the liver to contrast enhance before the scan sequence is initiated.

The rate of contrast injection should be adjusted so that the entire bolus is delivered within 1 to 2 min. Techniques for administration include a *biphasic rate* (total volume 150 to 180 ml delivered at 2.5 to 5.0 ml/s for 10 to 20 s, then 1 ml/s for 100 to 130 s) and a *uniphasic rate* (total volume 150 ml delivered at 2.5 ml/s for 60 s). Berland and Lee (7) have shown that the faster uniphasic rate produces earlier and greater peak contrast enhancement of the liver compared with the slower biphasic rate. Although no data on the influence of uniphasic and biphasic injections on the accuracy of CT detection of focal lesions have been published, lesion detection with a uniphasic technique theoretically should be better than, or at least equal to, that with a longer, less rapid, biphasic injection. Further studies addressing this issue should be available in the future.

Considerable attention has been given to the new nonionic, low-osmolar contrast agents, and many institutions now use them exclusively. Compared with ionic, high-osmolar agents, they are less cardiotoxic and are associated with fewer and less severe allergic and nephrotoxic reactions, but they are considerably more expensive (8). A recent paper by Nelson and coworkers (9) compared the degree of contrast enhancement of the liver following administration of three contrast agents: iothalamate-60 (Conray-60, Mallinkrodt, St. Louis, Mo.), iopamidol-300 (Isovue-300, Squibb Diagnostics, Princeton, N.J.), and iohexol-300 (Omnipaque-300, Winthrop, New York, N.Y.). There was no significant difference in maximal hepatic contrast enhancement between the three agents during BDCT. However, for delayed CT (images obtained 5 h postcontrast), maximal contrast enhancement was greater with iothalamate-60 and iopamidol-300 than with iohexol-300.

Delayed Iodine Scanning (DIS)
DIS consists of obtaining axial scans of the liver 4 to 6 h following administration of contrast containing a total iodine dose of at least 60 g. This dose of iodine has been shown to produce an increase in hepatic attenuation of 20 HU over baseline non-contrast-enhanced scans (10). The contrast load can be administered intravenously or intraarterially (e.g., following hepatic angiography or hepatic CT angiography or portography) (Fig. 3-2). Both ionic and nonionic contrast agents can be used, but hepatic enhancement following iohexol-300 is inferior to that produced by iothalamate-60 or iopamidol-300 (9).

CT Angiography (CT-A) and CT Portography (CT-AP)
CT-A and CT-AP consist of obtaining axial hepatic CT scans during simultaneous intraarterial infusion of contrast material. CT-A is performed by injecting contrast material into the common hepatic artery. Because hepatic neoplasms receive their blood supply from the hepatic artery, CT-A increases hepatic lesion detection by producing marked contrast enhancement of small hepatic tumors. The concentration, rate, and volume of contrast material administration are critical for obtaining good-quality scans. Initially, we performed CT-A by injecting a total of 12 ml of 30% contrast material at a rate of 1 ml/s during each consecutive 13-s cluster of three 2-s scans. However, hepatic perfusion abnormalities were common and made scan interpretation difficult in some cases (11) (Fig. 3-3). More recently, using a programmable power injector, we decreased the concentration of contrast material from 30% to 15% and increased the injection rate to 2 ml/s during each 13-s cluster of three 2-s scans (volume of 26 ml per cluster). This has improved the quality of the CT-A scans by reducing perfusion abnormalities (Fig. 3-4).

CT-AP is performed by acquiring axial hepatic CT scans during simultaneous injection of 100 to 150 ml of 60% contrast material at a rate of 2 to 3 ml/s into the superior mesenteric or splenic artery, thus returning the contrast material to the liver by means of the portal circulation. Since hepatic neoplasms receive their blood supply from the hepatic artery, contrast material entering the liver by means of the portal vein will not produce

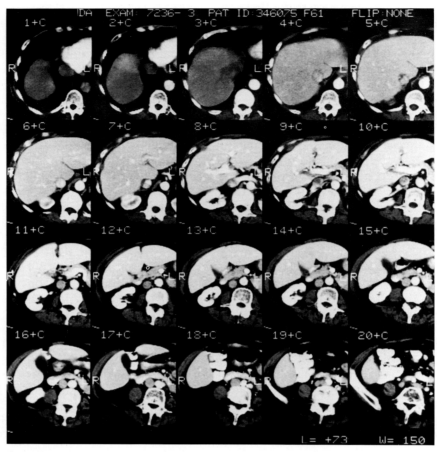

FIGURE 3-1A

enhancement of the neoplasms. However, hepatic parenchymal attenuation will increase significantly. Thus CT-AP increases detection of hepatic lesions by increasing the attenuation of normal hepatic parenchyma relative to focal neoplasms, i.e., by increasing their *relative contrast attenuation* (see Fig. 3-2).

The decision of whether to use CT-A or CT-AP varies from institution to institution. Both techniques are similarly accurate in detecting focal hepatic lesions. I prefer to use CT-A, finding it subjectively easier to look for small contrast-enhancing lesions rather than small nonenhancing lesions. If there is a replaced or anomalous hepatic artery, the hepatic artery supplying the portion of the liver with no known tumor is catheterized for CT-A. However, if selective catheterization of the hepatic artery is difficult, CT-AP is a good alternative.

Applications of BDCT, DCT, DIS, and CT-A/CT-AP
The liver can be evaluated from three different perspectives, depending on the clinical indications:

1. *Abdominal Survey.* The liver is only *part* of the evaluation of the entire abdomen. It is performed in patients with a known or suspected primary nonhepatic neoplasm in whom there is no clinical or laboratory evidence of hepatic disease.

2. *Liver Survey.* The liver is the *primary organ* to be evaluated. It is performed in patients with a known or clinically suspected primary or metastatic hepatic tumor or in nononcology patients with suspected liver disease on the basis of clinical and laboratory evaluation.

3. *Lesion Detection.* The goal is *precise* detection of the *number* and anatomic *location* of tumor nodules in a patient with known liver neoplasm. It is

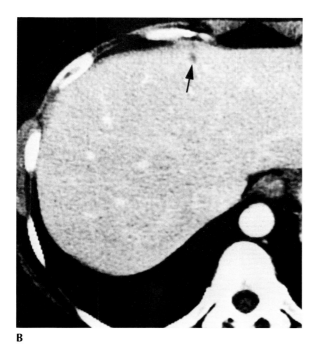

FIGURE 3-1
Bolus dynamic CT scans. (A) Normal bolus dynamic CT of the liver. CT scan consists of 20 consecutive 10-mm scans acquired during the injection of 150 ml of 60% contrast material. First image (1 + C) was acquired 20 s following the bolus injection of 2.5 ml/s. Note excellent contrast enhancement of hepatic parenchyma and hepatic vessels. (B) Colon carcinoma metastasis. Bolus dynamic CT shows a 5-mm hypodense lesion in the anterior aspect of the left lobe (arrow), proven at surgery to be a metastasis.

performed in patients who are candidates for surgical resection of a primary or metastatic hepatic tumor.

Abdominal Survey. Abdominal survey studies are performed for evaluation of patients with known or suspected neoplasms to detect primary or metastatic abdominal disease. Thus CT technique must be optimal for imaging the solid abdominal organs, as well as the retroperitoneum and gastrointestinal tract. BDCT is the best technique for performing an abdominal survey (2,4).

Liver Survey. Liver survey is performed for precise evaluation of the liver in patients in whom there is clinical or laboratory evidence of hepatic disease.

Primary neoplasm: Patients may be suspected of having a primary benign or malignant hepatic neoplasm on the basis of a variety of clinical symptoms and/or laboratory studies. The most common benign hepatic tumors are hemangiomas and focal nodular hyperplasia. Although these tumors can cause symptoms, they usually are detected incidentally during abdominal imaging performed for some unrelated reason. If hemangioma is suspected, a technetium-99m red blood cell scan will usually give a specific diagnosis (12). Other alternatives include MRI and angiography (13,14).

Hepatocellular carcinoma is the most common primary malignant hepatic tumor. It usually arises in patients with cirrhosis and is suspected clinically if the alpha-fetoprotein level is elevated. We use BDCT for liver survey in patients who are candidates for hepatic resection. It is an accurate method for tumor detection and assessment of resectability, and it can be used to guide percutaneous biopsy.

Metastatic neoplasm: Most liver surveys are performed in oncology patients in whom there is strong clinical or laboratory suspicion of hepatic metastases. If the examination is requested only to confirm the clinical diagnosis, sonography and guided biopsy are performed. If the patient is to be placed on a treatment protocol that requires sequential evaluation of the response of the liver metastases, BDCT is the modality of choice. Recent investigations have shown that the sensitivity of MRI and BDCT for hepatic lesion detection is similar (15,16). Thus, depending on the preference at individual institutions, MRI and BDCT can be used interchangeably for liver survey.

Lesion Detection. Lesion detection studies are performed for patients with a known primary or metastatic hepatic tumor who are candidates for hepatic resection. The imaging techniques have two goals: (1) definition of hepatic arterial anatomy for the surgeon, and (2) precise identification of the number and location of the lesions.

Most patients who are candidates for hepatic resection have already been determined to have a potentially resectable lesion, most often by BDCT. If BDCT has not been performed (the lesion may have been detected by sonography), we suggest that it be obtained, since it may display findings that

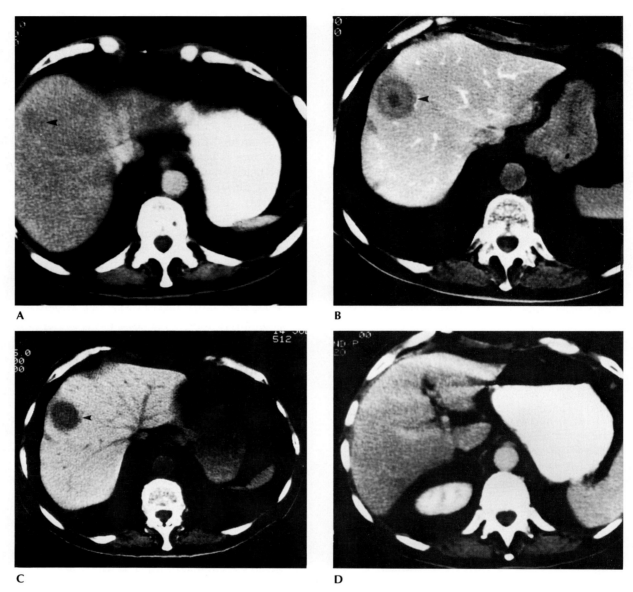

FIGURE 3-2
Sequential bolus dynamic, CT-AP, and DIS scans in a patient for potential resection of colon cancer metastasis. (A) Bolus dynamic scan shows ill-defined lesion in the dome of the liver (arrowhead). No other lesions were found. (B) CT-AP at same level as part A shows metastasis more clearly defined (arrowhead). (C) DIS at same level as part A (post CT-AP) shows metastasis (arrowhead). (D) Bolus dynamic scan at level of main portal vein appears normal. (E) CT-AP at same level as part D shows two small metastases (arrowheads). (F) DIS at same level as part D fails to show lesions seen on CT-AP (E). (G) Bolus dynamic scan through inferior right lobe appears normal. (H) CT-AP at same level as part G shows small metastasis (arrowhead). (I) DIS at same level as part G confirms metastasis.

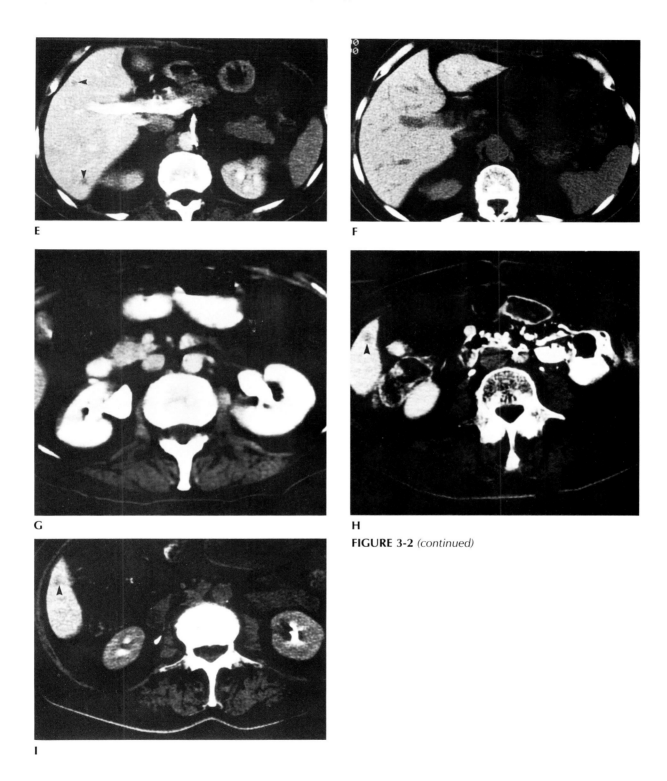

FIGURE 3-2 *(continued)*

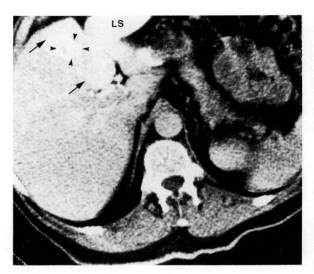

FIGURE 3-3
CT-A scan: colon carcinoma metastasis. Scan obtained during arterial injection of 30% contrast material at 1 ml/s shows a colon carcinoma metastasis in the medial segment of the left lobe (arrowheads), obscured by hypervascular surrounding perfusion defect in the medial segment (arrows) and in the lateral segment (LS).

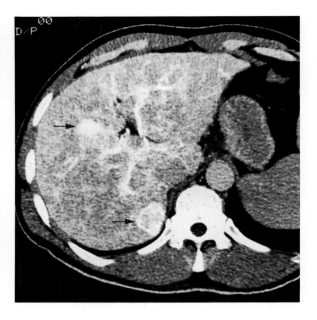

FIGURE 3-4
CT-A scan: hepatocellular carcinoma. Scan obtained during arterial injection of 15% contrast material at 2 ml/s shows two hypervascular tumor nodules (arrows) with no perfusion abnormalities.

would obviate hepatic resection. If MRI or BDCT have been performed as the initial imaging modality, the evaluation process proceeds as follows:

Hepatic angiography is used to define the arterial anatomy of the liver for the surgeon. It can be perfomed using standard film technique or digital image processing. I use standard film technique, since I expect the examination to provide not only arterial anatomy, but also to detect the lesion being studied, to detect additional unsuspected lesions, and to reveal invasion of the portal or hepatic veins. The latter two findings often obviate resection.

Precise identification of the number and location of the lesions is then determined by CT-A or CT-AP (see Fig. 3-2). Both have been shown to detect additional lesions not seen by BDCT or arteriography in 40 to 55 percent of patients (17,18).

Patients who are still considered to have a resectable hepatic lesion at the conclusion of BDCT, angiography, and CT-A or CT-AP are then rescanned without additional contrast material 4 to 6 h after CT angiography (Fig. 3-5). Since most patients receive sufficient contrast material during angiography and CT-A (60 g iodine), DIS is a

FIGURE 3-5
Sequential bolus dynamic, CT-A, and DIS scans in a patient for potential resection of a colon carcinoma metastasis. (A) Bolus dynamic scan near the top of the liver is normal. (B) CT-A at the same level as part A also appears normal. (C) DIS at the same level as part A obtained after CT-A shows two metastases in the liver (arrowheads). (D) Bolus dynamic scan obtained near the midliver shows a single lesion in the medial segment of the left lobe (arrowhead). Small arrow indicates portal vein branch. (E) CT-A scan obtained at same level as part D shows metastasis in medial segment (arrowhead). Small arrow indicates portal vein branch. (F) DIS obtained after CT-A confirms medial segment lesion (arrowhead), but shows two additional lesions in the right lobe (arrowheads) near the small portal vein branch (v).

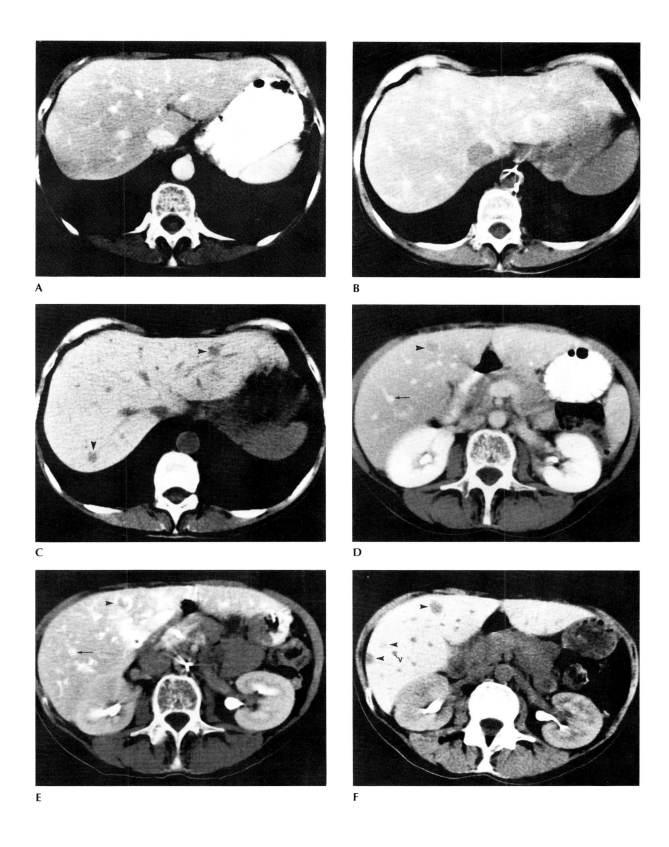

simple adjunctive technique. It is scheduled to follow the CT-A scan and can be performed while the patient is in the hospital following angiography and CT-A or prior to leaving the hospital if the arteriogram is performed as an outpatient study.

The role of MRI in the preoperative evaluation of patients prior to hepatic resection is addressed in other chapters in this book and in some recent papers (19,20).

RESULTS OF HEPATIC CT TECHNIQUES
BDCT

The accuracy of BDCT in detecting *patients* with hepatic neoplasms and in detecting the *number* of hepatic tumor nodules in each patient has been evaluated in several recent studies. Chezmar and coworkers (16) reported a study evaluating BDCT performed with a 150-ml contrast material bolus delivered at a rate of 2 to 3 ml/s in 28 patients with a total of 93 primary or metastatic tumor nodules. BDCT detected the presence of hepatic neoplasm in 26 of 28 patients (93 percent) and detected 86 of 93 individual tumor nodules (92 percent). The detection rate for tumor nodules less than 1 cm in diameter was 13 of 19 (68 percent), while for nodules greater than 1 cm, detection was 73 of 74 (99 percent).

We reported a series of over 500 patients with colon carcinoma in 1988 (5). In this series, BDCT was performed using a 150-ml bolus of contrast material delivered at a rate of 2.5 ml/s for 20 s and 1 ml/s for 100 s. The incidence of metastatic disease proven at surgery was 7.6 percent, and the accuracy of BDCT detection of patients with metastases was 87.5 percent.

A recent group of 20 patients with known primary or metastatic tumor who subsequently underwent hepatic resection were studied with BDCT using the same contrast enhancement technique described earlier (21). All 20 patients had known tumor. The detection rate of BDCT for the *number* of tumor nodules was 57 percent. This is similar to the rate of 66 percent reported by Sitzmann and colleagues (20), although the exact techniques of contrast enhancement were not elucidated by the authors of this report.

The lowest detection rate for BDCT for the *number* of tumor nodules was reported by Heiken and colleagues (15). In their series of 8 patients with 37 tumor nodules, BDCT detected only 14 lesions (38 percent). However, the contrast-enhancement technique employed was the drip-infusion method (bolus of 50 ml of 76 percent contrast material followed by drip infusion of 150 ml of 60 percent contrast material), and one patient had only a nonenhanced scan. This low detection rate again emphasizes the inadequacy of the drip-infusion technique [also see the report by Paushter and colleagues (6)].

DIS

Delayed iodine scanning (DIS) has been employed in several recent studies. In the study by Chezmar et al. (16) noted earlier, DIS detected 30 of 93 hepatic tumor nodules (86 percent), compared with 86 of 93 (92 percent) detected by BDCT (16). The detection rate of DIS for nodules less than 1 cm in diameter was 6 of 19 (67 percent), while for nodules greater than 1 cm, it was 24 of 74 (32 percent), compared with BDCT at 68 and 99 percent, respectively.

In another series from the same institution, Nelson et al. (19) reported that DIS detected 44 of 60 tumor nodules (73 percent). In the series by Heiken et al. (15), detection rate for DIS was 12 of 23 lesions (52 percent). In Freeny and Ryan's series (21), DIS detected 60 percent of tumor nodules, compared with 57 percent for BDCT (Figs. 3-3 and 3-5).

CT-A and CT-AP

There have been no published studies comparing the results of CT-AP and CT-A in the same group or in a matched group of patients. Thus it is not possible to compare these two different techniques of contrast administration accurately. However, CT-A and CT-AP both produce a substantial increase in the detection of the *number* of hepatic metastases or primary tumor nodules. The choice between the two techniques is thus based on institutional or individual preference at the present time.

Multimodality Approach

None of the CT techniques is 100 percent accurate in detection of tumor nodules. Thus a combination of techniques will yield the largest number of true-positive lesions, but also will increase the number of false-positive diagnoses. Thus there is a tradeoff when employing a combination of examinations.

The highest accuracy for detection of individual tumor nodules is achieved with a combination of CT and MRI. A complete discussion of MRI techniques is found in other chapters in this book. A recent series by Nelson et al. (19) indicates that the the most sensitive combination is CT-AP and MRI, yielding a sensitivity of 96 percent. A series by Freeny and Ryan (21) included sequential CT-A, DIS, and MRI. Sensitivity for lesion detection was 97 percent with this combination.

CONCLUSIONS

BDCT currently is the best CT technique for both *abdominal survey* and *liver survey*, yielding excellent results in detection of primary intraabdominal malignancy as well as in detection of *patients* with primary or metastatic hepatic tumor. However, these superior results are dependent on the use of the bolus technique for contrast material administration: acquisition of rapid-sequence axial scans (image repetition rate of six to nine scans per minute) during the initially simultaneous bolus injection of 150 to 180 ml of 60% contrast material injected within 60 to 120 s.

The techniques of contrast material administration can be altered to improve the CT detection rate for the *number* of individual hepatic tumor nodules. This can be accomplished by arterial infusion of contrast material (CT-A or CT-AP) and by obtaining delayed images 4 to 6 h following a dose of at least 60 g iodine (DIS). These techniques are best used in patients who are being considered for hepatic resection. Detection rates can be expected to increase from 57 to 66 percent for BDCT to 77 to 94 percent for CT-AP or CT-A.

A *multimodality approach* combining different CT and MRI techniques is the most accurate method for detecting the number of individual tumor nodules.

REFERENCES

1. Zeman RK, Clements LA, Silverman PM, et al: CT of the liver: A survey of prevailing methods for administration of contrast material. AJR 150:107, 1988.
2. Foley WD, Berland LL, Lawson TL, et al: Contrast enhancement technique for dynamic hepatic CT scanning. Radiology 147:797, 1983.
3. Foley WD: Dynamic hepatic CT. Radiology 170:617, 1989.
4. Alpern MB, Lawson TL, Foley WD, et al: Focal hepatic masses and fatty infiltration detected by enhanced dynamic CT. Radiology 158:45, 1986.
5. Ferrucci JT, Freeny PC, Stark DD, et al: Advances in hepatobiliary radiology. Radiology 168:319, 1988.
6. Paushter DM, Zeman RK, Scheibler PL, et al: CT evaluation of suspected hepatic metastases: Comparison of techniques for IV contrast enhancement. AJR 152:267, 1989.
7. Berland LL, Lee JY: Comparison of contrast media injection rates and volumes for hepatic dynamic incremental computed tomography. Invest Radiol 23:918, 1988.
8. Katayama H, Yamaguchi K, Kozuka T, et al: Adverse reactions to ionic and nonionic contrast media: A report from the Japanese committee on the safety of contrast media. Radiology 175:621, 1990.
9. Nelson RC, Chezmar JL, Peterson JE, Bernardino ME: Contrast-enhanced CT of the liver and spleen: Comparison of ionic and nonionic contrast agents. AJR 153:973, 1989.
10. Perkerson RB Jr, Erwin BC, Baumgartner BR, et al: CT densities in delayed iodine hepatic scanning. Radiology 155:445, 1985.
11. Freeny PC, Marks WM: Hepatic perfusion abnormalities during CT angiography: Detection and interpretation. Radiology 159:685, 1986.
12. Brodsky RI, Friedman AC, Maurer AH, et al: Hepatic cavernous hemangioma: Diagnosis with ^{99m}TC-labeled red cells and single photon emission CT. AJR 158:125, 1987.
13. Stark DD, Felder RC, Wittenberg J, et al: Magnetic resonance imaging of cavernous hemangioma of the liver: Tissue-specific characterization. AJR 145:213, 1985.
14. Freeny PC. Angiography of hepatic neoplasms. Semin Roentgenol 18:114, 1983.
15. Heiken JP, Lee JKT, Glazer HS, Ling D: Hepatic metastases studied with MR and CT. Radiology 156:423, 1985.
16. Chezmar JL, Rumancik WM, Megibow AJ, et al: Liver and abdominal screening in patients with cancer: CT versus MR imaging. Radiology 168:43, 1988.
17. Freeny PC, Marks WM: Computed tomographic arteriography of the liver. Radiology 148:193, 1983.
18. Matsui O, Takashima T, Kadoya M, et al: Liver metastases from colorectal cancers: Detection with CT during arterial portography. Radiology 165:65, 1987.

19. Nelson RC, Chezmar JL, Sugarbaker PH, Bernardino ME: Hepatic tumors: Comparison of CT during arterial portography, delayed CT, and MR imaging for preoperative evaluation. Radiology 172:27, 1989.
20. Sitzmann JV, Coleman JA, Pitt HA, et al: Preoperative assessment of malignant hepatic tumors. Am J Surg 159:137, 1990.
21. Freeny PC, Ryan JA: Preoperative hepatic imaging for lesion detection using bolus-dynamic CT, CT angiography, delayed iodine CT, and MR. Presented at the 76th Scientific Assembly and Annual Meeting of the RSNA, Chicago, November 29, 1990.

4
Hepatic Imaging Using High-Field MRI

W. DENNIS FOLEY

Detection of focal hepatic disease is critical in patients with suspected primary or secondary malignancy. MRI at high field strength (1.5 Tesla) is uniquely different to imaging at low to intermediate field strength (0.1 to 0.6 Tesla), since the field dependence of tissue relaxation parameters affects the choice of pulse sequence and timing parameters to produce the best lesion contrast (1). In addition, motion artifact-reduction techniques, use of contrast agents, and detection of extrahepatic disease are all factors that effect MRI image quality, lesion detectability, and the clinical utility of MRI in relation to CT scanning.

The earliest definitive clinical experience utilizing hepatic MRI was obtained at 0.6-Tesla field strength (2). This study demonstrated the superiority of a relatively short TE (20 ms), short TR (300 ms), multiple-excitation ($n = 16$) spin-echo pulse sequence in anatomic delineation and lesion detectability. This T1-weighted pulse sequence exploited the significant differences in T1 at 0.6 Tesla between normal liver and focal lesions. In addition, anatomic image quality or image signal-to-noise ratio was enhanced by the use of a relatively short TE (20 ms) and multiple excitations for each phase-encoding gradient step. The signal averaging inherent in the multiple excitation technique reduced motion artifacts by averaging and blurring without requiring additional artifact-reduction techniques. The relatively short TR (300 ms) and 1.5-cm slice thickness allowed the T1-weighted acquisition to be completed in 10 to 11 min of imaging time. Lesion characterization (differentiation of cyst, hemangioma, and metastasis) could, in many patients, be accomplished by an additional T2-weighted pulse sequence (3).

If all factors affecting image signal and noise are controlled, there is a linear increase in image signal-to-noise ratio with increasing field strength. This assumes equivalence in terms of magnetic field homogeneity and uniformity of radiofrequency and gradient power supplies. However, image quality is degraded by motion artifact, probably to a greater extent than at low to intermediate field strengths, and image contrast is affected by changes in tissue relaxation rates with changing field strength.

As field strength increases between 0.6 and 1.5 Tesla, there is an increase in T1 of both normal liver and focal lesions (1). Various investigators have either projected or demonstrated a decrease in hepatic lesion contrast at 1.0 and 1.5 Tesla in comparison with 0.6 Tesla when using the T1-weighted short TE (20 ms), short TR (300 ms), multiple-excitation technique (4,5). This indicates that in addition to lengthening of the T1 of both lesion and liver, there is convergence of these two values with increasing field strength. In comparative imaging trials at 1.0 and 1.5 Tesla, a T2-weighted pulse sequence with a TE of 75 to 100 ms, a TR of 2000 to 2500 ms, and two excitations for each phase-encoding gradient step has proven superior to the initial standard T1-weighted spin-echo pulse sequence (Fig. 4-1).

T2-weighted contrast may be accentuated by a slight decline in the T2 value of normal liver with increasing field strength. Measured T2 values of normal liver at midfield strength (0.35 to 0.5 Tesla)—45 to 55 ms—have been higher than those recorded at 1.5 Tesla (35 to 40 ms). This reduction in T2 value with increasing field strength has not been noted in other tissues. A possible explanation is greater susceptibility effect secondary to inhomogeneous distribution of iron in the reticuloendothelial system of normal liver.

While the signal-to-noise ratio of this T2-weighted pulse sequence is enhanced by the use of both high field and long TR, it is significantly degraded, relative to a T1-weighted pulse sequence, by the relatively long TE. In addition, there is minimal signal averaging with only two excitations per phase-encoding gradient step. Most vendors now offer a combination of various artifact-reduction techniques that are designed to improve image quality in hepatic MRI obtained at 1.5 Teslas, particularly the T2-weighted pulse sequences.

The earliest artifact-reduction techniques evaluated were respiratory gating, which significantly prolonged acquisition time and was thus clinically unacceptable (6). Respiratory-sorted phase encoding (RSPE) is a technique in which the magnitude of successively applied phase-encoded gradient steps is modulated by the degree of respiration (7). During maximum inspiration, the high-intensity signal arising from the subcutaneous abdominal wall fat, rather than projected in random fashion to overlay the internal abdominal anatomy, is displaced externally outside the field of view. In essence, RSPE seeks to register the anatomy between successive views. An important feature of the technique is that there is no time penalty, as there is with respiratory gating. The technique works best in patients with synchronous and relatively low-frequency respiration and is not able to cope well in patients who have markedly asynchronous respirations.

Gradient-moment nulling, or "flow compensation," is a first-order correction for soft-tissue or vascular motion that occurs between the 90- and 180-degree pulse of a spin-echo acquisition (8). In gradient-moment nulling (GMN), there is reshaping of the slice select and readout gradients, which are mathematically designed so that a phase shift of moving structures is completely nullified at the center of the readout echo. As with RSPE, no time penalty is involved with GMN. Clinical experience and controlled trials have demonstrated that GMN is better than RSPE in artifact reduction at 1.5 Tesla (9)(Fig. 4-2).

Most vendors now offer the combination of GMN and RSPE for artifact reduction. The combination is more efficacious than any single technique alone and is particularly valuable in the relatively long TE of T2-weighted pulse sequences, which, until recently, provided the best image contrast at 1.5 Teslas. The long TR of T2-weighted pulse sequences precludes the use of signal averaging as is used with the T1-weighted technique.

Vascular-motion artifacts within the plane of slice are significantly reduced by GMN. However, this is accompanied by positive signal within intrahepatic vessels, a factor that can result in diagnostic difficulty in distinguishing relatively high-intensity small peripheral hepatic lesions from small peripheral intrahepatic branch vessels.

The artifact-reduction techniques RSPE and GMN are complemented by presaturation of tissue planes outside the imaging volume that prevents artifactual signal from pulsatile flow in the aorta and inferior vena cava from being registered over the soft-tissue anatomy (Fig. 4-1).

In a recently reported study using a 1.5 Tesla imaging system, the T1-weighted spin-echo pulse sequence was modified by use of an asymmetrical fractional echo-sampling technique to result in a TE of 12 ms (10). The short TE significantly improved lesion-to-liver contrast of the T1-weighted spin-echo acquisition. Measured contrast-to-noise ratios of this T1-weighted sequence were superior to those of conventional T2-weighted spin-echo pulse sequences. This is a significant change from previous experience comparing T1- and T2-weighted pulse sequences for lesion detectability at high field. In essence, the short TE both improves signal-to-noise ratio and enhances T1-weighted contrast.

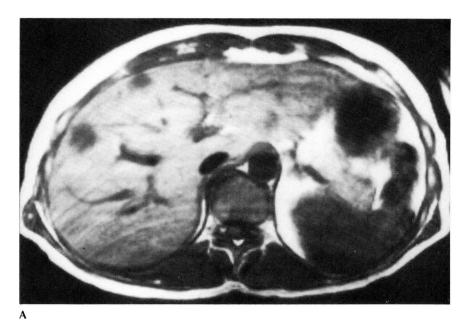

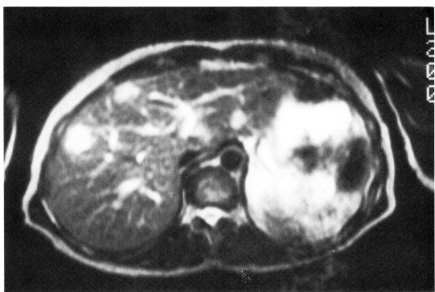

FIGURE 4-1
Multiple hepatic metastases imaged using standard T1-weighted (A) and T2-weighted (B) pulse sequences at 1.5 Tesla. All lesions are identified on each sequence. There is superior anatomic image quality on the T1-weighted image (TR/TE/NEX = 300/20/16), but better lesion contrast on the T2-weighted image (TR/TE/NEX = 2000/100/2). T2-weighted images acquired using presaturation, gradient-moment nulling (GMN), and respiratory-sorted phase encoding (RSPE).

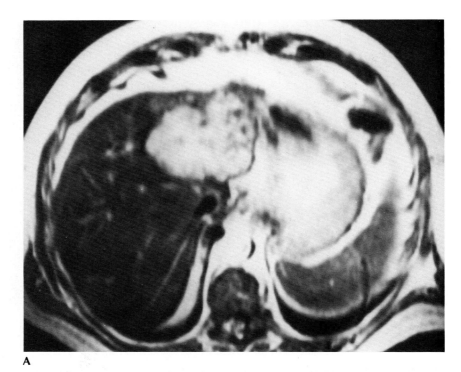

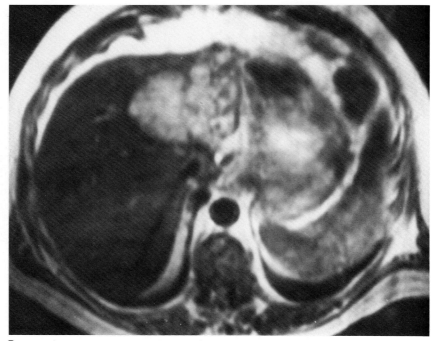

FIGURE 4-2
Left hepatic lobe metastases from colon carcinoma. Gradient-moment nulling (GMN) (A) is compared with respiratory-sorted phase encoding (RSPE) (B) using a T2-weighted acquisition (TR/TE/NEX = 2000/100/2). Image quality and contrast are superior using GMN.

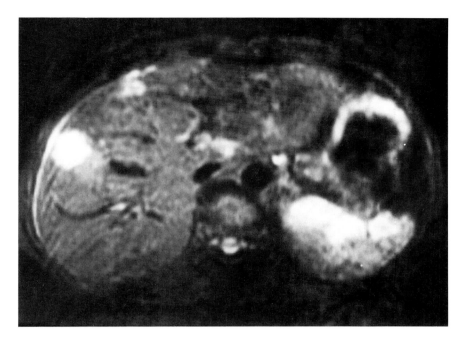

FIGURE 4-3
Same patient as in Figure 4-1. Short T1 inversion recovery sequence used. Image contrast is superior to the T2 acquisition demonstrated in Figure 4-1B. There is minimal signal from subcutaneous fat and little motion artifact. However, anatomic image quality is inferior to other sequences reflecting a lower signal-to-noise ratio.

INVERSION RECOVERY

Inversion recovery is an imaging sequence that is technically more difficult to implement than spin echo. An intrinsic advantage of inversion recovery is that T1- and T2-weighted contrast is additive. In addition, the inversion time can be selected such that the signal from subcutaneous fat is nullified using a pulse sequence denoted as STIR—short inversion time (TI) inversion recovery (11). Thus inversion recovery has potential advantages in terms of contrast and artifact reduction (Fig. 4-3). However, the TI chosen to nullify the signal from subcutaneous fat also lessens, to some extent, lesion contrast. Reported results using T2-weighted spin-echo and inversion-recovery pulse sequences at 1.5 Teslas have indicated virtual equivalence in lesion detectability. However, STIR images suffer from poor anatomic resolution and are not as useful as T2-weighted spin-echo images for distinction of hemangiomas and cysts from other focal hepatic lesions (12).

FAST-SCAN TECHNIQUES

While various motion compensation techniques, as discussed earlier, have been applied to T2-weighed pulse sequences at 1.5 Tesla, another approach has been to implement rapid data acquisition during one breath-hold. This has been done with gradient-recalled echo techniques in which rephasing is performed by reversal of the readout gradient without the use of a separate 180-degree refocusing pulse. This approach can significantly shorten TR. In addition, the flip angle can be varied in conjunction with the TR to produce a flip angle (the Ernst angle) that maximizes the signal-to-noise ratio. T2-weighted fast scan sequences are obtained with a relatively short flip angle (10 to 30 degrees) and relatively long TR (100 to 200 ms). With T2-weighted fast-scan techniques, there is positive enhancement of intravascular signal. This can result in diagnostic difficulty in distinguishing a peripheral lesion from a peripheral hepatic blood vessel (Fig. 4-4). T1-weighted

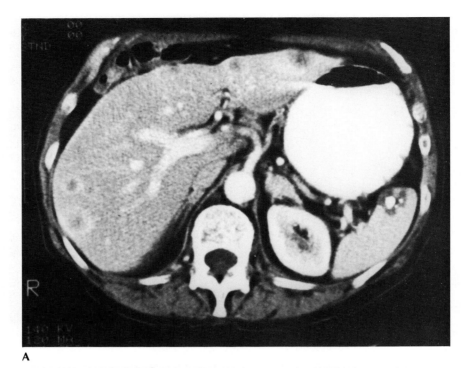

A

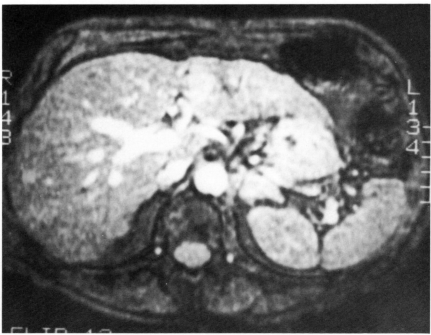

B

gradient-recalled echo pulse sequences are obtained with a flip angle approximating 90 degrees and with a relatively short TR and TE. These scans have better signal-to-noise ratios than T2-weighted fast scans and are not associated with the potentially confusing positive intravascular signal from peripheral hepatic vessels.

Although fast-scan techniques, dependent on selected TR, matrix, and number of excitations, can be obtained with reasonable image quality in approximately 12 s, the gains in artifact reduction (acquisition during a single breath-hold) are offset to a considerable extent by reduction in image signal-to-noise ratio. This reduction in SNR is due to the lack of a refocusing pulse (which normally counteracts magnetic field inhomogeneity), a relatively short TR (which results in incomplete T1 relaxation between acquisitions), and for T2-weighted sequences, the use of a narrow flip angle. T1-weighted gradient-recalled echo sequences are preferred and are being implemented in initial clinical trials evaluating the diffusible contrast agent Gd-DTPA in hepatic imaging.

In cerebral MRI, Gd-DTPA is an excellent contrast agent, since, in normal brain, it is confined to the intravascular space by an intact blood-brain barrier. However, in focal lesions in which the blood-brain barrier is disturbed, Gd-DTPA diffuses into the extravascular tissues. As with iodinated urographic contrast agents, Gd-DTPA rapidly diffuses into the extravascular space of normal thoracic and abdominal viscera. Following intravenous Gd-DTPA administration, there is rapid equilibration of the injected dose with the hepatic extravascular tissues, and an early peak hepatic enhancement is obtained. Maximum contrast enhancement with relatively hypovascular focal lesions is obtained with fast-scan acquisition within the first 2 min following Gd-DTPA administration (10). A T1-weighted fast-scan acquisition that allows multiple contiguous slice images to be obtained can be implemented using a long TR (110 ms) in combination with a short TE (5 ms) and a flip angle of 80 degrees. Initial studies indicate some improvement in lesion/liver contrast using gadolinium contrast-enhanced fast-scan acquisition over conventional spin-echo techniques (10). However, to date there has been no significant improvement in lesion detectability.

Acquisition within a single breath-hold using a spin-echo sequence rather than a gradient echo sequence has been accomplished using the asymmetrical fractional echo-detection scheme described earlier (13). With a TE of 10 ms, a TR of 275 ms, a section thickness of 12 mm, an interslice gap of 3 mm, a 128 × 128 matrix, and one excitation, a complete hepatic MRI study can be obtained in 23 s. This has the advantage of improved signal-to-noise ratio in comparison with gradient-echo sequences, but at the expense of a more prolonged imaging time. It is unlikely that the technique could be applied as a single-breath-hold technique to any significant segment of the clinical patient population.

COMPARATIVE SENSITIVITY OF HEPATIC MRI AT MIDFIELD AND HIGH FIELD:

Spin-echo MRI at midfield and high field has been compared. Lesion detectability using standard T1-weighted pulse sequences (TE = 20 ms) at midfield is equivalent in performance to T2-weighted pulse sequences at high field (14). These results have been obtained using identical pulse sequences and image-processing software in systems obtained from the same vendor but differing only in magnetic field strength.

CLINICAL APPLICATION OF HEPATIC CT AND MRI

Results of dynamic hepatic CT scanning with bolus contrast administration and spin-echo MRI at midfield and high field also have resulted in

---

FIGURE 4-4
Patient with metastatic breast carcinoma. Dynamic contrast-enhanced CT scan (A) is compared with gradient-recalled echo image (B). There is positive enhancement of inplane hepatic vessels on the MRI study. This may cause diagnostic difficulty in distinguishing peripheral focal lesions with increased signal intensity from intrahepatic vessels "on end" on a T2-weighted fast-scan sequence.

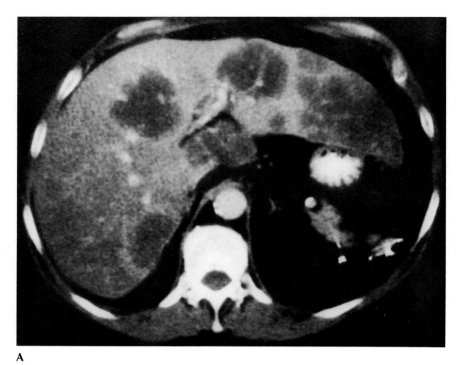

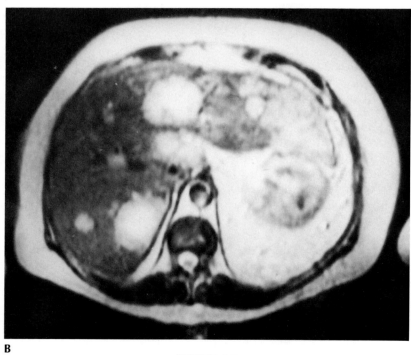

FIGURE 4-5
Hepatic metastases imaged using dynamic bolus contrast-enhanced CT (A) and T2-weighted MRI at 1.5 Tesla (B). There is equivalent sensitivity to focal hepatic lesions.

equivalent results in terms of hepatic lesion detectability. There is equivalent sensitivity of the dynamic CT technique with standard T1-weighted spin-echo pulse sequence (TE = 20 ms) at midfield and T2-weighted spin-echo pulse sequences at high field (Fig. 4-5). However, in both comparison studies, the CT technique resulted in significantly better sensitivity in detection of extrahepatic disease (15). Thus, in clinical practice, CT is still favored as the imaging technique of choice in oncologic patients suspected of having both hepatic and extrahepatic disease. MRI is reserved for patients with significant allergy to iodinated contrast agents or patients with equivocal or negative findings on CT scan who are strongly suspected of having focal hepatic disease. The equivocal findings on CT may be focal low-attenuation regions that could represent either metastatic disease or focal fatty liver. MRI can distinguish these possibilities. Focal lesions are hyperintense on T2-weighted pulse sequences and focal fatty liver isointense. Phase-contrast techniques improve discrimination between hepatic metastases and fatty liver by exploiting the difference in lipid content (16).

ADRENAL MASS CHARACTERIZATION

Patients with suspected hepatic metastatic disease may on occasion have a normal liver but isolated unilateral adrenal enlargement, the differential diagnosis of which is nonfunctioning adrenal adenoma or adrenal metastases. In lieu of percutaneous adrenal biopsy, MRI may be used to distinguish these two conditions. Rather than relying on measured adrenal/liver signal-intensity ratios, which are affected by the tissue composition of the liver (iron or fat), by the relative inhomogeneity within the image field, and by the magnetic field strength employed, measurement of T2 values in the adrenal have been found to be the most accurate MRI technique. Nevertheless, measured T2 values have resulted in only 80 percent true-positive discrimination between adrenal adenoma and adrenal metastases (17). Thus, in patients with normal bleeding and coagulation times, percutaneous adrenal biopsy is favored.

RETICULOENDOTHELIAL CONTRAST AGENTS

The utility of hepatic MRI at all field strengths may be improved by the development of superparamagnetic reticuloendothelial contrast agents (ferrite particles) being done in Boston and tested at the Massachusetts General Hospital. These contrast agents cause rapid dephasing of normal liver signal and enhanced contrast of lesion/liver, either using relatively long TRs in a T1-weighted pulse sequence or an equilibrium pulse sequence (short TE, long TR)(18). There is no time dependent effect of contrast enhancement as occurs with the diffusible gadolinium contrast agents. The initial results with the ferrite contrast agents suggest that they may produce improved detectability at midfield but that the effect on lesion detectability at high field, in comparison with conventional spin-echo pulse sequences, is not significant (19).

REFERENCES

1. Bottomley PA, Foster TH, Asgersinger RE, Pfeifer LM: A review of normal tissue NMR relaxation times and relaxation mechanisms from 1–100 MHz. Med Phys II:425, 1984.
2. Stark DD, Wittenberg J, Edelman RR, et al: Detection of hepatic metastases by magnetic resonance: Analysis of pulse sequence performance. Radiology 159:365, 1986.
3. Stark DD, Felder RC, Wittenberg J, et al: Magnetic resonance imaging of cavernous hemangioma of the liver: Tissue specific characterization. AJR 145:213, 1985.
4. Henkleman RM, Hardy P, Poon PY, Bronskill MJ: Optimal pulse sequences for imaging hepatic metastases. Radiology 161:727, 1986.
5. Foley WD, Kneeland JB, Cates JD, et al: Contrast optimization for the detection of focal hepatic lesions by MR imaging at 1.5 T. AJR 149:1155, 1986.
6. Runge VM, Clanton JA, Partain CL, James AE: Respiratory gating in magnetic resonance imaging at 0.5 T. Radiology 151:521, 1984.
7. Bailes DR, Gilderdale DJ, Bydder GM, et al: Respiratory order phase encoding (ROPE): Method for reducing respiratory motion artifacts on MR imaging. J Comput Assist Tomogr 9:835, 1985.
8. Pattany PM, Phillips JJ, Chin LC, et al: Motion artifact suppression technique (MAST) for MR imaging. J Comput Assist Tomogr 11:369, 1987.

9. Mitchell DG, Vinitski S, Burr DL, et al: Motion artifact reduction in MR imaging of the abdomen: Gradient moment nulling versus respiratory sorted phase encoding. Radiology 169:155, 1988.
10. Edelman RR, Siegel JB, Singer A, et al: Dynamic MR imaging of the liver with Gd-DTPA: Initial clinical results. AJR 153:1213, 1989.
11. Bydder GM, Steiner RE, Boumgart LH, et al: MR imaging of the liver using short TI inversion recovery sequences. J Comput Assist Tomogr 9:1084, 1985.
12. Dousset N, Weissleder RH, Hendrick RE, et al: Short TI inversion recovery imaging of the liver: Pulse sequence optimization in comparison with spin echo imaging. Radiology 171:327, 1989.
13. Mirowitz S, Lee JKT, Brown JJ, et al: Rapid acquisition spin echo (RASE) MR imaging: A new technique for reduction of artifacts and acquisition time. Radiology 175:131, 1990.
14. Steinberg HV, Alarcon JJ, Bernardino ME: Focal hepatic lesions: Comparative MR imaging at 0.5 and 1.5 T. Radiology 174:153, 1990.
15. Chezmar JL, Rumancik WM, Megibow AJ, et al: Liver and abdominal screening in patients with cancer: CT versus MR imaging. Radiology 168:43, 1988.
16. Rummeny E, Saini S, Stark DD, et al: Detection of hepatic metastases with MR imaging: Spin echo versus phase contrast pulse sequences at 0.6 T. AJR 153:1207, 1989.
17. Baker ME, Blinder R, Spritzer C, et al: MR evaluation of adrenal masses at 1.5 T. AJR 153:307, 1989.
18. Stark DD, Weissleder R, Elizondo G, et al: Superparamagnetic iron oxide: Clinical application as a contrast agent for MR imaging of the liver. Radiology 168:297, 1988.
19. Marchal G, VanHecke P, Demaerel P, et al: Detection of liver metastases with superparamagnetic iron oxide in 15 patients: Results of MR imaging at 1.5 T. AJR 152:771, 1989.

5

Midfield MRI of the Liver

DAVID D. STARK

MRI is under development worldwide for detection, differential diagnosis, staging, and treatment follow-up in patients at risk for cancer or metabolic disease of the liver. Major technical issues relevant to upper abdominal and liver MRI have been defined, and a variety of solutions are under development. Effective motion-suppression techniques and optimal pulse sequences have been identified for various clinical tasks. Although optimal techniques are different at low, middle, and high field strengths and performance varies among instruments from different manufacturers, there is now sufficient experience to match imaging techniques to specific clinical applications for each machine. This chapter reviews concepts governing assessment of MRI for detection of focal liver lesions and details results obtained on a mid field system at Massachusetts General Hospital.

TISSUE CONTRAST

Inherent tissue contrast available for detection of hepatic metastases has been carefully studied using a variety of systems operating at field strengths below 1 Tesla (Table 5-1). Compared to liver tissue, most tumors have an increased water content and have prolonged T1 and T2 relaxation times. Hydrogen density is correlated with T1 and water content. For the detection of liver metastases, it is significant that T1 contrast (the cancer/liver T1 difference) is on average greater than T2 contrast (at 0.35 to 0.6 Tesla; Table 5-1).

Lesions become detectable on MR images when the difference in signal intensity (contrast) between the lesion and surrounding liver is sufficient to distinguish the lesion as a real object and not an artifact or random fluctuation in pixel signal intensity (noise). A priori, it does not matter whether the lesion is bright or dark relative to liver. Therefore, it is the magnitude of contrast, relative to noise (CNR), that determines lesion detectability, and CNR can be measured to quantitate the performance of different imaging techniques (Table 5-2).

When tissue characteristics are known, mathematical theory can be used to calculate tissue signal intensities and image contrast (1,2). These calculations allow prediction of pulse-sequence performance under specified conditions. For example, calculations predict that T1-weighted images will outperform T2-weighted images for liver cancer detection at low and moderate field strengths (2) (Table 5-1). T1 weighting can be achieved using either spin-echo or inversion-recovery techniques. In general, T1 contrast causes lesions to be dark and T2 contrast causes lesions to be bright. It is undesirable to have both T1 and T2 influence image contrast, since lesions

TABLE 5-1. *Hydrogen Density and Relaxation Times of Liver and Cancer*

	Tissue	Moss (16)	Schmidt (20)	Stark*
Hydrogen density	Liver		0.62 ± .18	0.67 ± .20
	Cancer		0.68 ± .17	0.69 ± .18
Increase			9%	4%
T1 (ms)	Liver	533	350	499 ± 140
	Cancer	746	730	876 ± 334
Increase		40%	109%	76%
T2 (ms)	Liver	56	46	48 ± 1.1
	Cancer	68	68	78 ± 32
Increase		21%	49%	63%
Field strength		0.35 T	0.35 T	0.6 T

Note: Hydrogen density is scaled relative to the hydrogen density of fat.
*Based on 40 patients with hepatic metastases, fitting 4 or more spin-echo measurements for each relaxation time determination. Mean ± standard deviation.

may be isointense to surrounding liver. To maximize T1-dependent lesion/liver contrast, it is necessary to minimize T2-dependent contrast by reducing TE (1–5). T1-dependent contrast is ensured by setting TR less than the T1 of liver, limiting recovery of longitudinal magnetization. Alternatively, the inversion-recovery sequence begins with an extra 180-degree pulse to invert longitudinal magnetization, with differential rates of magnetization recovery introducing T1 contrast.

The reliability of mathematical predictions of image contrast has been confirmed by direct measurement of CNR on clinical images (Table 5-2). Interestingly, techniques such as the IR 1500/280/18, which maximize lesion/liver contrast, may not be the best sequence for lesion detection. In addition to contrast, morphologic features such as lesion size, location, and edge sharpness influence detectability. For example, large lesions that deviate nearby blood vessels and have sharp margins with adjacent liver are more easily detected than small, vaguely marginated lesions surrounded by solid liver parenchyma. The ability to detect lesions based on morphology is corrected with image quality or "anatomic resolution," which in turn is correlated with the signal-to-noise ratio (SNR) (Table 5-2).

NOISE AND MOTION ARTIFACTS

Theoretical predictions of contrast-to-noise ratios (CNR) do not consider the influence of ghost artifacts, the major determinant of noise on abdominal images (4). Therefore, techniques that suppress ghosting produce greater CNRs and have better lesion conspicuity than would be expected from contrast theory alone. This advantage is confirmed by clinical experience. For example, image contrast theory predicts that inversion-recovery (IR) sequences will slightly outperform short TR/short TE sequences with respect to lesion/liver CNR or lesion "detectability" (2). In actual clinical practice, the short TR/short TE spin-echo sequence is superior because of its ability to suppress motion artifacts (4,5) (Table 5-2). The advantage of fast spin-echo imaging is that short TR allows averaging of numerous acquisitions (N_{acq}, excitations) within a fixed scan time, reducing ghosts and image noise by $(N_{acq})^{1/2}$ (4). Additionally, TE is an independent factor determining the relative intensity of ghosts, which decrease as a function of $TE^{1/2}$. Minimizing TE increases signal from tissue while reducing the fraction of signal misregistered as ghost noise (4). Therefore, used together, short TR and short TE increase both SNR and T1-dependent image contrast, thus maximizing CNR.

Techniques that maximize CNR will maximize lesion detection in a *population* of patients. Individual variations in respiratory motion, tissue relaxation times, and liver fat content can significantly alter CNR and pulse-sequence performance in *individual* patients.

It is important to note that techniques developed for low and midfield systems (0.02 to 1.0 Tesla) may not be optimal at 1.5 Tesla due to dispersion:

TABLE 5-2. Quantitative Analysis of Pulse-Sequence Performance

				Performance Rank	
Pulse Sequence	n*	Liver SNR†	Cancer/Liver Magnitude CNR‡	CNR	Confidence Factor¶
SE 1500/30	7	19.9	1.9 ± 0.9	19	
SE 1500/30 PC§	7		3.0 ± 2.4	15	
SE 1500/60	7	13.3	3.5 ± 3.0	14	
SE 1500/90	6	9.5	5.5 ± 4.2	10	
SE 2000/30	27	17.2	2.4 ± 2.1	18	10
SE 2000/30 PC	25		4.2 ± 3.1	13	8
SE 2000/60	33	11.8	4.7 ± 3.6	11	9
SE 2000/60 PC	6		6.9 ± 2.7	7	
SE 2000/90	27	8.7	7.5 ± 5.3	5	7
SE 2000/120	5	6.0	7.7 ± 3.4	4	
SE 2000/180	4	3.7	4.2 ± 2.0	12	
IR 1500/450/30	33	16.5	6.2 ± 3.6	9	5
IR 1500/450/30 PC	1		1.6	20	
IR 1500/450/18	35	17.8	7.9 ± 4.2	3	3
IR 1500/280/18	30	11.3	7.2 ± 3.7	6	2
SE 500/30	37	25.5	6.4 ± 4.1	8	6
SE 500/30 PC	6		2.9 ± 2.1	17	
SE 260/30	32	24.8	8.1 ± 4.6	2	4
SE 260/30 PC	5		3.2 ± 0.9	15	
SE 260/18	39	27.4	10.3 ± 5.2	1	1

Note: Data are normalized to reflect a standard 9-min scan time for all pulse sequences.
*n = Number of patients studied; imaging performed at 0.6 Tesla.
†SNR, signal-to-noise ratio.
‡CNR, contrast-to-noise ratio, also known as signal-difference-to-noise ratio, SD/N; CNR = SD/N = $(S_{tumor} - S_{liver})$/noise.
§PC, phase contrast "opposed-phase image" obtained using the chemical shift imaging method of Dixon.
¶Confidence factor, the ratio of the mean CNR to its standard deviation, is calculated only when number of patients (n) is ≥25.

prolongation of tissue T1 relaxation as field strength increases (6–8). Theory suggests that T2-weighted images may offer superior CNR at 1.5 Tesla (2). However, clinical experience will be needed to determine the relative sensitivity of T1- and T2-weighted pulse sequences to motion artifacts at high field strength (9–11). Ultimately, selection of a technique for motion-artifact suppression may determine which pulse sequence is most effective for any particular machine.

PULSE-SEQUENCE OPTIMIZATION
Timing Parameters

Many published reports on MRI of liver tumors have been compromised by a limited choice of timing parameters, e.g., machine restrictions limiting the minimum TR to 500 ms and the minimum spin-echo TE to 30 ms. This SE 500/30 sequence gives an offsetting balance of T1 and T2 contrast that often results in poor image contrast (low CNR; Table 5-2) and poor lesion conspicuity. Excellent T1 contrast is available by means of inversion-recovery (IR) techniques; however, IR techniques require use of long TR, limiting the number of data acquisitions that can be averaged (12,13). As a result, scan time of IR images is typically long, and ghost artifacts obscure normal and pathologic hepatic anatomy. Furthermore, many imaging systems fail to acquire sufficient slices for anatomic coverage of the entire liver (18-cm craniocaudal length) on a single acquisition, necessitating repeat scanning (14–16).

Owing to manufacturer limitations in achieving the short TE capabilities necessary for T1-weighted spin-echo imaging, most early research emphasized the value of T2-weighted sequences for the detection of liver metastases (16–20). In general, these studies were biased by using scan times as long as 18 min for T2-weighted sequences, while spending only 5 min on T1-weighted images. Since SNR and image quality are proportional to the scan time, such comparisons are invalid.

STIR (short tau inversion-recovery) sequences have not been widely available but show promise for abdominal imaging due to suppression of signal from subcutaneous fat, reducing respiratory ghost artifacts (19,21). Furthermore, because of the short T1 (typically 100 ms), T1 and T2 contrast are additive and liver lesions appear bright. Although the CNR theory for STIR is straightforward, clinical evaluations are needed to determine efficacy of ghost noise suppression. STIR sequences use long TR and long TE, rendering heightened sensitivity to motion. STIR may be particularly valuable at 1.5 Tesla, but at midfield, SNR and CNR are inadequate for reliable liver lesion detection.

Gradient-Echo Imaging
Gradient-echo techniques (FLASH and others) have been implemented on several MRI systems with wide variations in pulse-sequence architecture (3,22–29). Although performance also varies, it is evident that fast (TR 30 to 300 ms) techniques are valuable for rapid anatomic surveys of high-contrast structures (3,24,29). Breath-hold imaging reduces noise by eliminating respiratory motion; however, since signal is proportional to imaging time, 10-s breath-hold images have much less signal than standard 10-min images. As a result of reduced SNR, anatomic resolution is reduced and low-contrast metastases are difficult to detect.

Gradient-echo images acquired with short TE and flip angles over 70 degrees show contrast dominated by tissue T1 differences (3,22). Conversely, images acquired with long TE (20 to 40 ms) and flip angles less than 40 degrees show contrast dominated by tissue T2 differences. Improved pulse sequences with ultrashort TE (10 ms or less) have been implemented at field strengths above 1.0 Tesla. These images show sufficient SNR and CNR for diagnostic use, but this has not yet been achieved at midfield.

Phase-Contrast Imaging
Phase-contrast (opposed-phase) images are obtained by moving the "gradient-induced echo" off center with respect to the "Hahn spin-echo" induced by the 180-degree pulse (30). Temporal displacement of the refocused echo by 5.4 ms corresponds to $1/|2(1-\omega)|$, where $1-\omega$ is the resonance-frequency difference between fat and water protons. This resonance-frequency difference is the product of the resonance frequency of the imaging system (25.1 MHz at 0.6 Tesla) and the chemical shift between fat and water protons expressed as parts per million (3.7 ppm). As a result of displacing the gradient and Hahn echoes by one-half precession cycle (5.4 ms × 93 Hz), the phases of fat and water magnetization are 180 degrees opposed at the time of the gradient-induced echo. Therefore, in the resulting "opposed-phase" image, pixel brightness is the net difference between fat and water magnetization.

Normal liver tissue contains less than 1 percent triglyceride by weight. Membrane lipids, which constitute 5 to 10 percent of the tissue weight, are not observable by any MRI technique due to the short T2 of highly ordered membrane lipids (31,32). Since membrane lipids contribute little or no signal to the hydrogen density observed by MRI, normal liver tissue and tissues such as cancer and spleen, which do not contain triglyceride, are effectively "pure water" tissues and show no difference in signal intensity between the conventional in-phase image and the Dixon phase-contrast or opposed-phase image. However, when fatty liver is present, the liver signal intensity will decrease on the opposed-phase image relative to liver signal intensity on the in-phase image. Since cancer signal intensity is unchanged, it follows that the signal intensity of cancer will increase relative to surrounding fatty liver (32,33).

Pulse-sequence timing-parameter (TR, T1, and TE) selection influences relaxation time "weighted" image contrast independent of chemical-shift–dependent image contrast introduced by using the Dixon method (33). Cancer/liver contrast is additive on T2-weighted opposed-phase pulse sequences, since both the T2 relaxation time difference and the MRI-observable fat content difference tend to decrease liver signal intensity relative to cancer. Conversely, T1-weighted opposed-phase pulse sequences show loss of cancer/liver contrast since the T1 relaxation time difference decreases cancer signal intensity while the MRI-observable fat content decreases liver signal intensity. Therefore, T2-weighted phase-contrast images equal or outperform T2-weighted conventional images in patients with normal and fatty livers, respectively (Table 5-2).

The clinical value of T2-weighted phase-contrast imaging in screening for hepatic metastases is based on the fact that 70 percent of patients with metastatic cancer show greater CNR on opposed-phase images than on corresponding in-phase T2-weighted images (32,33). This evidence of a high incidence of fatty infiltration in patients with cancer is consistent with older observations that fatty liver is a frequent finding in patients undergoing biopsy for metastatic cancer. Since triglyceride accumulates in only one of the two tissues of interest (liver but not cancer), triglyceride can be exploited as if it were a contrast agent. In individual patients with fatty liver, T2-weighted phase-contrast images may have greater CNR than conventional techniques. However, fatty infiltration also increases liver signal intensity on conventional T1-weighted images and similarly increases cancer/liver CNR over that seen in nonfatty livers. Therefore, conventional T1-weighted sequences usually outperform phase-contrast sequences. The ideal combination for cancer screening may be a T1-weighted conventional image and a T2-weighted phase-contrast image.

CNR Standardization
Unfortunately, performance of similar pulse sequences can vary from system to system, even at the same field strength. Contrast may vary when pulse-sequence architecture or slice geometry influences the "apparent" tissue relaxation times. For example, use of Gaussian pulses in conjunction with contiguous slices (Technicare 0.6-Tesla system) allows significant "cross-talk" between slices, effectively reducing the TR. Interestingly, this interaction may be a source of contrast on the short TR T1-weighted images and would be expected to decrease contrast when used in conjunction with long TR T2-weighted techniques.

To standardize clinical comparisons of different imaging systems and pulse-sequence techniques, a readily available contrast phantom that models physiologic motion is required. The normal spleen is an excellent model of liver cancer for several reasons: (1) the spleen has relaxation times (T1 and T2) as well as proton density similar to liver metastases, (2) the spleen is similar to cancer in containing little or no MRI-observable lipid, (3) the spleen is located on the same transverse sections as the liver, and (4) the spleen is a large homogeneous organ from which reproducible image-intensity data can be measured. The similarity of normal spleen to liver cancer has been confirmed on clinical images and indicates that pulse-sequence performance assessed using the spleen/liver CNR can substitute for cancer/liver CNR as a reliable predictor of pulse-sequence performance in the detection of liver cancer (33).

LIMITATIONS OF CT

The absolute accuracy of CT, MRI, or other imaging techniques for the detection of hepatic metastases is difficult to determine in clinical studies (34–43). However, for the clinical task of screening cancer patients at risk for hepatic metastases, CT outperforms scintigraphy and sonography and is the accepted "gold standard" (44). Unfortunately, recent data from several centers suggest that the sensitivity (true positive fraction, TPF) of contrast-enhanced CT for detecting individual hepatic *lesions* is only 34 to 37 percent and the sensitivity for identifying *patients* with one or more lesions is only 73 to 74 percent (37,40,42,43) (Fig. 5-1). Indeed, the false-negative rates for CT account for most of the unexpected late cancer deaths in patients who have previously undergone "curative" excision of primary cancers (44,45).

NEW CT TECHNIQUES

No consensus exists as to what constitutes a technically adequate CT examination (35,39,46). While most centers routinely use iodinated contrast material to improve lesion detection, in patients with

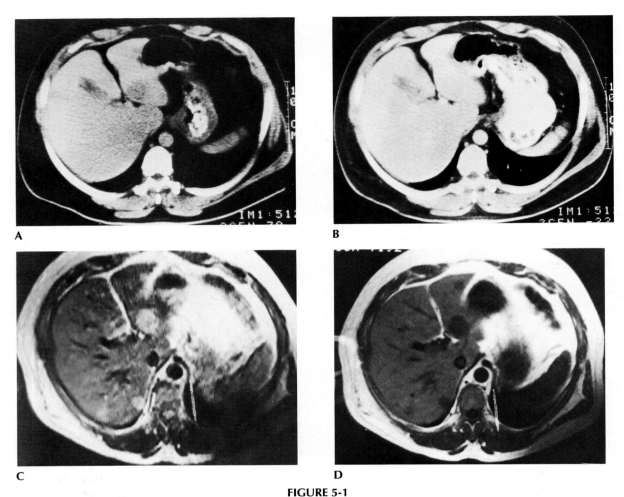

FIGURE 5-1

Adenocarcinoma on the colon. (A) CT scan shows lesion in the lateral segment of the left hepatic lobe. (B) CT repeated during intravenous injection of a 42-g bolus of iodine obscures the lesion. (C) SE 2000/60 image obtained the same week as the CT scan. A single high-intensity metastasis is seen in the left hepatic lobe. Additionally, two smaller, 1-cm metastases are well seen in the posterior segment of the right hepatic lobe. (D) SE 260/15 image shows higher SNR and less motion related blurring. An additional 1-cm lesion is now confidently identified in the anterior portion of the lateral segment of the left hepatic lobe. A total of four lesions are now confidently identified.

hypervascular metastases, iodinated contrast material obscures lesions (47). Therefore, under ideal circumstances, both noncontrast and contrast-enhanced scans would be performed routinely. Even accepting the inconvenience, cost, and risks associated with iodinated contrast material, experts disagree regarding the technique for contrast administration. Most centers infuse 40 g iodine over 2 or 3 min while performing rapid sequential scans with table incrementation through the liver (dynamic sequential bolus CT) (48,49). Infusion of an additional 20 g iodine with repeat scanning after a 4- to 6-h delay (delayed CT, DCT) may detect additional lesions (35). Other data suggest that lesion detection is maximized when contrast is administered by means of a hepatic artery catheter (CT angiography, CTA) (43,50–52). Such attempts to improve the performance of iodinated contrast agents have been offset by increased toxicity and invasiveness.

A technical limitation common to all CT techniques is the sequential single-slice data acquisition, requiring patient cooperation in breath-holding to duplicate the exact level of inspiration for each sequential scan. Scan-to-scan variations in breath-holding result in CT examinations that skip some anatomic levels while duplicating others.

COMPARATIVE ACCURACY OF MRI VERSUS CT

Our clinical results at the Massachusetts General Hospital using a midfield system (Technicare 0.6-Tesla) have previously been published (4). The accuracy of MRI relative to CT for the diagnosis of liver metastases was determined in a randomized, controlled comparative study including 135 subjects, 57 with cancer metastatic to the liver, 27 with benign cysts or hemangiomas, and 51 "normal controls" without focal liver disease. The sensitivity of a 1-h MRI "examination" consisting of four pulse sequences for detecting *individual metastatic deposits* was 64 percent, significantly greater than the 51 percent for CT ($p < 0.001$)(Fig. 5-2). The difference in sensitivity for identifying *patients with hepatic metastases* was less (MRI 82 percent versus CT 80 percent). Indeed, in clinical practice it is often more important to identify abnormal patients than to count individual lesions. For example, once the diagnosis of hepatic metastases is established, needless excision of primary pancreatic, breast, lung, and perhaps some colon cancers can be avoided. Furthermore, appropriate systemic chemotherapy is begun as soon as possible. Therefore, the most important task in hepatic imaging is to distinguish normal patients from abnormal ones (those with one or more liver lesions).

Perhaps even more important than sensitivity is the specificity of a diagnostic technique used to screen for the presence of disease (34). For example, since most patients do not have liver metastases, it is important not to have a high false-positive rate (low specificity). In patients without hepatic metastases, the specificity of MRI was 99 percent versus 94 percent for CT, and this difference was statistically significant at $p < 0.05$ (41). Analysis of these data using receiver-operating-characteristic (ROC) curves shows that MRI is a better test than CT for screening patients at risk to develop hepatic metastases.

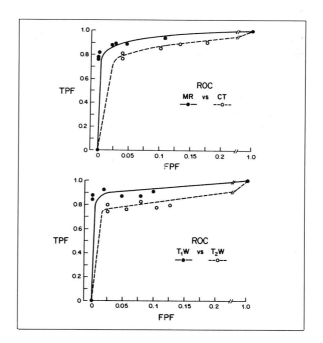

FIGURE 5-2
ROC curves in the diagnosis of metastatic liver cancer. True-positive fraction (TPF) shown on the coordinate, and the false-positive (FPF) on the abscissa. (A) ROC curves for the combined four pulse-sequence MRI examination (IR 1500/450/18, SE 250/15, SE 2000/60,120) and contrast-enhanced CT. Area under the MRI curve is greater than under the CT curve; therefore, MRI was superior for this test. (B) ROC curves for T1-weighted IR 1500/450/18 and T2-weighted SE 2000/120 pulse sequences. The T1-weighted sequence outperformed the T2-weighted sequence for detection of metastases.

Pulse-sequence performance assessed by the ability of radiologists to detect lesions has confirmed the validity of the CNR (Table 5-2) as an index of lesion conspicuity in a randomized trial designed to mimic the clinical situation of image interpretation (5,41). In clinical practice, significant differences are found between individual MRI pulse sequences for detection of individual lesions. The sensitivity of both T1-weighted SE (64 percent) and IR (65 percent) pulse sequence was significantly ($p < 0.001$) greater than either the TE 60-ms (43 percent) or TE 120-ms (43 percent) T2-weighted pulse sequences. Indeed, pulse-sequence performance assessed by the ability of a radiologist to detect lesions is quite similar to the rank order of CNR performance and pulse-sequence performance predicted by image contrast theory. These comparative data are valid for pulse-sequence performance on one particular machine (Technicare 0.6-Tesla). Similar results have been reported from centers using similar techniques on different machines (43,44). Certainly, the relative efficacy of pulse sequences will vary with different manufacturers and field strengths. However, this methodology is generally suitable for determining the best pulse sequence for any machine and any clinical application.

The Massachusetts General Hospital experience has shown that a single 10-min T1-weighted short TR/short TE pulse sequence is superior to contrast-enhanced CT for diagnosing focal liver lesions (41). However, it is important to note that extrahepatic lesions are still poorly detected by MRI and that CT is significantly more sensitive for detecting pancreatic ($p < 0.001$) and renal ($p < 0.05$) masses. Since extrahepatic lesions detectable by CT occur in 10 percent of patients at risk for hepatic metastases, the choice between CT and MRI is complex (14,34). When availability and cost of MRI and CT are comparable, the need to detect extrahepatic lesions must be balanced against the risk of CT contrast material (53) and the superiority of MRI for imaging the liver itself. Nevertheless, availability, cost, and habits of the referring clinicians may dominate scientific considerations.

REFERENCES

1. Hendrick RE: Image contrast and noise, in Stark DD and Bradley WG (eds): Magnetic Resonance Imaging. St. Louis, CV Mosby, 1988 pp 66–83.
2. Henkelman RM, Hardy P, Poon PY, Bronskill MJ: Optimal pulse sequence for imaging hepatic metastases. Radiology 161:727, 1986.
3. Hendrick RE, Kneeland B, Stark DD: Maximizing signal-to-noise and contrast-to-noise ratios in FLASH imaging. Magn Reson Imaging 5:117, 1987.
4. Stark DD, Hendrick RE, Hahn PF, Ferrucci JT Jr: Motion artifact suppression by fast spin echo imaging. Radiology 164:183, 1987.
5. Stark DD, Wittenberg J, Edelman RR, et al: Detection of hepatic metastases by magnetic resonance: Analysis of pulse sequence performance. Radiology 159:365, 1986.
6. Bottomley PA, Foster TH, Argersinger RE, Pfeifer LM: A review of normal tissue hydrogen NMR relaxation times and relaxation mechanisms from 10-100 MHz: Dependence on tissue type, NMR frequency, temperature, species, excision, and age. Med Phys 11:425, 1984.
7. Fullerton GD, Cameron KL, Ord VA: Frequency dependence of magnetic resonance spin-lattice relaxation of protons in biological materials. Radiology 151:135, 1984.
8. Johnson GA, Herfkens RJ, Brown MA: Tissue relaxation time: In vivo field dependence. Radiology 156:805, 1985.
9. Bailes DR, Gilderdale DJ, Bydder GM, et al: Respiratory ordered phase encoding (ROPE): A method for reducing respiratory motion artifacts in MR imaging. J Comput Assist Tomogr 9:835, 1985.
10. Ehman RL, McNamara MT, Pallack M, et al: Magnetic resonance imaging with respiratory gating: Techniques and advantages. AJR 143:1175, 1984.
11. Glover G: Physiological Motion and Gating in MRI. Presented at the 3rd Annual Meeting of the Society for Magnetic Resonance Imaging, San Diego, Calif., March 1985.
12. Bydder GM, Young IR: NMR imaging: Clinical use of the inversion recovery sequence. J Comput Assist Tomogr 9:659, 1985.
13. Doyle FH, Pennock JM, Banks LM, et al: Nuclear magnetic resonance imaging of the liver: Initial experience. AJR 138:193, 1982.
14. Hendrick RE, Nelson TR, Hendee WR: Optimizing tissue contrast in magnetic resonance imaging. Magn Reson Imaging 2:193, 1984.
15. Kneeland JB, Knowles RJR, Cahill PT: Multisection multiecho pulse magnetic resonance techniques: Optimization in a clinical setting. Radiology 155:159, 1985.
16. Moss AA, Goldberg HI, Stark DD, et al: Hepatic tumors: Magnetic resonance and CT appearance. Radiology 150:141, 1984.
17. Demas BE, Hricak H, Goldberg HI, Margulis AR: Magnetic resonance imaging diagnosis of hepatic metastases in the presence of negative CT studies. J Clin Gastroenterol 7:553, 1985.
18. Glazer GM, Aisen AM, Francis IR, et al: Evaluation of focal hepatic masses: A comparative study of MRI and CT. Gastrointest Radiol 11:263, 1986.
19. Ortendahl DA, Hylton N, Kaufman L, et al: Analytic tools for magnetic resonance imaging. Radiology 153:479, 1984.
20. Schmidt HC, Tscholakoff D, Hricak H, Higgins CB: MR image contrast and relaxation times of solid tumors in the chest, abdomen, and pelvis. J Comput Assist Tomogr 9:738, 1985.

21. Bydder GM, Steiner E, Blumgart FLH, et al: MR imaging of the liver using short TI inversion recovery sequences. J Comput Assist Tomogr 9:1084, 1985.
22. Buxton RB, Edelman RR, Rosen BR, et al: Contrast in rapid MR imaging: T1- and T2-weighting. J Comput Assist Tomogr 11:7, 1987.
23. Bydder GM, Young IR: Clinical use of the partial saturation and saturation recovery sequences in MR imaging. J Comput Assist Tomogr 9:1020, 1985.
24. Ferrucci JT: MR imaging of the liver. AJR 147:1103, 1986.
25. Haase A, Matthaei D, Hanicke W, Frahm J: Dynamic digital subtraction imaging using fast low-angle shot MR movie sequences. Radiology 160:537, 1986.
26. Hamm B, Wolf KJ, Felix R: Conventional and rapid MR imaging of the liver with gadolinium-DTPA in clinical use. Radiology 164:313, 1987.
27. Nelson RC, Chezmar JL, Steinberg HV: Dynamic and delayed CT versus short TE/TR spin-echo and fast field-echo MR for the detection of focal hepatic lesions. Radiology 161:331, 1986.
28. Ohtomo K, Itai Y, Yoshikawa K, et al: Hepatic tumors: Dynamic MR imaging. Radiology 163:27, 1987.
29. Provost TJ, Hendrick RE: Maximizing signal-to-noise and contrast-to-noise ratios in spin echo imaging using nonstandard flip angles. Magn Reson Imaging 4:105, 1986.
30. Dixon WT: Simple proton spectroscopic imaging. Radiology 153:189, 1984.
31. Heiken JP, Lee JKT, Dixon WT: Fatty infiltration of the liver: Evaluation by proton spectroscopic imaging. Radiology 157:707, 1985.
32. Lee JKT, Dixon WT, Ling D, et al: Fatty infiltration of the liver: Demonstration by proton spectroscopic imaging: Preliminary observations. Radiology 153:195, 1984.
33. Stark DD, Wittenberg J, Middleton MS, Ferrucci JT Jr: Liver metastases: Detection by phase-contrast MR imaging. Radiology 158:327, 1986.
34. Alderson PO, Adams DF, McNeil BJ: Computed tomography, ultrasound, and scintigraphy of the liver in patients with colon or breast carcinoma: A prospective comparison. Radiology 149:225, 1983.
35. Bernardino ME, Erwin BC, Seinberg HV, et al: Delayed hepatic CT scanning: Increased confidence and improved detection of hepatic metastases. Radiology 159:71, 1986.
36. Finlay IG, Meek DR, Gray HW, et al: Incidence and detection of occult hepatic metastases in colorectal carcinoma. Br Med J 284:803, 1982.
37. Freeny PC, Marks WM, Ryan JA, Bolen JW: Colorectal carcinoma evaluation with CT: Preoperative staging and detection of postoperative recurrence. Radiology 158:347, 1986.
38. Knopf D, Torres WE, Fajman WJ, Sones PJ: Liver lesions: Comparative accuracy of scintigraphy and computed tomography. AJR 138:623, 1982.
39. Miller DL, Vermess M, Doppman JL, et al: CT of the liver and spleen with EOE-13: Review of 225 examinations. AJR 143:235, 1984.
40. Reinig JW, Dwyer AJ, Miller DL, et al: Liver metastasis detection: Comparative sensitivities of MR imaging and CT scanning. Radiology 162:43, 1987.
41. Stark DD, Wittenberg J, Butch RJ, Ferrucci JT Jr: MR detection of hepatic metastases: A randomized, controlled comparison with CT. Radiology 165:399, 1987.
42. Sugarbaker PH, Vermess M, Doppman JL, et al: Improved detection of focal lesions with computerized tomographic examination of the liver using ethiodized oil emulsion (EOE-13) liver contrast. Cancer 54:1489, 1976.
43. Weyman PJ, Lee JKT, Heiken JP, et al: Prospective evaluation of hepatic metastases: CT scanning, CT angiography, and MR imaging. Radiology 161:206, 1986.
44. Borg SA, Rubin P, DeWys WD: Metastases and disseminated disease, in Clinical Oncology: A Multidisciplinary Approach, 6th ed. New York, American Cancer Society, 1983, pp 498–515.
45. Adson MA: Cannon Lecture—Hepatic metastases in perspective, AJR 140:695, 1983.
46. Freeny PC, Marks WM: Hepatic hemangioma: Dynamic bolus CT. AJR 147:711, 1986.
47. Bressler EL, Alpern MB, Glazer GM, et al: Hypervascular hepatic metastases: CT evaluation. Radiology 162:49, 1987.
48. Foley WD, Berland LL, Lawson TL, et al: Contrast enhancement technique for dynamic hepatic computed tomographic scanning. Radiology 147:797, 1983.
49. Freeny PC, Marks WM: Patterns of contrast enhancement of benign and malignant hepatic neoplasms during bolus dynamic and delayed CT. Radiology 160:613, 1986.
50. Ohishi H, Uchida H, Yoshimura H, et al: Hepatocellular carcinoma detected by iodized oil. Radiology 154:25, 1985.
51. Heiken JP, Lee JKT, Glazer HS, Ling D: Hepatic metastases studied with MR and CT. Radiology 156:423, 1985.
52. Yumoto Y, Jonno K, Tokuyama K, et al: Hepatocellular carcinoma detected by iodized oil. Radiology 154:19, 1985.
53. Wolf GL: Opinion: Safer, more expensive iodinated contrast agents: How should we decide? Radiology 150:557, 1986.

6

Ultralow-Field MRI of the Liver

RUEDI F. THOENI

Magnetic resonance imaging (MRI) has become an important technique in the large armamentarium of radiologic imaging. It has been enthusiastically embraced for evaluation of many organ systems and diseases and now is the most important method for assessing pathology of the central nervous system. Over the years, different magnetic field strengths have been used for various applications, with the middle and high fields most frequently employed for abdominal imaging (1–3). More recently, most commercial scanner research, development, and sales efforts have been devoted to the high-field superconductive systems with magnetic field strengths of up to 2.0 Tesla. Nevertheless, low-field units, which have been developed (4–7) and used, represent an attractive alternative, particularly for those institutions for which the high costs of a high-field system are not feasible. I will discuss the advantages and disadvantages of low-field MRI and report results on abdominal imaging with an ultralow magnetic field.

TECHNICAL AND LOGISTIC CONSIDERATIONS

Cost, service, and maintenance of a magnet increase with field strength if a magnet of equivalent aperture is considered. Superconductive magnets are most cost-effective at high field strengths of 0.25 Tesla or more, but at low field strengths, resistive and permanent magnets are preferable (8). Permanent and resistive magnets have similar siting requirements and production costs, but permanent magnets have the advantage of not requiring cooling water or electricity. Also, maintenance costs are higher for resistive magnets because they need a large power supply and heat exchanger. Permanent magnets can have open designs that increase patient comfort and eliminate failure of study due to claustrophobia. The transverse field in permanent magnets permits the use of solenoidal coils, which have fewer constraints on shaping and greater manufacturing tolerance. Also, low-field units, such as we have used for abdominal imaging at the University of California, San Francisco, can occupy a relatively small area that is no larger than 35 m^2 (or 350 ft^2) (9). These site requirements correspond to the size of a conventional fluoroscopy suite. Therefore, low purchase and installation costs, which include limited need for shielding and low overhead expenditures, represent advantages of low-field scanners.

In addition to economic advantages, imaging sequences also take advantage of some intrinsic characteristics of operation at low field strengths. Sensitivity to motion is decreased in the low field as compared with the middle and high fields, and therefore, many special techniques to suppress motion artifacts are not needed. Such techniques can increase imaging time, e.g., multiple averaging, or decrease the number of slices. Absolute background homogeneity is higher for low field strengths than for middle and high field strengths, and chemical-shift blurring and susceptibility artifacts are proportionally lower in the low magnetic field. Also, T1 relaxation times decrease with decreasing field strength (10,11). This results in higher signal-to-noise levels per unit time, improved lesion contrast, and improved contrast latitude.

CLINICAL APPLICATIONS OF LOW-FIELD MRI IN THE ABDOMEN

We became interested in applying these intrinsic characteristics of the low field to abdominal imaging after observing the usefulness of the low field for imaging the skeletal and central nervous systems. While T1-weighted images in the low field are available today, they were not feasible at the time our study was conducted. Therefore, our investigation was limited to T2-weighted spin-echo sequences in the low field, and these were compared with those obtained in the middle field (12). We were able to study 30 patients by low magnetic field strength (0.064 Tesla) and middle magnetic field strength (0.35 Tesla). Both units were manufactured by Diasonics (Toshiba). The middle field unit used a superconductive magnet and a quadrature coil, and the low-field scanner employed a permanent magnet with a solenoidal coil. T2-weighted spin-echo sequences were used with a TR of 2000 ms and a dual echo (TE 30/60–105). All images were analyzed using the following image parameters: the ratio of signal to noise, the ratio of signal difference between lesion and normal liver to noise, and the ratio of signal difference between lesion and normal liver to signal of liver, also called *contrast*. Lesion detection was determined, and all examinations were ranked for quality (ranking between 0 = nondiagnostic and 4 = excellent).

We found that for metastases and for hepatocellular carcinomas, signal-to-noise ratios and contrast-to-noise (CNR) ratios were persistently smaller in the low field than in the middle field. For metastases, contrast was higher in the low field than in the middle field (Fig. 6-1), but no appreciable difference was found for hepatocellular carcinomas (Table 6-1). These results were obtained by calculating the tissue parameters and were confirmed by individual ranking of the quality of the examinations for assessing liver vessels, lesion margins, and lesion contrast. Image qualities of 3+ and 4+ were more frequently assigned in the middle field (80 percent) than in the low field (50 percent) for evaluation of intrahepatic vessels, but lesion contrast was ranked at 3+ and 4+ in 88 percent of the patients in the low field and in 72 percent in the middle field. Rankings of 3+ and 4+ were given for assessment of liver lesions in 75 percent of patients in the low field and in only 37 percent of patients in the middle field if the second echo was analyzed. In comparison with the middle field, we found that lesions in the liver were better seen in the low field in 31 percent (Figs. 6-1 and 6-2), were equally well seen in 65 percent, and were more poorly visualized in only 4 percent (Table 6-2). Owing to the overall inferior signal-to-noise ratio in the low field, areas outside the liver received lower rankings in the low field than in the middle field. Only fluid-filled structures, such as the gallbladder and the stomach, showed similar quality rankings in middle and low fields.

The inferior image quality in the low field restricts the use of MRI in the abdomen to assessment of the liver. The low field is excellent for lesion detection in the liver and represents a cost-effective

TABLE 6-1. *Contrast in Low and Middle Fields for Primary and Secondary Liver Lesions*

Pathology	Contrast			
	Low, 2000/30	Middle, 2000/30	Low, 2000/105	Middle, 2000/60
Metastases	0.32 ± 0.18	0.27 ± 0.17	0.85 ± 0.60	0.43 ± 0.30
Hepatocellular carcinomas	0.23 ± 0.67	0.27 ± 0.17	0.42 ± 0.46	0.38 ± 0.20

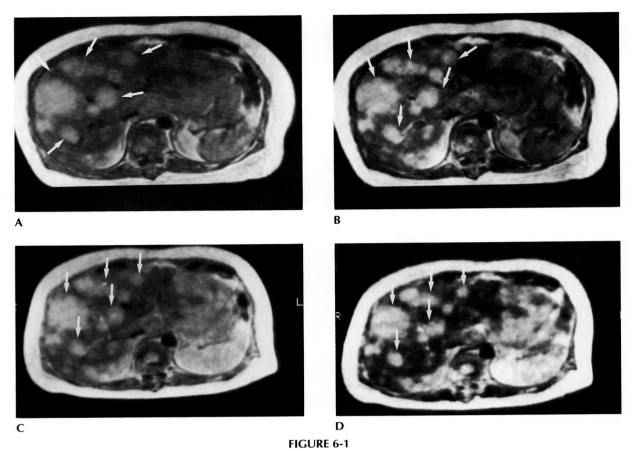

FIGURE 6-1
Patient with metastatic breast carcinoma. (A) Middle field: TR 2000 ms, TE 30 ms. Multiple lesions of increased signal intensity (arrows) are seen in the liver. (B) Middle field: TR 2000 ms, TE 60 ms. The signal intensity of the multiple metastatic lesions (arrows) is increased over those in part A. (C) Low field: TR 2000 ms, TE 30 ms. Similar to the middle field, lesions in the liver (arrows) are well outlined. (D) Low field: TR 2000 ms, TE 105 ms. Contrast for the multiple liver lesions (arrows) is higher in the low field than contrast observed in the middle field.

TABLE 6-2. Overall Results in the Low Field for Liver Lesions*

Area	Low Field Compared with Middle Field		
	Equal	Worse	Better
Liver	65	4	31
Abdomen	16	80	4

*Percent of patients ranked equal, worse, or better in low field as compared with middle field.

study for this purpose. Nevertheless, the present lack of good T1-weighted images and the lower signal-to-noise ratio and associated lower image resolution represent serious disadvantages of this method. It remains to be seen whether improved sequence design (14) (Fig. 6-3), including excellent T1-weighted sequences, will overcome the limitations imposed on the low field by presently available imaging sequences.

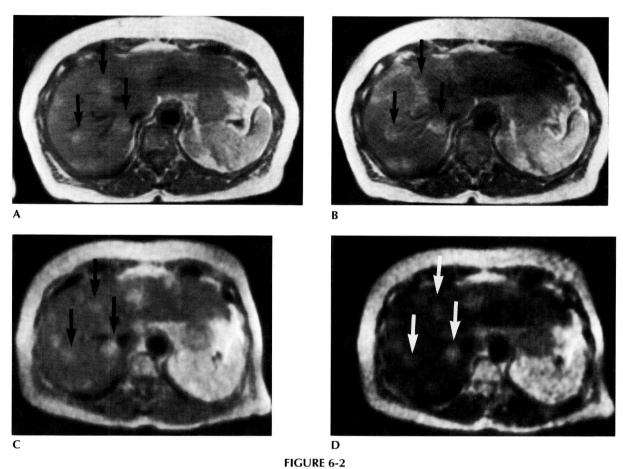

FIGURE 6-2
Patient with metastatic lung carcinoma to liver. (A) Middle field: TR 2000 ms, TE 30 ms. Lesions in the liver (arrows) are barely seen. (B) Middle field: TR 2000 ms, TE 60 ms. The second echo shows the lesions (arrows) to slightly better advantage. (C) Low field: TR 2000 ms, TE 30 ms. Multiple lesions (arrows) are seen throughout the liver and are better seen than in the middle field. (D) Low field: TR 2000 ms, TE 105 ms. Multiple liver lesions (arrows) are slightly better shown in the low than in the middle field.

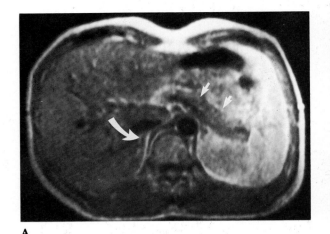
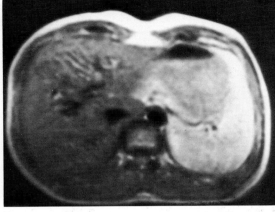
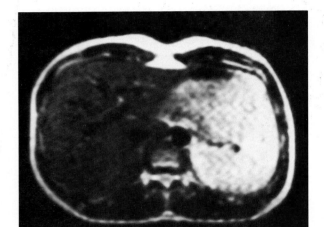

FIGURE 6-3
Normal volunteer. (A) *Recent improvements with imaging sequences have resulted in better image quality. Pancreas* (straight arrows) *and right adrenal gland* (curved arrow) *are clearly defined.* (B) *Low field: TR 2000 ms, TE 30 ms. Image quality is similar to that obtained with the T1-weighted image.* (C) *Low field: TR 2000 ms, TE 105 ms. The second echo shows acceptable image quality, but resolution is clearly inferior to what one could expect from images in the middle field.*

REFERENCES

1. Winkler ML, Thoeni RF, Luh N, et al: Hepatic neoplasia: Breath-hold MR imaging. Radiology 170:801, 1989.
2. Reinig JW, Dwyer AJ, Miller DL, et al: Liver metastases: Detection with MR imaging at 0.5 and 1.5 T. Radiology 170:149, 1989.
3. Steinberg HV, Alarcon JJ, Bernardino ME: Focal hepatic lesions: Comparative MR imaging at 0.5 and 1.5 T. Radiology 174:153, 1990.
4. Sepponen RE, Sipponen JT, Sivula A: Low field (0.02 T) nuclear magnetic resonance imaging of the brain. J Comput Assist Tomogr 9:237, 1985.
5. Fitzsimmons JR, Thomas RG, Mancuso AA: Communication: Proton imaging with surface coils on a 0.15-T resistive system. Mag Reson Med 2:180, 1985.
6. Smith MA, Best JJK, Douglas RHB, Kean DM: The installation of a commercial resistive NMR imager. Br J Radiol 57:1145, 1984.
7. Oldendorf W: Low field strength magnetic scanners. J Comput Assist Tomogr 9:1153, 1985.

8. Kaufman L, Arakawa M, Hale JD, et al: Low field MRI, in Margulis AR, Gooding CA (eds): Diagnostic Radiology. San Francisco, University of California, San Francisco, Radiology Research and Education Foundation, 1989, pp 97–104.
9. Kaufman L, Crooks LE, Arakawa M, et al: Prospects for increasing the accessibility of MRI. Admin Radiol 6:32, 1987.
10. Koenig SH, Brown RD, Adams D, et al: Magnetic field dependence of 1/T1 in tissue. Invest Radiol 19:76, 1984.
11. Rinck PA, Fischer HW, Elst LV, et al: Field-cycling relaxometry: Medical applications. Radiology 168:843, 1988.
12. Thoeni RF, Luh N, Winkler M, et al: Low-field MR imaging of the liver. Radiology 169(P):64, 1988.
13. Thoeni RF, Rothschild PA, Crooks LE, et al: Ultralow field MRI of the liver. Radiology (submitted).
14. Kaufman L, Kramer DM, Hake K, et al: Advances in low-field MRI, in Gooding CA (ed): Diagnostic Radiology. San Francisco, University of California, San Francisco, Radiology Research and Education Foundation, 1990, pp 213–226.

III. LESION DETECTION BY MRI AND CT: COMPARATIVE STUDIES

7

Hepatic Lesions Detected by MRI and CT Comparative Studies: The National Institutes of Health Experience

JOSEPH A. FRANK, ANDREW J. DWYER, DONALD L. MILLER, and JAMES W. REINIG

Evaluation of the liver for metastases is an essential part of the initial staging and follow-up of patients with various malignancies. Hepatic metastases are present in as many as 25 percent of malignancies (e.g., gastrointestinal, lung, breast, and melanoma) at the time of presentation (1). Over the past decade, there have been several clinical studies performed at the National Institutes of Health (NIH) comparing various imaging modalities in an attempt to define sensitivities for the detection of hepatic metastases (2–8). The focus of this chapter will be to summarize the NIH experience using contrast-enhanced computed tomography (CT) and magnetic resonance imaging (MRI) at middle and high field strengths in patients with known or suspected hepatic metastasis.

CONTRAST-ENHANCED CT, 1980–1984

In the early 1980s, CT was considered the most sensitive technique in detecting focal liver disease. Various contrast-enhanced CT techniques such as bolus dynamic, arterial portography de-

The authors would like to thank Anna Scheib for her help in preparing this manuscript. The authors would also like to acknowledge Drs. Alfred Chang, Paul Sugarbaker, and Barbara Ward and the rest of the radiologists and staff fellows at the NIH who have been involved in the studies presented within this chapter.

layed CT were developed to improve the delineation of hepatic metastases. Noncontrast CT (NCT) and CT enhanced with drip infusion of water soluble contrast material (WS-CT) were reported to detect less than half of surgically proven metastases (3). CT enhanced with the bolus administration of water-soluble contrast material (dynamic CT) also has been used in the evaluation and staging of patients with colorectal carcinomas and has been found to miss 27 percent of surgically proven metastases (9). Moreover, early experience suggested that these imaging modalities had a size threshold for detecting liver lesions above 2 cm (3). Therefore, there was a need for a more sensitive examination for detecting liver metastases.

In 1980, Vermess and coworkers (8) introduced an experimental intravenous liposoluble contrast material for CT, EOE-13. EOE-13 was an aqueous emulsion of iodinated esters of poppyseed oil that was phagocytized by the reticuloendothelial system, thereby increasing the density of the liver and spleen. In 1984, Miller et al. (2) summarized the experience at the NIH in 225 contrast-enhanced CT exams (179 patients) using EOE-13 (EOE-CT). EOE-13 resulted in an increase in visual contrast between normal parenchyma, on the one hand, and hepatic lesions and vascular structures, on the other hand, providing an excellent display of hepatic and splenic metastases (1–3,8).

In 1984, Sugarbaker et al. (3) reported on the results from 53 patients with 129 hepatic metastases in which NCT, WS-CT, and EOE-CT were compared with surgical findings. Noncontrast CT (NCT) demonstrated only 40.6 percent and WS-CT demonstrated only 33.6 percent, whereas EOE-CT detected 76.6 percent of surgically verified lesions in 30 patients. All lesions detected by NCT or WS-CT were seen by EOE-CT. Additionally, the threshold of lesion size detectable by EOE-CT was approximately one-half that of WS-CT and NCT. EOE-CT revealed 83 percent of the masses in the 1 to 2-cm range, whereas WS-CT and NCT showed 26 and 20 percent of these masses, respectively. Although EOE-13 appeared to be a highly effective CT contrast agent, it was unstable and had significant side effects, including fever, rigor, and headache (1,2). Pretreatment with intravenous steroids avoided some of the symptoms, and for this reason, EOE-13 remained an experimental contrast agent only used at a few institutions. At the NIH, EOE-CT was considered the "gold standard" for the evaluation of hepatic metastases.

COMPARISON OF CT AND MRI, 1984–1987

In 1984, MRI began at the NIH on a 0.26-Tesla Vista 2055 Picker International MRI unit. The early imaging results in the abdomen were poor because the standard T2-weighted spin echo (SE) pulse sequences (e.g., SE 2000/80) required long scanning times, were riddled with artifacts due to respiratory motion, and provided poor anatomic display.

A major advancement in MRI techniques occurred as a result of the work of Stark et al. (10), who demonstrated that the short echo time (TE) and short repetition time (TR) spin-echo (SE) pulse sequence with multiple repetitions produced near motionless images with excellent anatomic detail and markedly reduced artifacts. Since the T1 values of normal liver parenchyma and hepatic metastases may differ as much as 40 percent, the short TE/short TR heavily T1-weighted SE images also provide excellent lesion/liver contrast. The short TE/short TR SE technique provided the necessary tool required to perform a study comparing CT and MRI in the detection of liver metastases.

Reinig et al. (4) reported on a comparison of NCT, EOE-CT, and three different MRI pulse sequences in patients with known hepatic metastases from colorectal carcinoma, renal cell carcinoma, and melanoma. CT scans were performed both without (NCT) and with infusion of 0.25 ml/kg EOE-13 (EOE-CT) on a third-generation (General Electric 8800 or 9800) scanner with 10-mm contiguous slices. MRI was performed at 0.5 Tesla using a short TE/short TR spin-echo (SE 300/26) T1-weighted pulse sequence with eight repetitions, a T2-weighted SE 2000/80 with two repetitions, and a short inversion time (TI) inversion-recovery (IR) sequence (STIR) with a TI of 100 ms, a TR of 1500 ms, and a TE of 30 ms (IR 1500/100/30) with four repetitions.

The SE 300/26 scans were obtained in approximately 20 min to cover the entire liver. The T2-weighted and STIR sequences were obtained in 8 to 12 min each. Metastatic lesions appear as regions relatively dark compared with normal liver on the T1-weighted SE 300/26, NCT, and EOE-CT scans, whereas on the T2-weighted SE 2000/80 and STIR sequences lesions demonstrate high signal intensity compared with liver. The STIR pulse sequence, owing to the synergistic effect of T1 and T2 on signal intensity, produces images that are sensitive to pathology and contain muted but discernible anatomic detail (11,12). Individual lesions were numbered and measured to the nearest 0.5 cm and were only considered positive if visible on at least two of the five scanning techniques.

Table 7-1 summarizes the lesion-by-lesion analysis from the follow-up study in 25 patients with a total of 162 lesions and includes the sensitivities and 99 percent confidence interval for each of the modalities (13). EOE-CT revealed 87.6 percent of the lesions, whereas the SE 300/26 and IR 1500/100 sequences detected 95.7 and 90.2 percent of the lesions, respectively. Both NCT and SE 2000/80 scans were inferior, revealing only 49.6 and 52.9 percent of lesions, respectively. There was no significant difference at the 0.01 significance level in the sensitivities between EOE-CT and SE 300/26, IR 1500/100 and EOE-CT, and SE 300/26 and IR 1500/100 by a McNemar analysis.

The *threshold of visibility* of a lesion, defined as the lesion size at which 90 percent of the lesions were detected, was between 1 and 2 cm for the SE

TABLE 7-1. Hepatic Lesions Detected by Size and Imaging Technique*

Lesion Size (cm)	NCT	EOE-CT	MRI, SE 300/26	MRI, SE 2000/80	MRI, IR 1500/100
0.5	0/1	4/6	3/6	0/3	1/3
1.0	4/16	17/28	26/28	5/25	15/22
1.5	3/14	24/29	28/29	10/20	18/19
2.0	14/34	37/39	38/39	21/34	33/33
2.1–3.0	20/31	33/33	33/36	19/32	27/28
3.1–4.0	9/12	16/16	16/16	10/14	11/11
>4.1	8/9	10/10	10/10	8/11	9/9
Total	58/117	142/162	155/162	74/140	115/127
Percent sensitivity	49.6	87.6	95.7	52.9	90.6
99% CI†	0.38–0.63	0.78–0.92	0.89–0.98	0.41–0.65	0.82–0.96

*All patients did not have all studies owing to equipment failure, unavoidable scheduling error, or claustrophobia during MRI scanning leading to the early termination of the examination.
†99% CI = 99 percent confidence intervals.

300/26, IR 1500/100, and EOE-CT scans (4). However, the threshold of lesion visibility for the NCT and SE 2000/80 T2-weighted images was inferior; lesions 5 and 10 cm in diameter, respectively, were missed. The short TE/short TR SE sequence also was shown by Stark et al. (14) to have a sensitivity of 64 percent in the detection of hepatic lesions, whereas T2-weighted SE images and contrast enhanced CT had sensitivities of 43 and 51 percent, respectively. The lower sensitivity of the T2-weighted spin-echo images in the detection of liver metastases probably reflects a combination of motion artifacts seen with this sequence and the observation that some tumors have similar relaxation properties to the liver, making them indistinguishable from normal liver parenchyma.

Based on these studies, it was concluded that MRI using a short TE/short TR (i.e., T1-weighted) spin-echo sequence with multiple repetitions was at least equivalent if not superior to EOE-CT, the surgically corroborated "gold standard" in the evaluation of hepatic metastases. Moreover, discrimination of vascular structures from focal hepatic masses, which may be difficult on NCT and EOE-CT, was straightforward on the T1-weighted SE sequences. The major criticism of these studies (4,14) was the lack of surgical verification, hence the true sensitivity and false-positive rate of MRI had not been determined.

COMPARISON OF CT AND MRI WITH SURGERY, 1987–1990

A prospective evaluation in patients with isolated colorectal liver metastases was initiated in 1986 to correlate contrast-enhanced CT and MRI findings with operative findings. Patients were undergoing laparotomy for treatment protocols conducted by the National Cancer Institute Surgical Oncology Branch for either hepatic resection or placement of hepatic artery catheters for intraarterial chemotherapy. In each case, the MRI and CT scans were performed within 3 weeks of surgery. A summary of the imaging techniques follows in order to allow for a comparison with other studies (15,16).

The three contrast-enhanced CT scanning techniques consisted of EOE-13–enhanced CT, arterial portography CT (AP-CT), and delayed-scanning CT (DS-CT) (7). All CT studies were performed on a third-generation CT scanner (General Electric 9800) with 10-mm slice thickness at 7-mm intervals. EOE-CT was obtained in the manner reported (5–7). Arterial portography was performed after angiography with the catheter in the superior mesenteric artery, injecting 30 ml/min of diatrizoate meglumine or iopamidol using a mechanical injector. The dynamic technique included nine scans usually with 35 cc of contrast material and repeated three to four times to cover the liver. The dose of contrast material in DS-CT was 79 g iodine (220 to 380 ml). DS-CT was performed 4 to 6 h after infusion of the iodinated agent. Only 1 of the 20 patients in this study did not have DS-CT.

MRI was performed at 0.5 Tesla (Picker International, Vista 2055) using a T1-weighted short TE/short TR (e.g., SE 300/20) with eight repetitions and a T2-weighted SE 2000/80 with four repetitions using the motion-artifact-suppression technique (MAST). The addition of this gradient moment nulling technique for motion suppression was probably the second noninvasive means of decreasing motion artifacts and improving the diagnostic yield of long TE/long TR SE or IR images (17). For both imaging sequences, a 10-mm slice thickness and 128 phase-encoded steps were used. Only 1 of the 20 patients was not included in the study, because of the presence of 40 liver metastases, which would have made correlation to operative findings difficult. In these 19 patients, 9 had liver metastases resected as part of a lobectomy or wedge dissection, whereas 10 patients had nodules assessed by palpation at surgery. Seven patients also had intraoperative ultrasound using a 5-MHz mechanical sector real-time transducer (7).

In addition to the preceding imaging examinations, 16 of these patients had MRI performed at 1.5 Tesla (General Electric Signa) prior to surgery (J. W. Reinig, and J. A. Frank, unpublished results). MRI was performed using the following imaging sequences: a T1-weighted short TE/short TR spin-echo pulse sequence (SE 300/25) with six excitations and a T2-weighted SE 2000/80 with two excitations and respiratory compensation. An inversion-recovery (IR 2000/6000/20) sequence with two excitations and respiratory compensation was performed in only 10 of these patients owing to scheduling difficulties or time constraints. All scans at 1.5 Tesla were performed with 128 phase-encoded steps and a 7.5-mm slice thickness and 2.5-mm slice gap. Sixteen patients underwent a maximum of eight imaging studies for evaluation of hepatic metastases (Fig. 7-1). Scans were evaluated prospectively for size and location, and data were recorded on schematic maps of the liver. Statistical analysis of the true-positive and false-positive findings on a lesion-by-lesion basis was performed by using a McNemar test for paired data (7).

Figure 7-2 is a dot plot comparing the results of the contrast enhanced CT and 0.5- and 1.5-Tesla MRI examinations with operative findings. The closed circles represent lesions identified by each imaging modality that were found at surgery (i.e., true positive), and undetected lesions are open circles (i.e., false negative). Seventy-eight lesions were found at surgery, ranging in size from 0.1 to 13 cm. Table 7-2 lists the sensitivity of each imaging study. Ward et al. (7) reported the overall sensitivity for five imaging studies (i.e., enhanced CTs and 0.5-Tesla MRI) as follows: EOE-CT, 83 percent; AP-CT, 78 percent; DS-CT, 82 percent; SE 300/20 at 0.5 Tesla, 84 percent; and SE 2000/80 at 0.5 Tesla, 64 percent. The T2-weighted SE 2000/80 studies were significantly worse than the EOE-CT ($p < 0.001$), DS-CT ($p < 0.005$), and T1-weighted SE 300/20 ($p < 0.001$) studies by McNemar test. The sensitivity for lesions ≥ 2 cm demonstrated no significant difference between EOE-CT (96 percent), AP-CT (95 percent), DS-CT (96 percent), and SE 300/20 MRI at 0.5 Tesla (97 percent); however, the T2-weighted SE 2000/80 study (76 percent) did significantly worse.

A comparison of the results obtained at 1.5 Tesla, reveals that the overall sensitivity in detecting lesions was significantly worse for all three techniques (i.e., SE 300/25, SE 2000/80, and IR 2000/600) when compared with the contrast-enhanced CT and 0.5-Tesla T1-weighted SE 300/20 MRI scans. There was no difference in the sensitivity of these techniques at 1.5 Tesla when compared with the SE 2000/80 scans at 0.5 Tesla. For lesions ≤ 2 cm, the sensitivity of each study was equally reduced, with no significant difference between each of the studies.

The false-positive rate for each technique based on the total number of nodules detected is as follows: EOE-CT, 16 percent; AP-CT, 31 percent; and DS-CT, 9 percent. At 0.5 Tesla, the SE 300/20 MRI rate was 3 percent and the SE 2000/80 MRI rate was 9 percent, and at 1.5 Tesla, the SE 300/25 MRI rate was 5 percent, the SE 2000/80 rate was 8 percent, and the IR 2000/600 rate was 9 percent. The T1-weighted SE 300/20 images performed at 0.5 Tesla had the lowest false-positive percentage compared with "gold standard" EOE-CT. Moreover, when calculated on a per-patient basis the false-positive percentage for the T1-weighted SE 300/20 scans at 0.5 Tesla was significantly lower

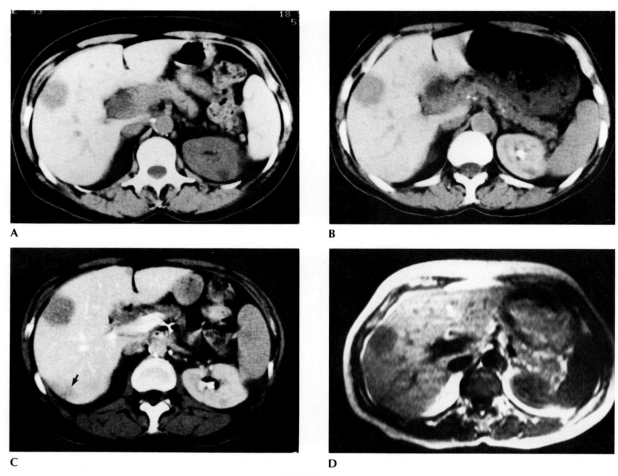

FIGURE 7-1

EOE-CT (A) and DS-CT (B) in a 44-year-old woman with metastatic colorectal carcinoma. Metastatic tumor appears hypointense compared with normal liver. (C) AP-CT lesion in right posterior lobe of liver (arrow) was not found at surgery and was considered to be a false-positive nodule. (D) T1-weighted SE 300/26 MRI image at 0.5 Tesla displaying colorectal metastases as low-signal-intensity lesion. T2-weighted SE 2000/80 (E) and IR 1500/100/30 (STIR) (F) images at 0.5 Tesla demonstrate the metastatic lesion as area of high signal intensity. [STIR image was not included as part of study by Ward et al. (7) and is presented here for illustration purposes.] At 1.5 Tesla, in the SE 300/25 (G) and IR 2000/600 (H) images, the lesion appears hypointense compared with normal parenchyma. On the T2-weighted SE 2000/80 scan (I), the lesion appears hyperintense.

than the rates for the contrast-enhanced CT studies (7), the IR 2000/600 MRI studies at 1.5 Tesla, and the T2-weighted images at both field strengths (Table 7-3).

Ward et al. (7) indicated that the T1-weighted SE 300/20 images obtained at 0.5 Tesla were as sensitive as EOE-CT for the detection of hepatic metastases from colorectal carcinoma and had the lowest false-positive rate. The SE 300/20 images at 0.5 Tesla were also the most sensitive in detecting hepatic lesions when compared with the SE 2000/80 images at 0.5 Tesla and all three pulse sequences performed at 1.5 Tesla. AP-CT had the highest false-positive rate, making it clinically useless.

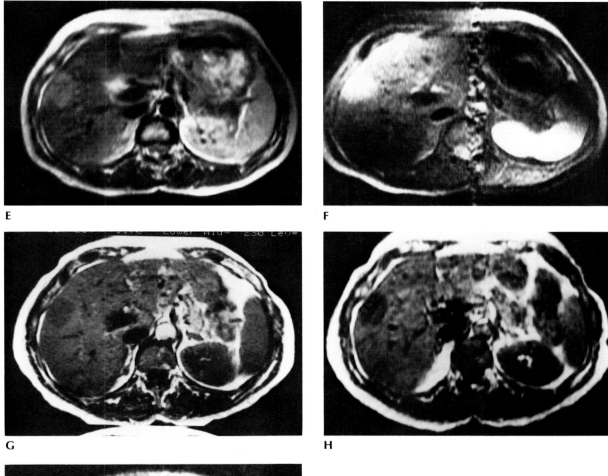

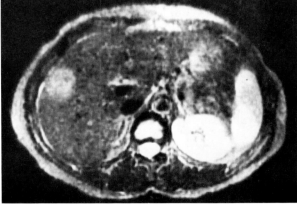

FIGURE 7-1 (continued)

These findings are contrary to those of Heiken et al. (15), who found AP-CT to be the most sensitive technique with the lowest false-positive rate in the detection of pathologically verified hepatic tumors when compared with DS-CT and three MRI pulse sequences (e.g., SE 300/15, SE 2100/35,90, proton-spectroscopic SE 1500/38,76) at 0.5 Tesla. The differences in the false-positive rates for AP-CT between the two studies may be due to streaming of the contrast media (5) or a result of the close pathologic examination of the liver that was performed ex vivo in Heiken et al. study. It is important to note that assessment of the liver at surgery has been reported to miss up to 6 percent of lesions found at autopsy (5). The discrepancy in the sensitivities of DS-CT found by Heiken et al. (52 percent) versus the NIH (82 percent) may reflect differences in the total iodine

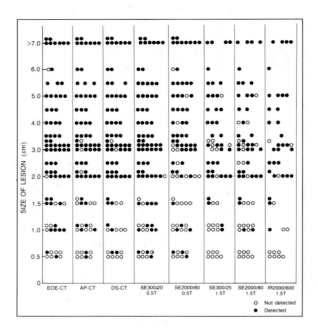

FIGURE 7-2
Dot diagram illustrating the size of nodules found at surgery and whether or not they were detected by each imaging modality. Lesion sizes were rounded off to the nearest 0.5 cm. Open circles represent lesions not detected, whereas closed circles are lesions detected by the scan.

dose administered to these patients (5,7,15). The decreased sensitivity observed by Heiken et al. for the T1-weighted SE 300/15 with four excitations (42 percent) may be due to an insufficient number of repetitions used for motion-artifact suppression (4–6,9,13), which would allow for better visualization of lesions from normal parenchyma.

Reinig et al. (6) reported the overall sensitivities for detection of hepatic metastases from colorectal carcinoma of the SE 2000/80 (72 percent), IR 2000/600/20 at 1.5 Tesla (90 percent), and SE 300/20 and SE 2000/80 at 0.5 Tesla to be higher than the results presented in Table 7-2. One obvious difference between the Reinig et al. study (6) and the results presented here is that comparison of imaging findings with surgically verified lesions would reflect the actual true-positive and false-positive rates for each modality. Futher, while there was some overlap of patients examined between the two studies, software updates at 1.5 Tesla improving respiratory compensation for the IR 2000/600/20 and SE 2000/80 sequences occurred after the completion of the study by Ward et al. (7). This significantly improved the image quality for those sequences and likely resulted in an increased sensitivity in the detection of hepatic metastases.

Steinberg et al. (16) evaluated focal hepatic lesions at 0.5 and 1.5 Tesla on MRI units from the same manufacturer, and found equality among the pulse sequences used at 0.5 and 1.5 Tesla, although the short TE/short TR SE sequence at 1.5 Tesla was significantly inferior. Based on the surgically verified results presented (see above), there would appear to be a relative inequality between the two magnetic field strengths. The differences between these studies may reflect the use of the greater number of excitations to obtain the T2-weighted (at 0.5 and 1.5 Tesla) and inversion-recovery images (at 1.5 Tesla) that should decrease motion artifacts and increased lesion detectability (16). Moreover, the similarities between the studies suggest that differences in the various MRI units play little, if any, role in the ability to detect hepatic lesions (5,6,16).

CONCLUSIONS

Our present approach for evaluating the liver for malignancy by MRI at 0.5 Tesla is as follows: (1) SE 300/10/8 (TR/TE/NEX) with 128 views (5.1 min), (2) IR 1850/100/4 with a TE of 30 ms and 128 views (16 min), and (3) SE 2000/80/4 with motion-suppression techniques and 128 views (17 min). All studies are performed with 10-mm contiguous slices. The total examination time for the MRI is usually 45 to 60 min depending on the size of the liver. Noncontrast CT of the abdomen is performed followed by an intravenous bolus dynamic scanning technique through the liver using a mechanical injector.

Future studies evaluating the sensitivity of an imaging modality or techniques (e.g., subsecond bolus-enhanced dynamic CT, new MRI pulse sequences with or without breath-holding techniques, or MRI contrast agents) in the detection of hepatic lesions should concentrate on determining the actual true-positive and false-positive rates. We should obtain prospective studies with surgical or autopsy verification to determine the actual sensitivity for an imaging modality and to delineate lesions based on size, location, and histology.

TABLE 7-2. Sensitivity of CT and MRI at 0.5 and 1.5 Tesla for Hepatic Lesions

	Sensitivity (%)[a]		
Exam	All	≥ 2cm	≤ 2 cm
EOE-CT	65/78 (83)	53/55 (96)	12/23 (52)
AP-CT	61/78 (78)	52/55 (95)	9/23 (39)
DS-CT[b]	61/74 (82)	53/55 (96)	8/19 (42)
MRI 0.5T			
SE 300/20[c]	65/77 (84)	54/55 (97)	11/22 (50)
SE 2000/80[c]	49/77 (64)	42/55 (76)	7/22 (32)
MRI 1.5T[d]			
SE 300/25[e]	37/61 (61)	33/42 (79)	4/19 (21)
SE 2000/80[f]	36/63 (57)	32/43 (74)	4/20 (20)
IR 2000/600[g]	30/43 (70)	27/30 (90)	3/13 (23)

[a]Number of true-positive/number of lesions found at surgery times 100.
[b]One patient did not have DS-CT, and therefore, 4 lesions not found at surgery excluded from the denominator.
[c]Incomplete MRI scan in one patient; therefore, lesion found at surgery excluded from analysis.
[d]Unpublished results, J.W. Reinig and J.A. Frank.
[e]Denominator reflects 16 of the 19 patients who went to surgery. In 3 patients, MRI was incomplete; therefore, 3 lesions found at surgery were excluded from the analysis.
[f]Denominator reflects 16 of the 19 patients who went to surgery. In 2 patients, MRI was incomplete; therefore, 2 lesions found at surgery were excluded from the analysis.
[g]Denominator reflects 10 of the 19 patients who went to surgery. In 3 patients, MRI was incomplete; therefore, 3 lesions found at surgery were excluded from the analysis.

TABLE 7-3. False-Positive Rate of CT and MRI at 0.5 and 1.5 Tesla

	False Positive Rate (%)	
Exam	Nodule Analysis*	Patient Analysis[†]
EOE-CT	12/77 (16)	9/19 (47)
AP-CT	27/88 (31)	12/19 (63)
DS-CT	6/67 (9)	5/18 (28)
MRI, 0.5 Tesla		
SE 300/20	2/67 (3)	2/19 (11)
SE 2000/80	5/54 (9)	4/19 (21)
MRI, 1.5 Tesla		
SE 300/25	3/39 (5)	2/16 (13)
SE 2000/80	3/39 (8)	3/16 (19)
IR 2000/600	3/33 (9)	3/10 (30)

*Number of false-positive lesions/total number of lesions detected by each imaging study.
[†]Number of patients with false-positive lesions/total number of patient studies. Only 18 patients were examined by DS-CT, 16 patients by 1.5-Tesla SE 300/25 and SE 2000/80, and 10 patients by 1.5-Tesla IR 2000/600.

REFERENCES

1. Miller DL, Rosenbaum RC, Sugarbaker PH, et al: Detection of hepatic metastases: Comparison of EOE-13 computed tomography and scintigraphy. AJR 141:931, 1983.
2. Miller DL, Vermess M, Doppman JL, et al: CT of the liver and spleen with EOE-13: Review of 225 examinations. AJR 143:235, 1984
3. Sugarbaker PH, Vermess M, Doppman JL, et al: Improved detection of focal lesions with computerized tomographic examination of the liver using ethiodized oil emulsion (EOE-13) liver contrast. Cancer 54:1489, 1984.
4. Reinig JW, Dwyer AJ, Miller DL, et al: Liver metastasis detection: Comparative sensitivities of MR imaging and CT scanning. Radiology 162:43, 1987.
5. Miller DL, Simmons JT, Chang R, et al: Hepatic metastasis detection: Comparison of three CT contrast enhancement methods. Radiology 165:785, 1987.
6. Reinig JW, Dwyer AJ, Miller DL, et al: Liver metastases: Detection with MR imaging at 0.5 and 1.5 T. Radiology 170:149, 1989.
7. Ward BA, Miller DL, Frank JA, et al: Prospective evaluation of hepatic imaging studies in the detec-

tion of colorectal metastases: Correlation with surgical findings. Surgery 105:180, 1989.
8. Vermess M, Doppman, JL, Sugarbaker P, et al: Clinical trails with a new intravenous liposoluble contrast material for computed tomography of the liver and spleen. Radiology 137:217, 1980.
9. Freeny PC, Mark WM, Ryan JA, Bolen JW: Colorectal carcinoma evaluation with CT: Preoperative staging and detection of postoperative recurrence. Radiology 158:347, 1986.
10. Stark DD, Wittenberg J., Edelman, RR, et al: Detection of hepatic metastases: Analysis of pulse sequences performance in MR imaging. Radiology 159:365, 1986.
11. Bydder GM, Steiner RE, Blumgart LH, et al: MR imaging of the liver using the short TI inversion recover sequence. J Comput Assist Tomogr 9:1084, 1985.
12. Dwyer AJ, Frank JA, Sank VJ, et al: Short-TI inversion-recovery pulse sequence: Analysis and initial experience in cancer imaging. Radiology 168:827, 1988.
13. Frank JA, Dwyer AJ: Magnetic resonance imaging of the liver, in Wilson MA, Ruzicka FF (eds): Modern Imaging of the Liver: Application of Computerized Tomography, Ultrasound, Nuclear Medicine, and Magnetic Resonance Imaging. New York, Marcel Dekker, 1989.
14. Stark DD, Wittenberg J, Butch RJ, Ferrucci JT Jr: Hepatic metastases: Randomized, controlled comparison of detection with MR imaging and CT. Radiology 165:399, 1987.
15. Heiken JP, Weyman PJ, Lee JKT, et al: Detection of focal hepatic masses: Prospective evaluation with CT, delayed CT, CT during arterial portography, and MR imaging. Radiology 171:47, 1989.
16. Steinberg HV, Alarcon JJ, Bernardino ME: Focal hepatic lesions: Comparative MR imaging at 0.5 and 1.5 T. Radiology 174:153, 1990.
17. Pattnay PM, Phillips JJ, Chiu LC, et al: Motion artifact suppression technique (MAST) for MR imaging. J Comput Assist Tomogr 11:369, 1987.

8

Emory Experience with Both CT and MRI in the Detection of Focal Liver Disease

MICHAEL E. BERNARDINO

During the early 1980s, computed tomography (CT) became the screening procedure of choice for the detection of focal liver disease at many institutions. This was primarily due to the fact that CT equipment was dramatically improved, offering both high-resolution and faster scanning (less than 5-second slices per dynamic scanning mode). Also, many different modes of intravenous contrast administration were tested to increase liver/lesion contrast. Two or three modes of contrast administration became mainstays at most radiology departments (1–3). These scanner/contrast combinations were able to detect focal liver disease with reliability at an earlier level than had been previously noted with sonography (which requires a skilled operator) or nuclear medicine (larger, more centrally located lesions). Again, while CT was used to detect focal liver disease, it actually became the screening, staging, and physical examination of the 1980s. More and more physicians relied on the CT study to determine whether there was abdominal disease and, if so, its extent, before seeing the patient. Because of this, CT scanners proliferated and their cost decreased. Thus a multitude of factors increased the use of abdominal CT.

Magnetic resonance imaging (MRI) was introduced in the early 1980s, but it became more of a factor in the mid-1980s. MRI offered superb soft-tissue contrast without the use of a contrast agent, which was needed to improve the sensitivity of CT. Many early studies comparing CT, which was a more mature diagnostic modality, with MRI were reported (4–7). However, these early papers suffered from poor standardization of techniques, and many were retrospective in analysis. They had varying results and came to different conclusions. Glazer et al. (4), using a 0.35-Tesla Diasonics MRI imager, detected a few less lesions with MRI than with CT. Their CT scanning was performed with a high-quality GE 9800 scanner utilizing the dynamic sequential bolus technique. Interestingly, they did detect more extrahepatic disease with CT than with MRI (Fig. 8-1). This should not be surprising in view of the fact that respiratory motion, vascular motion, and the lack of a bowel contrast agent make the detection of upper abdominal disease outside the liver difficult by MRI. Another report, by Stark et al. (5), demonstrated that a low-to-middle field strength, T1-weighted spin echo imaging (more T1-weighted than in the Glazer et al. paper) gave increased signal-to-noise ratios and contrast between tumor and normal surrounding liver. Later, using this same extremely short TR/TE spin echo sequence, Stark et al. demonstrated that their MRI unit, a 0.6-Tesla Technicare unit, outperformed CT at their institution. There was a problem with

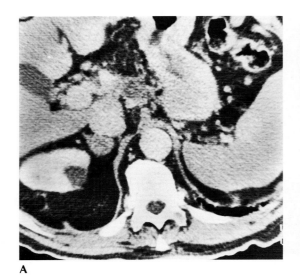 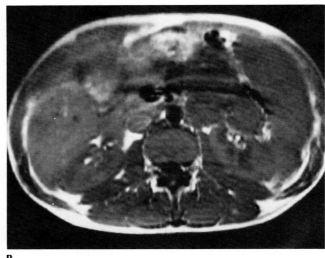

FIGURE 8-1
(A) CT section demonstrates a right renal cyst, right adrenal metastasis, and numerous periportal nodes. These findings were difficult to detect with earlier MRI scanners. They were obscured by motion artifacts due to respiration, blood flow, and bowel peristalsis.
(B) MRI section shows significant respiratory and bowel motion. Large retroperitoneal nodes cannot be easily seen.

the paper in that the CT studies were not standardized as to technique. Some patients received contrast material, some did not, and the amount of contrast material administered varied throughout.

In another paper, Foley (8) demonstrated that the same spin echo sequences that had worked so well for Stark et al. did not provide superior results at 1.5 Tesla (Fig. 8-2). The short TR/TE spin echo sequences missed the majority of lesions at the higher field strength because they became isointense. Although the paper did not directly compare CT to MRI, it did raise questions as to whether MRI data varied with field strength, sequence, or manufacturer's specifications. Thus the early MRI data asked as many questions as they answered. The purpose of this communication is to review the Emory experience at both 0.5 and 1.5 Tesla and to compare our data with the previous literature.

0.5 TESLA

In reviewing the work of Glazer et al. and Stark et al., I felt that a major difference between the two papers was a result of the varied spin echo sequences used by each group. However, this could not explain the entire magnitude of variance between the results. Both groups used different magnets and CT scanners, and CT contrast administration techniques were different. Thus we felt that any prospective study would have to standardize these techniques. Also, inherently, data from one institution can be biased because of the equipment and expertise of the individuals involved. Therefore, we developed a study in which patient entry would be applicable to the "real world," while MRI techniques would be the same at more than one institution (9). At the low field strength, we chose two T1-weighted techniques (short TR/TE spin echo and inversion recovery) to evaluate the liver for focal liver disease detection and screening (thus agreeing with Stark et al. that T1 sequences are needed at the lower-to-middle field strengths). The number of data acquisitions, matrices, and slices were standardized between both Emory and New York University, as well as the magnet, which was a similar 0.5-Tesla Philips superconductive Gyroscan. The

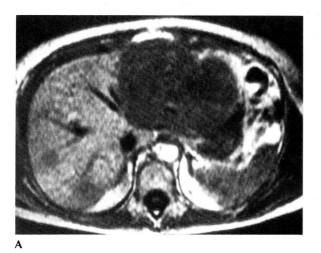 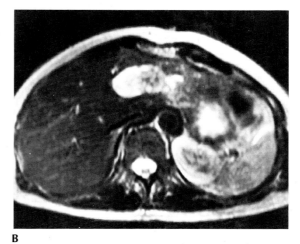

FIGURE 8-2
(A) MRI image performed at 0.5 Tesla utilizing a TR 300/TE 20-ms sequence demonstrates good contrast between the low-intensity hepatic tumors and the surrounding normal hepatic parenchyma. (B) MRI image at 1.5 Tesla using a TR 2000/TE 100-ms sequence demonstrates high-intensity metastases in the lateral segment of the left hepatic lobe. Many clinical investigators came to different conclusions as to which was the optimum pulse sequence for hepatic lesion detection because of the differences in magnet field strength and machine capability.

CT technique was similar, as was the amount of contrast material. It was a dynamic sequential bolus CT performed on either a GE 9800 CT scanner or Siemens DR-3. Delayed iodine scans were obtained in as many patients as possible. In order to eliminate reader bias, a system was developed in which the scans were randomized and read by the opposite institution (Emory read N.Y.U. scans and N.Y.U. read Emory scans). No history was given. The results were then graded by the home institution. The data were then combined and the information analyzed.

Of the 59 patients who were entered into the study, 32 were disease-free by both modalities. Ninety-three lesions were detected in the remaining 27 patients. There was no significant difference in the detection rate between the two CT techniques, either alone or in combination with the two MRI techniques at the highest confidence level of 3. Dynamic CT detected 90 percent of the lesions, delayed CT detected 83 percent, inversion-recovery MRI detected 90 percent, spin echo MRI detected 81 percent, combined MRI detected 91 percent, and combined CT imaging detected 96 percent (Fig. 8-3).

Seventy-four of the lesions were greater than 1 cm in size. Dynamic CT detected 97 percent; delayed CT, 92 percent; inversion-recovery MRI, 97 percent; spin echo MRI, 68 percent; combined MRI 90 percent; and combined CT, 97 percent. There was no statistical difference among the modalities, either separate or combined. When lesions less than 1 cm were considered, 19 were noted. Dynamic CT detected 63 percent; delayed CT, 56 percent; inversion-recovery MRI 63 percent; spin echo MRI, 37 percent; combined MRI, 63 percent; and combined CT, 89 percent. The major problem with the data in this paper, as with most papers that deal with liver lesion detection, is verification. The livers were not sliced at 1-cm or less intervals, and it is impossible to determine whether the total amount of disease was actually detected. Also, false-positive results were noted more often with MRI owing to motion and vascular artifacts. However, some of these could have been present (true-positive MRI) and undetected by CT (false-negative CT).

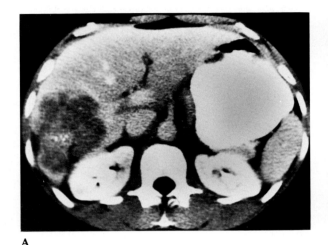
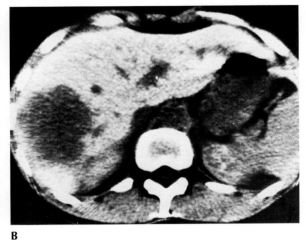
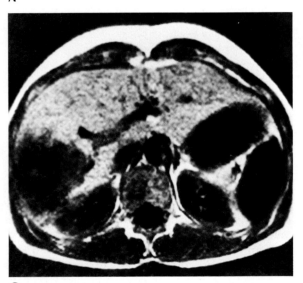

FIGURE 8-3
(A) *Dynamic contrast CT scan of the liver demonstrates a lesion in the right hepatic lobe. In the central portion of the lesion there is high density due to calcium.* (B) *Delayed iodine CT shows the same lesion.* (C) *Inversion-recovery, TR 14000/TI 400/TE 20 ms MRI study demonstrates the low-intensity lesion in the right hepatic lobe. In our study there was no statistical difference in lesion detection comparing low- to middle-field MRI with CT.*

A major point of the paper, however, is the fact that extrahepatic disease was more likely detected by CT. Thus T1-weighted MRI alone would not be adequate to screen the upper abdomen for disease. Also, in 4 of the 59 patients (7 percent), no liver metastases were detected. However, these patients did have extrahepatic disease that was not seen by MRI. Thus, while MRI was accurate at staging the liver, it was not accurate in determining total disease in the upper abdomen, a very important point. If MRI is to succeed and become the screening procedure of choice, it must adequately evaluate areas besides the liver to justify the disparity in cost between it and CT (Emory MRI $1000, CT $495).

1.5 TESLA

Because of the varied results of pulse performances at a higher field strength (10–12), we decided to duplicate the previous study at the higher field strength using pulse sequences that are commonly available to most imagers (13).

Therefore, inversion recovery was not used at the higher field strength, since many of the imagers at the time of the study did not offer this sequence or the sequence did not operate optimally on one of the test-site imagers at the study's inception. A combination of T1- and T2-weighted SE sequences was used and compared with dynamic sequential bolus and delayed CT. Sixty-nine patients were entered into this study. Again, the referral population of the study might be considered somewhat "skewed" because these are the routine types of patients seen at tertiary-care centers. Also, there were minor differences from the previous study in that not all the diagnostic modalities or sequences were performed on each patient. This was due to machine time availability. Thirty-four of the 69 patients had noncontrast CT performed on three different types of CT scanners, either a 9800 GE with HiLight detectors, a Siemens DR 3, or a Philips LX scanner. Contiguous 8- or 10-mm axial sections were obtained. Sixty-eight of the 69 patients had dynamic incremental contrast scans after an intravenous injection of 150 to 180 cc iodinated 60 percent contrast solution. The rates of injection of the iodinated solution were slightly different between the two institutions. One institution used 2 to 3 cc/s continuous injections, while at the other institution biphasic injections of 5 cc/s for 10 seconds, followed by 1 cc/s were used. Seven to 11 scans were obtained per minute, beginning 30 to 45 seconds after the injection. Twenty-five of the 69 patients had delayed CT scans performed. This was primarily due to either machine availability or patient availability. All delayed iodine scans were obtained after a total of 60 gm iodine was injected, and these patients were imaged 4 to 6 hours after the contrast material injection.

The MRI imagers for the study were different. General Electric and Philips 1.5-Tesla superconducting magnets were used. Sixty-five patients underwent T1 spin echo sequences with TEs of 20 and TRs of 250 to 300 ms. Sixty-seven of the 69 patients underwent T2-weighted spin echo sequences. A TR of 2000 was used with either a TE of 80 or 100 ms. Two to four data acquisitions were obtained. Flow compensation was performed on 32 of these patients. Twenty-three of these 32 studies were repeated with respiratory compensation. The remaining 35 T2-weighted MRI studies were performed without flow compensation, respiratory compensation, or presaturation. Scans were randomized for interpretation purposes. The interpreters were blinded as to patient name or disease. Scans from one institution were sent to the other institution for reading and were graded by the home institution. Consensus rating of all CT and MRI cases by the home institution (based on surgical follow-up, imaging follow-up, and clinical follow-up) determined the "gold standard" for each case. This is an inherent weakness of the study; all livers were not pathologically sectioned.

Again, lesions were characterized as to definite, maybe, or not present on a 3 through 1 scoring system. The presence and location of the lesions were marked on a liver map with a maximum of 5 lesions per hepatic segment (maximum 20 per liver). Surgical exploration confirmed the presence of disease in 5 patients, percutaneous biopsy in 8, imaging and/or clinical follow-up in 46. Of the 46, 18 were positive and 28 were negative. Forty-three of the 46 patients had clinical or imaging follow-up of over 6 months.

The sensitivity for the individual lesion detection at the highest confidence level of 3 was 51 percent for noncontrast CT, 70 percent for dynamic CT, 71 percent for delayed CT, 47 percent for T1-weighted spin echo MRI, and 77 percent for T2-weighted spin echo MRI (Fig. 8-4). It should be noted that these data are based on a varied number of lesions. This was due to the fact that not all patients received all sequences. The noncontrast CT total possible number of lesions was 138; dynamic CT totaled 262, delayed CT totaled 129, T1-weighted spin echo MRI totaled 243, and the T2-weighted spin echo MRI totaled 265. There was no statistical difference between dynamic CT, delayed CT, and spin echo T2-weighted MRI for lesion detection. When lesions were categorized as to size, dynamic CT, delayed CT, and T2-weighted spin echo MRI remained the most sensitive for detection of lesions greater than 1 cm. Again, no statistical difference could be found between the sensitivities of these three methods. However, in the detection of lesions less than 1 cm in size, T2-weighted spin echo MRI was significantly more sensitive ($p < 0.006$) than the four other methods (Fig. 8-5). For lesions less than 1 cm in size, noncontrast CT had the possibility of

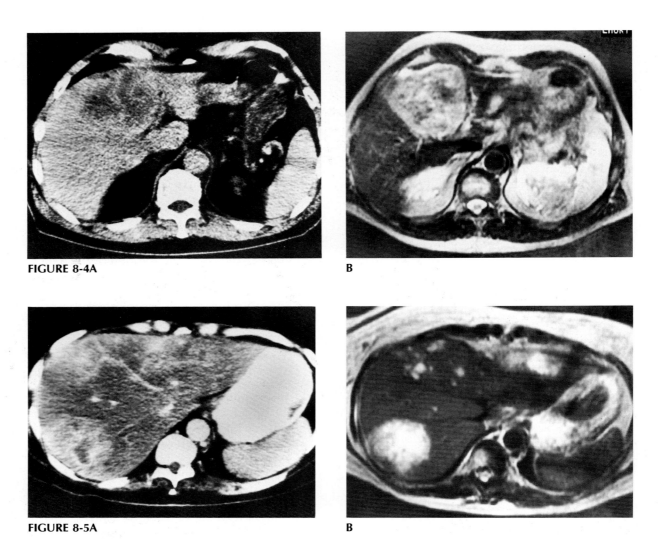

FIGURE 8-4
(A) *Dynamic contrast CT study shows solitary lesion in the medial segment of the left hepatic lobe. (B) MRI examination of the liver at TR 2000/TE 100 ms demonstrates the same lesion. For lesions greater than 1 cm in size, MRI and CT were equal at 1.5 Tesla in the detection of hepatic masses.*

FIGURE 8-5
(A) *CT section demonstrates multiple metastases within the liver. (B) T2-weighted spin echo MRI at TR 2000/TE 100 ms demonstrates more lesions within the liver. Many of the newly detected, high-intensity masses are less than 1 cm in size.*

detecting 20 lesions, but detected only 5 percent; dynamic CT had the possibility of detecting 48 lesions, but detected only 27 percent; delayed CT had the possibility of detecting 32 lesions, but detected only 31 percent; spin echo T1-weighted MRI had the possibility of detecting 28 lesions, but detected only 18 percent; and T2-weighted spin echo MRI had the possibility of detecting 48 lesions, but detected only 63 percent.

The overall sensitivity for detection of patients with disease was 89 percent for dynamic CT versus 86 percent for spin echo T2-weighted MRI.

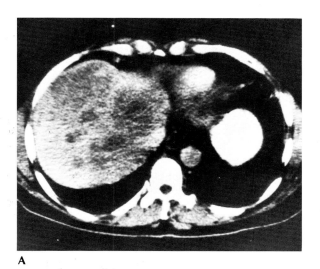 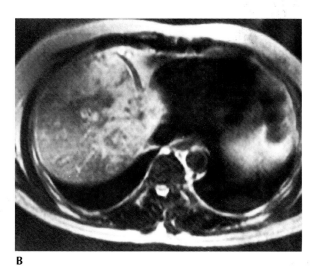

FIGURE 8-6
CT (A) and MRI (B) sections demonstrate multiple hepatic metastases. However, there are slightly more metastases demonstrated by CT than by MRI.

There were 6 patients in whom CT diagnosed disease and MRI did not (Fig. 8-6) and 2 patients in whom MRI diagnosed diseases and CT did not. As in the previous study, CT was superior to MRI in the detection of extrahepatic disease. In 7 patients, significant extrahepatic disease was prospectively identified on CT alone. These included 5 cases of retroperitoneal masses/lymph nodes and 2 cases of basilar lung nodules. In 3 patients, MRI identified adrenal masses that CT did not.

This study is interesting in that CT and MRI were roughly equivalent for detection of focal liver lesions. However, for lesions less than 1 cm in size, CT did not perform as well as MRI. This should not be surprising in view of the fact that small lesions probably become isodense, even with the best techniques, when intravenous contrast material is administered. The "fade in" contrast effect masks many small lesions. Also, imaging at 1.5 Tesla requires methods to decrease motion artifacts, which are more prevalent at the higher field strength. Very few of these motion-reduction techniques were utilized in this study. Thus MRI performed well despite the fact that flow compensation, presaturation, and respiratory compensation were not used. One could argue that MRI should perform far better in the future. Again, T1-weighted spin echo MRI sequences did not perform as well at the higher field strength, which is confirmatory of the previous work of Foley (8). The T2 sequence was the superior sequence for imaging at the higher field strength. It is possible, however, that rapid acquisition T1-weighted spin echo MRI (shorter TRs and TEs) will improve these results (14). Also, inversion-recovery MRI at the higher field strength may be just as successful as some other authors have indicated in their work (12).

The problem of poor, unreliable extrahepatic disease detection continues to plague MRI. As in this study, many of the lesions were missed with MRI. Predominantly, these misses were due to motion artifacts, lack of a bowel contrast agent, and vascular artifacts. These problems must be solved consistently before MRI screening at the higher field strength is to become routine.

Our two studies were done over a number of years. The data inherently have become outdated with each new software upgrade on the MRI units. Thus the MRI units should be viewed as in continuous evolution, with the preceding data being a worst-case scenario. Also, it should be noted that the data presented for both CT and MRI are inherently suspect because there is no true "gold standard." The preceding data are based on detection of a lesion or lesions. They probably do not give a true picture of *total disease extent*. As published by Nelson et al. (15), there is a

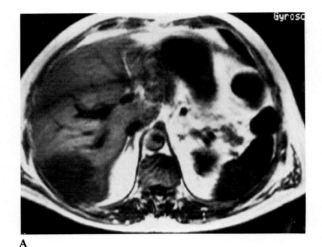

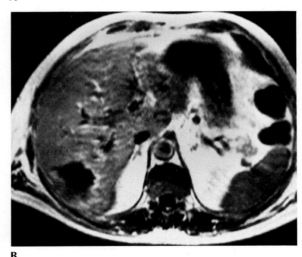

FIGURE 8-7
(A) *MRI section at TR 300/TE 315 ms demonstrates a hypointense lesion in the right hepatic lobe.* (B) *After administration of 1 ml/kg of gadolinium-DTPA, the lesion in the right hepatic lobe is again noted. However, there is a hyperintense blush on the periphery of the mass with increased signal noted in the surrounding hepatic parenchyma. Also, increased contrast is noted between the normal hepatic parenchyma and the tumor. MRI contrast agents have great promise for improving hepatic lesion detection.*

15 to 20 percent increase in sensitivity when more invasive diagnostic techniques are utilized, such as CT portography. This increase in sensitivity is primarily in the area of lesions less than 2 cm in diameter. Of the two modalities, it is my belief that MRI has more potential with the development of MRI contrast agents (16–19). However, should a good-quality CT contrast agent be developed, it is possible that CT sensitivity will improve to equal that of future MRI sensitivity (Fig. 8-7). In any case, I believe that the future of MRI is bright, and I hope that more studies will be performed on a multi-institutional basis, since I believe that there is less bias in such data.

REFERENCES

1. Foley WD: Dynamic hepatic CT. Radiology 170:617, 1989.
2. Bernardino ME, Erwin BC, Steinberg HV, et al: Delayed hepatic CT scanning: Increased confidence and improved detection of hepatic metastases. Radiology 159:71, 1986.
3. Platt JF, Glazer GM: IV contrast material for abdominal CT: Comparison of three methods of administration. AJR 151:275, 1988.
4. Glazer GM, Aisen AM. Francis IR, et al: Evaluation of focal hepatic masses: A comparative study of MRI and CT. Gastrointest Radiol 11:263, 1986.
5. Stark DD. Wittenberg J, Butch RJ, et al: Hepatic metastases: Randomized, controlled comparison of detection with MR imaging and CT. Radiology 165:399, 1987.
6. Nelson RC, Chezmar JL, Steinberg HV, et al: Focal hepatic lesions: Detection by dynamic and delayed computed tomography versus short TE/TR spin echo and fast field echo magnetic resonance imaging. Gastrointest Radiol 13:115, 1988.
7. Reinig JW, Dwyer AJ, Miller DL, et al: Liver metastasis detection: Comparative sensitivities of MR imaging and CT scanning. Radiology 162:43, 1987.
8. Foley WD: Hepatic MR imaging at 1.5 T. Radiology 168:326, 1988.
9. Chezmar JL, Rumancik WM, Megibow AJ, et al: Liver and abdominal screening in patients with cancer: CT versus MR imaging. Radiology 168:43, 1988.
10. Reinig JW, Dwyer AJ, Miller DL, et al: Liver metastases: Detection with MR imaging at 0.5 and 1.5 T. Radiology 170:149, 1989.
11. Shuman WP, Baron RL, Peters MJ, et al: Comparison of STIR and spin-echo MR imaging at 1.5 T in 90 lesions of the chest, liver, and pelvis. AJR 152:853, 1989.
12. Steinberg HV, Alarcon JJ, Bernardino ME: Comparative MR imaging at 0.5 and 1.5 Tesla in the evaluation of focal hepatic lesions. Radiology 174:153, 1990.
13. Vassiliades VG, Foley WD, Alarcon JJ, et al: Hepatic Metastases: CT versus MR Imaging at 1.5 T. Presented at the 75th Scientific Assembly and Annual Meeting of the RSNA, Chicago, Ill., November 1989. Gastrointest Radiol (in press).

14. Mirowitz SA, Lee JKL, Brown JJ, et al: Rapid acquisition spin-echo (RASE) MR imaging: A new technique for reduction of artifacts and acquisition time. Radiology 175:131, 1990.
15. Nelson RC, Chezmar JL, Sugarbaker PH, et al: Hepatic tumors: Comparison of CT during arterial portography, delayed CT, and MR imaging for preoperative evaluation. Radiology 172:27, 1989.
16. Unger EC, Winokur T, MacDougall P, et al: Hepatic metastases: Liposomal Gd-DTPA-enhanced MR imaging. Radiology 171:81, 1989.
17. Jones EC, Chezmar JC, Nelson RC, et al: Variability of Hepatic Enhancement with Regard to Time and Location in Gd-DTPA Enhanced Dynamic MR Imaging. Presented at the 75th Scientific Assembly and Annual Meeting of the Radiological Society of North America, Chicago, Ill., November 1989.
18. Saini S, Stark DD, Hahn PF, et al: Ferrite particles: Superparamagnetic MR contrast agent for enhanced detection of liver carcinoma. Radiology 162:217, 1987.
19. Rocklage SM, et al: Synthesis and Characterization of Biomimetic Manganese Piridoxal-5'-Phosphate for MR Imaging. Presented at the Sixth Annual Meeting of the Society of Magnetic Resonance in Medicine, New York, 1987.

IV. SPECIAL MRI TECHNIQUES FOR LIVER LESION IMAGING

9

STIR MRI of the Liver

WILLIAM P. SHUMAN,
ALBERT A. MOSS, and
RICHARD L. BARON

Spin-echo imaging has been shown to be reasonably sensitive for focal pathology in the parenchyma of the liver. Heavily T1-weighted images appear to have optimal sensitivity for low to middle field strengths, while heavily T2-weighted images have optimal sensitivity at higher field strengths (1,2). However, the spin-echo technique carries an intrinsic disadvantage, since, in spin echo, T1 and T2 are subtractive from each other with regard to their effects on tissue brightening. While it is true that this subtractive effect can be minimized by selecting TR and TE values to weight images, even in heavily T1-weighted images, some T2 effect does subtract from tissue conspicuity. Conversely, even in heavily T2-weighted images, some T1 effect does detract from the brightening of pathology; this decreases lesion conspicuity below that which could be obtained if "pure" T2 images were possible (3).

In MRI, pathology can be differentiated from normal tissue because most pathology has a longer T1 *and* a longer T2 than normal tissue, presumably due to increased water content and different magnetic environment of the increased water content. One might thus postulate that an optimal MRI sequence for creating contrast between normal and pathologic tissues would be one that *adds* T1 and T2 together rather than the subtractive effect found in spin echo. Short TI inversion recovery (STIR) is just such a sequence.

STIR PHYSICS

In STIR, the 90 to 180-degree pulse of a spin-echo sequence is preceded by an inverting 180-degree pulse. After the inverting 180-degree pulse, it is possible to take advantage of the difference in longitudinal recovery times (T1) of the fat (quick) and water (slow) spins to produce fat suppression. If the time between the inverting 180-degree pulse and the subsequent 90-degree pulse (the TI time) is appropriately selected, the inverted longitudinal magnetization of fat spins will have recovered from negative values to zero on their way to positive values. The 90-degree pulse will thus see no longitudinal magnetization from fat spins to flip into the transverse plane. Since the fat spins will have recovered to zero more quickly than water spins, the water spins will still have some residual negative longitudinal magnetization that will be flipped into the transverse plane by the 90-degree pulse. The net effect is fat signal suppression.

However, there is an additional fringe benefit with STIR: marked brightening of pathology relative to normal tissue. With STIR, tissue that has a long T1 will have much residual negative longitudinal magnetization to flip into the transverse plane. If this tissue *also* has a long T2, the vector in the transverse plane will remain large and produce a bright signal when refocused by the final 180-degree pulse. Thus tissue with a long T1 *and* a long T2 (most pathology) produces a very bright signal compared with tissue that has a shorter T1 and a shorter T2 (most normal tissue). Suppression of fat signal further enhances any pathology that may be surrounded by fatty tissues. The net effect is very high conspicuity for pathology, since it becomes very bright relative to surrounding normal tissue (3).

STIR is not only unique when compared with spin-echo imaging but is unique when compared with more traditional types of inversion recovery (long TI inversion recovery, which is T1-weighted) (4). In traditional inversion recovery, the TI is relatively long. After the inverting 180-degree pulse, longitudinal magnetization has had time to recover through zero into the positive direction by the time of the 90-degree pulse. This means that in traditional inversion recovery, long T1 tissue (which recovers slowly) appears very dark and short T1 tissue (which recovers quickly) appears very bright; the net effect is one of heavy T1 weighting.

Bydder et al. (3) originally described the STIR technique in 1985 and demonstrated images obtained at low field strength. Since then, numerous reports have discussed the use of STIR at low and middle field strengths in various tissues of the body, especially liver, spine, and lymph nodes (5–7). More recently, the use of STIR has been reported at higher field strengths (1.0 and 1.5 Tesla) (8,9). At higher field strengths, the T1 increases for all tissues; however, the difference between the T1 of fat and that of water is slightly greater than at lower field strengths. One might postulate that there could be even greater conspicuity produced with STIR at these higher field strengths. Since fat signal has been suppressed, chemical-shift artifacts observed at higher field strengths in spin-echo imaging are not seen with STIR.

In the liver, one might postulate that STIR would produce high conspicuity of focal pathology. Since fat is normally scattered throughout the parenchyma of the liver, suppression of signal from this fat might further increase the conspicuity for focal pathology. In addition, increased lesion conspicuity with STIR may uncover some regions of focal pathology where abnormal cells are scattered among normal hepatocytes. In theory, therefore, STIR may have the potential for adding incremental information in liver MRI.

STIR TECHNIQUE

Since the intensity of signal in STIR depends on the differential relaxation times between fat and water, the overall signal produced by STIR is less than in spin echo. This means that STIR is more sensitive to pulse-sequence technique; optimizing pulse-sequence parameters with STIR is important. First, the 180-degree pulse needs to be reasonably precise (and hard), since there are two 180-degree pulses in STIR and any imprecision will result in substantial loss of signal. This requires fairly uniform 180-degree pulses across the body part and uniform magnetic field. In addition, selecting the optimal TI is critical. Some previous reports on STIR have used an arbitrarily selected TI—between 100 and 150 ms at lower field strengths and between 150 and 170 ms at higher field strengths. However, it is possible to "tune" the TI for each individual patient and each individual body part (9). Tuning the TI to maximize fat suppression is important because the optimal TI will vary from patient to patient depending on loading of the body coil by different body sizes. It also will vary between body parts in the same patient, possibly due to differences in fat composition. Therefore, discovering the optimal TI for each body part in each patient will help optimize the image. This can be done by observing the center frequency spectral display during the prescan process (Fig. 9-1). This center frequency spectral display shows the heights of the fat and water peaks for any given TI, TE, and TR combination. By selecting a TR and TE and varying the TI up and down, one can discover the TI that produces the lowest fat peak and use that TI for subsequent imaging in that region of that patient. This will optimize fat suppression. Using this technique, we find that the optimal TI for fat suppression at 1.5 Tesla on our scanner varies between 150 and 170 ms depending on the individual patient. Our most commonly used TI values turn out to be 155 and 160 ms.

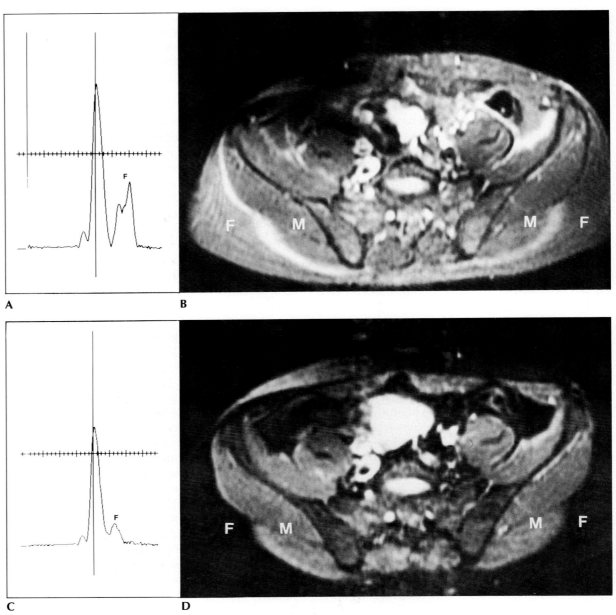

FIGURE 9-1
TI tuning technique using center frequency spectral display. (A) Spectral display with a TI of 110 ms. Note height of fat peak (F). (B) Image obtained with a TI of 110 ms corresponding to part A. Note that intensity of signal from subcutaneous fat (F) and muscle (M) is comparable. (C) Spectral display with a TI of 150 ms. Note lower fat peak (F). (D) Image obtained with a TI of 150 ms corresponding to part C. Note that intensity of signal from subcutaneous fat (F) has been suppressed so that it is much less than muscle (M).

Other imaging parameters are selected as follows: A relatively long TR is used to maximize brightening due to long tissue T1, and a relatively long TE is used to maximize tissue brightening due to long tissue T2. We have found that the combination of a TR of 2000 ms, a TE of 40 ms, and a TI of 160 ms is the most commonly used sequence to optimize fat suppression and lesion conspicuity with STIR. Generally, two repetitions (NEX = 2) are used in order to produce adequate signal so that motion-induced artifacts do not dominate the image. However, if surface coils are used, or when imaging is performed in a portion of the body where there is little motion, a single repetition (NEX = 1) may be adequate. If a single repetition is used, further improvement of signal-to-noise ratio may be achieved by a narrow-bandwidth imaging (bandwidth of 4). Narrow-bandwidth imaging is particularly compatible with STIR because the chemical-shift artifacts accentuated in spin echo by narrow-bandwidth imaging is not present in STIR. An additional advantage of narrow-bandwidth single-repetition imaging is that twice as many slices can be achieved in the same amount of time. For example, using single-repetition narrow-bandwidth imaging, 16 slices can be obtained in 8 minutes (1.5 Tesla). However, if motion-induced artifacts are anticipated as a significant problem (such as in the region of the liver), two-repetition imaging may be required and only 8 slices can be achieved in 8 minutes.

STIR: SENSITIVITY AND LESION CONSPICUITY

At least five published reports have indicated that STIR is more sensitive than spin echo in the liver or produces more conspicuous focal lesions. STIR was originally reported by Bydder et al. (3) in 1985 in an article that illustrated STIR imaging in 20 patients. Working at 0.12 Tesla, Bydder et al. pointed out that STIR produced high contrast between normal liver and focal abnormality and suggested that STIR may be valuable in screening for metastatic liver disease (Fig. 9-2). Working at 0.5 Tesla, additional theoretical analysis and evaluation of STIR lesion conspicuity in the liver were provided by Dwyer et al. (10). These authors analyzed signal-difference-to-noise ratios in 43 patients with STIR and several types of spin echo and found STIR sequences superior both in subjective and measured objective parameters. They felt that STIR represented a near ideal pulse sequence for screening for cancer in various areas of the body, including the liver. Further documentation came from Paling et al. (8), who analyzed signal-difference-to-noise ratios in 20 consecutive patients with known liver metastases. At 1.0 Tesla, STIR produced greatest signal-difference-to-noise ratios in 18 of the 20 patients when compared with five different spin-echo sequences, including phase contrast. High-field-strength (1.5-Tesla) STIR has been evaluated for detection of focal pathology by Albert et al. (11). They compared STIR with T1-weighted and heavily T2-weighted spin-echo sequences and found STIR more efficient in detecting liver metastases than any spin-echo sequence at the higher field strength.

At the University of Washington we have prospectively evaluated 41 proven liver lesions with both STIR (using 2000/145-170/40) and a double-echo spin-echo (2000/20/80) MRI at 1.5 Tesla. Sequences were evaluated separately by two radiologists and then in conjunction, and the total number of lesions detected was counted for each sequence. In addition, lesions were blindly graded for conspicuity using a 0-4 scale. When individual lesions received the same score with T2-weighted spin echo and STIR, the lesion conspicuity was subjectively directly compared and the more conspicuous chosen. In this series, all lesions detected by spin-echo imaging also were detected by STIR. In addition, STIR detected three lesions that were clearly missed by spin echo (Fig. 9-3). Two of these three were biopsied and represented cellular infiltration of tumor among normal hepatocytes. When lesions were compared for conspicuity, STIR showed a higher conspicuity score (greater conspicuity) than spin echo in 66 percent of cases and equal conspicuity in 34 percent. In no case was STIR less conspicuous than any spin-echo sequence. While it is acknowledged that subjective conspicuity scales are open to bias, visual assessment of lesions detected by MRI has been shown useful and practical, although less accurate than quantitative methods such as contrast-to-noise ratios (12). Subjective scales such as these are frequently used in radiologic comparison studies that use ROC methodology.

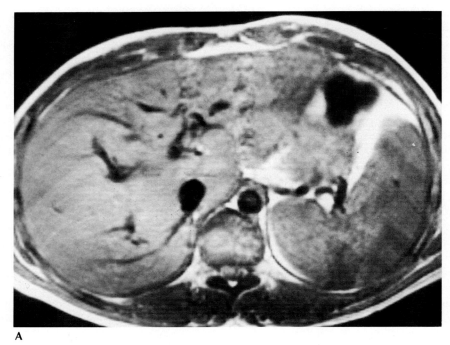

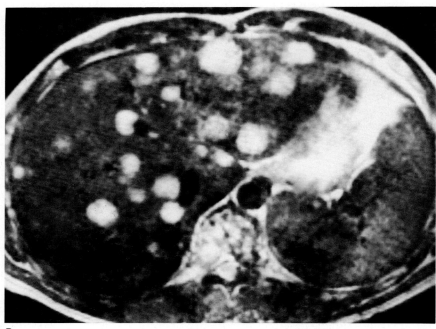

FIGURE 9-2
Metastatic melanoma to liver. (A) Mixed-weighted (2000/20) image. Lesions barely discernible. (B) T2-weighted image (2000/80). Multiple bright foci of metastases evident. (C) STIR image. Metastatic foci are very bright. Note additional lesion in spleen (arrow). *(D) CT at same level. Metastases in liver and spleen* (arrow).

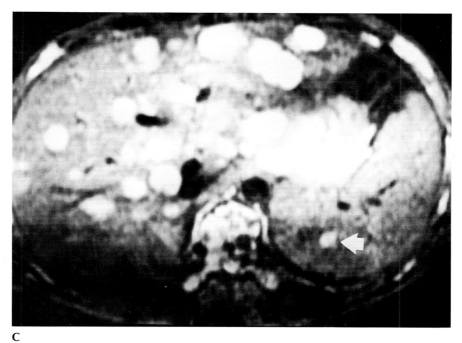

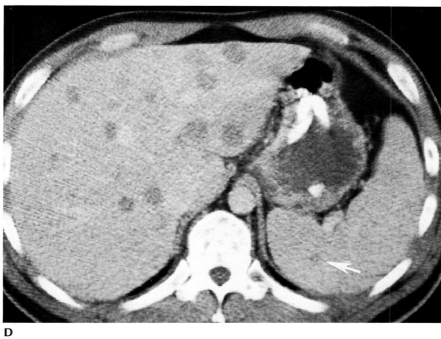

FIGURE 9-2 *(continued)*

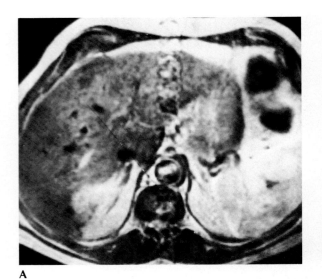 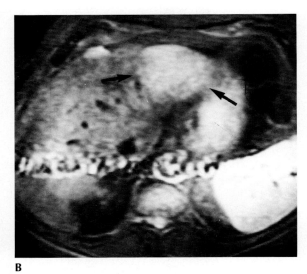

FIGURE 9-3
Patient with breast carcinoma and biopsy-proven metastasis in the lateral segment of the left lobe of the liver seen only with STIR. (A) T2-weighted image (2000/80). Small motion artifact is evident, but no lesion is seen in left lobe. (B) STIR demonstrates large region of moderate brightening in left lobe. Biopsy taken from this area showed tumor cells among normal hepatocytes.

The sum of all these reports suggests that STIR sensitivity may be slightly greater than that of any single spin-echo sequence or combination of spin-echo sequences. There is no doubt, however, that STIR creates significantly greater lesion conspicuity than spin echo in the majority of focal lesions in the liver.

STIR VOLUME OF ABNORMALITY

In their original article on STIR, Bydder et al. (3) reported that lesions appeared more extensive with STIR. In our comparison of individual lesions on both spin-echo and STIR imaging at the University of Washington, we also noticed that a substantial proportion of lesions appeared larger on STIR than on spin-echo imaging (9) (Fig. 9-4). As with Bydder's group, we wondered what might cause this discrepant appearance in volume with STIR imaging.

One of the unfortunate characteristics of STIR is that all types of pathology appear equally bright. Whether additional water in tissue is due to edema, inflammation, or malignant degeneration, all appear very bright on STIR. Thus tumor surrounded by edema will likely appear larger on STIR than on spin echo because STIR is able to pick up both gross and minimal amounts of edema. STIR is unable to distinguish between marked brightening caused by the tumor and marked brightening caused by adjacent edema; it all appears to be the same lesion. Tumor extending into adjacent tissue by microscopic infiltration also appears very bright on STIR; it is indistinguishable from peritumoral edema. In our series, each lesion detected by either spin echo or STIR was measured in its greatest width, length, and height to the nearest 0.5 cm using hand-held calipers. We then calculated the volume for each lesion assuming a prolate ellipse on each sequence and compared the volume on the largest spin-echo sequence with the volume on STIR. Since there is considerable inherent error in volume calculations based on hand-held caliper measurements, spin-echo and STIR volumes were arbitrarily categorized as being similar in size if they were less than 20 percent different. Differences in volume of more than 20 percent were categorized

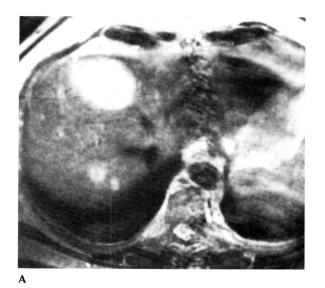 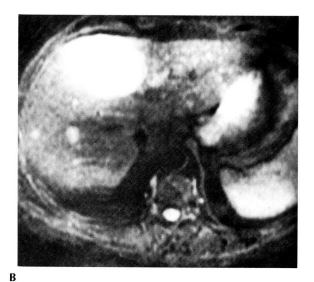

FIGURE 9-4
Liver metastases from colon carcinoma. (A) T2-weighted image (2000/80) shows large lesion anteriorly. (B) STIR image. Anterior lesion appears larger than in T2 image.

as being dissimilar. Using this approach, lesions appeared more than 20 percent larger on STIR than spin echo in 14 (34 percent) of the 41 lesions.

In this particular series, spatially correlated biopsies of discrepant tissue (tissue that appeared abnormal on STIR but normal on spin echo) could not be obtained. We have, however, noted a similar phenomenon in extremity sarcomas, where tumor volume was greater on STIR than spin echo. In extremity sarcomas, we were able to biopsy the discrepant tissue in eight patients. In two (25 percent), the discrepant tissue was additional malignant tumor, detected only by STIR. In the remaining six patients, the discrepant tissue was additional edema adjacent to tumor, detected only by STIR.

At least two series have reported now that in an individual lesion STIR detects a greater volume of abnormality than does spin echo in about 20 to 30 percent of cases (3,9). Why this is true remains conjectural, but in the majority of cases it appears due to greater sensitivity by STIR to peritumoral edema. The possibility remains, however, that STIR also picks up additional tumor missed by spin echo, most of which may represent microscopic infiltration into normal hepatic tissue.

LIMITATIONS OF STIR

There is no doubt but that the STIR sequence produces lower overall signal intensity for any given tissue than does spin echo. Because of this, the signal-to-noise ratio in STIR images is poorer than in spin-echo images, even though conspicuity for individual lesions may be greater. With a lower signal-to-noise ratio, motion-induced artifacts are more prominent in STIR than in spin echo. However, STIR can be utilized in conjunction with saturation pulses, respiratory gating, and narrow bandwidth to decrease motion-induced artifacts. Some manufacturers have combined gradient moment nulling (MAST or FLOW COMP), which further reduces artifacts on STIR imaging. In addition, there is a greater susceptibility to artifacts and a greater sensitivity to inhomogeneity of the magnetic field with STIR than with spin echo. The number of slices that can be obtained in any given amount of time with STIR is slightly less than with spin echo; this may limit its utility as a screening sequence.

CLINICAL USE OF STIR

Because of overall low signal-to-noise ratios and poorer spatial resolution relative to spin-echo images, STIR imaging rarely is used alone in liver evaluation. However, STIR can be extremely useful when employed as an adjunct to spin-echo imaging. In any circumstance where maximal sensitivity is important (such as counting the number and location of lesions in a patient being considered for liver resection), we feel the incremental sensitivity of STIR over spin echo makes its use important. In addition, the dramatic lesion conspicuity produced by STIR is useful when demonstrating abnormalities to referring clinicians. Occasionally, the detection of a greater volume of abnormality by STIR may be clinically useful. Radiation therapists who wish to treat all tissue at risk for containing tumor may rely heavily on STIR images for radiation therapy planning. Finally, a normal STIR examination may be clinically useful because it increases confidence in the absence of an abnormality.

Our current liver evaluation typically involves a T1-weighted coronal localizer sequence followed by an axial double-echo spin-echo sequence with mixed and T2-weighted images. The final sequence is an axial STIR, which adds either 8 or 16 minutes to the imaging time depending on the number of repetitions used. STIR can be spatially localized to any abnormality detected on spin echo or can include all the liver if the entire liver is being screened. With this approach, STIR sequences are used as an adjunct to spin echo in approximately 95 percent of our liver MRI studies.

REFERENCES

1. Stark DD, Wittenberg J, Edelman R, et al: Detection of hepatic metastases: Analysis of pulse sequence performance in MR imaging. Radiology 159:365, 1986.
2. Foley WD, Kneeland JB, Cates JD, et al: Contrast optimization for the detection of focal hepatic lesions by MR imaging at 1.5 T. AJR 149:1155, 1987.
3. Bydder GM, Steiner GM, Blumgart LH, et al: MR imaging of the liver using short TI inversion recovery sequences. J Comput Assist Tomogr 9:1084, 1985.
4. Bydder GM, Young IR: MR imaging: Clinical use of the inversion recovery sequence. J Comput Assist Tomogr 9:659, 1985.
5. Porter BA, Neumann EB, Olson DO, et al: STIR Imaging of Lymphadenopathy: Advantages over Conventional Spin-Echo Techniques. Presented at the Annual Meeting of the Radiological Society of North America, Chicago, Ill., November 1987.
6. Wiener SN, Rzeszotarski MS: Thick Section STIR: A Screening Technique for Vertebral Metastases. Presented at the Annual Meeting of the Radiological Society of North America, Chicago, Ill., November 1987.
7. Unger EC, Moldofsky P, Hartz WH, et al: MR Imaging of Bone Marrow Disease Using STIR. Presented at the Annual Meeting of the Radiological Society of North America, Chicago, Ill., November 1987.
8. Paling MR, Abbitt PL, Mugler JP, Brookeman JR: Liver metastases: Optimization of MR imaging pulse sequences at 1.0 T. Radiology 167:695, 1988.
9. Shuman WP, Baron RL, Peters MJ, Tazioli PK: Comparison of STIR and spin-echo MR imaging at 1.5 T in 90 lesions of the chest, liver, and pelvis. AJR 152:853, 1989.
10. Dwyer AJ, Frank JA, Sank VJ, et al: Short TI inversion recovery pulse sequence: Analysis and clinical experience in cancer imaging. Radiology 168:827, 1988.
11. Albert S, Cheung YY, Leeds NE: T2-Weighted Inversion Recovery Imaging of Liver Metastases at High Field. Presented at the 88th Annual Meeting of the American Roentgen Ray Society, San Francisco, California, May 1988.
12. Glazer GM, Woolsey EJ, Borrello J, et al: Adrenal tissue characterization using MR imaging. Radiology 158:73, 1986.

10

Chemical-Shift Imaging of the Liver

JOSEPH K. T. LEE

There are at least three different ways to perform chemical-shift imaging of the liver (1–4). The first involves selective excitation or selective saturation of a particular resonant frequency and requires MRI imagers with excellent field homogeneity. The second type employs phase-encoding gradients in two dimensions and is too time-consuming for routine clinical imaging. The third type, called the *phase-contrast technique*, is a modification of the conventional SE technique. It can produce separate water and fat images with good spatial resolution within a reasonable imaging time (less than 30 min) using commercially available MRI imagers. This technique exploits the difference in rate of precession between protons in water molecules and protons in fatty acid molecules. Because there is a difference in resonant frequency of 3 parts per million (50 Hz in a 0.3-Tesla field) between water and fat protons, the MRI signal can be considered to be a vector sum of the magnetizations of fat protons precessing at one frequency and water protons precessing at a slightly higher frequency. Conventional MRI data are obtained, with both sets of protons contributing to the SE. The magnetizaton vectors of water and fat are pointing in the same direction (i.e., are in phase), and this image is called the *in-phase image* or a *water-plus-fat image*. A second set of data is acquired with the time of the read gradient or the 180-degree pulse modified so that the signal is acquired when the water and fat magnetizations point in opposite directions (i.e., are out of phase). The resulting image is called an *opposed image* or a *water-minus-fat image*. These two images can be added to produce a water image or subtracted to yield a fat image. Figure 10-1 is a schematic diagram illustrating the difference between the in-phase and the opposed-phase sequences at a 0.35-Tesla field strength.

CLINICAL APPLICATIONS

Fatty Infiltration

Conventional spin-echo and inversion-recovery techniques have proved to be insensitive for detection of fatty infiltration of the liver (5–7). In experimental models, the signal intensity for the liver was shown to increase only minimally despite massive increases in liver triglyceride content (6). It is certainly rare for even lobar fatty infiltration to be clearly visible as an area of high intensity on spin-echo (SE) sequences (7) (Fig. 10-2).

In contradistinction to conventional SE sequences, the phase-contrast technique (also called *proton-spectroscopic imaging*) is a sensitive method for detecting fatty infiltration of the liver. With this technique, diffuse and focal fatty liver can be distinguished from normal liver both visually and

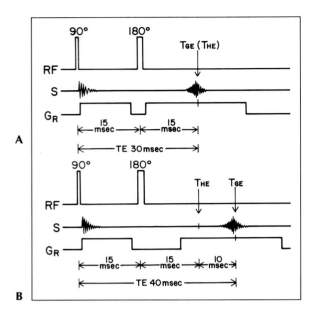

FIGURE 10-1
A schematic diagram illustrating the difference between in-phase (A) and opposed-phase (B) sequences at a 0.35 Tesla field strength (T_{GE} = time of gradient echo; T_{HE} = time of Hahn's echo; RF = radiofrequency; G_R = read-out gradient). (From Lee JKT, Koehler RE, Heiken JP: MRI technique, in Lee JKT, Sagel SS, Stanley RJ (eds): Computed Body Tomography with MRI Correlation. New York, Raven Press, 1989. Reprinted by permission.)

quantitatively (8,9). On an opposed image in which pixel brightness is a net difference between water and fat magnetizations, normal liver has an intermediate signal intensity greater than that of muscle, whereas fatty liver generally has a lower signal intensity equal to or less than that of muscle (Fig. 10-3). In one study, the signal intensity of the liver in 16 of 18 patients with diffuse fatty infiltration was similar to or less than that of back muscle. In 2 patients with a diffuse fatty liver, the hepatic signal intensity was greater than that of back muscle on the opposed image, although it was less than the hepatic signal intensity on the corresponding in-phase image. In normal liver the lipid signal fraction is less than 10 percent whereas in fatty liver it is greater than 10 percent and usually exceeds 20 percent. This technique is particularly helpful in differentiating between focal fatty infiltration and metastases, because such a distinction occasionally can be difficult with CT (Figs. 10-4 and 10-5).

Neoplasms
On relatively T2-weighted opposed images, primary and secondary hepatic malignancies appear as focal hyperintense areas relative to the adjacent normal hepatic parenchyma (10,11) (Fig. 10-6). Whereas primary hepatomas and metastases usually have a high signal intensity similar to that of the spleen, normal liver parenchyma has a signal intensity intermediate to that of the spleen and paraspinal muscle. In an original study performed on a 0.35 Tesla at our institute, the opposed images either showed more lesions or provided better contrast than contrast-enhanced CT or conventional T2-weighted spin-echo examinations in nearly half the patients with proven hepatic metastases (10). Of interest, more than half these patients had coexisting fatty infiltration, which may account for the increased sensitivity of the opposed image in detecting hepatic metastases.

Our recent study of patients performed on a 0.5-Tesla unit confirmed that opposed images are more sensitive than conventional T2-weighted SE images for detecting hepatic metastases. However, the short TR/short TE (TR of 325 ms, TE of 15 ms) SE sequence not only provided better conspicuity, but also depicted more lesions than the opposed images in a significant number of patients (11). This is not surprising because the opposed image is relatively T2-weighted (TR of 1500 ms, TE of 38 and 68 ms), and prior studies have shown that a T1-weighted SE sequence is superior to a T2-weighted SE sequence in the detection of hepatic metastases at low to middle magnetic field strengths (12,13). Although somewhat controversial (14), both theoretical and clinical studies have indicated that T2-weighted SE sequences are superior to T1-weighted SE sequences for detecting hepatic metastases at higher magnetic field strengths (12,15). It would be interesting to determine whether T2-weighted opposed imaging is better than T1-weighted SE imaging at higher field strengths. Likewise, it would be interesting to compare the accuracy of opposed images and T2-weighted SE imaging at higher field strengths.

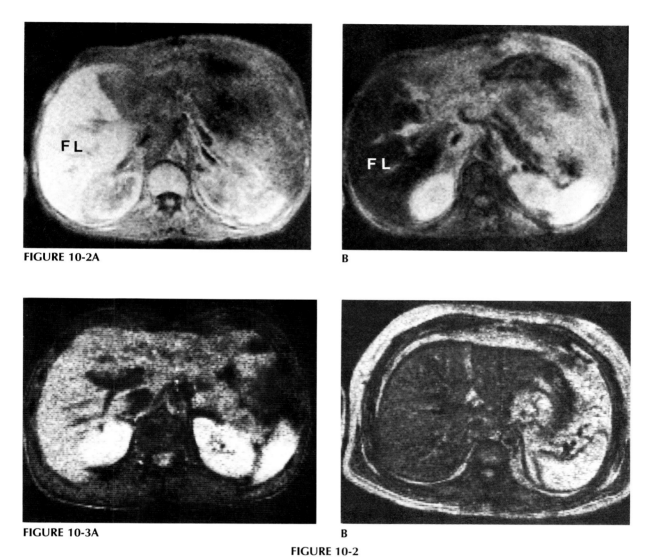

FIGURE 10-2
Lobar fatty infiltration. Fatty liver (FL) is manifested as a higher signal area on T1-weighted sequence (A) and lower signal on T2-weighted sequence (B).

FIGURE 10-3
Normal versus fatty liver on the opposed image. Note that normal liver in (A) has a signal intensity intermediate between the spleen and paraspinal muscle, whereas fatty liver (B) has a signal intensity similar to that of paraspinal muscle. (Part A from Lee JKT, Dixon WT, Ling D, et al: Fatty infiltration of the liver: Demonstration by proton spectroscopic imaging. Preliminary observations. Radiology 153:195, 1984. Reprinted by permission.)

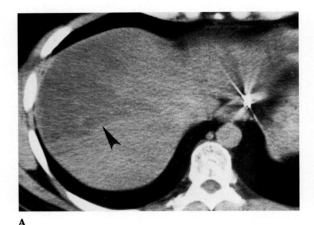
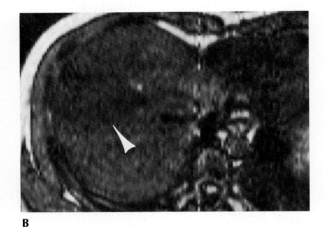

FIGURE 10-4
Focal fatty infiltration of the liver. (A) Contrast-enhanced CT scan demonstrates an irregularly shaped area of lower attentuation (arrowhead). This may represent either a focal area of fatty infiltration or a neoplasm. (B) Opposed image shows the corresponding area to have a lower signal intensity (arrowhead) than the adjacent liver parenchyma, indicating fatty infiltration rather than a neoplasm.

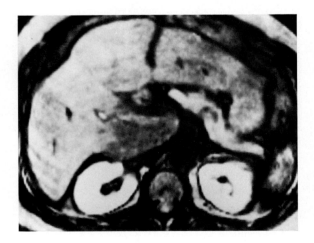

FIGURE 10-5
Focal fatty infiltration of the caudate lobe. Opposed image shows a low signal caudate lobe compatible with fatty infiltration in this patient with cirrhosis. The caudate lobe has a lower attenuation than the rest of the liver on a prior CT study, raising the possibility of focal fat versus neoplasm.

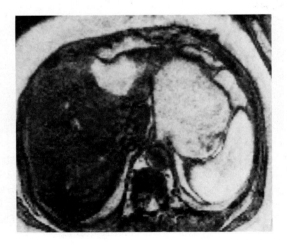

FIGURE 10-6
Hepatic metastasis from primary breast carcinoma. Note that the metastasis has a signal intensity similar to that of the spleen and much higher than that of adjacent liver parenchyma.

LIMITATIONS

Several theoretical limitations of this phase-contrast technique deserve comment. Partial misregistration of protons attached to the fatty acid molecule may cause a slight underestimation of the amount of hepatic fat present. This inaccuracy may arise because the protons in the CH_3 group at the end of each fatty acid molecule have precessional properties different from those of both water molecules and the CH_2 groups of the fatty acid molecule. Therefore, the protons of the CH_3 group contribute to both the apparent water and lipid signals. In addition, interference from other proton-containing compounds in the liver, such as glycogen and lactate, have not been taken into account. The fact that the lipid in the hepatic cell membrane is not measured with this technique is not a drawback, since one would not expect the lipid content of the cell membrane to be altered in fatty infiltration or other hepatic disorders. Also, it should be kept in mind that the lipid fraction measured with this technique represents the percentage of total hepatic signal derived from the protons in fatty acid protons imaged and not the weight per volume of lipid, which is the conventional method of expressing fatty infiltration of the liver.

CONCLUSIONS

Chemical-shift imaging of the liver using the phase-contrast technique allows imaging of hepatic water independent of hepatic fat. Whereas pure water and pure fat images can be constructed from a set of in-phase and opposed images, opposed images are usually the only ones required to make a diagnosis of fatty infiltration.

Although primary and metastatic hepatic malignancies can be identified easily on T2-weighted opposed images, the opposed images are usually no better than T1-weighted SE imaging (short TR/short TE) for detection of hepatic metastases. The major role of chemical-shift imaging of the liver at intermediate field strength is in the differentiation of focal fatty infiltration of the liver from metastases, both of which appear as focal areas of low attentuation on CT studies.

REFERENCES

1. Dixon WT: Simple proton spectroscopic imaging. Radiology 153:189, 1984.
2. Rosen BR, Wedeen VJ, Brady TJ: Selective saturation NMR imaging. J Comput Assist Tomogr 8:813, 1984.
3. Sepponen RE, Sipponen TJ, Tanttu JI: A method for chemical-shift imaging: Demonstration of bone marrow involvement with proton chemical shift imaging. J Comput Assist Tomogr 8:585, 1984.
4. Brateman L: Chemical shift imaging: A review. AJR 146:971, 1986.
5. Doyle FH, Pennock JM, Banks LM, et al: Nuclear magnetic resonance imaging of the liver: Initial experience. AJR 138:193, 1982.
6. Stark DD, Bass NM, Moss AA, et al: Nuclear magnetic resonance imaging of experimentally induced liver disease. Radiology 148:743, 1983.
7. Stark DD, Goldberg HI, Moss AA, Bass NM: Chronic liver disease: Evaluation by magnetic resonance. Radiology 150:149, 1984.
8. Heiken JP, Lee JKT, Dixon WT: Fatty infiltration of the liver: Evaluation by proton spectroscopic imaging. Radiology 157:707, 1985.
9. Lee JKT, Dixon WT, Ling D, et al: Fatty infiltration of the liver: Demonstration by proton spectroscopic imaging. Preliminary observations. Radiology 153:195, 1984.
10. Lee JKT, Heiken JP, Dixon WT: Detection of hepatic metastases by proton spectroscopic imaging: Work in progress. Radiology 156:429, 1985.
11. Schertz LD, Lee JKT, Heiken JP, et al: Proton spectroscopic imaging (Dixon method) of the liver: Clinical utility. Radiology 173:401, 1989.
12. Henkelman RM, Hardy F, Poon PY, Bronskill MJ: Optimal pulse sequence for imaging hepatic metastases. Radiology 161:727, 1986.
13. Stark DD, Wittenberg J, Butch RJ, Ferrucci JT: Hepatic metastases: Randomized, controlled comparison of detection with MR imaging and CT. Radiology 165:399, 1987.
14. Reinig JW, Dwyer AJ, Miller DL, et al: Liver metastases: Detection with MR imaging at 0.5 and 1.5 T. Radiology 170:149, 1989.
15. Foley WD, Kneeland JB, Cates JD, et al: Contrast optimization for the detection of focal hepatic lesions by MR imaging at 1.5 T. AJR 149:1155, 1987.
16. Lee JKT, Koehler RE, Heiken JP: MRI techniques, in Lee JKT, Sagel SS, Stanley RJ (eds): Computed Body Tomography with MRI Correlation. New York, Raven Press, 1989.

11

Steady-State MRI of the Liver

STEVEN E. HARMS,
DUANE P. FLAMIG, AND
KARL A. GLASTAD

Physiologic motion has been the major limitation in producing consistently high quality MRI images of the liver. A number of methods have been developed to compensate for motion and reduce artifacts, including cardiac and respiratory gating, signal averaging (1), gradient moment nulling (2–4), presaturation (5,6), and phase-ordered respiratory compensation (7). All these techniques compensate for the motion artifacts on the image, but the motion itself continues throughout the sequence.

Another approach to reducing motion artifacts—producing images faster than physiologic motion—can be accomplished by echo planar imaging with substantial changes in imager hardware or by steady-state pulse sequences using existing hardware (8). With scan times as short as 30 ms, echo planar imaging can acquire image data fast enough to freeze cardiac motion and is certainly adequate for liver imaging. CT scans (with scan times on the order of 1 to 2 ms) can reliably reduce motion effects for routine liver imaging. Using CT for a model, steady-state pulse sequences have produced images with scan times similar to CT (9–11). As expected, steady-state sequences using conventional imaging hardware to produce scan times of 3 s or less are quite effective in reducing motion artifacts that often limit routine MRI sequences.

This chapter reviews the multiple steady-state sequences available for fast-scan imaging of the liver. The contrast behavior and the potential of steady-state sequences in routine liver evaluations are discussed.

STEADY-STATE SEQUENCES

A pulse sequence becomes steady state when the transverse and longitudinal magnetizations are in equilibrium from one repetition to the next. The repetition times are shorter than either the T1 or T2 of the tissues. The sequence does not depend on relaxation to occur between repetitions in order to produce a signal; instead, there is a continual exchange of transverse and longitudinal magnetizations. Steady state is the fastest method for producing the multiple projections needed for conventional Fourier imaging acquisition.

The contrast behavior of steady-state sequences is not easily extrapolated from that usually seen in spin-echo or long TR gradient echo sequences. In order to understand the potential of steady state, the various steady-state pulse sequences and their attributes are explored. Sequences that are employed with production software on conventional imagers are shown in Table 11-1. The GRASS sequence is diagramed in Figure 11-1A. Using a full echo, echo times of 10 ms can

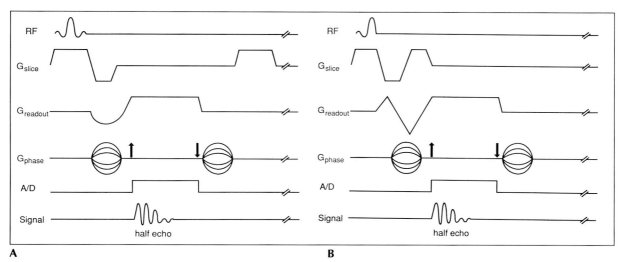

FIGURE 11-1
Pulse-sequence examples. Pulse-sequence diagrams of two types of steady-state sequences that can be used to produce rapid images of the liver. Conventional GRASS (A) is compared with turbo GRASS (B), our adaptation of the GRASS sequence. Turbo GRASS uses truncated sinc pulses to reduce the slice-selection gradient area so that gradient moment nulling can be applied with a shorter echo time.

TABLE 11-1. *Commercially Available Steady-State Sequences*

GRASS
FISP
FLASH
Spoiled GRASS
SSFP/CE-FAST/PSIF

TABLE 11-2. *Recently Introduced Steady-State Sequences*

Turbo FLASH
Turbo GRASS
FASTER
FATS
Steady-state spin echo
Missing pulse
Stimulated echo
ROAST

be achieved with a TR of 23 ms. With half-Fourier echoes, a TE of 5 ms can be attained. Constant amplitude gradient spoilers are used for the GRASS sequence. This sequence is unbalanced and does not employ gradient moment nulling in the version depicted. Production FISP is very similar to GRASS. Classical or original FISP uses a balanced sequence that resulted in phase-cancellation errors in routine imaging. Classical FISP has resurfaced on an experimental sequence called ROAST, which adjusts for the phase errors, but to date has not been used for liver imaging. FLASH uses gradient spoilers to produce more T1 contrast. RF rather than gradient spoiling is used for spoiled GRASS. RF spoiling breaks up the steady state of very long T2 fluids while maintaining a steady state for shorter T2 tissues. Since the high signal from the long T2 fluids is reduced by RF spoiling, spoiled GRASS produces T1-like contrast. SSFP, CE-FAST, and PSIF are similar sequences in which the gradient spoilers are used to reduce the signal contribution from the gradient echo while capturing the RF echo produced by sequential RF pulses (12,13). These sequences produce a fluid-weighted appearance.

Some recently discussed sequences that are not yet commercially available are listed in Table 11-2. Turbo FLASH utilizes much shorter echo and repetition times to produce images in as little as 300 ms. Inversion pulses can be added in front of a string of FLASH repetitions to produce more T1 contrast. Turbo GRASS (Fig. 11-1B) is our adaptation of a shortened GRASS sequence with gradient moment nulling. This sequence reduces the TE with the use of truncated sinc pulses that reduce the gradient needed for slice selection and gradient moment nulling. The TE for a 6-mm-thick Turbo GRASS slice is 6 ms. For a 10-mm slice, the TE can be reduced to less than 5 ms. FASTER and FATS have no role in liver imaging, since they are used only for nonselective three-dimensional acquisitions (14). Steady-state spin echo produces improved contrast compared with gradient-echo sequences but suffers from a loss in signal-to-noise ratio (SNR). Similar effects are also seen from missing-pulse (15) and stimulated-echo (16,17) sequences. Although ROAST can produce fluid-enhanced contrast in the cervical spine, this sequence doubtfully could be utilized for liver imaging because of the need for two excitations.

ARTIFACTS

Images obtained in less than 3 s with a gradient-echo sequence are sufficient for substantially reduced artifacts due to bowel and respiratory motion. The multiple pulse sequences such as spin echo, SSFP, missing pulse, and stimulated echo continue to produce significant artifacts from respiratory motion. Cardiac and vascular motion remain problematic even on gradient-echo sequences. Gradient moment nulling is required for GRASS sequences to produce sufficient reduction in vascular artifacts. A very short echo time (1 ms) may obviate the need for gradient moment nulling. Vascular artifacts are most severe on SSFP/CE-FAST/PSIF, where short T2 tissues have a reduced SNR compared with long T2 fluid, and two widely separate RF pulses are needed to produce the RF-generated echo. Any sequence requiring more than one RF pulse per signal acquisition will tend to have more motion artifacts. For this reason, spin-echo and stimulated-echo sequences have more problems with motion artifacts than a well-compensated gradient-echo sequence. Gradient moment nulling likely will be required to produce reasonable liver images with steady-state sequences that use more than one RF pulse.

CONTRAST

Even though motion-artifact-free steady-state images of the liver can be reliably generated, a problem of insufficient contrast remains when compared with conventional spin-echo sequences. Most pathology is only slightly darker than normal liver on turbo GRASS or GRASS images. Hemangiomas are not "lightbulbs," cysts are not dark, and tumors cannot be distinguished from even the most obvious benign disease seen on spin-echo images. Figures 11-2 and 11-3 demonstrate the relative lack of contrast and specificity of steady-state sequences for liver pathology compared with conventional sequences.

As the sequence uses shorter TE and TR values, steady-state contrast behavior becomes more dominant. Increasing the flip angle usually improves T1 weighting in long TR sequences; however, in a very short TE/TR GRASS sequence where steady-state contrast dominates, no contrast differences are seen with a variation in flip angle (Fig. 11-4). Since transverse and longitudinal magnetizations are in equilibrium in the steady state, little effect is gained by changing the flip angle. The major effect of flip angle on the steady state is to change the SNR of the image. RF spoiling can break up the steady state from long T2 fluids and produce a more T1 contrast image. Very little fluid is present in the liver, and RF spoiling has no visible effect (Fig. 11-5). One method that has effectively changed the contrast of a steady-state sequence is the addition of an inversion pulse at the beginning of a string of turbo FLASH repetitions. A relatively long inversion time is added to the sequence that significantly increases the scan time. Acquiring projections at different times following the inversion pulse produces projections of varying T1 weighting. The weighting and contrast of the image are somewhat ambiguous, since they are made up of all these projections with many different effective T1 values. This method likely will not be competitive with the contrast or specificity provided by a good spin-echo image.

A major attribute of steady-state sequences is their ability to obtain good visualization of

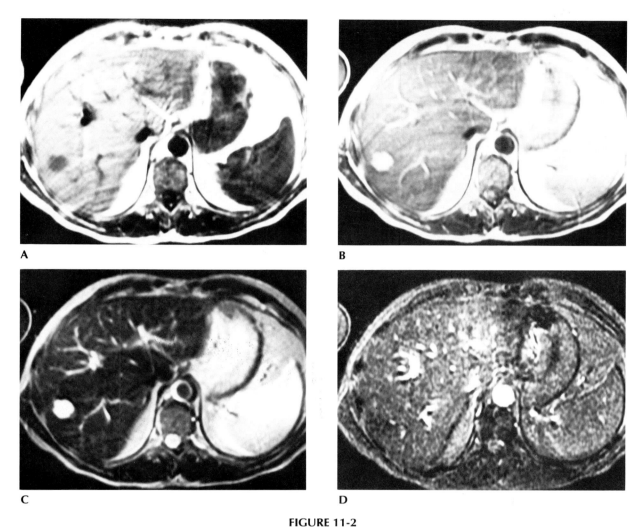

FIGURE 11-2

Hemangioma. A classic appearance for a hemangioma is shown with the lesion being homogeneous low intensity on the heavily T1-weighted SE 10/300 image (A) and high intensity on the fat-suppressed, flow-compensated SE 30/2000 (B) and SE 80/2000 (C) images. (D) A GRASS 5/33 image through the same area does not demonstrate the lesion.

vessels, an effect particularly evident on thin-section gradient-echo images with gradient moment nulling. For this reason, we have made a steady-state sequence part of our routine liver imaging protocol. Hepatic and portal veins, splenic vein, vena cava, and major arteries are routinely well visualized. An example of the capability of these flow-sensitive images is shown in Figure 11-6. Since many patients with liver disease also have surgically produced shunts to relieve portal hypertension, a vascular-weighted steady-state sequence is useful in identifying and characterizing vascular shunts.

Steady-state images can be rapidly acquired in sequence through a fixed location to obtain dynamic images. When combined with a bolus of gadolinium contrast material, dynamic imaging is a powerful new way to characterize lesions by MRI

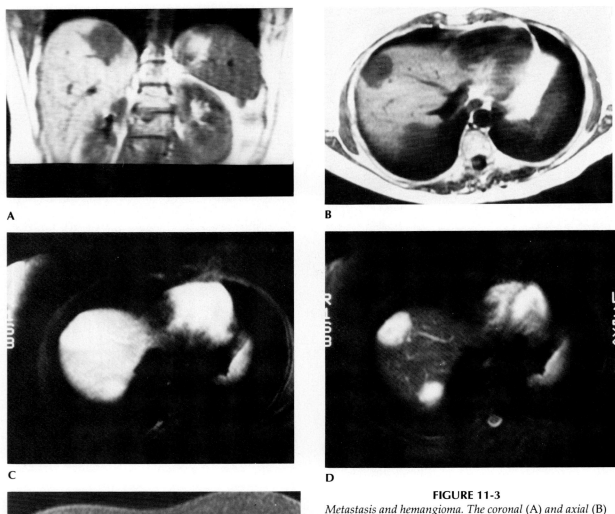

FIGURE 11-3
Metastasis and hemangioma. The coronal (A) and axial (B) heavily T1-weighted SE 10/300 images show two well-defined low-intensity masses. The anterior mass is a vascular metastasis, and the posterior lesion is a hemangioma. These lesions have high intensity on the fat-suppressed, flow-compensated SE 30/2000 (C) and SE 80/2000 (D) images. (E) The lesions are subtle and remain indistinguishable on the turbo GRASS 6/23 image.

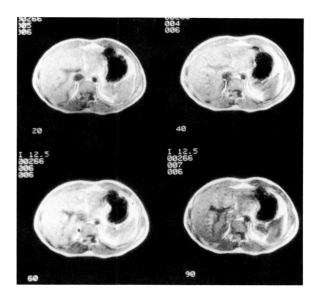

FIGURE 11-4
Flip-angle adjustment. A GRASS 5/33 sequence is used at various flip angles to demonstrate the effect of flip-angle adjustment on image contrast and SNR. Images with flip angles of 20, 40, 60, and 90 degrees are labeled. When the steady state is used, adjustments in flip angle produce no difference in contrast. The major effect of flip-angle variation is on the SNR of the image.

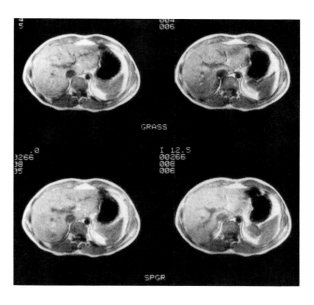

FIGURE 11-5
Effect of RF spoiling. A GRASS 5/33 sequence is used without RF spoiling (top two images) and with RF spoiling (bottom two images). There is no demonstrable effect of RF spoiling on liver image contrast. The lack of any change is probably due to the lack of long T2 fluids in this anatomic region. The major effect of RF spoiling is to break up the steady state of long T2 fluids. RF spoiling has little effect on the steady state of shorter T2 tissues.

(18). Occasionally this dynamic bolus tracking provides insight about lesions that is not possible with conventional sequences (Fig. 11-7). However, this method is not practical for routine screening purposes.

New liver-specific contrast agents use magnetic susceptibility primarily as a contrast mechanism (19,20). Because of the increased sensitivity of gradient-echo sequences to magnetic susceptibility effects, these sequences could reduce the dose of liver-specific contrast agent necessary for adequate liver imaging (21). Liver-specific contrast agents may overcome many of the inherent contrast defects that are problems with current steady-state methods. The very rapid and reliable acquisitions possible with these steady-state sequences may offset the added expense of the contrast agent.

SUMMARY

Steady-state imaging is rapidly emerging as a method for reducing motion artifacts and producing high-quality, reliable images of the liver. A great deal of progress has been made toward understanding the contrast mechanism of steady-state imaging sequences. Although the right combination for optimal liver contrast has not yet been discovered, there is potential for a breakthrough. In the words of Yogi Berra, "We must be making all the wrong mistakes."

As liver-specific contrast agents emerge, the need for inherent liver contrast in a sequence is less critical. Instead, rapid acquisitions and sensitivity to magnetic susceptibility effects are dominant concerns in pulse-sequence selection. With the use of liver-specific contrast agents, steady-state imaging may become the workhorse sequence of future liver MRI diagnosis.

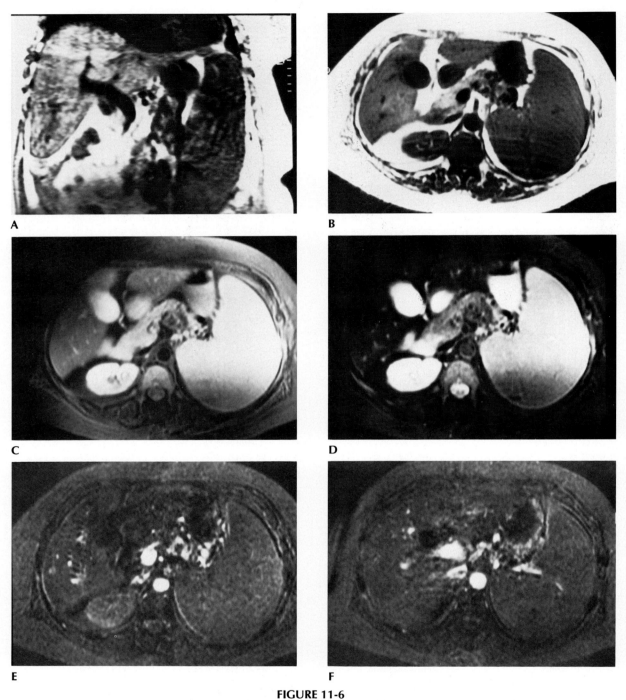

FIGURE 11-6

Splenic vein thrombosis. T1-weighted SE 10/300 coronal (A) and axial (B) images show extensive small, round, low-signal-intensity venous collaterals in the splenic hilum. The fat-suppressed, flow-compensated SE 30/2000 (C) and SE 80/2000 (D) images show the extensive collaterals as low intensity. These findings are evidence of splenic vein thrombosis. Further information on the extent of the thrombosis is provided by the turbo GRASS 6/23 images, where flowing blood is shown as high intensity. (E) The turbo GRASS image at the level of the splenic vein thrombosis shows the high-intensity small venous collaterals without visualization of the normal splenic vein. (F) Another turbo GRASS image at another level shows good flow in the portal vein.

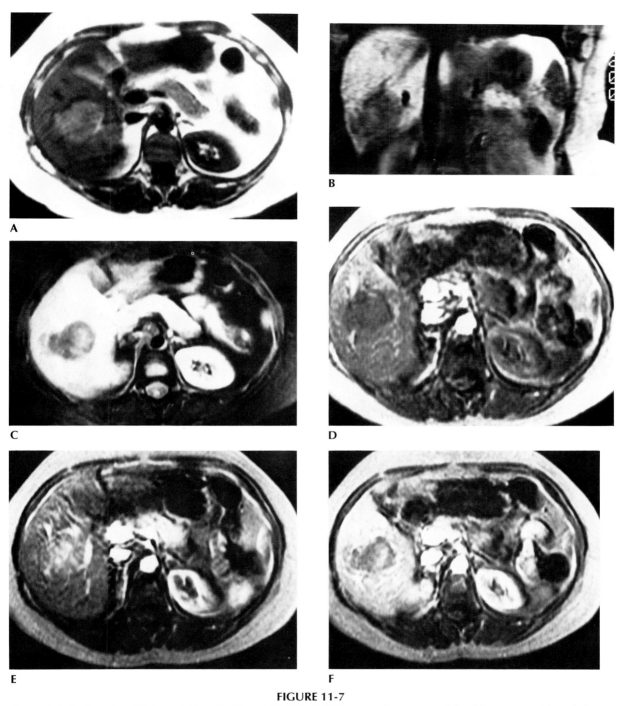

FIGURE 11-7

Dynamic bolus tracking. (A) *An axial heavily T1-weighted SE 10/300 image shows a well-defined liver mass with slightly increased intensity compared with surrounding liver.* (B) *A fat-suppressed coronal SE 10/300 image shows the mass as decreased intensity relative to surroundings.* (C) *The fat-suppressed, flow-compensated SE 30/2000 and SE 80/2000 (not shown) images also show a low-intensity mass. These findings are evidence of a fatty liver mass. Hepatomas commonly have increased fat, but other liver processes also can have fat. A turbo GRASS 5/23 image is performed through the mass with a bolus injection of gadolinium-DTPA. The initial image* (D) *shows a low-intensity mass that enhances immediately on the early bolus image* (E) *and washes out on the late image* (F). *Note the renal enhancement pattern on the dynamic images.*

REFERENCES

1. Stark DD, Hendrick RE, Hahn PF, Ferrucci JT Jr: Motion artifact reduction with fast spin-echo imaging. Radiology 164:183, 1987.
2. Haacke EM, Lenz GW: Improving MR image quality in the presence of motion by using rephasing gradients. AJR 148:1251, 1987.
3. Mitchell DG, Vinitske S, Burk DL Jr, et al: Motion artifact reduction in MR imaging of the abdomen: Gradient moment nulling versus respiratory-sorted phase encoding. Radiology 169:155, 1988.
4. Duerk JL, Pattany PM: Analysis of imaging axes significance in motion artifact suppression technique (MAST): MRI of turbulent flow and motion. Magn Reson Imaging 7:251, 1989.
5. Felmlee JP, Ehman RL: Spatial presaturation: A method for suppressing flow artifacts and improving depiction of vascular anatomy in MR imaging. Radiology 164:559, 1987.
6. Edelman RR, Atkinson DJ, Silver MS, et al: FRODO pulse sequence: A new means of eliminating motion, flow, and wraparound artifacts. Radiology 166:231, 1988.
7. Dixon WTY, Brummer ME, Malko JA: Acquisition order and motional artifact reduction in spin warp images. Magn Reson Med 6:74, 1988.
8. Saini S, Stark DD, Rzedzian RR, et al: Forty-millisecond MR imaging of the abdomen at 2.0 T. Radiology 173:111, 1989.
9. Raval B, Mehta S, Narayana P, et al: Feasibility of fast MR imaging of the liver at 1.5 T. Magn Reson Imaging 7:203, 1989.
10. Unger EC, Cohen MS, Gatenby RA, et al: Single breath-holding scans of the abdomen using FISP and FLASH. J Comput Assist Tomogr 12:575, 1988.
11. Winkler ML, Thoeni RF, Luh N, et al: Hepatic neoplasia: Breath-hold MR imaging. Radiology 170:801, 1989.
12. Gyngell ML: Application of steady-state free precession in rapid 2DFT NMR imaging: Fast and CE-fast sequences. Magn Reson Imaging 7:463, 1988.
13. Merboldt KD, Bruhn H, Frahm J, et al: MRI of "diffusion" in the human brain: New results using a modified CE-FAST sequence. Magn Reson Med 9:423, 1989.
14. Harms SE, Flamig DP, Fisher CF, Fulmer JM. New method for fast MR imaging of the knee. Radiology 173:743, 1989.
15. Patz S, Wong STS, Roos MS: Missing pulse steady-state free precession. Magn Reson Med 10:194, 1989.
16. Hasse A, Frahm J, Matthaei D, et al: MR imaging using stimulated echoes (STEAM). Radiology 160:787, 1986.
17. Foo TKF, Perman WH, Poon CSO, et al: Magn Reson Med 9:203, 1989.
18. Hamm B, Wolf K-J, Felix R: Conventional and rapid MR imaging of the liver with Gd-DTPA. Radiology 164:313, 1987.
19. Saini S, Stark DD, Hahn PF, et al: Ferrite particles: Superparamagnetic MR contrast agent for the reticuloendothelial system. Radiology 162:211, 1987.
20. Saini S, Stark DD, Hahn PF, et al: Ferrite particles: Superparamagnetic MR contrast agent for enhanced detection of liver carcinoma. Radiology 162:217, 1987.
21. Majumdar S, Zoghbi SS, Gore JC: Influence of pulse sequence on the relaxation effects of superparamagnetic iron oxide contrast agents. Magn Reson Med 10:289, 1989.

V. FAST IMAGING

12

Fast-Scan MRI of the Abdomen

JENS FRAHM

State-of-the-art high-field MRI systems allow routine use of fast-scan MRI techniques characterized by low-flip-angle gradient-echo sequences such as FLASH. Thus measuring times are reduced to a few seconds while maintaining image quality similar to that obtained with conventional spin-echo sequences. This chapter briefly outlines the basic ideas underlying major fast-scan MRI techniques. Relaxation-times contrast and flow properties are related to the specific conditions encountered in the abdomen. Recommended imaging strategies entirely focus on single-breath-hold acquisitions covering measuring times from about 2 to 25 s. While longer examinations are completely disregarded, the unavoidable trade-offs in image quality associated with even faster acquisitions in the subsecond (0.5 to 1.0 s) or high-speed regime (<0.1 s) are discussed.

FAST-SCAN MRI TECHNIQUES

In studies of the central nervous system (CNS), clinical applications of MRI take advantage of both T1-weighted and T2-weighted images for the detection and characterization of pathology. Although in the past imaging data were obtained using spin-echo MRI techniques, clinical experience is based on tissue contrast that is independent of a particular imaging technique. Thus present knowledge may be completely transferred to the use of corresponding fast-scan MRI protocols. In fact, fast-scan sequences are now available that provide access to the same contrast but within only a fraction of the imaging time of a spin-echo examination. Low-flip-angle gradient-echo sequences such as FLASH (1,2) yield proton density, spin-lattice relaxation time, and flow contrast, while steady-state free-precession (SSFP) echo sequences such as CE-FAST (3-5) allow acquisition of T2-weighted fast-scan images.

In general, the quality of gradient-echo images has been considerably improved over the past 5 years. This is predominantly due to technological progress in the manufacture of both more homogeneous whole-body magnets and stronger magnetic field gradient systems with reduced eddy currents. These achievements translate into longer free induction decay (FID) signals and shorter gradient-echo times that not only improve the signal-to-noise ratio (SNR) but also markedly decrease the sensitivity to signal losses by tissue susceptibility differences and motion.

Financial support by the Bundesminister für Forschung und Technologie (BMFT) of the Federal Republic of Germany (Grant 01 VF 8606/6) is gratefully acknowledged.

The FLASH Sequence

Basically, the FLASH sequence combines low-flip-angle RF excitation with the acquisition of a gradient-recalled echo (1,2). This gradient echo is derived from the FID by reversal of the frequency-encoding read gradient. The repetition time of the sequence, i.e., the time required for excitation and detection of the data of one phase-encoded projection, may be as short as desired or as the system hardware allows, e.g., 3 to 4 ms for high-speed imaging or about 10 ms for conventional fast-scan applications.

The speed of the FLASH sequence is due to the fact that a low-flip-angle excitation leaves a major part of the longitudinal magnetization untouched. On the contrary, a 90-degree excitation reads the entire magnetization at once and therefore requires a waiting period for magnetization recovery. After a few excitations, FLASH sequences establish a dynamic steady state of the longitudinal magnetization in which the loss of magnetization by excitation is fed back through T1 relaxation. Transverse magnetizations are either absent (e.g., short T2, low flip angles, motion) or are spoiled by RF (6,7) or gradient (8) means. The degree of saturation controls the image contrast as a function of repetition time or flip angle.

The CE-FAST Sequence

In addition to proton density and T1 contrast, CE-FAST sequences (3-5) predominantly emphasize tissues with long T2 relaxation times. In fact, in the presence of signal contributions with long T2 relaxation times, and provided that a number of further conditions are fulfilled that lead to phase stability of the MRI signal from one repetition cycle to the next, repetitive RF pulse sequences create a steady state of both the longitudinal and transverse magnetizations. Corresponding SSFP imaging applications result in two types of MRI signals, the SSFP-FID following RF pulses and the SSFP-echo preceding RF pulses, that both differ from the conventional FID signal. The CE-FAST sequence acquires a gradient echo of the SSFP-echo signal. Excellent T2 contrast is due to the fact that the SSFP-echo represents a complex overlap of spin echoes and stimulated echoes from preceding RF pulses with effective echo times that are multiples of the RF pulse-repetition time. Fast-scan MRI sequences as well as applicational aspects are described in detail in reference 9.

FAST-SCAN MRI: CNS VERSUS ABDOMEN

The current speed and quality of both T1-weighted FLASH and T2-weighted CE-FAST images are sufficient to replace conventional spin-echo sequences in routine clinical studies of the CNS. Combined fast-scan MRI protocols allow high-quality brain imaging in less than 10 min, yielding patient comfort as well as high patient throughput (10). Unfortunately, the protocol outlined for brain imaging can not be completely transferred to abdominal studies because the CE-FAST sequence suffers from a strong sensitivity to motion (11). In fact, even slow motion of the cerebrospinal fluid in the ventricles may cause signal voids in CE-FAST images. The occurrence of motion in the presence of the imaging gradients introduces phase variations from one repetition cycle to the next that completely destroy steady-state conditions of the transverse magnetization. Thus abdominal applications of the CE-FAST sequence in general do not yield satisfactory images. In the absence of motion, very low SNRs are expected for most abdominal organs owing to their short T2 relaxation times (liver $\approx$ 30 to 35 ms, muscle $\approx$ 25 to 30 ms) as compared with brain tissue ($\approx$ 150 to 200 ms), so that pathology with long T2 relaxation times would yield good T2 contrast.

FIGURE 12-1

Proton density and T1 contrast as a function of flip angle in fast-scan MRI of the upper abdomen: 26-s single-breath-hold multislice FLASH MR images (TR of 100 ms, single excitation) of a normal volunteer. The spatial resolution corresponds to a data matrix of 256 × 256 pixels covering a field of view of 350 mm with a slice thickness of 6 mm. Two images were selected out of a series of eight images acquired simultaneously. The flip angle increases from 10 degrees (top) to 60 degrees (bottom) as indicated.

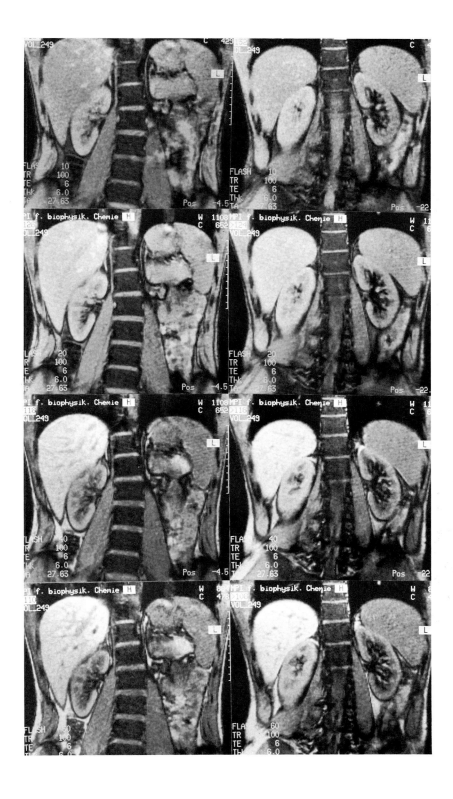

On the contrary, FLASH sequences are rather motion-insensitive, in particular for gradient-echo times of 6 ms or below, and therefore allow the acquisition of excellent proton density and T1-weighted images of the upper abdomen within breath-hold imaging times. Studies of healthy volunteers (20 to 30 years of age) were carried out at 2.0 Tesla on a Siemens Magnetom equipped with a conventional 10 millitesla per meter gradient system. All images were acquired using a circularly polarized body coil. Informed consent was obtained prior to the investigation.

RESULTS AND DISCUSSION
Single-Breath-Hold FLASH MRI
For a given repetition time, the contrast of FLASH images is controlled by a variation of the flip angle. The series of images shown in Figure 12-1 illustrates corresponding contrast variations using single-breath-hold images of the upper abdomen within total imaging times of 26 s. This duration is considered to be the maximum value applicable to studies of cooperative patients. The images represent two of eight coronal images at different levels that were acquired simultaneously using a repetition time of 100 ms and a data matrix of 256 × 256 pixels. The slice thickness is 6 mm. There are no motion artifacts visible, so that spine, liver, spleen, and kidneys are clearly depicted.

Proton-density contrast is obtained at flip angles of only 10 degrees (Figure 12-1, top images), yielding isointense signals from almost all tissues. An increase to 20 degrees leads to an increase in both SNR and T1 contrast. A flip angle of 40 degrees results in an optimized SNR (at a TR of 100 ms) and a fully developed T1 contrast, e.g., between liver and spleen or muscle and fat. A further increase of the flip angle to 60 degrees (Figure 12-1, bottom images) only slightly improves contrast at the expense of overall signal strength and slice profile quality due to saturation.

Shorter imaging times are available by a number of different strategies. The most obvious modifications are a reduction of the number of phase-encoding steps from 256 to 192 or 128 and by a reduction of the number of simultaneously acquired slices while maintaining spatial resolution. Figure 12-2 demonstrates that similar proton density and T1 contrast as in Figure 12-1 are available when adjusting the range of flip angles to a reduced repetition time of 40 ms (left column of images) or 15 ms (right column). Since the FLASH sequence used exhibits a minimum repetition cycle of 12-ms duration, the number of slices is reduced from eight (TR of 100 ms) to three (TR of 40 ms) and one (TR of 15 ms). Accordingly, the flip angle required for strong T1 contrast reduces from 40 to 60 degrees (TR of 100 ms) to 30 degrees (TR of 40 ms) and 20 degrees (TR of 15 ms).

Imaging times vary from 10 to 20 s for the three-slice sequence depending on the number of phase-encoding steps and/or signal averaging. Of course, single-slice acquisitions may be performed even faster. A repetition time of 15 ms leads to an imaging time of 3.8 s per 256 × 256 image (7.7 s for two excitations, as in Fig. 12-2, right column). In contrast to multislice applications, where blood signals are partially or even completely saturated, single-slice images exhibit strong signals from blood vessels due to a steady inflow of unsaturated spins from neighboring sections. Flow signals may be especially emphasized by imposing very strong saturation onto stationary tissue signals, as shown for a flip angle of 30 degrees (TR of 15 ms) in Figure 12-2.

On the other hand, blood flow may be a source of ghosting artifacts in the phase-encoding dimension of abdominal images. This problem predominantly occurs with transverse image orientations due to high-speed pulsatile flow in the aorta and vena cava. The effect is demonstrated in Figure 12-3, where the intensities of misregistered flow signals increase with flip angle (20 to 60 degrees). The artifacts lead to both signal overlap and cancellation depending on the phase of the flow signal relative to that of stationary tissue. An easy solution to the problem is spatial presaturation (12) of flowing spins on one or both sides of the imaging plane. The image in the lower right of Figure 12-3 was acquired by dual-side saturation using 4-cm-thick sections with a distance of about 1.5 cm to the volume covered by the multislice acquisition. The images were obtained from a single breath-hold within a total imaging time of 26 s (TR of 100 ms). The number of images had to be reduced from eight to five when incorporating the extra RF pulses for flow suppression.

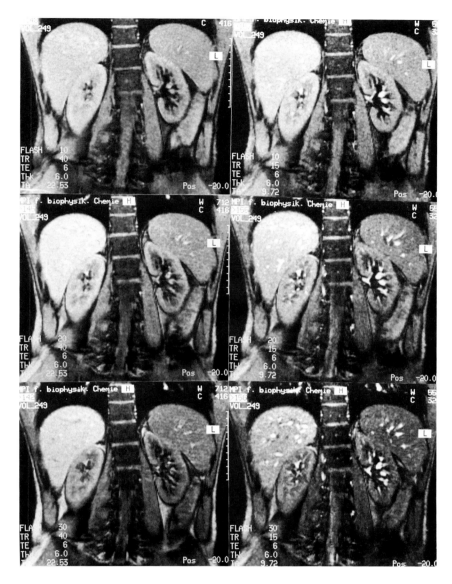

FIGURE 12-2
Proton density and T1 contrast as a function of flip angle and repetition time in fast-scan MRI of the upper abdomen: 20-s single-breath-hold multislice FLASH MR images (left column, TR of 40 ms, three images, two excitations) and 7.5-s single-breath-hold single-slice FLASH MR images (right column, TR of 15 ms, two excitations) *of a normal volunteer. Other parameters are as in Figure 12-1. The flip angle increases from 10 degrees (top)* to *30 degrees (bottom) as indicated.*

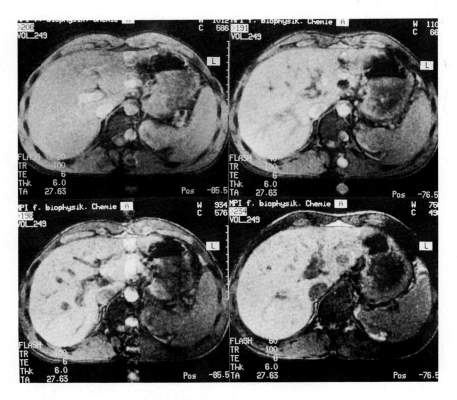

FIGURE 12-3
Flow artifacts and flow suppression in fast-scan MRI of the abdomen: 26-s single-breath-hold multislice FLASH MR images (TR of 100 ms, eight images, single excitation) of a normal volunteer. Other parameters are as in Figure 12-1. The flip angle increases from 20 degrees (upper left) to 60 degrees (lower left) as indicated. The lower right image stems from a corresponding multislice acquisition (TR of 100 ms, 60 degrees, five images, single excitation) with the use of flow suppression on either side of the imaging plane (sections of 4 cm thickness). In order to incorporate spatial presaturation RF pulses into the imaging sequence, the number of slices has to be reduced from eight to five while keeping the repetition time constant.

So far, a reduction of the imaging time has been accomplished without sacrificing spatial resolution. In fact, the detection of small lesions in patients clearly benefits from the high resolution accessible with breath-hold images. At field strengths of 1.0 to 2.0 Tesla, such images are obtainable with a good SNR using a slice thickness of only 4 to 6 mm and a FOV of 300 to 400 mm that is covered by a conventional data matrix of 256 × 256 pixels. Figure 12-4 shows an example of a space-occupying lesion in the left kidney that is well delineated in zoomed sections of the original single-breath-hold images. Since the study was a multislice acquisition, the lesion can be accurately followed through neighboring planes from the same set of images.

FAST-SCAN MRI STRATEGIES FOR ABDOMINAL IMAGING

Single-breath-hold imaging using FLASH MRI sequences yields high-quality images of the upper abdomen with access to proton density, T1, and flow contrast. No tradeoffs in image resolution, SNR, or contrast have to be made to gain imaging

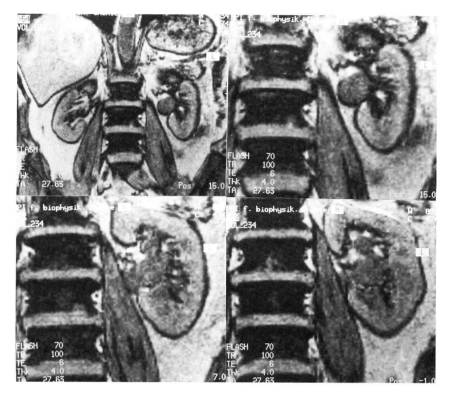

FIGURE 12-4
T1-weighted single-breath-hold multislice FLASH MR images (TR of 100 ms, 70 degrees, single excitation, 26 s) of a patient with a space-occupying lesion in the left kidney. Other parameters are as in Figure 12-1. The image on the upper right is a zoomed section of the image on the upper left. The lower images represent corresponding sections through neighboring planes from the same set of multislice images.

speed. In fact, imaging times from 2 to 25 s include a number of possible strategies for patient studies that allow a matching to the breath-holding capabilities of individual patients. Under these circumstances, the physiologic requirements to effectively freeze motions in the images are easily fulfillable, as demonstrated in Figures 12-1 to 12-4.

Table 12-1 summarizes potential strategies for single-breath-hold imaging of the abdomen. Variations in the number of simultaneously acquired slices, in the spatial resolution, and in the number of excitations are related to typical imaging times. In a similar way, Table 12-2 describes the available contrast for typical sets of repetition times, flip angles, and acquisition modes. While spin-density contrasts require a certain minimum imaging time due to the use of low flip angles in conjunction with relatively long repetition times (>60 ms), T1 and flow contrast are available almost independent of a predetermined imaging time. In general, the visibility of the vasculature may be switched on or off as desired. Blood flow is best visualized in strongly T1-weighted single-slice acquisitions, whereas flow presaturation is preferably combined with multislice acquisitions. Additional information regarding lesion detection and characterization may be obtained from dynamic contrast agent studies that are fully compatible with single-breath-hold FLASH MRI.

TABLE 12-1. Fast-Scan MRI Strategies for Abdominal Imaging: Imaging times

Data Matrix	Repetition Time (ms)	No. of Slices	No. of Excitations	Imaging Time(s)
256 × 256	100	8	1	26
192 × 256	100	8	1	19
128 × 256	200	16	1	26
256 × 256	40	3	2	20
256 × 256	40	3	1	10
192 × 256	40	3	2	15
128 × 256	80	6	1	10
256 × 256	15	1	2	7.7
256 × 256	15	1	1	3.8
256 × 256	25	2	1	6.4
128 × 256	15	1	1	1.9
128 × 256	50	4	1	6.4

Note: Best results are obtained on state-of-the-art high-field MRI units. The achievable image quality is demonstrated in Figures 12-1 to 12-4 using a field of view of 350 mm and a slice thickness of 6 mm. The given number of slices is based on a repetition cycle of about 12 ms for the acquisition of one phase-encoded projection. A decrease in this value and a concomitant increase in the number of slices for the same imaging time is possible at the expense of the signal-to-noise ratio by increasing the receiver bandwidth.

TABLE 12-2. Fast-Scan MRI Strategies for Abdominal Imaging: Contrast Capabilities

Contrast	Repetition Time (ms)	Flip Angle (degrees)	Slice Mode
Proton density	200	10–20	Multi
	100	10	Multi
T1	200	70	Multi
	100	40–60	Multi
	40	20–30	Multi
	15	20	Single
Flow	100	70	Single
	40	40	Single
	15	30	Single

Note: Imaging parameters as in Table 12-1.

HIGH-SPEED MRI OF THE ABDOMEN?

It has been stated that no reasonable images of the upper abdomen may be obtained unless peristaltic motions have been frozen by means of ultrafast or instant acquisitions. In view of the present results, however, it is clear that high-speed techniques are not required for abdominal imaging. In fact, the most obvious and unavoidable achievement of a high-speed acquisition is a considerable loss in image quality. This applies to all currently available techniques, such as echo-planar imaging (13,14), subsecond FLASH (15,16), and high-speed STEAM (17,18). While abdominal applications should not accept a sacrifice in spatial resolution and SNR, the only potential justification for a low-resolution, limited SNR image may be cardiac MRI. However, even in heart studies, images from a single cardiac cycle are only required for patients with severe arrhythmias precluding the derivation of a useful ECG trigger signal for cine MRI studies.

Since longer imaging times result in better images, abdominal studies should exploit the fact that motions are slower than in the heart. In cases where breath-hold scans are not possible, it has been proposed to match a FLASH sequence to the time scale of peristaltic motions. The required imaging times of about 0.5 to 1.0 s yield single-slice images with a data matrix of only 128 × 128 pixels and a slice thickness of 10 mm. Although the images are of good quality at first glance, it should be noted that their typical pixel size is up to a factor of 10 larger than that of a typical breath-hold image (256 × 256 matrix, 4-mm slice thickness). This extent of image blurring is a distinct disadvantage, in particular since subsecond images were originally intended to minimize blurring effects by freezing motion.

One interesting aspect of subsecond images is the possible separation of contrast manipulation and imaging (15). Since the inherent contrast of the FLASH images may be kept to proton-density differences by the use of very low flip angles (5 to 10 degrees), a preceding spin-echo 90-degree (x')–180-degree(y')–90-degree$(-x')$ sequence may impose T2 contrasts onto the longitudinal equilibrium magnetization. Alternatively, a preceding 180-degree inversion pulse followed by an appropriate delay may generate inversion-recovery T1 contrasts. In fact, T1 contrast inversion between liver and spleen is easily accomplished by adjusting the inversion delay to null out the signal intensities of either organ.

CONCLUSIONS

There is no doubt that conventional spin-echo imaging will be steadily replaced by fast-scan MRI techniques. This not only applies to abdominal investigations, where a certain speed is required to overcome the motion problem, but also to studies of the CNS. In both cases, total investigational times may become as short as 10 min using high-field MRI systems.

In general, a clinical user of fast-scan MRI sequences is free to make his or her own compromise between SNR, spatial resolution, and measuring time. It should be noted, however, that image information is sacrificed if the acquisition becomes faster than necessary. For abdominal applications, single-breath-hold imaging turns out to be an optimum. For example, a 20-s breath-hold scan may give the best results in the form of high-quality multislice images for a cooperative patient. If only shorter measuring windows are accessible, then the use of a smaller number of slices maintains image quality with reduced measuring times of a few seconds. The unavoidable penalty in image quality introduced with ultrafast acquisitions may be acceptable for single-cardiac-cycle imaging.

REFERENCES

1. Haase A, Frahm J, Matthaei D, et al: FLASH imaging: Rapid NMR imaging using low flip-angle pulses. J Magn Reson 67:258, 1986.
2. Frahm J, Haase A, Matthaei D: Rapid NMR imaging of dynamic processes using the FLASH technique. Magn Reson Med 3:321, 1986.
3. Hawkes RC, Patz S: Rapid Fourier imaging using steady-state free precession. Magn Reson Med 3:9, 1987.
4. Gyngell ML: The application of steady-state free precession in rapid 2DFT NMR imaging—FAST and CE-FAST sequences. Magn Reson Imaging 6:415, 1988.
5. Gyngell ML: The steady-state signals in short-repetition-time sequences. J Magn Reson 81:474, 1989.
6. Darasse L, Mao L, Saint-Jalmes H: Spoiling Techniques in Very Fast TR Imaging. Presented at the Society of Magnetic Resonance in Medicine 5th Annual Meeting, Montreal, August 1986.
7. Zur Y, Bendel P: Elimination of the Steady State Transverse Magnetization in Short TR Imaging. Presented at the Society of Magnetic Resonance in Medicine 6th Annual Meeting, New York, August 1987.
8. Frahm J, Hänicke W, Merboldt KD: Transverse coherences in rapid FLASH NMR imaging. J Magn Reson 72:304, 1987.
9. Frahm J, Gyngell ML, Hänicke W: Rapid scan techniques, in Stark DD, Bradley WJ Jr (eds): Magnetic Resonance Imaging. St. Louis, Mosby, 1991.
10. Bruhn H, Gyngell ML, Merboldt KD, et al: A Fast Scan Protocol for MRI of Brain Lesions in Less than 10 Minutes. Presented at the Society of Magnetic Resonance in Medicine 9th Annual Meeting, New York, August 1990.
11. Patz S, Hawkes RC: The application of steady-state free precession to the study of very slow fluid flow. Magn Reson Med 3:140, 1986.
12. Frahm J, Haase A, Merboldt KD, et al: Flow Effects in Rapid FLASH NMR Images. Presented at the Society of Magnetic Resonance in Medicine 5th Annual Meeting, Montreal, August 1986; Frahm J, Merboldt KD, Hänicke W, Haase A: Flow suppression in rapid FLASH NMR images. Magn Reson Med 4:372, 1987.
13. Ordidge RJ, Howseman A, Coxon R, et al: Snapshot imaging at 0.5 T using echo-planar techniques. Magn Reson Med 10:227, 1989.
14. Rzedzian RR, Pykett IL: Instant images of the human heart using a new, whole-body MR imaging system. AJR 149:245, 1987.
15. Haase A: Snapshot FLASH MRI: Applications to T1, T2, and chemical-shift imaging. Magn Reson Med 13:77, 1990.
16. Frahm J, Merboldt KD, Bruhn H, et al: 0.3-Second FLASH MRI of the human heart. Magn Reson Med 13:150, 1990.
17. Frahm J, Haase A, Matthaei D, et al: Rapid NMR imaging using stimulated echoes. J Magn Reson 65:130, 1985.
18. Frahm J, Merboldt KD, Hänicke W, et al: High-Speed Single Cardiac Cycle STEAM MRI of the Human Heart. Presented at the Society of Magnetic Resonance in Medicine 9th Annual Meeting, New York, August 1990.

13

Ultrafast MRI of the Liver

SANJAY SAINI and
MARK S. COHEN

Magnetic resonance imaging (MRI) techniques that reduce scan times to less than a second provide the long-awaited potential of eliminating motion artifacts from MRI images of the abdomen. These rapid imaging techniques include ultrafast pulse sequences with which a fully resolved MRI image can be obtained in less than 100 ms. In this chapter we will review the technical basis of ultrafast MRI and assess the results of a preliminary clinical investigation on a prototype scanner designed by Advanced NMR Systems (Instascan, Woburn, Mass.). Comparison with competing rapid imaging techniques including gradient-echo pulse sequences (scan time tens of seconds) and turbo FLASH (scan time approximately 1 s) will not be discussed herein.

PRINCIPLES

The theoretical concept of ultrafast echo-planar MRI was first advanced by Mansfield in 1977 (1). Although initial clinical images were obtained as early as 1983 (2), diagnostic-quality ultrafast MRI images with scan times of 40 to 100 ms were not obtained until more recently (3–7).

Spatial Resolution
Ultrafast pulse sequences produce MRI images with a single excitation. In comparison, for conventional pulse sequences, the total number of excitations equals the number of phase-encoding steps selected, which is typically 128 or 192 or 256. With single-shot ultrafast MRI, phase encoding after the solitary excitation is performed by rapidly oscillating the frequency-encoding and phase-encoding gradients, which generates a series of gradient-recalled echoes. Special hardware and software adaptations are necessary to perform this rapid gradient switching. As a result, two phase encoding lines, each with 128 or 256 frequency-encoding points, can be generated per millisecond. However the total number of phase-encoding steps in ultrafast MRI pulse sequences is limited by the signal decay (defined by T2 or T2*) during the period of data acquisition. As a result, the ensuing ultrafast MRI images usually have fewer phase-encoding steps than are typically present in conventional MRI images. This, coupled with physical limitations of gradient-switching rates and gradient amplitudes, places some restrictions on the in-plane resolution of single-shot ultrafast MRI images.

With the earliest implementations of Instascan, most of the attention was placed on temporal resolution at a cost in spatial resolving power, so that the typical single-shot images had spatial resolutions of 3 × 3 mm. To overcome these limitations in spatial resolution, Rzedzian, Weisskoff, and others have developed ultrafast MRI techniques utilizing either multiple excitations (mosaic or MESH methods) (8), conjugate-synthesis techniques (9), or combinations of these two methods (10,11). As a result, the spatial resolutions in single-shot techniques are now four times better (1.5 × 1.5 mm), and with two excitation pulses, 0.8 × 1.5 mm pixels can be obtained, giving spatial resolution comparable to conventional imaging. These recent improvements of Instascan have been developed such that a special MRI scanner is not required; an otherwise conventional General Electric Sigma system can be modified to perform ultrafast MRI.

Tissue Contrast

With respect to pulse-sequence design, ultrafast MRI is quite similar to conventional MRI with the availability of spin-echo (SE), gradient-echo (GE) and inversion-recovery (IR) pulse sequences. Thus the resulting MRI image contrast has many similarities to conventional MRI. For example, in the SE scan pulse sequence, all spatial encoding is performed under a conventional Hahn spin echo (12), and therefore, image contrast is identical to that of conventional scanning. The singular difference being that because it is possible to acquire images after one excitation pulse, the TR is effectively infinite. Since the contributions of T1 relaxation time to image contrast are TR-dependent, infinite TR images are acquired without any residual T1 information, resulting in both better contrast in T2-weighted scans and better signal-to-noise ratios. Furthermore, as in conventional MRI, the T2 contrast can be varied freely by adjusting the echo time, TE (short TE: proton density; long TE: T2-weighted). When T1 weighting is desired, inversion-recovery scan methods may be used (13), which offer excellent and readily controlled T1 contrast behavior. T1 contrast also can be introduced into ultrafast MRI images when repetitive imaging (with interscan times less than 5 times tissue T1 time) is performed at a single anatomic level. However, just as T2 contrast is superior in ultrafast MRI images (in comparison to conventional MRI images), T1 contrast is not as striking on the ultrafast T1-weighted images.

Three-Dimensional Imaging

While conventional MRI allows the acquisition of high-quality thin sections, the signal-to-noise ratio in single-shot methods is generally poor when slice thickness is less than 5 mm. One method to overcome this limitation is to use ultrafast three-dimensional imaging or volume-encoding methods. For example, in three-dimensional imaging, a separate excitation is required for each slice (or partition), and the resulting signal-to-noise ratios are much higher (it is typically increased by the square root of the number of partitions). Thus a 16-partition three-dimensional scan will have four times the signal-to-noise ratio of a comparable single-slice acquisition. Using three-dimensional implementations of Instascan, 2-mm-thin slices in the brain, 3-mm slices in the body (14), and 2-mm sections in the heart (15) have been acquired that have both good signal-to-noise ratio and good spatial resolution. The 10- to 48-s acquisition times are long compared to the single-shot scans, however, and it is not yet known how effective such methods will be in a clinical setting. Recently, the three-dimensional technique has been applied also to gradient-echo acquisitions (16). In this mode, sixteen 2-mm sections are acquired in as little as 1 s.

Chemical Shift

An important feature of single-shot imaging in the clinical setting is the need for chemical-shift resolved scanning. For this, water and fat must be imaged separately. In practice, water-only scans are likely to be used. Three major techniques are utilized for lipid suppression. In the original Instascan implementation Rzedzian (9) used a slice-selective 90-degree pulse followed by a water selective 180-degree pulse to form each image. This method, unfortunately, is incompatible with multislice imaging. Quite nearly as effective is the use of a lipid-selective 90-degree pulse, followed by a gradient-crusher pulse, preceding each scan (17). It is this fat-suppression technique that is now used for Instascan. Finally, where T1-weighted scans are desirable, an Instascan implementation of the STIR technique (18) is also extremely effective.

HEPATIC ECHO-PLANAR MRI

In the upper abdomen, ultrafast MRI techniques offer the potential of providing motion-free, high-contrast T2-weighted images. In a preliminary report, we demonstrated that SE ultrafast MRI images obtained with the Instascan technique on a prototype 2.0-Tesla (85.1-MHz) MRI scanner were of uniform quality (7). While organ boundaries were less sharp than on conventional MRI images, high tissue contrast routinely permitted the identification of the common bile duct in the porta hepatis. The large difference in the resonance frequency of water and lipid protons also allowed independent imaging of water and lipid protons simply by varying the frequency of the narrow-bandwidth 180-degree refocusing pulse. Thus, on water images, fatty tissue, including subcutaneous fat, retroperitoneal fat, mesentery, and fatty bone marrow, was of low signal intensity. As a result, chemical-shift artifacts that are normally exaggerated at high field were absent on ultrafast MRI images. Tissues with long T2 relaxation times (gallbladder, CSF) appeared hyperintense. In comparison to the liver, hepatic metastases (Fig. 13-1), hemangiomas (Fig. 13-2), and cysts also appeared hyperintense. These tumors could be discriminated because liver cysts remained bright even on images obtained with TE times of >150 ms. Indeed, since liver was isointense to background noise on these images, <5-mm liver cysts were readily detected. Cavernous hemangiomas also were hyperintense but faded out at relatively shorter TE times. Furthermore, hemangiomas showed marked heterogeneity, while cysts were of uniform signal intensity. Liver metastases were less hyperintense than cysts and hemangiomas and faded on TE times of >30 ms. They also demonstrated marked lesion heterogeneity and peritumoral edema.

The major limitation of ultrafast MRI images was inability to distinguish retroperitoneal adenopathy from the gastrointestinal tract (Fig. 13-3). With nonincremental dynamic (images every 1 s) imaging technique, physiologic motion (bowel peristalses) can be exploited as a source of tissue contrast. However, early experience suggests that this approach is of limited value because the TR of 1 s reduces T2 tissue contrast. Thus it is highly unlikely that ultrafast MRI images will eliminate the need for a gastrointestinal contrast agent.

CONCLUSION

The clinical utilization of MRI has been limited due to the degradation of conventional MRI images by physiologic motion and the lack of an adequate bowel contrast agent (19). Ultrafast MRI offers considerable promise in overcoming one of

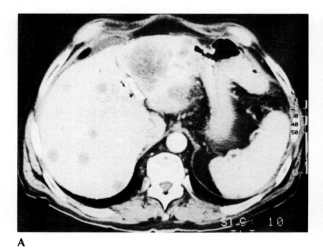
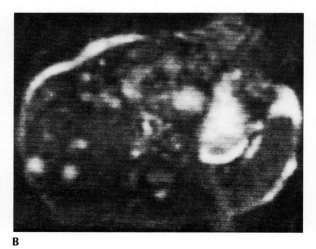

A   B

FIGURE 13-1
Liver metastases from carcinoma of the pancreas. (A) Contrast-enhanced CT scan. (B) Ultrafast MRI image; TR: infinity; TE: 90 ms; 1-cm slice; 64 × 128 data matrix; approximately 100-ms scan time. Several hyperintense liver metastases are seen. Note the good correlation with accompanying CT scan. The image demonstrates low in-plane resolution but high lesion/liver contrast because the liver is of low signal intensity. Note the presence of ascites on both images.

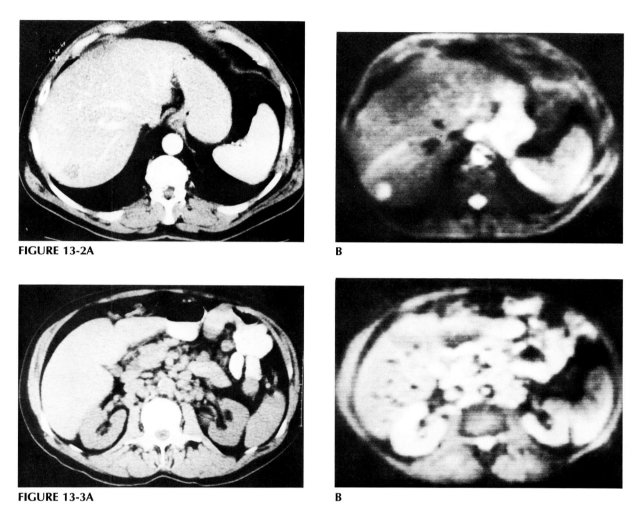

FIGURE 13-2
Hepatic hemangioma. (A) Contrast-enhanced CT scan. (B) Ultrafast MRI image; TR: infinity; TE: 60 ms; 1-cm slice; 64 × 128 data matrix; approximately 70-ms scan time. The 1.5-cm lesion is well seen on both images. On the ultrafast MRI image, the hemangioma demonstrates high signal intensity. Differentiation from metastases is performed with more T2-weighted images (longer TEs), where the metastases lose signal intensity before hemangiomas.

FIGURE 13-3
Retroperitoneal lymphadenopathy from Hodgkin's lymphoma. (A) Non-contrast-enhanced CT scan. (B) Ultrafast MRI image; TR: infinity; TE: 30 ms; 1-cm slice; 64 × 128 data matrix; approximately 40-s scan time. Note the difficulty in distinguishing retroperitoneal lymphadenopathy from bowel loops and gallbladder. This suggests the need for a gastrointestinal contrast agent even for this imaging technique.

these impediments. In comparison to conventional acquisitions, the single-shot scanning techniques are hundreds or thousands of times more rapid and are therefore largely immune to the problems of motion artifacts that traditionally have plagued MRI. Therefore, these new imaging techniques dramatically broaden the range of applications that will be routinely accessible for MRI to include simplified cardiac imaging, dynamic imaging with contrast agents, and kinematic imaging. While the dynamic visualization of moving or rapidly changing structures is a relatively obvious application of single-shot imaging, there are also important applications in extremely motion-sensitive methods such as diffusion imaging (20, 21). In the case of abdominal imaging in general and liver imaging in particular, the clinical utilization of MRI will undoubtedly witness increasing clinical applications with greater availability of rapid imaging techniques. How the 100-ms ultrafast methods compared with the 1-s fast pulse sequences in a clinical setting will be the focus of intense debate in the coming years.

REFERENCES

1. Mansfield P: Multi-planar image formation using NMR spin echoes. J Physiol C10:L55, 1977.
2. Rzedzian RR, Mansfield P, Doyle M, et al: Real-time NMR clinical imaging in pediatrics. Lancet 1:1281, 1983.
3. Rzedzian RR, Pykett IL: Instant images of the human heart using a new, whole-body MR imaging system. AJR 149:245, 1987.
4. Pykett IL, Rzedzian RR: Instant images of the body by magnetic resonance. Magn Reson Med 5:563, 1987.
5. Crooks LE, Arakawa M, Hylton NM, et al: Echo-planar pediatric imager. Radiology 166:157, 1988.
6. Stehling MJ, Howseman AM, Ordridge RJ, et al: Whole-body echo-planar MR imaging at 0.5 T. Radiology 170:257, 1989.
7. Saini S, Stark DD, Rzedzian RR, et al: Forty-millisecond MR imaging of the abdomen at 2.0 T. Radiology 173:111, 1989.
8. Rzedzian RR: High-speed, high-resolution spin-echo imaging by mosaic scan and MESH, in Book of Abstracts, Society for Magnetic Resonance in Medicine, Montreal, 1987.
9. Rzedzian RR: A method for instant whole-body MR imaging at 2.0 Tesla and system design considerations in its implementation, in Book of Abstracts, Society for Magnetic Resonance in Medicine, Montreal, 1987.
10. Weisskoff RM, Dalcanton JJ, Cohen MS: High-resolution 64-msec instant images of the head. Magn Reson Imaging 8:93, 1990.
11. Cohen MS, Weisskoff RM: Ultra-fast imaging. Magn Reson Imaging (in press).
12. Hahn EL: Spin-echoes. Phy Rev 80:580, 1950.
13. Weisskoff RM, Cohen MS, Rzedzian RR: Fat suppression techniques: A comparison of results in instant imaging, in Book of Abstracts, Society for Magnetic Resonance in Medicine, Amsterdam, 1989.
14. Cohen MS, Rohan ML: 3D volume imaging with Instascan, in Book of Abstracts, Society for Magnetic Resonance in Medicine, Amsterdam, 1989.
15. Cohen MS, Brady TJ: Unpublished observations.
16. Cohen MS, Dalcanton JJ, Weisskoff RM, Rohan ML: Kinematic imaging of the knee using instant MRI, in Book of Abstracts, Society of Magnetic Resonance in Medicine, New York, 1990.
17. Weisskoff RM: Improved hard-pulse sequences or frequency-selective presaturation in magnetic resonance. J Magn Reson 86:170, 1990.
18. Bydder GM, Young IR: MR imaging: Clinical use of the inversion recovery sequence. J Comput Assist Tomogr 9:659, 1985.
19. Ferrucci JT: MR imaging of the liver. AJR 147:1103, 1987.
20. McKinstry RC, Weisskoff RM, Cohen MS, et al: Instant MR diffusion/perfusion imaging. Magn Reson Imaging 8:401, 1990.
21. Turner R, Le Bihan D: Single-shot diffusion imaging at 2.0 Tesla. J Magn Reson 86:445, 1990.

14

MRI Fluoroscopy: Applications of Ultrashort TR Real-Time MRI

STEPHEN J. RIEDERER

X-ray fluoroscopy is a well-recognized method in radiology for facilitating the preparation of a radiographic procedure. The method is real-time, provides a high number of images per second, and enables the radiologist to interactively position the patient. The original motivation for this MRI fluoroscopy project was to provide a similar imaging method in magnetic resonance. Specifically, the goals were (a) an image acquisition time of 500 ms or less, (b) continuous, arbitrarily long image acquisition, and (c) an image reconstruction time of about 150 ms or less. The purpose of this chapter is to discuss how we at the Mayo Clinic have developed an imaging technique that meets these specifications (1,2). In developing this technique, we have been the first to propose and study the concepts of ultrashort repetition times (TR) in MRI image acquisition (3) as well as the first to develop dedicated instrumentation for performing MRI image reconstruction in real time (4). It is important to stress that these concepts of ultrashort TR and real-time reconstruction can each be exploited separately or together in a variety of applications.

In the next section I present some of the technical details of MRI fluoroscopy. These include the data acquisition, image reconstruction, and some of the considerations for performing interactive MRI. The bulk of this chapter is then devoted to a discussion of the applications of the MRI fluoroscopy technique. This includes continuous and snapshot imaging as well as interactive techniques. Finally, I close this chapter with a general discussion of the potential advantages and limitations of MRI fluoroscopy techniques, as well as speculation on possible new directions.

MRI FLUOROSCOPY TECHNIQUE

Data Acquisition

Image quality in MRI fluoroscopy or, for that matter, in any imaging method is dictated by the quality of the acquired data. Recall the first two goals discussed at the outset: short acquisition time and continuous imaging capability. At the time this project was initiated in 1987, the state of the art in conventional MRI made use of TRs of 20 ms or more in conjunction with 128 or more phase encodings per image. This provided an image acquisition time of 2.5 s, considerably longer than the 500-ms goal. The only possible alternative was the echo-planar imaging (EPI) technique of Mansfield (5,6), which made use of custom gradient coils. Thus, given the constraint of attempting to implement MRI fluoroscopy acquisition on an MRI system with conventional (< 1 G/cm) gradients, there were several possible options: (a) modify a conventional pulse sequence to enable TRs of less than 20 ms and employ fewer than 128 phase-encoding views, (b) attempt to implement EPI on a system with conventional gradients, or (c) use some hybrid of the first two options.

In fact, the first option has proved to be the method of choice given the constraint of standard gradients, and details of this sequence will be discussed presently. The second option, the EPI approach, runs into fundamental limitations as a consequence of the relatively small gradient strength. Briefly, the smaller the available readout gradient amplitude, then the longer is the duration of the readout of a line of data. For resolution in the phase-encoding direction of 64 encodings or more, the total readout duration for all lines begins to approach 100 ms. Although such readouts are permitted by the data-acquisition hardware, typically, the T2 relaxation times of the materials of interest and the limited homogeneity of the principal magnetic field cause the available signal to decay away. In short, one is only sampling noise, and the images are of inadequate quality. It should be noted that modern EPI systems are possible primarily because of gradient technology enabling 4 G/cm gradients. Moreover, the image-acquisition times of about 30 ms are used not so much because such times are desired per se, but rather such times are necessary to ensure that adequate signal is present over the entire readout duration.

The third option, the hybrid approach, also has been considered. The principal difficulty with this technique is that some groups of echoes in the raw data space are acquired at different echo times than other groups of echoes. This causes discontinuities in the phase of the raw data, similar to that caused by motion of an object under study during the scan. Just as for the motion case, this leads to smearing and ghosting in the phase-encoded direction in the reconstructed image. The extent of these artifacts can be reduced by dynamically changing the echo times during the scan (7), but not enough for this method to be viable.

The first option, that of reducing the TR in a standard limited flip angle pulse sequence, was implemented on our commercial General Electric 1.5-Tesla Signa MRI scanner. In general, this implementation required that all gradient and RF pulses be narrower in duration and higher in amplitude than for a standard sequence. A considerable reduction in TR time can be obtained simply by modifying the characteristics of the echo. For example, in a standard sequence, 256 samples of the signal are acquired with a 32-kHz bandwidth. Echo duration is 8 ms. The fluoro sequence acquires half the number of samples at twice the bandwidth. This results in an echo duration of only 2 ms, enabling a 6-ms reduction in the TR.

With the standard gradients of our commercial MRI unit, the minimum possible TRs are 7.1 and 6.3 ms and are the minimum practical limits for the GRASS and FLASH pulse sequences, respectively. As might be expected, the gradients become the limiting factor. The readout gradient amplitude limit prevents additional increases in bandwidth and proportionate decreases in the echo duration. Perhaps more important, the finite rise times of each gradient pulse now comprise a considerable fraction of the TR interval. With standard technology, the typical rise time is 500 μs from 0 to 1 G/cm. With five such ramps per TR interval, a reduction in the rise time of 100 μs would enable a fivefold, or 500-μs, reduction in the TR interval.

In addition to reduction of the TR, the acquisition time for one image is reduced in proportion to the number of phase encodings or "views" used. I have acquired images with as few as 32 phase encodings, but for most applications, the resultant spatial resolution is inadequate. There are several possible modifications to standard phase encoding that can maintain resolution while enabling a reduction in the number of repetitions required. One such method is the use of a fractional number of excitations in which the phase encodings that are used do not span symmetrical areas of k-space (8). If pushed to the extreme, the method will require some retrospective phase correction. However, it has been my experience that a so-called 3/4 NEX acquisition can be used without such correction. For example, with this approach, an image acquired using data from 96 repetitions will have resolution closely resembling one formed from a standard 128 repetitions.

A second technique that can enable a reduction in the number of required phase encodings is the use of a nonsquare or rectangular field of view (FOV). In general, the number of phase encodings necessary is proportional to the desired FOV along the phase-encoding direction. If the object under study does not have an approximately circular cross section, then the rectangular FOV can be exploited by performing the phase encoding along the smaller dimension of the object. In imaging the abdomen, this would be anteroposterior.

Examples of a standard MRI image and one acquired with the ultrashort TR technique are shown in Figure 14-1. Figure 14-1A was formed with a TR/TE of 20/9 ms, 256 resolutions along the horizontal (frequency-encoded direction), 192 phase encodings acquired along the vertical, and a 40 × 40 cm FOV. Image-acquisition time was 3800 ms. On the other hand, Figure 14-1B was formed using a TR/TE of 10.1/5.8 ms in GRASS sequence, 128 phase encodings, and all other parameters the same. Image-acquisition time was only 1280 ms. Because of the reduced number of readout points, the resolution along the horizontal direction is degraded two times in the high-speed image (Fig. 14-1B). Nonetheless, Figure 14-1B has nearly comparable quality to Figure 14-1A. This example demonstrates that high-resolution images are possible with subsecond acquisition times.

Reconstruction

The third goal stated at the outset for the MRI fluoroscopy technique was an image-reconstruction time of 150 ms or less. The intent of this was to enable the image formed from the MRI fluoroscopy acquisition to be displayed virtually instantaneously after acquisition was completed. Because the acquisition was designed to operate continuously, it was necessary that the reconstruction be performed repeatedly as well. The result is that images are reconstructed and displayed at a rate of approximately six per second. It should be stressed that the time between the display of successive images, approximately 160 ms, is distinct from the image-acquisition time. As discussed in the preceding section, the latter quantity is dictated by the TR and the number of phase encodings used per image.

A schematic of the MRI fluoroscopy reconstruction apparatus and a timing diagram for the reconstruction are shown in Figure 14-2. Referring first to Figure 14-2A, the device is designed to be attached to an arbitrary MRI system. Specifically, the detected NMR signals are accessed immediately after they are digitized and, as shown at the upper left, are directed to a first-in, first-out (FIFO) memory. The purpose of the memory is to store all data that might be acquired during the 160 ms used for reconstruction. The principal element of the reconstruction instrumentation is a dedicated array processor (AP).

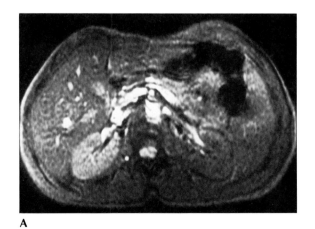 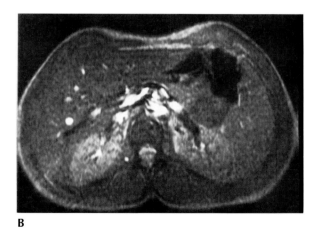

A B

FIGURE 14-1

(A) *Standard GRASS image formed with a TR/TE of 20/9 ms, 256 resolutions along the horizontal (frequency-encoded direction), 192 phase encodings acquired along the vertical, and a 40 × 40 cm FOV. Image-acquisition time was 3800 ms. (B) Ultrashort TR image formed with a TR/TE of 10.1/5.8 ms and 128 phase encodings. Image-acquisition time 1280 ms.*

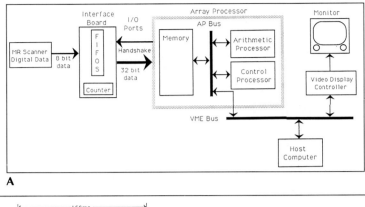

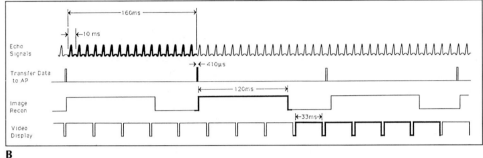

FIGURE 14-2
(A) *System schematic of real-time MRI image reconstruction device. The principal element of the reconstruction instrumentation is a dedicated array processor.* (B) *Timing diagram for continuous real-time MRI fluoroscopic image reconstruction. (From Wright RC, Riederer SJ, Farzaneh F, et al: Real-time MR fluoroscopic data acquisition and image reconstruction. Magn Reson Med 12:407, 1989. Reprinted by permission.)*

Referring next to Figure 14-2B, the acquired echo signals are shown in the first line, each separated from the next by the TR used, here assumed to be 10 ms. After 16 echoes (shown in bold) have been acquired and stored in the FIFO memory, they are rapidly transferred into the array processor by means of a high-speed input port. Immediately thereafter, the fast Fourier transform (FFT) of each individual echo is taken. Next, these 16 echoes are incorporated with whatever number of echoes was measured previously so that an image with the desired resolution can be formed. For example, if 64 phase encodings per image are being used, then the 16 echoes transferred to the AP will be incorporated with the immediate $64 - 16$, or 48, echoes previously measured. Transformation is performed in the phase-encoding direction, the magnitude is formed, and the final result is directed to the display controller shown in Figure 14-2A, which converts the reconstructed magnitude values into a video-format image. The timing for this is shown in the bottom two lines of Figure 14-2B, which in bold lines shows schematically the newly reconstructed video signals. The time from measurement of any of the 16 echoes of the top line of Figure14-2B until the appearance of the image formed from those echoes (and the requisite number of preceding echoes) is, on average, 200 ms. This can be considered the average data latency from acquisition to display.

Many variations of the preceding process are possible. If more than 64 phase encodings are used per image, then the update simply includes correspondingly more than the 48 preceding echoes. The updates are done at the same rate of one reconstruction every 160 ms. However, the spatial resolution is improved and the temporal resolution is degraded. This design has essentially decoupled the image-reconstruction time from the data-acquisition time and resolution. Within broad limits, characteristics of the image acquisition can be altered substantially with little or no effect on the speed of the image reconstruction.

Modifications for Interactive MRI
If interactive MRI is to be performed in real time, then in addition to considerations for high-speed data acquisition and reconstruction, as discussed previously, capability must be provided to enable the operator to alter parameters during the scan. This depends largely on the specific capabilities of the unit used for acquisition. With some systems, all scan parameters are selected and fixed prior to the scan, and once the scan begins, no modifications are possible. On the other hand, under ideal conditions for interactive MRI, the scan can operate continuously and the operator can modify parameters at the keyboard or some alternative input/output device and the pulse sequence will be modified within several repetitions.

Many features of the imaging sequence can conceivably be altered interactively. These include which section is being imaged, the spatial and contrast characteristics of the image, the position of saturation pulses, and so on. Of course, TR, TE, and the nutation angle are also potentially adjustable. My colleagues and I have recently shown how oblique angulation and T1 contrast can be interactively modified in real time (9).

APPLICATIONS

I have thus far demonstrated the utility of two fundamental concepts of MRI: (1) ultrashort (<10-ms) repetition times for image acquisition and (2) high-speed MRI image reconstruction. These two concepts can be used separately or in conjunction with each other in many possible applications. In this section I discuss several possible applications.

Continuous MRI Fluoroscopy
Application of the continuous short TR MRI sequence results in a real-time sequence with an image-presentation rate of about 5 images per second. Because of the relatively poor contrast with continuous ultrashort TR scans, this technique is best used for visualization of morphology or distinguishing materials having very large contrast differences. This technique can be used to observe dynamic phenomena such as peristalsis, respiratory motion, or the temporal characteristics of administered contrast media.

Continuous Interactive MRI Fluoroscopy
The technique of continuous imaging just discussed can be coupled with interactive manipulation of scan parameters to enable real-time interactive imaging. For example, by allowing the operator to adjust the offset frequency and combination of gradient waveforms, the irradiated slice and obliquity of the slice can be adjusted in real time. An example of this is given in Figure 14-3. The goal of this procedure is to visualize the origin of the portal vein. The results in Figure 14-3 are stills taken from the continuous real-time sequence. Figure 14-3A is one of the initial images in the sequence and clearly shows the inferior vena cava, superior mesenteric vein, aorta, and the origin of the superior mesenteric artery. Shortly after this image was formed, the slice of irradiation was positioned more superiorly and an axis of rotation along the anteroposterior direction was selected. Next, the section was rotated so that the left side of the image was placed more cranially and the right side more caudally. After a 30-degree rotation, the linear extent of the portal vein is clearly depicted in Figure 14-3B (*arrow*). Having selected the slice at the desired oblique angulation, at this point one could turn to an alternative MRI procedure to, say, generate an MRI angiogram or quantitatively estimate flow.

Snapshot MRI
To address the aforementioned reduced contrast intrinsic to continuous ultrashort TR imaging, Farzaneh (10) and Haase (11) have independently proposed the technique of "snapshot" ultrashort TR imaging. The concept here is to precede the data acquisition with a contrast-preparation phase. A comparison of standard inversion recovery (IR) and T1-weighted snapshot pulse sequences is given in Figure 14-4. In both cases, the contrast preparation consists of a 180-degree inversion pulse followed by a TI waiting period. In the standard IR sequence (Fig. 14-4A), only one phase-encoding view is measured per inversion pulse. However, for the snapshot case (Fig. 14-4B), the entire image is measured in the

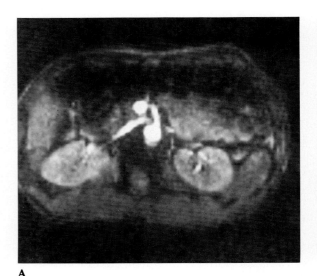
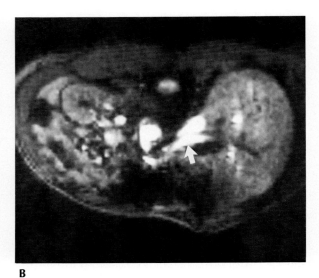

FIGURE 14-3
Still images taken from a real-time interactive setting of oblique angulation. (A) Initial axial image clearly showing major blood vessels in the abdomen. (B) Image formed after rotating the imaged slice 20 degrees about the anteroposterior axis. Left side of image is positioned cranially and right side is caudal. Rotation was performed to visualize the linear extent of the portal vein (arrow).

data-acquisition phase. Acquisition time for the image is the repetition time in data acquisition multiplied by the number of phase-encoding views used. For example, for a TR of 7.1 ms and 128 phase-encoding views, the image-acquisition time is 900 ms. This time is clearly adequate for acquiring an entire image during a breath-hold.

The principal disadvantage of snapshot short TR imaging is a reduced signal-to-noise ratio (SNR) as compared with a spin-echo–based acquisition following the same contrast-preparation phase. For example, in the standard IR sequence in Figure 14-4A, essentially the full contrast difference created by the inversion pulse is measured by the spin echo. The only reduction in the prepared signal is due to the nonzero echo time of the spin echo, a reduction of typically 10 to 15 percent. On the other hand, with the snapshot sequence (Fig. 14-4B), a limited nutation angle is used during each repetition of the readout. Accordingly, to first order the signal magnitude behaves in proportion to the sine of the nutation angle. For angles of 30 degrees or less, the measured signal will be reduced by 50 percent or more compared with

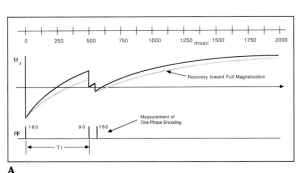
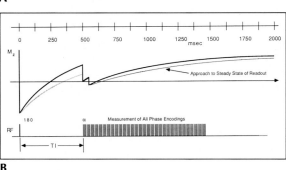

FIGURE 14-4
Schematics of standard inversion recovery (A) and T1-weighted snapshot GRASS (B) pulse sequences.

that made available by the preparation. Nutation angles larger than 30 degrees will cause an approach to steady state that is too rapid to enable full utilization of the prepared contrast. Thus, to summarize, standard spin-echo–based acquisitions offer relatively high SNRs and contrast-to-noise ratios (CNRs). This is at the expense of acquisition times of tens of seconds to several minutes. On the other hand, the snapshot technique provides acquisition times of about 1 s, but with SNRs appreciably smaller than the spin-echo–based approach.

A comparison of the two techniques is presented in Figure 14-5. Figure 14-5A is a transaxial image of the liver and spleen acquired with a standard inversion recovery technique using a TR/TI/TE of 1500/150/20 ms with 128 × 256 resolution. Acquisition time for the 2 NEX scan was 8 minutes. This TI was selected to best null out the fat signals, and the resultant image has a good SNR but nonetheless still portrays some ghosting indicative of incomplete suppression of motion. Figure 14-5B shows a result acquired using the snapshot technique diagramed in Figure 14-4B. Following the 180-degree inverting pulse an effective TI time of 150 ms was used. The subsequent data acquisition was done with 128 phase encodings with a TR/TE of 7.1/3.5 ms and a 30-degree nutation angle. Image-acquisition time was 900 ms. Although this has more noise than the conventional result in Figure 14-5A, contrast between liver and spleen is good, the fat signal is suppressed, and there are essentially no artifacts due to motion.

Snapshot short TR imaging gives the operator additional scan parameters besides the traditional TR, TE, and TI. Unlike standard spin-echo imaging, the magnetization in snapshot imaging is in general not measured in the steady state. Consequently, every phase encoding potentially measures a different degree of signal and contrast. This would be analogous in standard IR imaging if the TI time, for example, were changed during the scan. Returning to the snapshot case, the order of phase encodings can have a major effect on the contrast of the image. If the

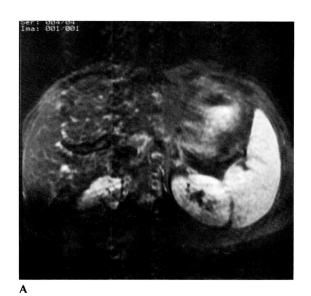
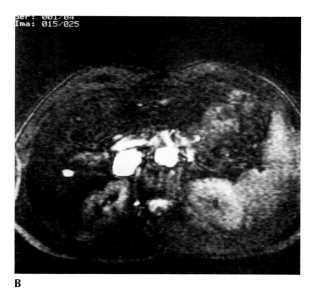

A   B

FIGURE 14-5
(A) *Transaxial image of the liver and spleen acquired with a standard inversion recovery technique using a TR/TI/TE of 1500/150/20 ms with 128 × 256 resolution. Acquisition time was 8 minutes. TI was selected to best null out the fat signals.* (B) *Ultrashort TR snapshot GRASS result acquired with an effective TI of 150 ms. Data acquisition was done with 128 phase encodings, a TR/TE of 7.1/3.5 ms, and a 30-degree nutation angle. Image-acquisition time was 900 ms.*

encodings for the low spatial frequencies are measured first, then the overall image contrast is determined principally by that set up in the contrast-preparation phase. On the other hand, if the standard sequential ordering of phase encodings is used, then at the time of the measurement of the low spatial frequency views, the magnetization will have partly reverted to its steady state. Overall image contrast will be less determined by the contrast-preparation phase. This has been described recently by Holsinger and Riederer (12).

The results in Figure 14-5 illustrate the tradeoff between standard spin-echo–based and snapshot imaging. The method of choice will only be determined after clinical evaluation.

Continuous Snapshot MRI

The concepts of the preceding two sections can be combined to yield the method of continuous snapshot MRI. With this technique, the standard ultrashort TR continuous fluoroscopy pulse sequence is initially operating. Then, at his or her discretion, the operator can apply a 180-degree inversion pulse. After the pulse, the magnetization recovers according to the T1 relaxation time of each material. After an operator-selected delay, the continuous short TR readout is initiated and images are reconstructed continuously. The resultant image sequence dynamically portrays the recovery toward equilibrium. With the dynamic contrast behavior visible on the display, it may be possible to detect features more readily than in static images, in much the same way that a cine movie loop can be used to more clearly see features of the object than individual constituent images from which the cine loop is formed. This technique is still under investigation.

DISCUSSION

I have discussed the development of the project that we at the Mayo Clinic have called "MRI fluoroscopy" and have presented several initial applications. The two central concepts that I have demonstrated are the advantages of the use of ultrashort (<10-ms) repetition times in the data acquisition and real-time image reconstruction. These two concepts can be used individually or separately in a variety of applications.

The principal advantage of ultrashort TRs is a reduction in the image-acquisition time compared with present techniques. With a TR of 7.1 ms and 128 phase-encoding views, the image-acquisition time is 900 ms. With a TR of 6.3 ms and 96 phase encodings, the image-acquisition time is 600 ms. Ultrashort TRs can be used in continuous acquisition, as was originally conceived with MRI fluoroscopy, or to read out in a burst the magnetization that has been prepared in some contrast-preparation phase.

Real-time image reconstruction is primarily an engineering accomplishment, as opposed to a new MRI data-acquisition technique. Before the advent of fast acquisition times, its practical utility was perhaps not that high. However, with image-acquisition times now in the range of 1 s or less, high image reconstruction is an important element of real-time MRI. With the technique described here, the data latency—the time from measurement to display—averages 200 ms. What the observer sees on the screen is that which has occurred at most about 200 ms earlier.

Ultrashort TRs and real-time image reconstruction were combined to yield the technique of continuous MRI fluoroscopy. With the additional capability to manipulate scan parameters, this opens up the technique of interactive MRI. It is expected that this may be useful in manipulating the slices for specialized MRI examinations of the abdomen, such as vascular procedures.

Snapshot MRI is a technique for generating high-contrast images with acquisition times ranging from 200 to 2000 ms. The exact value depends on the TR used as well as the number of phase encodings. In comparison with standard spin-echo imaging, the snapshot technique suffers from a diminished signal-to-noise ratio, but the short acquisition time enables the gathering of image data during a single breath-hold. The snapshot technique has been in use only since 1989, and hence some future developments may restore some of the SNR loss, perhaps at the expense of somewhat increased scanning time. Such development and detailed clinical evaluation will determine its ultimate place in MRI.

The focus of this chapter has been on acquisition techniques that employ a sequence of ultra short TRs. As mentioned earlier, the other principal acquisition technique is the echo-planar method of Mansfield, which allows image-acquisition times of about 30 ms. Recent results generated with this method have been impressive, but it too has its disadvantages, the principal one being the requirement for very high homogeneity of the magnetic field. Regardless of the ultimate role of these fast scan methods, it is fair to say that advances in fast scan MRI in the past year have shown the feasibility of the acquisition of diagnostic MRI images during a breath-hold.

REFERENCES

1. Riederer SJ, Tasciyan T, Farzaneh F, et al: MR fluoroscopy: Technical feasibility. Magn Reson Med 8:1, 1988.
2. Farzaneh F, Riederer SJ, Lee JN, et al: MR fluoroscopy: Initial clinical studies. Radiology 171:545, 1989.
3. Farzaneh F, Lee JN, Tasciyan T, et al: A Short TR Pulse Sequence for MR Fluoroscopy. Presented at the 6th Annual Meeting of the Society of Magnetic Resonance Imaging, Boston, February 1988.
4. Wright RC, Riederer SJ, Farzaneh F, et al: Real-time MR fluoroscopic data acquisition and image reconstruction. Magn Reson Med 12:407, 1989.
5. Mansfield P: Multi-planar image formation using NMR spin echoes. J Physiol (Lond) 10:L55, 1977.
6. Pykett IL, Rzedzian RR: Instant images of the body by magnetic resonance. Magn Reson Med 5:563, 1987.
7. Farzaneh F, Riederer SJ: Hybrid Imaging with the Use of Gradient-Recalled Echoes. Presented at 74th Annual Meeting of the Radiology Society of North America, Chicago, November, 1988.
8. MacFall JR, Pelc NJ, Vavrek RJ: Correction of spatially dependent phase shifts for partial fourier imaging. Magn Reson Imaging 6:143, 1988.
9. Holsinger AE, Wright RC, Riederer SJ, et al: Real-time interactive magnetic resonance imaging. Magn Reson Med 14:547, 1990.
10. Farzaneh F: Ph.D. dissertation, Department of Biomedical Engineering, Duke University, 1989.
11. Haase A: Snapshot FLASH MRI. Magn Reson Med 13:77, 1990.
12. Holsinger AE, Riederer SJ: The importance of phase encoding order in ultrashort TR snapshot GRASS imaging. Magn Reson Med (in press).

15

Magnetization-Prepared Rapid Gradient-Echo (MP-RAGE) MRI

EDUARD E. DE LANGE,
JOHN P. MUGLER, III, and
JAMES R. BROOKEMAN

At the 1989 annual meeting of the Society of Magnetic Resonance in Medicine, Haase et al. introduced a new pulse-sequence technique called snapshot FLASH magnetic resonance imaging (MRI) (1,2). This technique, which has also been called turbo FLASH or snapshot GRASS, is characterized by a combination of two distinct pulse-sequence segments. The first segment is used to prepare the magnetization for tissue contrast, and the second, which is a fast gradient-echo sequence, is used for data acquisition. With the newly developed pulse-sequence technique, generically named *Magnetization-Prepared RApid Gradient-Echo* (MP-RAGE) imaging, MRI images with high tissue contrast are obtained in extremely short imaging times and virtually without motion artifacts. Preliminary evaluation indicates that the technique may be particularly useful in evaluating the liver for focal disease.

THE MP-RAGE PULSE SEQUENCES

Gradient-echo pulse sequences are characterized by the fast sampling of data, yielding high speed MR images with signal-to-noise ratios (SNR) comparable to spin-echo (SE) images; however, contrast-to-noise ratios (CNR) are generally lower (3,4). By changing TR, TE, and the flip angle, image contrast can be manipulated somewhat, but in general, contrast relationships between tissues are complex, and gradient-echo images are neither T1- nor T2-weighted in the sense of SE imaging (3).

A rapid gradient-echo (RAGE) image obtained with a short TR, short TE, and a small flip angle displays contrast that is essentially dominated by the proton density of the tissues (5). When such a RAGE sequence is preceded by pulses to prepare the magnetization [magnetization-preparation (MP) pulses], the spin-density contrast can be transformed to T1-weighted or T2-weighted contrast.

To acquire a T1-weighted MP-RAGE image, a single nonselective 180-degree pulse is used to prepare the magnetization (Fig. 15-1). The 180-degree inversion pulse rotates the longitudinal magnetization from the positive z axis to the negative z axis. If a time delay follows the inversion pulse to allow T1 relaxation to occur and this delay is followed by the RAGE sequence for the image acquisition, the image displays T1 inversion-recovery contrast. The inversion delay time between the MP pulse and the start of the RAGE sequence basically determines the image contrast and SNR.

To acquire a T2-weighted MP-RAGE image, a combination of three nonselective pulses (90, 180, and 90 degrees) is needed to prepare the magnetization (2,5). The first 90-degree pulse

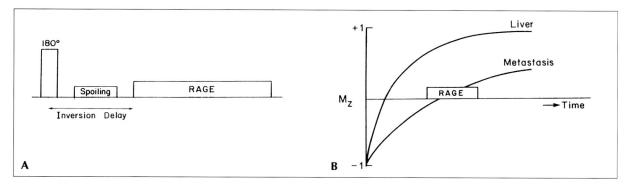

FIGURE 15-1
T1-weighted MP-RAGE sequence. (A) To provide T1-contrast, a nonselective 180-degree pulse is employed for magnetization preparation (MP). After a certain inversion delay, the rapid gradient-echo (RAGE) sequence is employed for image acquisition. A spoiler gradient before the RAGE sequence is used to dephase any residual transverse magnetization resulting from an imperfect inversion pulse. (B) The 180-degree MP pulse rotates the longitudinal component of the magnetization (M_z) to the negative z axis. During the inversion delay time, T1-relaxation of the tissues occurs. (The T1 of the liver is shorter than the T1 of metastasis.) If the RAGE sequence is employed as the longitudinal magnetization of the metastasis passes through the xy plane, an image is acquired on which the liver is bright and the metastasis is black.

rotates the magnetization from the positive z axis to the transverse plane. As with SE imaging, a time interval is allowed for T2 decay to occur and T2-dependent contrast to develop between different tissues (Fig. 15-2). The 180-degree pulse is applied to refocus the static field inhomogeneity contributions to the dephasing of the magnetization in the transverse plane (i.e., to perform a spin-echo). When the transverse magnetization is refocused (after twice the interval between the first 90-degree pulse and 180-degree pulse), the second 90-degree pulse is applied to restore the refocused magnetization to the z axis, thereby "storing" the T2 contrast of the tissues in the form of longitudinal magnetization. The interval between the two 90-degree pulses is the period during which the T2 contrast develops between tissues and is labeled TE_{prep}. When both 90-degree pulses are applied about the x axis (in the rotating frame) and the 180-degree pulse is applied about the y axis, the longitudinal magnetization encoded by T2 decay is rotated to the negative z axis (i.e., driven inversion) (6). We found that this technique provides greater contrast between liver lesions and normal liver than does the technique described by Haase (5), in which all preparation pulses are applied about the same axis, causing longitudinal magnetization to rotate to the positive z axis (i.e., driven equilibrium). The RAGE sequence is also used to acquire the T2-weighted images.

A particular advantage of the MP-RAGE technique is that it can be implemented on most current MRI imagers with only minor modifications to the machine hardware and software. This is because the gradient strengths and switching times required are much less demanding on the MRI system than those required for other techniques, such as echo-planar imaging. We implemented the sequences on our Magnetom 63SP 1.5-Tesla scanner (Siemens Medical Systems, Iselin, N.J.) with maximum gradient strengths of 10 millitesla per meter and gradient switching times of about 0.6 ms. Implementation of the sequences is not restricted to high-field MRI systems, and similar sequences could be implemented on lower-field systems as well. However, the intrinsically lower SNR and shorter T1 values may be a drawback to the effective use of this technique at low field strength.

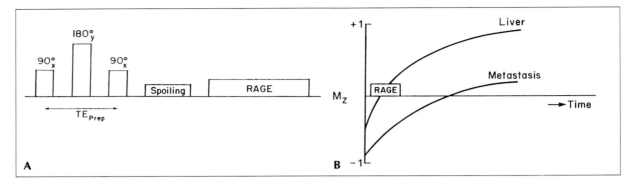

FIGURE 15-2
T2-weighted MP-RAGE sequence. (A) For the T2-contrast a combination of three nonselective pulses is needed. The first 90-degree pulse about the x axis rotates the magnetization to the xy plane. After time is allowed for T2 contrast to develop between tissues, the 180-degree pulse about the y axis is applied to refocus the dephasing spins. When the spin-echo is obtained, a second 90-degree pulse is applied about the x axis to "store" the T2 contrast in the form of longitudinal magnetization along the negative z axis. The interval between the two 90-degree pulses (TE_{prep}) is the period during which T2 contrast develops. A spoiler gradient is applied to dephase any residual transverse magnetization resulting from imperfect pulses. (B) After the longitudinal magnetization is encoded by T2 contrast and rotated to the negative z axis, the RAGE sequence is employed for data sampling. However, since T1 relaxation occurs after the longitudinal magnetization is encoded, T1 contrast adds to T2 contrast. Since the T2 of the liver is shorter than that of metastasis, the T2-encoded longitudinal magnetization is less than that of metastasis. If the RAGE sequence is employed as the magnetization of the liver passes through the xy plane, the liver will be black and the metastasis will be bright (magnitude reconstruction).

TWO-DIMENSIONAL MP-RAGE IMAGING OF THE LIVER

The MP-RAGE pulse sequences described by Haase et al. were primarily developed to permit real-time determination of MRI parameters (1,5). These pulse sequences included the use of very short RAGE acquisitions sufficient for T1 and T2 calculations, but provided images that had insufficient SNRs and CNRs for clinical liver evaluations. We improved the technique to yield fast and clinically useful imaging of the liver.

For the two-dimensional (2D) MP-RAGE sequences, each image is sampled as a single slice using the RAGE sequence with one acquisition. To obtain images of high quality, the acquisition period needs to be long enough to provide an adequate SNR. However, lengthening the data-acquisition period also increases artifacts from motion, since sampling of data occurs during the cardiac and respiratory (if breath-holding is not employed) cycles.

For our T1-weighted images we chose an acquisition time of less than 1 s to adequately limit motion artifacts during quiet respiration. Employing both theoretical calculations and experimental measurements in normal volunteers (7), we found that an inversion delay of 350 ms, a TR of 7.1 ms, a TE of 3.7 ms, and a flip angle of 10 degrees provided a reasonable compromise for generating strong T1 contrast. The flip-angle choice represents a tradeoff between increased SNR and CNR and increased artifacts due to the buildup of steady coherences, both of which occur with increased flip angles. We used the liver/spleen contrast as a model for liver/lesion contrast in these optimization studies. Also, to obtain isotropic in-plane voxel dimensions, we employed an asymmetrical field-of-view (FOV) of 350 × 700 mm with an image matrix of 128 × 256. The resulting acquisition time for the RAGE sequence was approximately 900 ms.

For the MP-RAGE sequences, data sampling occurs during a T1 transient, and therefore, T1 decay adds to the prepared contrast. This is particularly a problem when the goal is to encode T2 contrast, since the T1 decay during the RAGE acquisition may destroy the T2 contrast developed with the preparation. However, when T2-weighted MP-RAGE images are obtained with the driven inversion preparation, as is the case with our technique, the T1 and T2 decays can complement each other. A similar situation arises with the short tau inversion recovery (STIR) technique. To achieve the desired contrast effect from the T2 preparation pulses, the RAGE acquisition time must be substantially shorter than that used for the T1-weighted images and also must be approximately the same as or shorter than the T1 of normal liver. For the T2-weighted MP-RAGE sequence we use a TR of 4.5 ms and only 64 phase-encoding steps to achieve an acquisition time of 290 ms. A TE of 2.4 ms is used, and the flip angle is 10 degrees. Images are obtained as a single acquisition, using an asymmetrical FOV of 300 × 600 mm.

Since in general the RAGE acquisition occurs during a T1-dependent transient, the resulting image contrast may be complex. Modifications of the RAGE sequence may be beneficial to improve T1- and T2-weighted contrast. Potential modifications include the use of reordered phase encoding (8) and/or a "multishot" approach that acquires the image data by concatenating several prepare-acquire cycles (9).

To determine the effectiveness of the 2D MP-RAGE technique compared with SE imaging in depicting liver lesions, we evaluated 15 patients with a variety of focal lesions in the liver (metastases, hemangiomas, and cysts). In all patients, T1-weighted and T2-weighted MP-RAGE images were obtained and correlated with conventional T1- and T2-weighted SE imaging. The parameters of the MP-RAGE sequences were given in the previous paragraph. For the T2-weighted MP-RAGE sequences, a TE_{prep} of 40 ms was used, since this technique provided essentially no signal from normal liver and relatively high signal from the lesions. However, the optimal TE_{prep} for liver lesions is yet to be determined, and it is likely that two or more TE_{prep} values will be needed to optimally characterize lesions. For the T1-weighted SE technique, a TR/TE 600/15 sequence was used with four acquisitions, a matrix of 128 × 256, FOV of 420 × 420 mm, and a total acquisition time of 5.1 min. For the T2-weighted SE technique, a multiecho sequence (SE 2800/40/80/120/160) was used with two acquisitions, a matrix of 128 × 256, FOV of 420 × 420 mm, and an acquisition time of 12.0 min. Images were obtained during quiet respiration for all pulse sequences, and straps were applied across the patient's abdomen to reduce motion artifacts (Figs. 15-3 and 15-4). CNRs of the largest lesion in each patient were calculated for all pulse sequences using corresponding transverse images and were normalized for slice thickness, voxel size, and imaging times. Mean CNRs of the T1-weighted MP-RAGE images were significantly greater than those of any of the other sequences. Mean CNRs of the T2-weighted MP-RAGE images were approximately equal to those of the SE sequences. The MP-RAGE images displayed no artifacts from respiratory motion, whereas artifacts were present on most of the SE images, particularly on the SE 2800/80/120/160 images. These findings indicate that the 2D MP-RAGE technique allows high-speed imaging of the liver without significant motion artifacts from respiration and provides T1-weighted images depicting liver lesions with significantly greater conspicuity than does the conventional SE technique (10).

DYNAMIC MP-RAGE IMAGING OF THE LIVER

Recent studies have indicated that dynamic evaluation of lesions of the liver may be more useful than conventional MRI in differentiating malignant lesions, such as metastases or hematomas, from benign hemangiomas (11). In these studies, gadolinium-DTPA was used for tissue enhancement, and rapid SE or gradient-echo techniques were used to acquire the images. The usefulness of these techniques is limited, since intervals between images are relatively long and tissue contrast may be relatively low. Besides, images may be blurred from motion artifacts due to respiration.

Since the MP-RAGE technique provides high-quality images with high contrast and virtually no motion artifacts, this new technique may be particularly suitable for dynamic liver imaging. We are currently investigating the use of dynamic T1-weighted MP-RAGE technique for the evaluation of hepatic lesions.

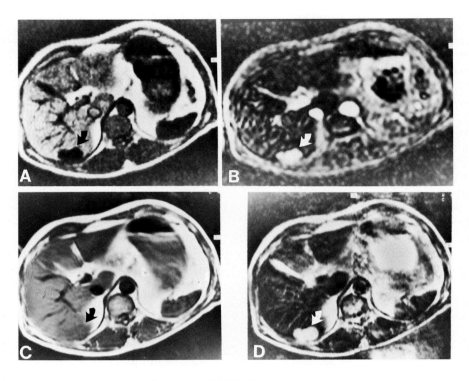

FIGURE 15-3
*MP-RAGE and SE images of liver metastasis. (A) Transverse T1-weighted MP-RAGE image obtained in approximately 1250 ms. Using an inversion delay of 350 ms between the 180-degree MP pulse and the start of the RAGE sequence, the liver displays relatively high signal intensity. The acquisition time of the RAGE sequence is approximately 900 ms. The lesion (arrow) displays low signal intensity. Conspicuity of the lesion is excellent, and there are virtually no motion-induced artifacts from respiration.
(B) Corresponding T2-weighted MP-RAGE image obtained in approximately 330 ms. Using a driven inversion preparation with a TE_{prep} of 40 ms, the normal liver displays low signal intensity. Owing to its long T1 and T2, the lesion (arrow) displays high signal intensity. There is excellent contrast between the lesion and the normal liver and no noticeable artifacts from motion. The acquisition time of the RAGE sequence is approximately 290 ms. (C) Corresponding conventional SE 600/15 image obtained in approximately 5 min. The lesion (arrow) is slightly hypointense compared with the liver and poorly visualized because of poor contrast. (D) SE 2800/120 image obtained in 12.0 min. The metastasis (arrow) displays relatively high signal intensity compared with the liver. Note considerable artifacts from respiratory motion.*

Dynamic imaging requires fast acquisitions of images at short intervals. To effectively use the MP-RAGE technique, certain limitations have to be taken into account. As explained earlier, the T1-weighted MP-RAGE sequence consists of a 180-degree inversion pulse to prepare T1 contrast, and after a certain delay to allow T1 relaxation to occur (350 ms in our case), the RAGE sequence is employed for data sampling to provide the image. At the end of the RAGE sequence, which is at approximately 1200 ms after the start of the preparation, T1 relaxation is incomplete. If a second MP-RAGE sequence were employed before sufficient longitudinal relaxation has occurred, an image would be

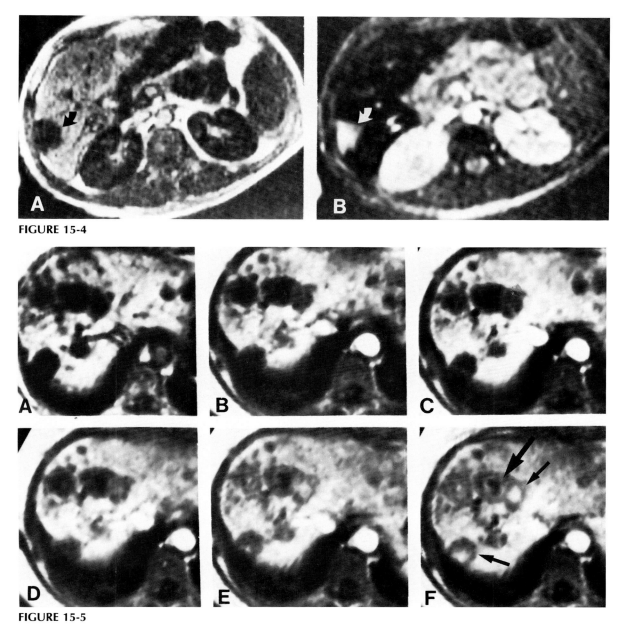

FIGURE 15-4
(A) T1-weighted MP-RAGE and (B) T2-weighted MP-RAGE images of a hemangioma (arrows). On both images there is high contrast between the lesion and the surrounding liver. There are no noticeable artifacts from respiratory motion.

FIGURE 15-5
Dynamic MP-RAGE imaging of the liver in a patient with multiple metastases from carcinoma of the ovary. Consecutive single slice images are obtained at the same level during quiet respiration of the patient. (A) The lesions are black on the nonenhanced images. Images obtained at 5 s (B), 10 s (C), 15 s (D), 20s (E) and 2 min (F) after the appearance of gadolinium-DTPA in the aorta. Some lesions enhance chiefly in the periphery (large arrow). Other lesions demonstrate more enhancement of the center (small arrows).

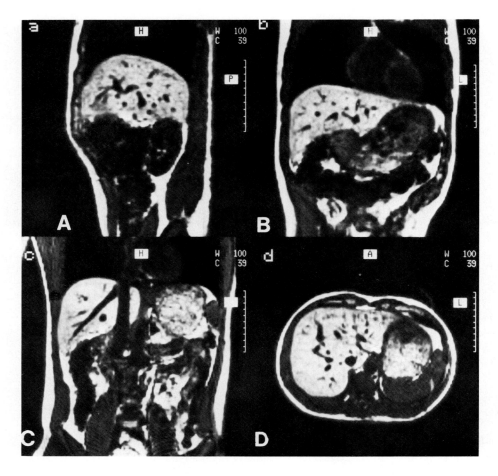

FIGURE 15-6
Three-dimensional T1-weighted MP-RAGE technique. (A) Sagittal, (B,C) coronal, and (D) transverse images of the abdomen of normal volunteer obtained from one data set. The slice thickness of all images is 2.7 mm. The structures of the upper abdomen are clearly depicted without distortion from respiratory motion.

obtained with significantly less T1 contrast than the first. Therefore, to obtain a second image with similar tissue contrast as the first, an additional delay is needed *after* the RAGE sequence to allow sufficient recovery of the longitudinal magnetization. In our preliminary studies, we used 3 s for this additional delay prior to the next MP-RAGE sequence. In practice, sequential images can be obtained approximately every 5 s. In our experience, this appears to be sufficient for high-speed dynamic imaging of liver lesions (Fig. 15-5). Through further optimization of this approach, we expect to obtain similar quality images at intervals of less than 3 s.

THREE-DIMENSIONAL MP-RAGE IMAGING OF THE LIVER

Recently we developed a novel three-dimensional (3D) MP-RAGE technique that employs a magnetization-preparation, data-acquisition, and magnetization-recovery cycle as the basic sequence element (12). This technique can provide high-quality three-dimensional image sets of the abdomen with minimal respiratory artifacts in as little as 7 min. The advantage of the three-dimensional volume technique over a two-dimensional technique is that thin, contiguous slices can be obtained with high SNRs and CNRs.

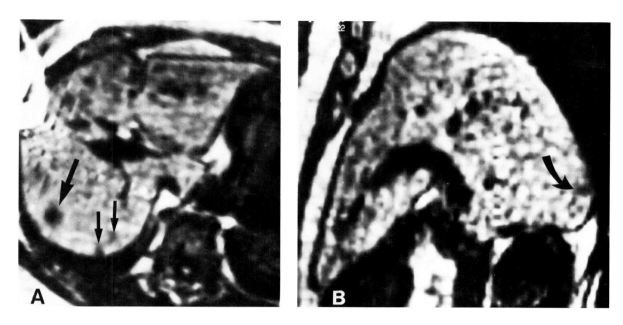

FIGURE 15-7
Three-dimensional T1-weighted MP-RAGE images of a patient evaluated for liver metastases. (A) Transverse (2.3-mm-thick) and (B) sagittal (3.3-mm-thick) images from the same three-dimensional data set. On the transverse image three metastases can be identified. Only the largest (large arrow) was seen on the initial CT scan. Each of the two smaller lesions (small arrows) measures 3 mm in diameter. One of these is also seen on the sagittal image, where the lesion has caused some bulging of the liver margin (curved arrow). The two small metastases were identified in retrospect on the CT scan.

The 3D MP-RAGE sequence also begins with a magnetization-preparation period as described earlier for the two-dimensional technique. After the longitudinal magnetization is encoded with the desired contrast during the MP period, a RAGE sequence is used to sample the prepared magnetization. However, with the three-dimensional technique, only a fraction of the desired three-dimensional k-space (spacial frequency space) volume is acquired by a given RAGE acquisition. Time is allowed after the RAGE acquisition for additional T1 recovery of the magnetization, after which the prepare-acquire-recovery cycle is repeated for the next fraction of the k-space volume. The duration of the three-dimensional sequence depends on the amount of k-space needed to image the region of the body. In the case of liver imaging, we currently use an image matrix of 128 (420 mm) × 128 (300 mm) × 256 (600 mm), which yields voxels of 3.3 × 2.3 × 2.3 mm. Respiratory triggering is used to initiate each MP-RAGE cycle during the same period of the respiratory cycle, and the approximate imaging time is 7 to 12 min. In our experience, this technique provides high-resolution images of the liver (Fig. 15-6) and allows the detection of very small lesions (Fig. 15-7).

CONCLUSION

The MP-RAGE sequence technique is a newly developed method providing images with high T1 or T2 tissue contrast obtained at high speed. Since the images are virtually free of respiratory motion artifacts, this technique may be particularly suitable for liver imaging. Preliminary experiments indicate that the pulse sequences may become an important means of detecting focal liver disease with MRI.

REFERENCES

1. Haase A, Matthaei D, Bartkowski R, et al: Inversion-recovery snapshot FLASH MR imaging. J Comput Assist Tomogr 13:1036, 1989.
2. Kiefer B, Deimling M, Finelli D: Ultrafast measurement of T1- and T2-weighted images with "snapshot" FLASH, in Book of Abstracts, vol 1, Society of Magnetic Resonance in Medicine, 1989, p 367.
3. Unger EC, Cohen MS, Gatenby RA, et al: Single breath-holding scans of the abdomen using FISP and FLASH at 1.5T. J Comput Assist Tomogr 12:575, 1988.
4. Frahm J, Haase A, Matthaei D: Rapid NMR imaging of dynamic processes using the FLASH technique. Magn Reson Med 3:321, 1986.
5. Haase A: Snapshot FLASH MRI: Applications to T1, T2, and chemical-shift imaging. Magn Reson Med 13:77, 1990.
6. Conturo TE, Beth AH, Kessler RM, et al: Cooperative T1 and T2 effects on contrast and T2 sensitivity with improved signal to noise using a new driven inversion spin-echo (DISE) sequence, in Book of Abstracts, vol 2, Society of Magnetic Resonance in Medicine, 1987, p 807.
7. Mugler JP III, Brookeman JR: Optimization of pulse-sequence parameters in "Snapshot-FLASH" imaging. Magn Reson Imaging. 8(S1):115, 1990.
8. Mugler JP III, Spraggins TA: Improving image quality in snapshot FLASH and 3D MP RAGE sequences by employing reordered phase encoding, in Works-in-Progress, Society of Magnetic Resonance in Medicine, 1990, p 1310.
9. Edelman RR, Atkinson DJ, Wallner B, et al: Breath-hold abdominal STIR and T2-weighted imaging using an interleaved ultrafast gradient-echo sequence, in Works-in-Progress, Society for Magnetic Resonance Imaging, 1990, p 35.
10. de Lange EE, Mugler JP III, Brookeman JR: Magnetization-prepared rapid gradient-echo (MP RAGE) MR imaging of the liver, in Book of Abstracts, Liver Imaging Symposium, Massachusetts General Hospital, Harvard Medical School, Boston, Mass., 1990.
11. Hamm B, Fisher E, Taupitz M: Differentiation of hepatic hemangiomas from metastasis by dynamic contrast-enhanced MR imaging. J Comput Assist Tomogr 14:205, 1990.
12. Mugler JP III, Brookeman JR; Three-dimensional magnetization-prepared rapid gradient-echo imaging (3D MP RAGE). Magn Reson Med 15:152, 1990.

VI. TISSUE CHARACTERIZATION: PRIMARY AND SECONDARY MALIGNANCY

16

Radiologic-Pathologic Correlation in Liver Tumors

PABLO R. ROS

This chapter reviews the major benign and malignant hepatic tumors in the adult, emphasizing the underlying microscopic and gross pathologic features that are responsible for the radiographic appearance of these focal liver masses. Of the entire classification of benign and malignant hepatic tumors, the discussion includes only those which are important due to their frequency, number of radiologic signs, and interest because of significant prognostic and clinical management implications. Rare tumors, pediatric neoplasms, and secondary malignancies are not considered due to space limitations.

Pathologic correlation is of paramount importance in understanding the appearance of liver neoplasms. Multiple imaging modalities are now available that allow preoperative information not only about the vascularity of masses [using angiography, blood-pool scintigrams, enhanced computed tomography (CT), gadolinium magnetic resonance imaging (MRI), and color Doppler], but also other parameters, such as the presence or absence of Kupffer cells in technetium-labeled sulfur colloid and iron oxide (ferrite)–enhanced MRI, the presence or absence of calcifications (by ultrasound, plain films, and CT), the presence or absence of capsule (MRI, CT, and ultrasound), possible presence of central fibrosis (MRI), and the presence or absence of necrosis and hemorrhage (CT, ultrasound, MRI, etc.). Before cross-sectional imaging, the basic parameters of radiologic-pathologic correlation were primarily applicable to pulmonary and musculoskeletal radiology, where excellent correlation could be obtained with plain films only. Now, these correlations are also available to abdominal viscera. The liver, a large, solid organ that has many neoplasms with dramatic differences in prognosis, is thus an ideal type for radiologic-pathologic correlation.

BENIGN HEPATIC TUMORS IN THE ADULT

Hemangioma

Hemangioma is the most common benign tumor of the liver. Its incidence in large autopsy series ranges from 0.5 to 10 percent, with a uniform geographic distribution. It is predominantly seen in women (M:F ratio of 1:5) of all ages and rarely seen in young children (1,2).

Hemangioma can range in size from a few millimeters to several centimeters, and although it is generally solitary, it may be multiple (approximately 10 percent). A hemangioma can have a central area of fibrosis, and occasionally, the tumor is entirely fibrosed. Microscopically, it is composed of vascular channels lined by endothelium (Fig. 16-1). Hemangioma is usually asymptomatic; rupture and hemoperitoneum are very rare.

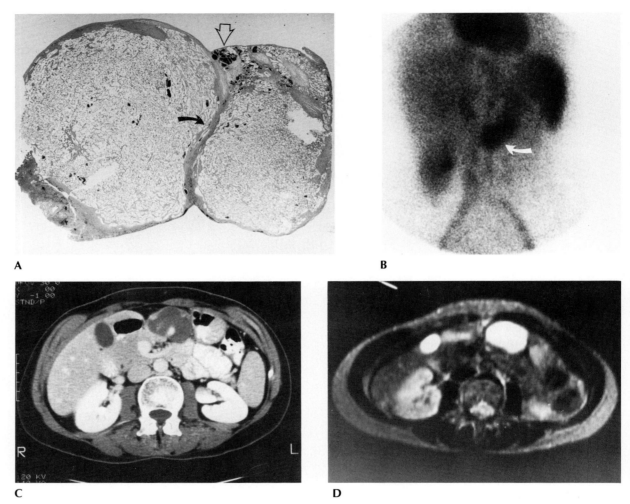

FIGURE 16-1

Subgross imaging correlation in hemangioma. (A) Subgross photomicrograph demonstrates typical features of hemangioma, such as its spongy network of vascular channels (some of them still filled with blood after specimen preparation), fibrous septation (arrows), and large peripheral feeding vessel (open arrow). (B) Planar-tagged blood cell scintigraphy demonstrates uptake in the midepigastrium corresponding with hemangioma (white arrow). (C) Enhanced dynamic CT demonstrates a predominately hypodense mass arising from the anteroinferior edge of the left lobe of the liver, which corresponds with area of increased uptake seen in part B. Note the intensely enhancing peripheral feeding vessel that correlates with the one seen on subgross photograph (A). (D) Axial T2-weighted image (TR 2500/TE 80) demonstrates the marked hyperintensity of the lesion typical of hemangioma.

Hemangioma may appear on plain films as an upper abdominal mass if it is very large. Calcification due to calcium deposition in an area of fibrosis or due to phleboliths may be seen. Blood-pool studies with erythrocytes labeled with technetium-99m (^{99m}Tc) demonstrate the delayed filling of the initial defect (Fig. 16-1). This noninvasive procedure has high specificity (3). Single-photon-emission CT (SPECT) is a very sensitive modality for identification of small hepatic hemangiomas using in vitro labeled red blood cells (RBC) with ^{99m}TC, and it may detect lesions as small as 1.5 cm (4).

The usual sonographic features are those of a hyperechoic, sharply marginated mass with a homogeneous internal pattern. However, the ultrasonographic appearance can vary from hypoechoic to mixed, depending on the size, degree of fibrosis, presence of internal hemorrhage, and degree of cystic internal change. High-level echoes with acoustical shadowing can be seen due to areas of calcification.

Unenhanced CT demonstrates a hypodense, well-marginated mass, usually near the surface of the liver, with central areas of markedly decreased attenuation corresponding to fibrosis or cystic change. Calcification with irregular borders may be present. CT offers another fairly specific method of diagnosis when dynamic studies are performed (Fig. 16-1). Typically, there is contrast enhancement from the periphery to the center with isodense filling compared with the rest of the liver in delayed phases (5).

Prior to MRI, angiography was considered to be the most specific diagnostic method for hemangioma. The hepatic artery is normal in caliber owing to a lack of high-velocity arteriovenous shunting, and there are no tumoral vessels or early venous return. The presence of early pooling of contrast with a persistent, very prolonged stain is characteristic of this entity and is responsible for the so-called "cotton wool" appearance of hemangioma (6).

MRI may demonstrate hemangioma with a high degree of sensitivity and specificity (7–9). The lesion has a very high signal intensity in T2-weighted images and a low signal intensity in T1-weighted images, probably reflecting the large amount of slowly flowing blood within the intricate vascular channels of this tumor (1,2,7–9) (Figs. 16-1 and 16-2). Differentiation from vascular metastasis (i.e., renal cell carcinoma, neuroendocrine tumors, etc.) is unlikely on MRI (Fig. 16-3).

Focal Nodular Hyperplasia

There is uncertainty about the nature of focal nodular hyperplasia (FNH), and regenerative, hamartomatous, and neoplastic theories have been postulated. This condition, although rare, is twice as common as hepatocellular adenoma (HCA). It is more frequent in women, but the sex ratio is not as striking as in HCA. It may affect all ages, but it predominates in the third to fifth decades of life. FNH is probably related to the use of contraceptive steroids.

Grossly, FNH is a solitary and firm nodular mass frequently measuring less than 3 cm in diameter (Fig. 16-4). It usually has a central stellate scar, and there are no areas of hemorrhage or necrosis. FNH is sharply demarcated by compressed liver; however, there is no true capsule. Microscopically, it is formed by normal hepatocytes abnormally arranged (Fig. 16-4).

In 75 percent of the cases, FNH is discovered incidentally. Alpha-fetoprotein and liver function tests are within normal limits. On plain film, FNH may be pedunculated and project as an extrahepatic noncalcified mass.

In approximately 50 percent of cases, there is normal accumulation of sulfur colloid (Fig. 16-4). In 10 percent of cases, there is hyperconcentration of the radionuclide, indicating increased vascularity and possible higher concentrations of Kupffer cells. FNH produces a defect in the scintigram in 40 percent of cases.

Ultrasonographically, FNH appears as a well-demarcated, hyperechogenic lesion (10) (Fig. 16-4). Homogeneous hypoechogenicity is rarely seen. Its echogenicity reflects the solid nature of FNH without central hemorrhage. By CT, there is frequently a hypodense mass with a hyperdense or isodense appearance following contrast injection (Fig. 16-5). A central hypodense and irregular zone can be seen corresponding with the central fibrotic scar, and calcification is rare (10).

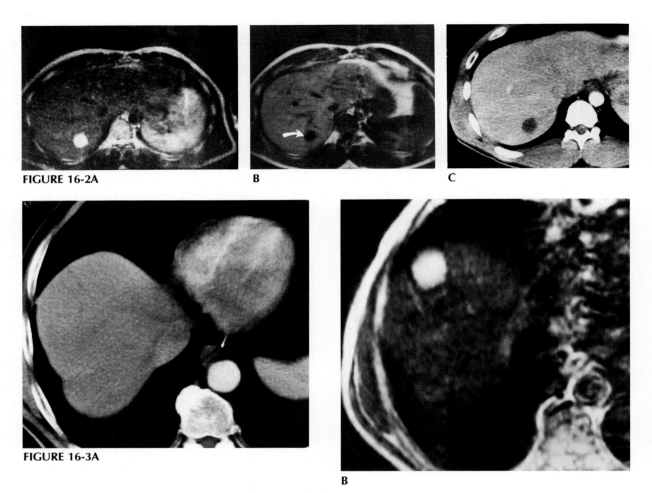

FIGURE 16-2
MRI-CT correlation in hemangioma. (A) T2-weighted image (TR 2500/TE 100) shows the typical marked hyperintensity of a hemangioma. Note that the intensity is brighter than that of the spleen. (B) T1-weighted image (TR 330/TR 20) shows that the lesion is markedly hypointense (arrow). (C) Corresponding enhanced CT demonstrates a nonspecific hypodense lesion. CT has low specificity for hemangioma even using a single-level dynamic technique. To diagnose a hemangioma, the most specific methods currently available are MRI and red blood cell scintigraphy.

FIGURE 16-3
Islet cell carcinoma mimicking hemangioma. (A) T2-weighted image (TR 2100/TE 80) shows a markedly hyperintense and well-limited lesion in the dome of the liver in this patient known to have an islet cell neoplasm of the pancreatic head. (B) Correlating CT section after contrast enhancement failed to demonstrate the same lesion. The only mimickers for hemangioma using MRI and heavily T2-weighted images are hypervascular metastases, as demonstrated in this example.

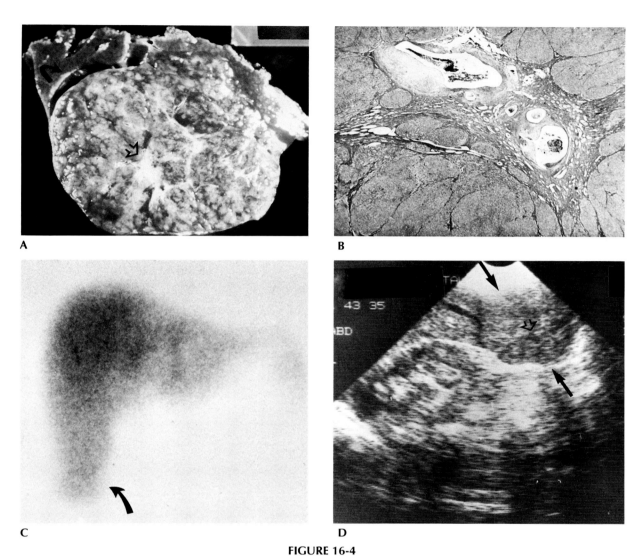

FIGURE 16-4
Pathologic imaging correlation in FNH. (A) Cut section of an FNH demonstrates its central scar (open arrow) and its nodular internal nature without significant areas of necrosis and hemorrhage. Also note the large draining vein (curved arrow) and the pedunculated appearance of this relatively small tumor. (B) Photomicrography of the central scar demonstrates its inhomogeneity with large vascular structures and smaller biliary canaliculi. The fact that the central scar in FNH is composed of not only fibrous tissue, but also vascular and biliary elements may play a role in its MRI appearance. (C) Sulfur colloid technetium-labeled liver/spleen scan demonstrates uptake in this pedunculated FNH originating in the inferior margin of the right lobe of the liver (arrow). (D) Corresponding ultrasound demonstrates the hyperechogenic nature of FNH and its lobulated contour. The scan can be seen as a hypoechoic area (open arrow).

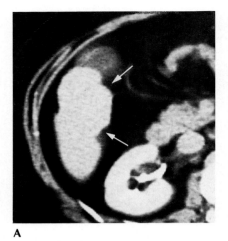
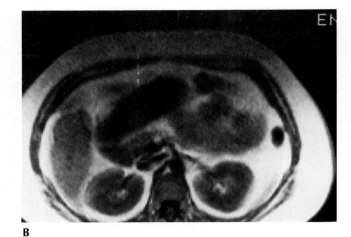

FIGURE 16-5
CT-MRI correlation to FNH. (A) Enhanced CT. There is an isodense FNH in the inferior portion of the right lobe of the liver that is only noticed by an abnormality in contour (arrows). (B) T1-weighted image (TR 500/TE 30) shows isointensity of the tumor with the rest of the liver parenchyma. (C) T2-weighted image (TR 2500/TE 80) demonstrates hyperintensity (arrow) within the FNH corresponding with the central scar. The remainder of the tumor is isointense also in T2-weighted image with a normal liver parenchyma.

Angiographically, 80 to 90 percent of cases are hypervascular. The radiations from the center to the periphery (centrifugal vascular supply) constitute the classic "spoke wheel" pattern seen in up to 70 percent of cases (Fig. 16-6). A very intense and homogeneous stain in the capillary phase without avascular zones is a reliable differential finding in distinguishing FNH from HCA, since avascular zones are frequently seen in HCA.

By MRI, FNH appears isointense in T1 and generally isointense or slightly hyperintense in T2 images. The central scar may remain hyperintense in T2 images (11,12) (Fig. 16-5).

Hepatocellular Adenoma
This tumor was extremely rare prior to 1960, when its incidence increased due to the widespread use of contraceptive steroids. It usually affects women of childbearing age, making it the most frequent tumor of the liver in women using contraceptive steroids. It is rarely seen in men.

HCA is usually solitary, encapsulated, and large (average size 8 to 10 cm). It is frequently subcapsular in location or pedunculated, facilitating local resection. Its cut surface is light brown to yellow, reflecting its high content of fat and glycogen. HCA often presents with foci of hemorrhage or necrosis (Fig. 16-7). Microscopically,

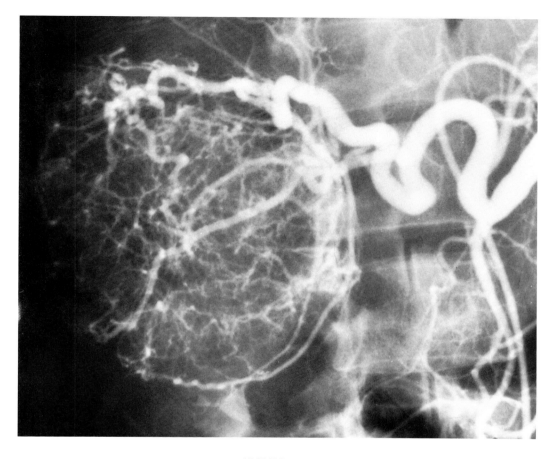

FIGURE 16-6
Angiography of FNH. Selective hepatic arteriogram demonstrates a hypervascular lesion with radiating vessels from the periphery to the center forming the so-called "spoke wheel" pattern.

HCA is composed of sheets and cords of hepatocytes mimicking normal liver; however, there are no portal or central veins or bile ducts (Fig. 16-7). The vascular supply is received through the capsule. Kupffer cells are present in HCA, and there can be fewer than, as many as, or even more than in normal liver parenchyma (13) (Fig. 16-7).

HCA may be discovered incidentally as an asymptomatic hepatic mass, or it may produce right upper quadrant pain. Rupture and subsequent hemoperitoneum are not uncommon, and the possibility of this complication is the main reason for its resection upon serendipitous discovery. The incidence of rupture is related mainly to the position of the adenoma within the liver. Alpha-fetoprotein levels are normal, as are liver function tests. Foci of hepatocellular carcinoma within HCA have been described in a very small number of cases.

The plain-film findings of HCA depend on the size of the tumor. Since HCA is commonly a large mass at the time of discovery, it frequently presents as a nonspecific soft-tissue mass without calcification (Fig. 16-8). The mass effect alters the normal liver contour, since HCA usually protrudes partially from the liver surface. Sometimes HCA can present as a right lower quadrant mass if the tumor is pedunculated. Fluid may be identified

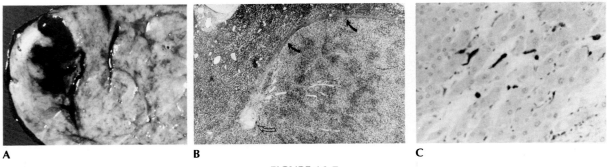

FIGURE 16-7
Pathology of adenoma. (A) *Close-up of a cut adenoma demonstrates internal hemorrhage as well as fracture line. Rupture of adenomas is frequent because they are soft tumors rich in fat and glycogen.* (B) *Photomicrography demonstrates the lighter color of the adenoma compared with the normal liver. Note the capsule* (curved arrows), *as well as a peripheral feeder* (open arrow), *branching toward the center of the adenoma.* (C) *In this high-power photomicrograph there is evidence of Kupffer cells* (dark stain) *that are present in all adenomas.*

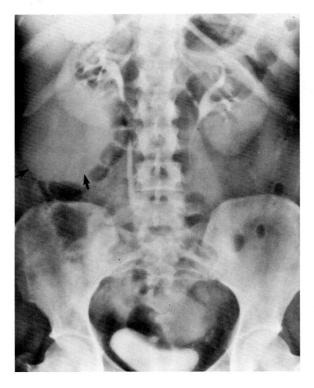

FIGURE 16-8
Plain-film findings in adenoma. Supine abdomen from an excretory urogram revealing a mass effect in the right upper quadrant displacing the air-filled hepatic flexure (arrows).

in cases of HCA rupture. Sulfur colloid scintigraphy commonly demonstrates a defect in the liver parenchyma. Although it has been described that HCA does not accumulate technetium-99m sulfur colloid, uptake can be present in a significant proportion of cases (14) (Fig. 16-9). Therefore, accumulation of activity by a hepatic tumor cannot be used as a definitive criterion to exclude HCA in favor of FNH. The most likely responsible factor for the usual lack of uptake of sulfur colloid in HCA appears to be the altered blood flow and not the absence of Kupffer cells (13).

The findings of HCA by ultrasonography are generally nonspecific. HCA may present as a well-defined, echogenic, intrahepatic mass with a central, single, large, anechoic space or multiple, small, irregular, anechoic areas. The echogenicity of HCA is due to the presence of fat and glycogen within the hepatocytes of HCA. The areas of anechogenicity correspond with areas of hemorrhage, recent or old. HCA can appear homogeneously echogenic, corresponding to tumor without internal hemorrhage.

On CT, HCA usually appears as a well-defined mass within the liver due to the presence of a capsule. It is commonly located near the surface of the liver. The density is variable from hypodense (due to fat and glycogen) in unenhanced studies to isodense in enhanced studies (15).

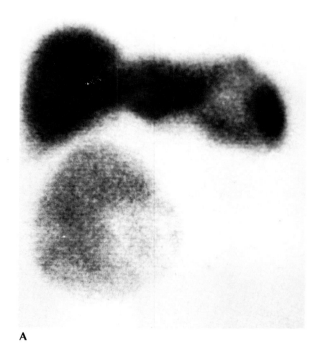
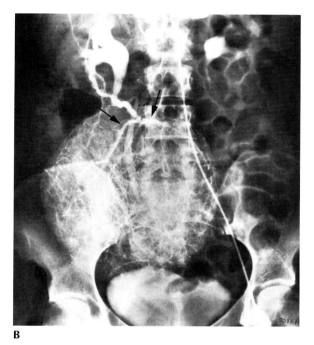

FIGURE 16-9
Adenoma, scintigraphy-angiographic correlation. (A) *Liver/spleen sulfur colloid scan disclosing uptake in a large, markedly pedunculated adenoma attached by a fibrovascular pedicle to the right lobe of the liver. The areas of inhomogeneity within the adenoma correspond to internal hemorrhage.* (B) *Correlating angiogram shows the hypervascular nature of adenoma as well as its large peripheral feeding vessels* (arrows).

Unenhanced CT may demonstrate areas of increased density within a hypodense lesion corresponding to recent intratumoral hemorrhage (Fig. 16-10), a characteristic finding in HCA. Occasionally, HCA can appear as a hepatic lesion with attenuation near water due to massive necrosis. CT is able to identify hemoperitoneum secondary to the rupture of an HCA.

HCA is a hypervascular tumor with large vessels on its periphery and centripetal flow. There is no arteriovenous shunting or vascular (portal or hepatic veins) invasion (Figs. 16-9 and 16-11). In the capillary phase, there is an intense stain that may have central avascular areas. This is a helpful sign because it indicates the presence of areas of hemorrhage, common in HCA.

By MRI, HCA appears as a well-defined hyperintense mass in T1- and T2-weighted images due to the fatty nature of this tumor (Fig. 16-12). Areas of fresh blood can easily be depicted and confirm the hemorrhagic nature of HCA.

Nodular Regenerative Hyperplasia (Nodular Transformation)

Nodular regenerative hyperplasia (NRH) (also known as *nodular transformation*) is characterized histologically by diffuse involvement of the liver by hyperplastic nodules composed of cells resembling normal hepatocytes (16) (Fig. 16-13). NRH occurs equally in men and women and is reported in all ages and races. Associated diseases include myeloproliferative syndromes, lymphoproliferative syndromes, and miscellaneous disorders. Various drugs also have been implicated, including steroids (particularly oral contraceptives), antineoplastics, and others (16). The etiologic role of these diseases and drugs and the exact incidence of NRH in these disorders are uncertain.

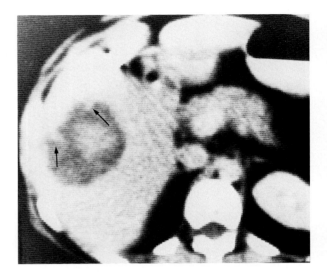

FIGURE 16-10
CT findings in adenoma. Enhanced CT demonstrates a hypodense lesion due to the presence of fat within the adenoma. A central area of increased density indicates recent hemorrhage. Hypervascular feeders (arrows) are seen in the periphery of the adenoma correlating with findings seen in Fig. 16-7B.

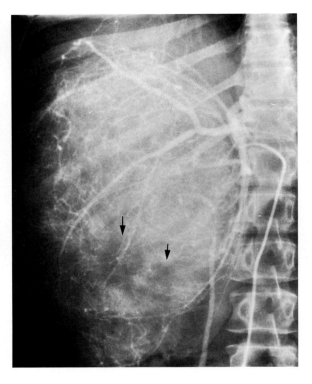

FIGURE 16-11
Angiographic findings in adenoma. The typical appearance of adenoma is seen as a very large tumor with large peripheral feeding vessels and centripetal flow. The avascular areas (arrows) indicate central hemorrhage.

Grossly, the nodules range in size from a few millimeters to large masses. Portal areas (bile ducts, portal veins, and hepatic artery branches) may be trapped within the nodules. No significant fibrosis is found in or around the nodules, an important feature distinguishing NRH from cirrhosis and from FNH of the liver (17). Large nodules, viewed out of context of the diffuse nodularity, can mimic HCA histologically. Patients with NRH may be asymptomatic or may present as idiopathic portal hypertension with varices, splenomegaly, or ascites.

The radiologic features of NRH reflect its composition by cells resembling normal hepatocytes and Kupffer cells, which may be present within or between the nodules (18). The nodules may take up ^{99m}Tc-sulfur colloid and have variable echogenicity on sonography. They are often hypodense on CT without significant enhancement. Central hemorrhage within a large nodule may occur. Angiographically, the nodules are vascular and may fill from the periphery with hypovascular areas due to hemorrhage. These findings may resemble some features of FNH, HCA, or metastases.

MALIGNANT HEPATIC TUMORS IN THE ADULT

Hepatocellular Carcinoma (HCC)
Typical HCC, although rare in the United States, is one of the most frequent primary visceral malignancies in the world, with over 1 million new cases per year. It has a bimodal geographic and age distribution: It is rare in the industrialized world and relatively frequent in other areas (sub-Saharan Africa and Asia). In low-incidence areas, HCC has a male predominance of 2.5:1, is more commonly seen in the 70- to 80-year-old range, and is rarely found in people younger than 40 years of age. In high-incidence areas, the age of presentation is 30 to 40 years of age and is male-predominant (8:1).

Grossly, there are three major forms: (1) massive or a single large mass (Fig. 16-14), (2) nodular

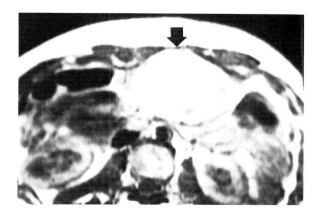

FIGURE 16-12
MRI appearance of adenoma. T1-weighted image (TR 600/TE 20) shows marked hyperintensity in an adenoma (arrow). Central inhomogeneity is due to hemorrhage.

or multifocal (Fig. 16-15), and (3) diffuse or cirrhotomimetic. Regardless of its gross appearance, HCC is a "soft" tumor that will frequently necrose and hemorrhage. If there is massive necrosis, HCC can appear cystic. Vascular invasion (portal vein, hepatic veins, and inferior vena cava) is common. Conversely, biliary invasion is uncommon. A gross variant, the "encapsulated" HCC, may have a better prognosis due to greater resectability than other types of HCC. Histologically, the majority of HCCs (or typical HCCs) are well-differentiated, with malignant hepatocytes arranged in cords or trabeculae, and frequently produce bile.

In low-incidence areas, the onset of symptoms is insidious. In high-incidence areas, HCC has a very aggressive course and may present with rupture and massive hemoperitoneum; jaundice is infrequent. Owing to the production of hormones and pseudohormones by HCC, there are frequently paraneoplastic manifestations. Liver function tests are usually abnormal but indistinguishable from cirrhosis, and alpha-fetoprotein levels are consistently elevated. HCC is also associated with hemochromatosis.

On plain roentgenograms, the findings are that of a nonspecific right upper quadrant mass of variable size. Unlike fibrolamellar carcinoma, calcification is almost never present in HCC (19). In patients with HCC and hemochromatosis, there are degenerative changes in joints. Scintigraphy with ^{99m}Tc-sulfur colloid demonstrates a defect in a diffusely diseased liver (20). Gallium-67 accumulates in the majority of HCCs.

By ultrasound, the appearance of HCC is variable from hypoechoic to echogenic (21). The hyperechoic HCC correlates with either fatty metamorphosis or marked sinusoidal dilatation. Ultrasonography is able to detect very small HCCs (2 to 3 cm), and it is advocated as the screening method for HCC in high-risk patients in combination with alpha-fetoprotein levels. On sonograms, it is possible to noninvasively evaluate the presence of tumoral thrombi in portal and hepatic veins, as well as in the inferior vena cava (22).

CT demonstrates a hepatic mass generally of decreased attenuation, with rapid enhancement in dynamic scans (23). Typical HCC commonly appears with large central areas of markedly decreased density corresponding to necrosis (Fig. 16-14). HCC can appear cystic on both sonograms and CT scans, making differentiation from a cystic mass [cystadenoma/cystadenocarcinoma, echinococcal cyst, and simple cyst (bile duct cyst, abscess, etc.)] difficult. In patients with hemochromatosis, a very dense liver is identified with an irregular contour, atrophy of the right lobe, prominence of the caudate lobe, and ascites—all signs of cirrhosis secondary to iron deposition. The foci of HCC are seen as localized areas of hypodensity in the hyperdense liver. CT is helpful in the identification of encapsulated HCC (24). In these cases, a thin rim of low density is seen surrounding the HCC in precontrast studies, and this enhances after the administration of contrast material.

Typical HCC is a very hypervascular tumor with abnormal vessels, arteriovenous shunts, and vascular invasion (25,26) (Fig. 16-16). Extension of HCC into the portal vein, hepatic veins, and inferior vena cava is characteristic (27), resulting in the "threads and streaks" sign secondary to growth of HCC inside the portal vein. Portal hypertension and esophageal varices are possible due to portal invasion by HCC.

HCC has a variable appearance on MRI. Low-, iso-, high-, and mixed-intensity patterns are seen (28,29) (Fig. 16-14). If there is steatosis in the HCC,

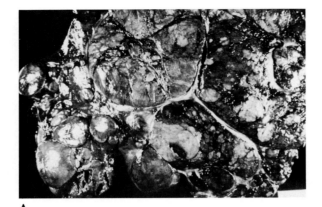

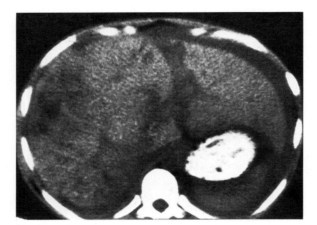

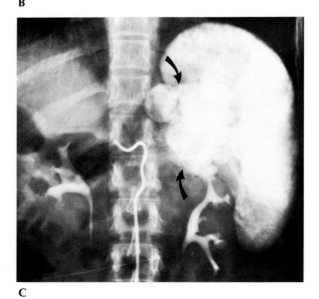

it has high intensity; however, if fibrosis predominates, there is low intensity. A low-intensity ring indicative of encapsulated HCC is detected more frequently on MRI than on CT.

Fibrolamellar Carcinoma

Fibrolamellar carcinoma (FLC) is now considered by many pathologists to be a distinct entity rather than a subtype of HCC. This distinction is justified by clinical, radiologic, and pathologic features (30). Although this neoplasm constitutes a minority of all hepatocellular malignancies (only 2 percent), it is significant because it involves young adults and has a better prognosis than typical HCC.

FLC is found in adolescents and young adults without any sexual predominance. No association with oral contraceptive use has been found. Clinically, FLC usually presents with pain, malaise, and weight loss; jaundice is only occasionally detected. A palpable mass is seen in two-thirds of patients. Alpha-fetoprotein levels are normal in most patients.

On gross examination, FLC is usually a sharp, firm, circumscribed mass with scalloped borders (Fig. 16-17). Occasionally, satellite nodules of tumor are present (multifocal FLC). On cut section, FLC has fibrous septa radiating from a central scar, thus mimicking the gross appearance of FNH. Histologically, FLC is characterized by abundant fibrosis arranged in lamellae and interspersed with neoplastic cells.

FIGURE 16-13

Nodular regenerative hyperplasia (NRH). (A) Cut section of a specimen demonstrates multiple nodules of variable size of NRH. Fibrous brands can be seen throughout the specimen. (B) CT scan shows multiple hypodense nodules distributed throughout the liver, indicating the diffuse nature of this process. No associated ascites. From Dachman AH, Ros PR, Goodman ZD, et al: Nodule regenerative hyperplasia of the liver: Clinical and radiologic observations. AJR 148:717, 1987. Copyright © by American Roentgen Ray Society. Reprinted by permission.) (C) Venous phase of an arteriogram in this patient with NRH demonstrates marked collateral circulation at the hilus of the spleen as well as splenomegaly. Owing to the diffuse involvement of the liver, patients with NRH have severe portal hypertension.

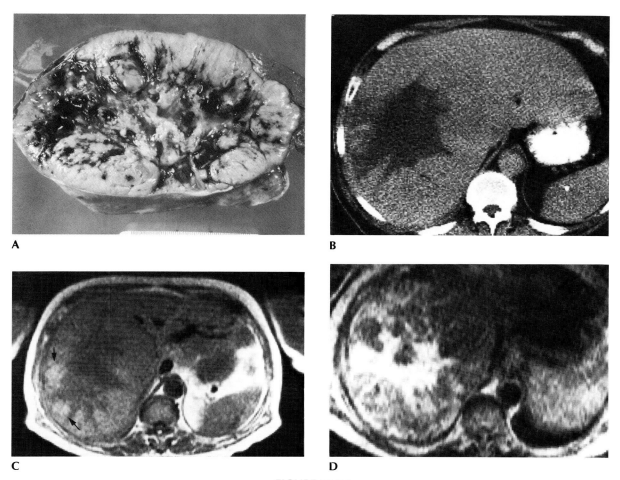

FIGURE 16-14

Massive or single HCC. (A) Cut-specimen photograph demonstrates a large HCC. Note that only the periphery of the tumor corresponds with viable tissue, while large portions of the center contain hemorrhage and liquefactive necrosis. (B) CT demonstrates a large central stellate hypodense area. The nature of this central hypodense area cannot be determined by CT alone. (C) T1-weighted image (TR 500/TE 30) shows the mass to be isointense with normal liver parenchyma, distorting normal liver vasculature, and a hypointense central area corresponding to the CT. Note the higher intensity in the periphery of the tumor (arrows) due to hemorrhage, frequently seen in HCC, that was not easily recognized as such on CT. (D) T2-weighted image (TR 2500/TE 100). The central area of the tumor has high signal intensity, therefore representing necrosis and not fibrosis. The fact the MRI can frequently distinguish fibrosis from liquefactive necrosis on T2-weighted images may be used to determine the etiology of hepatic neoplasms.

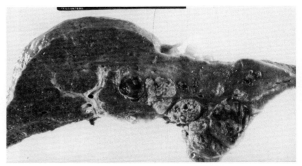

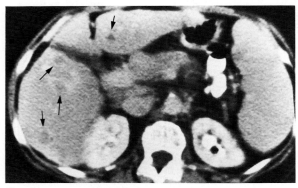

FIGURE 16-15
Nodular or multifocal HCC. (A) Cut specimen demonstrates multiple nodules of HCC in its multifocal or nodular form. Note hemorrhage and necrosis in some of the nodules. In addition, a micronodular, cirrhotic liver can be seen in the uninvolved areas. HCC frequently arises, in the Western hemisphere, in a cirrhotic liver. (B) Enhanced CT demonstrates multiple foci of HCC. HCC in its multifocal form may appear as multiple nodules of similar size without a primary or larger nodule. Therefore, HCC should be considered in differential diagnosis of metastatic disease (arrows).

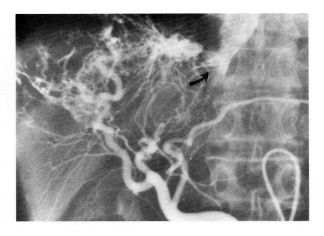

FIGURE 16-16
Angiography of HCC. Hypervascular tumor in the dome of the liver characterized by neovascularity as well as a large AV shunting. Note in this arterial phase image the shunt filling of the most superior portion of the inferior vena cava (arrow).

On plain films, FLC may present as an upper abdominal mass with calcification. The sonographic and CT findings reflect the homogeneous nature of FLC and its prominent fibrosis (30,31). Sonographically, FLC appears as a homogeneously echogenic mass that may have areas of high-level echoes and acoustical shadowing due to calcification.

On unenhanced CT, FLC is a hypodense mass with a lobulated contour (Fig. 16-17). A central area of further decreased density or calcification corresponds with the central scar that may calcify. CT scan after contrast injection reveals marked enhancement. Sulfur colloid scintigraphy shows FLC as a defect in a normal liver pattern. Unlike HCC, there is no evidence of cirrhosis. On angiography, FLC appears as a hypervascular tumor with a prominent stain and frequently demonstrates compartmentalization in the capillary phase.

Radiologically, multifocal FLC can appear as multiple lesions seen as defects on sulfur colloid scintigrams, as echogenic masses on sonograms, and as hypodense masses on CT scans (32).

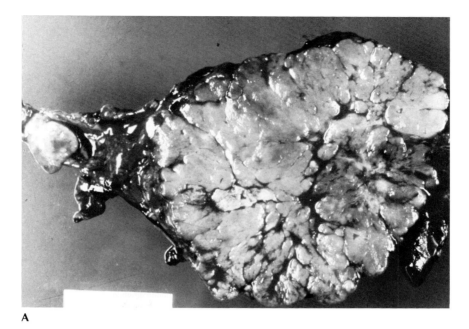

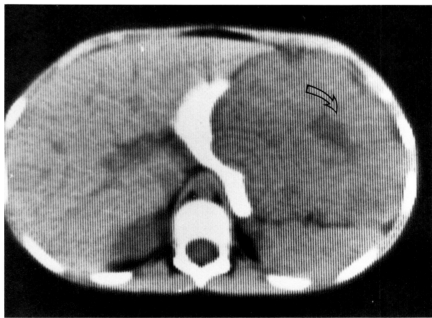

FIGURE 16-17

Fibrolamellar carcinoma (FLC). (A) Gross cut photograph of this FLC shows nodular appearance due to the presence of multiple fibrous septa that radiate from central scars. This appearance is similar to that of FNH. (B) Unenhanced CT demonstrates the lobulated contour and hypodense nature of FLC. Note the central hypodense area corresponding to the fibrotic scar.

REFERENCES

1. Glazer GM, Aisen AM, Francis IR, et al: Hepatic cavernous hemangioma: Magnetic resonance imaging. Radiology 155:417, 1985.
2. Itai Y, Ohtomo K, Furui S, et al: Noninvasive diagnosis of small cavernous hemangioma of the liver: Advantage of MRI. AJR 145:1195, 1985.
3. Moinuddin M, Allison JR, Montgomery JH, et al: Scintigraphic diagnosis of hepatic hemangioma: Its role in the management of hepatic mass lesions. AJR 145:223, 1985.
4. Tumeh SS, Benson C, Nagel JS, et al: Cavernous hemangioma of the liver: Detection with single photon emission computed tomography. Radiology 164:353, 1987.
5. Freeny PC, Marks WM: Hepatic hemangioma: Dynamic bolus CT. AJR 147:711, 1986.
6. Takayasu K, Moriyama N, Shima Y, et al: Atypical radiographic findings in hepatic cavernous hemangioma: Correlation with histologic features. AJR 146:1149, 1986.
7. Ferrucci JT: MR imaging of the liver. AJR 147:1103, 1986.
8. Ros PR, Lubbers PR, Olmsted WW, Morillo G: Hemangioma of the liver: Magnetic resonance–gross morphologic correlation. AJR 149:1167, 1987.
9. Stark DD, Felder RC, Wittenberg J, et al: Magnetic resonance imaging of cavernous hemangioma of the liver: Tissue-specific characterization. AJR 145:213, 1985.
10. Welch TJ, Sheedy PF II, Johnson CM, et al: Focal nodular hyperplasia and hepatic adenoma: Comparison of angiography, CT, US and scintigraphy. Radiology 156:593, 1985.
11. Butch RJ, Stark DD, Malt RA: Case report: MR imaging of hepatic focal nodular hyperplasia. J Comput Assist Tomogr 10:874, 1986.
12. Schiebler ML, Kressel HY, Saul SH, et al: MR imaging of focal nodular hyperplasia of the liver. J Comput Assist Tomogr 11:651, 1987.
13. Goodman ZD, Mikel UV, Lubbers PR, et al: Kupffer cells in hepatocellular adenomas. Am J Surg Pathol 11:191, 1987.
14. Lubbers PR, Ros PR, Goodman ZD: Accumulation of technetium-99m sulfur colloid by hepatocellular adenoma: Scintigraphic-pathologic correlation. AJR 148:1105, 1987.
15. Mathieu D, Bruneton JN, Drouillard J, et al: Hepatic adenomas and focal nodular hyperplasia: Dynamic CT study. Radiology 160:53, 1986.
16. Stromeyer FW, Ishak KG: Nodular transformation (nodular "regenerative" hyperplasia) of the liver: A clinicopathologic study of 30 cases. Human Pathol 12:60, 1981.
17. Mones JM, Saldana MJ, Albores-Saavedra J: Nodular regenerative hyperplasia of the liver: Report of three cases and review of the literature. Arch Pathol Lab Med 108:741, 1984.
18. Dachman AH, Ros PR, Goodman ZD, et al: Nodular regenerative hyperplasia of the liver: Clinical and radiologic observations. AJR 148:717, 1987.
19. Teefey SA, Stephens DH, Weiland LH: Calcification in hepatocellular carcinoma: Not always an indication of fibrolamellar histology. AJR 149:1173, 1987.
20. Kudo M, Hirasa M, Takakuwa H, et al: Small hepatocellular carcinomas in chronic liver disease: Detection with SPECT. Radiology 159:697, 1986.
21. Holm J, Jacobsen B: Accuracy of dynamic ultrasonography in the diagnosis of malignant liver lesions. J Ultrasound Med 5:1, 1986.
22. Shimamoto K, Sakuma S, Ishigaki T, Makino N: Intratumoral blood flow: Evaluation with color Doppler echography. Radiology 165:683, 1987.
23. Hayashi N, Yamamoto K, Tamaki N, et al: Metastatic nodules of hepatocellular carcinoma: Detection with angiography, CT, and US. Radiology 165:61, 1987.
24. Muramatsu Y, Takayasu K, Moriyama N, et al: Peripheral low-density area of hepatic tumors: CT-pathologic correlation. Radiology 160:49, 1986.
25. Sumida M, Ohto M, Ebara M, et al: Accuracy of angiography in the diagnosis of small hepatocellular carcinoma. AJR 147:531, 1986.
26. Takayasu K, Shima Y, Muramatsu Y, et al: Angiography of small hepatocellular carcinomas: Analysis of 105 resected tumors. AJR 147:525, 1986.
27. Mathieu D, Guinet C, Bouklia-Hassane A, Vasile N: Hepatic vein involvement in hepatocellular carcinoma. Gastrointest Radiol 13:55, 1988.
28. Ebara M, Ohto M, Watanabe Y, et al: Diagnosis of small hepatocellular carcinoma: Correlation of MR imaging and tumor histologic studies. Radiology 159:371, 1986.
29. Itoh K, Nishimura K, Togashi K, et al: Hepatocellular carcinoma: MR imaging. Radiology 164:21, 1987.
30. Friedman AC, Lichtenstein JE, Goodman Z, et al: Fibrolamellar hepatocellular carcinoma. Radiology 157:583, 1985.
31. Francis IR, Agha FP, Thompson NW, Keren DF: Fibrolamellar hepatocarcinoma: Clinical, radiologic and pathologic features. Gastrointest Radiol 11:67, 1986.
32. Titelbaum DS, Burke DR, Meranze SG, Saul SH: Fibrolamellar hepatocellular carcinoma: Pitfalls in nonoperative diagnosis. Radiology 167:25, 1988.

17

MRI of Hepatic Metastatic Disease

JACK WITTENBERG

In the Western world, detection and characterization of hepatic metastases and their differentiation from hemangiomas and cysts are the most common challenges in hepatic tumor imaging. The incidence of hepatic metastases is considerable, ranging from 1 to 24 percent at the time of diagnosis of a variety of common primary tumors (1). Necropsy studies have demonstrated hepatic metastases in more than half the patients with primary malignancies having portal venous drainage (2). Alternatively, hemangiomas may be found in up to 7 percent of the adult population (3). In other areas of the world, particularly Southeast Asia and Japan, the high incidence of hepatocellular carcinoma enlarges the scope of differential diagnoses of common hepatic tumors.

In order for MRI to be considered a considerable advance in hepatic tumor assessment, it must be capable of a substantial incremental increase in accuracy not only of detection, but also of differential diagnosis. Emerging consensus indicates that such accuracy in tissue-specific characterization may, in fact, be available.

DIFFERENTIATION OF METASTASES FROM HEMANGIOMAS AND CYSTS

Morphologic Criteria

It is probably fair to say at this point in the routine care of patients that decisions about the etiology of these masses are most commonly based on a visual assessment of morphologic patterns along with a qualitative assessment of the intensity of the signal itself. This is apparently true regardless of pulse sequences or magnet strengths employed (4–6). Furthermore, with notable exceptions (7,8), it is T2-weighted pulse sequences that give the most valuable information in making these decisions.

Most lesions are hypointense on T1-weighted pulse sequences and variably hyperintense on more heavily weighted T2 sequences (4). Figure 17-1 demonstrates the spectrum of morphologic and signal-intensity characteristics that were retrospectively developed among a group of patients with metastatic tumors and/or common benign tumors. In total, over 300 metastatic lesions in 98 patients with a variety of primary tumors (colon, 60 percent; pancreas, 13 percent; lung, 5 percent; and breast, 4 percent) were compared with 37 hemangiomas and 50 cysts in 24 and 7 patients, respectively. The examinations were all performed on a superconducting magnet operating at 0.6 Tesla. T1-weighted images were generated from both spin-echo 260–330/14–20 (TR/TE) and inversion recovery 1500/15/450 (TR/TE/TI) pulse sequences, while T2-weighted images were derived from progressively more heavily weighted spin-echo pulse sequences, 2000–2350/60–120–180. It is notable that aside from a single

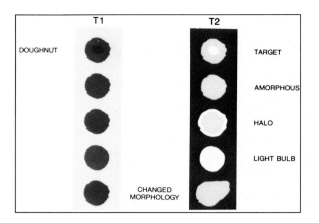

FIGURE 17-1
Diagram of T1- and T2-weighted morphologic features. Typical appearance of all masses is illustrated, and those with specific features are labeled. Morphologic patterns describe a characteristic T1- or T2-weighted pattern or, as with changed morphology, a combined T1- and T2-weighted pattern. The most common, but not necessarily exclusive, correlative pulse-sequence pattern is indicated for each characteristic pattern. (From Wittenberg J, Stark DD, Forman BH, et al: Differentiation of hepatic metastases from hepatic hemangiomas and cysts by using MR imaging. AJR 151:79, 1988. Copyright © by American Roentgen Ray Society. Reprinted by permission.)

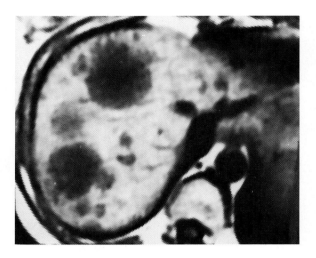

FIGURE 17-2
Doughnut sign. Multiple metastases, the largest two of which demonstrate the lower central signal intensity.

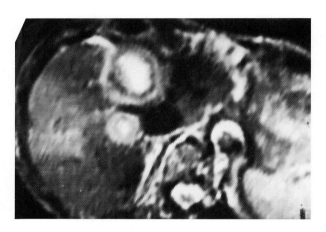

FIGURE 17-3
Target sign. Two metastases with central increased signal intensity, in this case surrounded by a well-defined high-signal-intensity rim.

morphologic pattern (doughnut), the T1-weighted masses were imaged simply as having a homogeneous low-signal-intensity appearance. Conversely, there was a variety of morphologic and signal intensity characteristics that typified T2-weighted lesions. For ease of communication, the following descriptors were established for the patterns, categorized by the pulse sequence or sequences on which they were observed:

T1-Weighted Pulse Sequences

1. *Doughnut:* A low-signal-intensity mass containing a distinct, regularly or irregularly rounded region of even lower signal intensity, usually placed centrally (Fig. 17-2). The total extent of the central area rarely exceeded one-half the total area of the lesion.

T2-Weighted Pulse Sequences

2. *Target:* A mass with a central, smooth or irregularly rounded high-signal-intensity region surrounded by a rind of tissue whose high intensity was less than that of the central area of the mass (Fig. 17-3). The outer margin of the lesion varied considerably from indistinct to distinct, occasionally having a rim of high signal intensity.

3. *Amorphous:* A mass of variably increased signal intensity whose contents were featureless and inhomogeneous (Fig. 17-4). The outer margins tended to be irregularly rounded and indistinct.

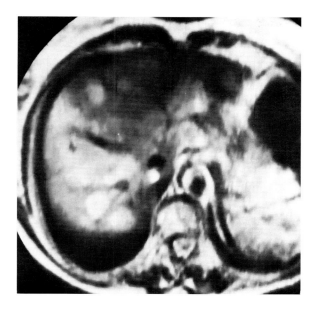

FIGURE 17-4
Amorphous sign. (From Wittenberg J, Stark DD, Forman BH, et al: Differentiation of hepatic metastases from hepatic hemangiomas and cysts by using MR imaging. ATR 151:79, 1988. Copyright © by American Roentgen Ray Society. Reprinted by permission.)

4. *Halo:* A mass with a distinct, but not necessarily smooth circumferential rim of high signal intensity that varied in thickness from 2 to 10 mm and encircled the periphery of a lesion whose inner contents were of lower signal intensity (Fig. 17-5).

5. *Lightbulb:* A round or elliptically shaped mass that usually had smooth and distinct margins and whose largely homogeneous contents had a very high signal intensity, similar to that of gallbladder or cerebrospinal fluid (Fig. 17-6).

Combined T1- and T2-Weighted Pulse Sequences

6. *Changed morphology:* A mass that was considerably altered in both shape and size on alternative pulse sequences. This occurred when an irregularly rounded lesion observed on a T1-weighted image appeared considerably larger, more geometrically shaped and hyperintense on T2-weighted images, usually with its base abutting a surface of the liver (Fig. 17-7).

Pathologic correlation available on some of these lesions combined with assumptions based on observed signal intensities permits specula-

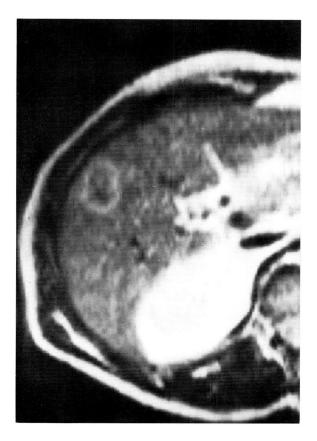

FIGURE 17-5
Halo sign.

tion as to the histologic underpinnings of these patterns. The doughnut and target patterns were seen more frequently with larger lesions and/or those metastases associated with primary lesions prone to necrosis. The central area of high signal intensity on T2-weighted pulse sequences is most consistent with a necrotic, partially liquified central zone. The signal intensity of the halo sign with T2 weighting suggests a greater water content than that of adjacent normal liver parenchyma, perhaps because of an edematous reaction incited by infiltration of tumor cells. The lightbulb sign in hemangiomas and cysts can be attributed to the considerable fluid in a slow-flowing or static cavity, respectively. The same sign in metastatic disease may be the result of complete tumor necrosis or a highly vascularized mass. The changed morphology is best explained

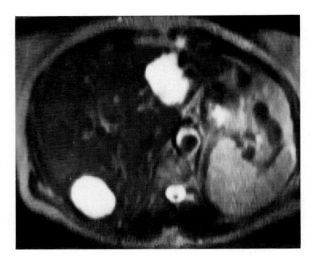

FIGURE 17-6
Lightbulb sign. The signal intensity of both metastases is similar to that of cerebrospinal fluid. The outline of the more anterior lesion is somewhat more irregular than the usual hemangioma. (From Wittenberg J, Stark DD, Forman BH, et al: Differentiation of hepatic metastases from hepatic hemangiomas and cysts by using MR imaging. AJR 151:79, 1988. Copyright © by American Roentgen Ray Society. Reprinted by permission.)

by the presence of lesion-surrounding edema, possibly due to tumor compromise of circulation of more peripheral tissues.

The frequency of these morphologic patterns in this study is given in Table 17-1. Amorphous, target, and halo morphologies were specific T2-weighted signs of metastases and were present in 45, 27, and 13 percent, respectively, of the 98 patients. Change in morphology, an observation made using both T1- and T2-weighted sequences, also was a specific morphologic pattern and was present in 12 percent of patients with metastatic disease. Neither the doughnut nor the lightbulb signs were tissue-specific; the former was present largely, but not exclusively, with metastatic disease, and the latter always was present with cysts or hemangiomas but also in 9 percent of patients with metastatic disease. The source of the primary tumor among the patients whose metastatic disease was characterized by the lightbulb sign was islet-cell tumors (3), sarcomas (2), carcinoid (1), adenocarcinoma of the pancreas (1), adenocarcinoma of the uterus (1), and unknown (1). Perhaps significant is that the first six of these primary tumors are ones whose metastases are frequently hypervascular.

Overall, 92 percent of the 98 patients with metastases had at least one of the specific morphologic patterns. Ohtomo et al. (6) reported an identical frequency in distinguishing patients with hemangiomas from those with hepatic metastases. Li et al. (9) compared the morphologic patterns observed in 24 hemangiomas with those of 91 metastatic tumors using a 0.35-Tesla superconducting magnet. They found that 26.0 percent of metastatic lesions in 23 percent of patients were indistinguishable from hemangiomas. All 18 hemangiomas smaller than 4 cm were confidently differentiated from metastases, while 5 of the 6 that were larger had irregular outlines or inhomogeneous internal structure. Similar to our observations, they found T2-weighted sequences to be the most accurate. They found that metastases with hemangioma-like morphology originated from primary tumors whose metastases are classically hypervascular (carcinoid, pheochromocytoma, and islet-cell tumor). These accuracy rates compare favorably with the 76.9 percent of patients with metastatic lesions described by Freeny and Marks (10) that had CT enhancement patterns atypical for hemangioma.

Particularly in view of the lack of a need for intravenous enhancement, MRI would seem to be the preferred imaging examination to distinguish metastatic tumor from common benign lesions. If a lesion that has other than lightbulb characteristics is discovered in such a tumor suspect, it can be assumed to be malignant. An ultasound examination should follow the observation of the lightbulb sign to exclude the presence of a cyst. In those patients with known primary lesions, particularly those associated with hypervascular metastases, a dynamic contrast-enhanced CT or ^{99m}Tc red blood cell flow study may be performed followed by a biopsy in other than typically enhancing lesions. In patients lacking a primary tumor, the former options could reasonably be tempered with a follow-up MRI examination in 3 to 6 months. It should be acknowledged that regardless of imaging technique, the accuracy for characterization of lesions less than 1 cm will be less because of partial volume effects.

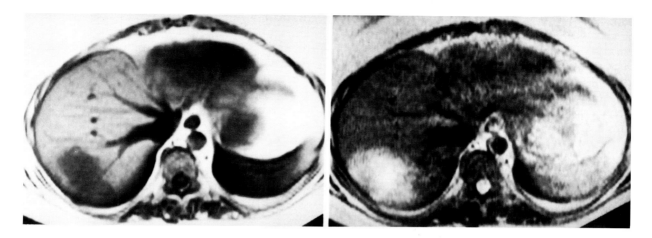

FIGURE 17-7
Changed morphology sign.

TABLE 17-1. Morphologic Patterns Observed on MRI Images in 129 Patients with Hepatic Disease[a]

		Findings	
Morphology of Lesion[b]	Pulse Sequence[c]	Metastatic Disease (n = 98)	Benign Disease (n = 31)
Amorphous	T2W	44 (45%)	0
Doughnut	T1W	27 (28%)	2 (6%)
Target	T2W	26 (27%)	0
Halo	T2W	13 (13%)	0
Change in morphology	T1W and T2W	12 (12%)	0
Lightbulb	T2W	9 (9%)	31 (100%)
Total:		131[a]	33[a]

[a]In 35 patients, more than one morphologic pattern was observed.
[b]See text for a description of each morphologic sign.
[c]T1W = T1-weighted; T2W = T2-weighted.

Source: From Wittenberg J, Stark DD, Forman BH, et al: Differentiation of hepatic metastases from hepatic hemangiomas and cysts by using MR imaging. *AJR* 151:79, 1988. Copyright © by American Roentgen Ray Society. Reprinted by permission of Williams & Wilkins.

Quantitative Criteria

Two studies have evaluated the utility of quantitative data to distinguish mestastases from hemangiomas and differ in their conclusions. Egglin et al. (11), using a 0.6-Tesla superconducting magnet, compared calculated T1 and T2 relaxation times, contrast-to-noise ratios, and signal-intensity ratios measured on spin-echo pulse images. They found by ROC analysis that lesion/liver signal-intensity ratio at 2350/180 was the most accurate in distinguishing hemangiomas from metastases. Utilizing a lesion/liver signal-intensity ratio of 3.5 as the cutoff between hemangiomas and cancer, a specificity of 93 percent and a sensitivity of 89 percent could be achieved using quantitative data alone. While prospectively untested in this analysis, it was felt that quantitative techniques could provide a valuable adjunct to morphologic analysis, particularly for radiologists with less developed skills than expert observers. This thesis was not verified in the study by Li et al. (9) using a 0.35-Tesla superconducting magnet. They found that lesion/liver signal-intensity ratios calculated from both T1-weighted (500/28–30) and T2-weighted (2000/28–150) images contributed very little incremental information beyond that available from morphologic analysis in discriminating between hemangiomas and metastases. Furthermore, their data suggested that more heavily T2-weighted sequences provide no gain in characterization, although admittedly their experience with the latter was small. As with many MRI studies, differences in magnet strength, pulse sequences utilized, and clinical experience make a definitive conclusion impossible. However, the observations of Egglin et al. (11) warrant the performance of a prospective study testing the added utility of quantitative information.

DIFFERENTIATION OF METASTASES FROM PRIMARY HEPATIC TUMORS

Morphologic Criteria

Differentiation of patients with primary hepatic tumors from those with metastases may be less of a problem clinically than radiographically, since the latter most often present with a known primary tumor. However, this problem is more than a theoretical one in endemic areas, where hepatocellular carcinoma complicating cirrhosis accounts worldwide for more than 1 million cases a year (12). Since this distinction is frequently not possible clinically or with available imaging techniques, definite MRI differentiation could make an important contribution.

Tumor encapsulation, steatosis, and a proclivity for vascular invasion seen in hepatocellular carcinoma, singularly or in combination, permit its differentiation from metastases in most instances (7,8,13). A tumor capsule composed of dense fibrous tissue may be identified in 24 to 44 percent of patients with hepatocellular carcinoma (7,8). This finding has not been reported to occur with metastases, although Rummeny et al. (14) have observed it in the rare hepatic adenoma. Characteristically, it is represented on T1-weighted images by a thin hypointense structure surrounding the tumor (7,8) and a double layer of both hypo- and hyperintensity on T2-weighted images (8). On the latter sequences, the outer layer of hyperintensity is thought to be caused by compressed blood vessels and ducts. The steatosis found in 10 to 47 percent of hepatocellular carcinomas is another feature that should be strongly considered as a clue to diagnosis (7,8). This is best appreciated by the relatively bright appearance of steatosis on T1-weighted sequences as a consequence of its shortened T1 relaxation time. Unlike the tumor capsule, this appearance has been observed in the unusual metastases containing fat, blood, or melanin (Fig. 17-8A). However, lipomas or pseudolipomas rarely involve the liver, and hemorrhagic complications of hepatic tumors are more likely to cause focal intralesional abnormalities rather than the diffuse homogeneous appearance of hepatocellular carcinoma seen on T1-weighted pulse sequences. The shortening of the signal intensity in metastatic melanoma is thought to be a consequence of the paramagnetic effect of melanin. A clue to identification, in addition to the presence of a known primary tumor, is that all lesions that are present do not necessarily have this characteristic appearance (Fig. 17-8B). Alternatively, with hepatocellular carcinoma, if the dominant lesion demonstrates high signal intensity, the satellite lesions invariably demonstrate this property. Finally, gross evidence of vascular invasion into either the portal or hepatic veins may be identified on an MRI scan with hepatocellular carcinoma. Rummeny et al. (13) noted this in 6 of 21 patients (29 percent) with hepatocellular carcinoma but not in metastases or other primary hepatic tumors. While it is likely that such invasion does occur at a histologic level in metastases, it remains unresolved by noninvasive imaging techniques.

Careful analysis of the morphologic configuration and signal intensity of the central portion of an inhomogeneous tumor may provide a final differential clue between metastases and primary hepatic tumors. The central necrotic area of a metastasis, while often irregularly shaped, invariably maintains an irregularly rounded, nonradiating configuration, giving rise to the doughnut and target descriptions. The central scar present in a variety of both benign and malignant primary hepatic tumors has a distinctly different appearance (15). Cleft scars have irregular, geometrically shaped borders, while stellate scars demonstrate thin radiating septae projecting to the periphery of the tumor from the similarly configured center. These configurations are apparent on both T1- and T2-weighted images, although their signal intensity varies according to the histologic nature of the scar-forming tissue. In those tumors with collagen-based scars, their appearance is hypointensive relative to

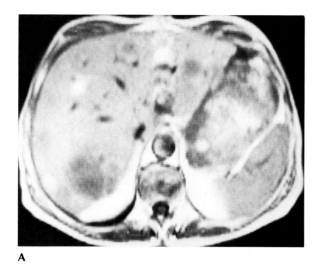
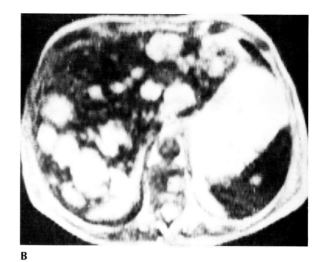

FIGURE 17-8
Melanoma metastases. (A) T1-weighted scan demonstrates several hepatic lesions, some of which have a signal intensity greater than normal liver parenchyma. (B) Ferrite-enhanced delayed scan demonstrates a considerable number of lesions not apparent in (A). Presumably the two higher-intensity lesions apparent with T1 weighting were appreciated because of a paramagnetic effect of a chemical form of melanin not present in the other lesions.

the liver on *both* T1- and T2-weighted sequences (15). Metastases that demonstrate the hypointense center on T1-weighted sequences (doughnut sign) always show a hyperintense signal (target sign) on T2-weighted sequences. The remaining descriptors of metastatic disease considered as specific when compared with hemangiomas and cysts are not as reliable for differentiation from primary hepatic tumors. Peritumoral edema, which gives rise to the charged morphology sign, was noted in 6 of 21 patients (29 percent) with hepatocellular carcinoma and in 2 of 7 patients (28 percent) with cholangiocarcinoma. Furthermore, the lack of malignant specificity for tumors with the halo sign has been established by our observation in a patient with an hepatic adenoma.

Quantitative Criteria
Comparisons of both calculated T1 and T2 values have failed to permit differentiation of metastases from hepatocellular carcinoma. Using midfield systems, both Ohtomo et al. (6) and Ebara et al. (7) demonstrated sufficient statistical overlap to invalidate this approach in individual patients. Rummeny et al. (13) added proton-density measurement to the preceding calculations with a 0.6-Tesla system and similarly concluded that quantitative assessment was not contributory in differentiating a variety of primary hepatic tumors from metastases. Similarly, the lesion/liver signal intensity that Egglin et al. (11) found valuable for differentiating hemangiomas from metastases demonstrated hepatocellular carcinoma to be indistinguishable from a wide variety of metastases. A single study performed at 1.5-Tesla strength has demonstrated that T2 values lack specificity in discriminating metastases from both malignant and benign primary hepatic tumors (16).

INTRAVENOUS CONTRAST ENHANCEMENT
Gadolinium-DTPA has shown progressive promise in elaborating enhancement patterns of hepatic tumors. Since the original description by Carr et al. (17) of intratumoral enhancement, improved injection techniques (18) combined with dynamic scanning (16,19–21) have provided clues to tumor etiology (16,20,21). As with enhanced CT, gadolinium-DTPA enhancement patterns reflect the degree of tumor vascularity, flow dynamics,

and vascular perfusion (16,20,21). Hemangiomas demonstrate early-phase bright enhancement, and most, but not all (21), show continued high signal enhancement with delayed imaging. However, as with CT, some of these MRI characteristics have already been demonstrated with metastases from breast (16), colon, and carcinoid primaries (21).

Iron oxide in the form of AMI-25 (Feridex, Advanced Magnetics, Cambridge, Mass.) is a particulate intravenous superparamagnetic contrast agent which, by virtue of its retention in Kupffer cells, has been shown clinically to improve detection of hepatic tumors (23) (Fig. 17-8B). Recently, Hahn et al. (24) have investigated the potential for this agent to provide etiologic information as well. They compared the effect on the signal-intensity characteristics of tumors during the circulatory phase (first 12 minutes after injection) with the retention phase (1 to 2 hours after administration). In both phases, there was significantly greater accumulation of AMI-25 by hemangiomas than by malignant neoplasms, resulting in a substantially greater loss of signal intensity of the former. Two hypotheses, not mutually exclusive, were apparent: (1) the delayed retention of AMI-25 in vascular channels that characterize the imaging of hemangiomas, and (2) the possibility of iron particle uptake by macrophages in hemangiomas. Either metastases or benign tumors capable of phagocytosis could exhibit sufficient signal loss to be confused with hemangiomas. Vascular tumors will predictably show signal loss in the circulatory phase; however, in those investigated, this was considerably less than with hemangiomas, and their retention-phase signal differences permitted further differentiation. Finally, the authors point out that interpretation of only post-contrast images interferes with recognition of the most characteristic feature of hemangiomas, the very prolonged T2. Given the demonstrable improvement in lesion detection (24), these results warrant further trials with both rapid early and delayed imaging techniques to exploit the potential of AMI-25 to refine differential diagnoses.

An alternative mechanism for exploring the superparamagnetic qualities of iron oxides for hepatic imaging is just emerging. Ultrasmall iron oxide particles (USIOP) of sufficiently small size (average diameter 11 nm) to cross the capillary endothelium have been developed (25), thereby creating a potential for employing these novel particulate pharmaceuticals for MRI receptor imaging. Such a strategy has been successfully accomplished in imaging asialoglycoprotein (ASG) receptors in the rat liver (26). Experiments with an ASG-targeted agent labeled with USIOP demonstrate selective accumulation in the liver (but not in the spleen) of particles bound to hepatocyte surface membranes. In vivo imaging demonstrates a signal-intensity decrease in the liver considerably larger than that observed with AMI-25 at equal doses. While the ultimate utility of this agent remains to be demonstrated for the same receptors in humans, its importance lies in the demonstration that specific receptor and potentially antibody-directed imaging may be feasible with this powerful new agent.

REFERENCES

1. Gilbert HA, Kagan AR: Metastases: Incidence, detection, and evaluation without histologic confirmation, in Weiss L (ed): Fundamental Aspects of Metastases. Amsterdam, North-Holland, 1976.
2. Scharschmidt BF: Hepatic tumors, in Wyngaarden JB, Smith LH (eds): Cecil's Textbook of Medicine. Philadelphia, Saunders, 1985.
3. Ishak KG, Rabin L: Benign tumors of the liver. Med Clin North Am 59:995, 1975.
4. Wittenberg J, Stark DD, Forman BH, et al: Differentiation of hepatic metastases from hepatic hemangiomas and cysts by using MR imaging. AJR 151:79, 1988.
5. Thoeni RF: MRI assists diagnoses of focal liver disease. Diagn Imaging October:102, 1989.
6. Ohtomo K, Itai Y, Furui S, et al: Hepatic tumors: Differentiation by transverse relaxation time (T2) of magnetic resonance imaging. Radiology 155:421, 1985.
7. Ebara M, Ohto M, Watanabe Y, et al: Diagnosis of small hepatocellular carcinoma: Correlation of MR imaging and tumor histologic studies. Radiology 159:371, 1986.
8. Itoh K, Nishimura K, Togashi K, et al: Hepatocellular carcinoma: MR imaging. Radiology 164:21, 1987.
9. Li KC, Glazer GM, Quint LE, et al: Distinction of hepatic cavernous hemangiomas from hepatic metastases with MR imaging. Radiology 160:613, 1986.
10. Freeny PC, Marks WM: Patterns of contrast enhancement of benign and malignant hepatic neoplasms during bolus dynamic and delayed CT. Radiology 160:613, 1986.

11. Egglin TK, Rummeny E, Stark DD, et al: Hepatic tumors: Quantitative tissue characterization with MR imaging. Radiology 176:107, 1990.
12. Weissleder R, Stark DD: MRI of the liver, in Silverman PM, Zeman RK, (eds): CT and MRI of the Liver and Biliary System. New York, Churchill-Livingstone, 1990.
13. Rummeny E, Weissleder R, Stark DD, et al: Primary liver tumors: Diagnosis by MR imaging. AJR 152:63, 1989.
14. Rummeny E, Saini S, Wittenberg J, et al: MR imaging of liver neoplasms. AJR 152:493, 1989.
15. Rummeny E, Weissleder R, Sironi S, et al: Central scars in primary liver tumors: MR features, specificity and pathologic correlation. Radiology 171:323, 1989.
16. Van Beers B, Demeine R, Pringot J, et al: Dynamic spin-echo imaging with Gd-DTPA: Value in the differentiation of hepatic tumors. AJR 154:515, 1990.
17. Carr DH, Brown J, Bydder GM, et al: Gadolinium-DTPA as a contrast agent in MRI: Initial clinical experience in 20 patients. AJR 143:215, 1984.
18. Hamm B, Wolf KJ, Felix R: Conventional and rapid MR imaging of the liver with Gd-DTPA. Radiology 164:313, 1987.
19. Saini S, Stark DD, Brady TJ, et al: Dynamic-spin echo MRI of liver cancer using gadolinium-DTPA: Animal investigation. AJR 147:357, 1986.
20. Ohtomo K, Itai Y, Yoshikawa K, et al: Hepatic tumors: Dynamic MR imaging. Radiology 163:27, 1987.
21. Edelman RR, Siegel JB, Singer A, et al: Dynamic MR imaging of the liver with Gd-DTPA: Initial clinical results. AJR 153:1213, 1989.
22. Freeny PC, Marks WM, Patterns of contrast enhancement of benign and malignant hepatic neoplasms during bolus dynamic and delayed CT. Radiology 160:613, 1988.
23. Stark DD, Weissleder R, Elizondo G, et al: Superparamagnetic iron oxide: Clinical application as a contrast agent for MR imaging of the liver. Radiology 168:297, 1988.
24. Hahn PF, Stark DD, Weissleder R, et al: Clinical application of superparamagnetic iron oxide to MR imaging of tissue perfusion in vascular liver tumors. Radiology 174:361, 1990.
25. Weissleder R, Elizondo G, Wittenberg J, et al: Ultrasmall superparamagnetic iron oxide: Characterization of a new class of contrast agents for MR imaging. Radiology 175:489, 1990.
26. Weissleder R, Reimer P, Lee AS, MR receptor imaging: Ultrasmall iron oxide particles targeted to asialosyloglycoprotein receptors. AJR (in press).

18

Hepatocellular Carcinoma: CT and MRI

KUNI OHTOMO,
YUJI ITAI, and
YASUHITO SASAKI

Computed tomography (CT) has been widely accepted as an indispensable modality for the diagnosis of hepatic masses, including hepatocellular carcinoma (hepatoma) (1–3). With recent technical improvements, MRI has been applied for imaging of the abdomen. However, its clinical role is not yet established. In this short review, we present CT and MRI appearances of hepatoma, with particular reference to radiologic-pathologic correlation including some pitfalls of differential diagnosis.

MACROSCOPIC CLASSIFICATION

Hepatoma is classified into three types macroscopically: diffuse, massive, and nodular. Tumor extent of ill-defined diffuse hepatomas is not clearly demonstrated on CT and MRI (Fig. 18-1). In massive hepatomas, CT usually shows a mass only partially. Although the number of the cases studied is limited, MRI demonstrates a massive lesion more clearly because of its excellent soft-tissue contrast (Fig. 18-2).

Nodular hepatomas have some distinct CT and MRI appearances that are useful for differential diagnosis. At CT scanning, nodular hepatomas mostly appear as hypodense masses surrounded by more hypodense rims. They are also seen as areas of low density on late postcontrast CT scans. Late enhancement is shown within the hypo-

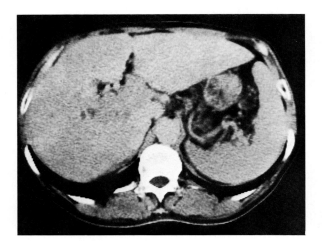

FIGURE 18-1
Diffuse hepatoma. Contrast CT shows tumor thrombus within the dilated portal vein. Tumor extent is not directly visualized.

dense rims and internal septal strands. About 50 to 60 percent of nodular hepatomas are iso- or hyperintense on T1-weighted MRI images, and over 90 percent are hyperintense on T2-weighted images. Hypointense rims are seen around the masses on T1-weighted images, and these rims are sometimes seen as double rings on T2-weighted images,

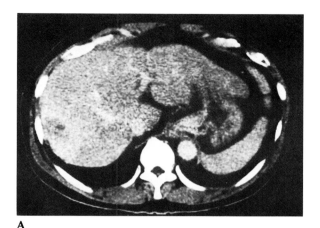
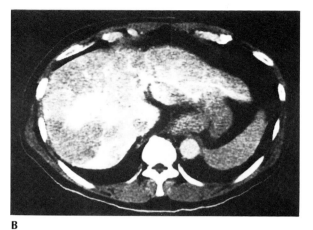
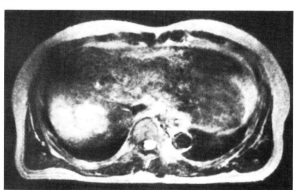

FIGURE 18-2
Massive hepatoma. (A) Contrast CT shows a small ill-defined low-density area in the right lobe of the liver. (B) CT obtained during arterial portography reveals a larger filling defect, the size of which corresponds to that of a hyperintense mass shown on a T2-weighted MRI image (C) Spin echo (SE) (TR/TE: 2000/90 ms).

that is, hypointense inner rings and hyperintense outer rings (Fig. 18-3). The inner ring corresponds to pure fibrotic capsule and the outer to compressed liver parenchyma containing prominent vascular spaces (4).

MICROSCOPIC CLASSIFICATION

Hepatomas are classified into four subtypes: trabecular, pseudoglandular, compact, and scirrhous. These subtypes may coexist within a single nodular mass. Within these types, MRI appearances of pure pseudoglandular hepatomas mimick those of cavernous hemangiomas (5,6). They appear homogeneously hyperintense on T2-weighted images (Fig. 18-4). This high intensity is probably due to serous fluid within pseudoglandular structures.

Compact hepatomas consist of dominant cellular components and lack sinusoid-like vascular spaces. These masses sometimes appear hypovascular on hepatic arteriography and dynamic CT. Well-differentiated hepatomas (Edmondson I) have been reported to be hypovascular. CT obtained after iodinated oil (Lipiodol) by means of a catheter introduced into the hepatic artery (Lipiodol CT) usually shows no or little deposits of iodinated oil within these hypovascular hepatomas.

SECONDARY CHANGES

Hepatomas manifest various secondary changes within the masses. They include fatty degeneration, hemorrhage, and necrosis. Fatty components within nodular hepatomas are seen as areas of low density (CT numbers under 0 HU) on CT and of high intensity on T1-weighted MRI images (Fig. 18-5). Initially, fatty degeneration was suggested as the only cause of high intensity on T1-weighted images (7). However, recent studies have revealed that nodular hepatomas without fatty degeneration may also appear hyperintense on T1-weighted images (Fig. 18-6). Further study

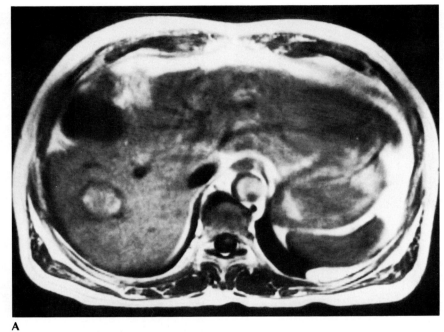
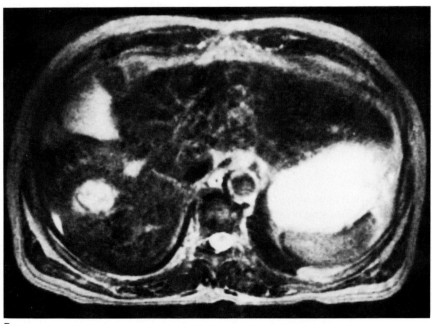

FIGURE 18-3
Nodular hepatoma. A mass in the right lobe appears hyperintense on T1-weighted (A: SE, 600/17) and T2-weighted (B: SE,2000/90) images. A hypointense rim around the mass is hypointense on the T1-weighted image and is seen as a double ring on the T2-weighted image.

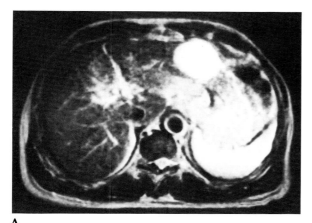
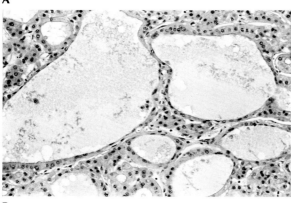

FIGURE 18-4
Pseudoglandular hepatoma. (A) A mass in the lateral segment is homogeneously hyperintense on a T2-weighted image (SE,2000/90). (B) Dense and homogeneous pseudoglandular structures are seen within the mass microscopically (H & E stain; original magnification × 50). (From Ohtomo K, Itai Y, Matuoka Y, et al: Hepatocellular carcinoma: MR appearance mimicking cavernous hemangioma. J Comput Assist Tomogr 14:650, 1990. Reprinted by permission.)

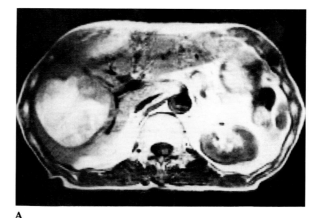
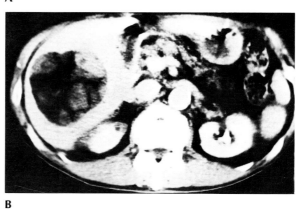

FIGURE 18-5
Nodular hepatoma with fatty degeneration. A mass in the right lobe contains fatty components that are hypodense on plain CT (A) and hyperintense on a T1-weighted image (B: SE,600/17).

is needed to determine pathologic causes of high intensity on T1-weighted images apart from fatty degeneration.

Recent hemorrhage within hepatomas may also be hyperintense on T1-weighted images. On T2-weighted images, hemorrhagic areas usually contain high and low intensities. This mixed intensity probably corresponds to the presence of various metabolites of hemoglobin. Old hemorrhage within hepatomas is hypointense on T1-weighted and T2-weighted images due to magnetic susceptibility of hemosiderin.

External rupture is one of the most serious complications of hepatomas. CT demonstrates hemoperitoneum or regional hyperdense hematoma (Fig. 18-7). MRI also shows the extent of hemorrhage. However, CT is more suitable for this kind of emergency.

In comparison with necrosis, which causes hyperintensity on T2-weighted images, hepatomas with coagulation necrosis appear hypointense on T2-weighted images. Coagulation necrosis is generally seen within hepatomas that have been effectively treated by embolization (Fig. 18-8). Since recurrent foci are seen as areas of high intensity

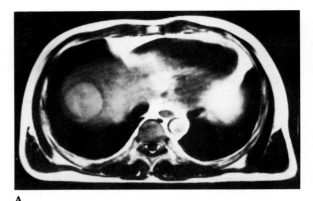

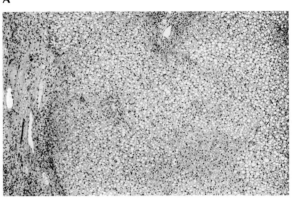

FIGURE 18-6
Nodular hepatoma without fatty degeneration. (A) A mass in the right lobe is hyperintense on a T1-weighted image (SE,600/17). (B) Microscopic examination reveals fatty deposits within the surrounding cirrhotic liver (H & E stain; original magnification × 10) and no fatty degeneration within the mass.

on T2-weighted images, MRI has been reported to be useful for follow-up of patients with hepatomas treated by embolization (8).

DYNAMIC STUDY

Dynamic CT using a bolus injection of iodinated contrast material has played an important role in the diagnosis of hepatomas. Dynamic MRI study is also obtainable in conjunction with serial quick scannings and a bolus injection of gadolinium(Gd)-DTPA (9). Patterns of enhancement of these two examinations are essentially the same because of correspondence of the pharmacokinetics of these

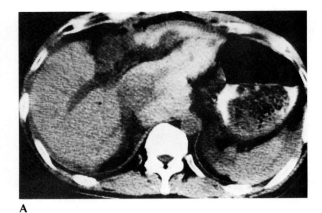

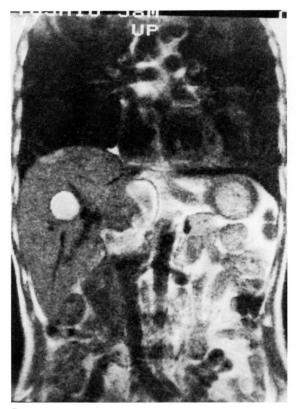

FIGURE 18-7
Ruptured nodular hepatoma. (A) Hyperdense hematoma derived from a ruptured hepatoma in the caudate lobe is seen within the lesser sac on plain CT. (B) A T1-weighted coronal image also reveals the extent of the hematoma around the mass (SE,600/17).

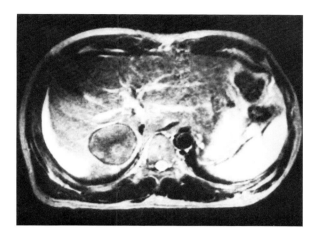

FIGURE 18-8
Nodular hepatoma treated by embolization. A mass in the right lobe is iso- and hypointense on a T2-weighted image (SE,2000/90). This mass has been treated by transcatheter arterial embolization, and a hepatic arteriogram (not shown) that was obtained at the same period with the MRI examination reveals no tumor stain. A thick hypointense rim around the mass probably corresponds to a capsule with reactive granulation.

two contrast materials. Nodular hepatomas usually manifest dense and transient enhancement of early phases of dynamic studies.

Dynamic study is also useful because cavernous hemangiomas show characteristic enhancement, i.e., dense and spreading (high-density fill-in or high-intensity fill-in) (Fig. 18-9). However, we have had one nodular hepatoma that showed dense and spreading enhancement (Fig. 18-10). This case shows that there is no rule without exception.

Another more critical shortcoming of dynamic study is slice misregistration due to different level breath-holding. This problem is more critical in small masses. To overcome this shortcoming, analysis of late phases is quite important. In our experience, MRI is more suitable to analyze the late phase because faint enhancement is more clearly demonstrated on MRI than on CT. When the hemangioma pattern is defined as hypointense on precontrast T1-weighted images and iso- or hyperintense on postcontrast images, 90 percent of hepatomas and hemangiomas are correctly classified without dynamic study (10).

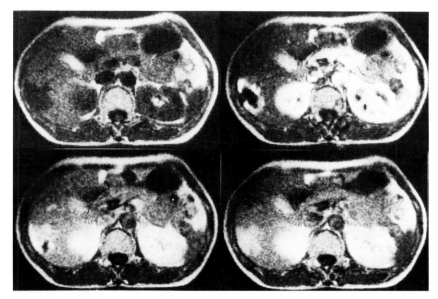

FIGURE 18-9
Cavernous hemangioma. Dynamic MRI using a bolus injection of 0.05 mmol/kg Gd-DTPA reveals dense spreading enhancement and complete high-intensity fill-in (spin-echo images, TR/TE 100/20 ms; upper right: precontrast; upper left: immediately after; lower left: 2 min after; lower right: 5 min after the administration of Gd-DTPA). (From Ohtomo K, Itai Y, Yoshikawa K, et al: Hepatic tumors: Dynamic MR imaging. Radiology 163:27, 1987. Reprinted by permission).

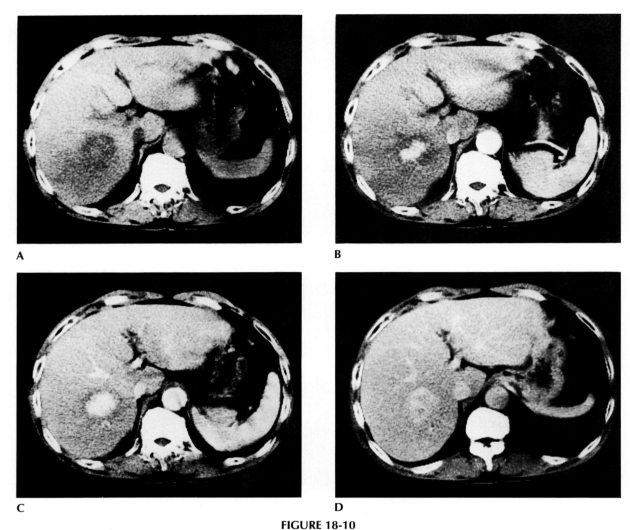

FIGURE 18-10
Nodular hepatoma. Dense spreading enhancement is revealed within a mass in the right lobe. (A) Precontrast CT. (B) Immediately after. (C) One minute after. (D) Five minutes after the administration of iodinated contrast material.

PITFALLS OF DIFFERENTIAL DIAGNOSIS: TUMOR-LIKE CONDITIONS

Adenomatous hyperplasias have been suggested to be one of the precursors of hepatomas. They are hypovascular on hepatic arteriography and are not seen as filling defects on CT obtained during arterial portography because they usually receive blood from the portal venous system. Adenomatous hyperplasias are hyperintense on T1-weighted images and hypointense on T2-weighted images. MRI appearances of adenomatous hyperplasias differ from those of typical nodular hepatomas, although hypovascular hepatomas cannot be ruled out. Malignant foci accompanying adenomatous hyperplasia have been reported to appear hyperintense within the surrounding hypointense hyperplastic lesion on T2-weighted images (11).

Round fatty infiltrations are hypodense on CT. Little enhancement is revealed on postcontrast CT. They are hyperintense on T1-weighted images and isointense on T2-weighted images. Pathologic examination is needed for the final diagnosis, especially when they are discovered among patients with risk factors for hepatomas (diffuse liver disease, hepatitis-B antigen carrier, and/or slight elevation of serum alpha-feto-protein level).

CONCLUSION

CT is quite useful for the detection and differentiation of hepatomas. MRI cannot replace CT at the present time, although the latter provides additional information on pathologic features of nodular hepatomas. Accumulated clinical experience shows that there is no rule without exception.

REFERENCES

1. Itai Y, Araki T, Furui S, et al: Differential diagnosis of hepatic masses on computed tomography, with particular reference to hepatocellular carcinoma. J Comput Assist Tomogr 5:834, 1985.
2. Araki T, Itai Y, Furui S, et al: Dynamic CT densitometry of hepatic tumors. AJR 135:1037, 1980.
3. Itai Y, Moss A, Goldberg HI: Transient hepatic attenuation difference of lobar or segmental distrbution detected by dynamic computed tomography. Radiology 144:835, 1982.
4. Itoh K, Nishimura K, Togashi K, et al: Hepatocellular carcinoma: MR imaging. Radiology 164:21, 1987.
5. Stark DD, Felder RC, Wittenberg J, et al: Magnetic resonance imaging of cavernous hemangioma of the liver: Tissue-specific characterization. AJR 145:213, 1985.
6. Ohtomo K, Itai Y, Matuoka Y, et al: Hepatocellular carcinoma: MR appearance mimicking cavernous hemangioma. J Compt Assist Tomogr 14:650, 1990.
7. Ebara M, Ohto M, Watanabe Y, et al: Diagnosis of small hepatocellular carcinoma: Correlation of MR imaging and tumor histologic studies. Radiology 159:371, 1986.
8. Yoshioka H, Nakagawa K, Shindou H, et al: MR imaging of hepatocellular carcinoma following transcatheter hepatic chemo-embolization (abstract in English). Nippon Acta Radiol 49:119, 1989.
9. Ohtomo K, Itai Y, Yoshikawa K, et al: Hepatic tumors: Dynamic MR imaging. Radiology 163:27, 1987.
10. Okada Y, Itai Y, Ohtomo K, et al: MR imaging of cavernous hemangioma of the liver: Differentiation with T1-weighted images with Gd-DTPA. Radiology 173(P):271, 1989.
11. Matsui O, Kadoya M, Kameyama T, et al: Adenomatous hyperplastic nodules in the cirrhotic liver: Differentiation from hepatocellular carcinoma with MR imaging. Radiology 173:123, 1989.

19

Differentiation of Malignant Liver Tumors by Subsecond Dynamic CT

R. LANGER, M. LANGER, C. ZWICKER,
F. ASTINET, and R. FELIX

Different types of malignant liver tumors show similar contrast medium enhancement patterns in conventional CT studies. The purpose of this prospective study was to determine specific criteria of contrast medium enhancement for the differentiation of liver malignancies using bolus-enhanced subsecond dynamic CT (angio-CT).

PATIENTS AND METHODS

Sixty patients with different primary and secondary malignant hepatic tumors were included in our prospective study. These included 25 patients with hepatocellular carcinoma (HCC), 14 patients with cholangio- and gallbladder carcinoma (CAC), and 21 patients with metastases of different primaries. All tumors were proven histologically by surgery or percutaneous ultrasound- or CT-guided biopsy. The CT scanner used was the Somatom Plus (Siemens, Erlangen, FRG), with a continuous tube rotation, a scanning time of 0.7 or 1 s, 170 to 250 mA, an interscan delay of 1 s or more, and a high-resolution screen matrix of 1024 × 1024 pixels. The slice thickness chosen was 10 mm. The contrast material was applied by a computer-triggered injector.

All patients were examined using the following protocol:

1. Unenhanced CT study of the whole liver, 0.7- or 1-s scanning time per slice.
2. Fast single-level dynamic CT (angio-CT) at the level of the largest tumor mass with an injection of 80 ml Iopromide 370 (flow rate 4 ml/s). The angio-CT scan series was started 10 s after the beginning of the contrast medium injection. Fifteen scans were obtained with an interscan delay of 1 s, followed by single scans every 10 s up to 1 min and 2, 3, and 5 min after the start of contrast medium application. In patients with suspected multifocal hepatocellular carcinoma, two contrast medium boluses at two different table positions were applied (2 × 60 ml Iopromide 370, flow rate 4 ml/s).
3. Incremental bolus-enhanced CT of the whole liver and entire abdomen during a continuous contrast medium injection of 100 ml contrast material with a flow rate of 1 or 2 ml/s.

All angio-CTs were analyzed quantitatively using time-density curves with regions of interest (ROIs) placed in normal liver tissue, abdominal aorta, and the most vascularized part of the tumor.

In addition two ratios were calculated, based on sequential computer-assisted image analysis:

$$T = \frac{\text{time to peak (lesion)} - \text{time to peak (aorta)}}{\text{time to peak (liver)} - \text{time to peak (aorta)}}$$

$$D = \frac{\text{relative maximum enhancement (tumor)}}{\text{relative maximum enhancement (liver)}}.$$

Time to peak measurement was normalized to the time to peak of the abdominal aorta in order to minimize the effects of circulatory factors.

T values of less than 1 indicate a faster tumor contrast enhancement compared with normal liver tissue; T values of greater than 1 indicate a slower enhancement. D quantifies the maximum enhancement of the lesion in comparison with the normal liver. D was measured in the most enhanced portions of the tumors.

Statistical analysis was carried out with the student's t test for unpaired groups. Image quality of the tumor delineation was determined qualitatively for all studies (unenhanced, angio-, and incremental dynamic studies).

RESULTS

Twenty-four of the HCCs were hypervascular during the arterial phase (Fig. 19-1); one was hypovascular. T was 0.34 ± 0.3, and D was 1.3 ± 0.3 (Table 19-1). The low T is due to a short time to peak (Fig. 19-2) in the most hypervascularized parts of the tumors compared with normal liver tissue. The maximum enhancement of the tumor was slightly higher than in the surrounding liver parenchyma.

All bile duct and gallbladder carcinomas were hypovascular (Fig. 19-3) and demonstrated a substantially slower time to peak ($T = 3.2 \pm 1.7$) and a reduced maximum enhancement of the tumor in relation to the liver parenchyma. The differences between both entities were statistically significant with a confidence level of $p < 0.05$ (student's t test).

For metastases, a considerable variability of T was present due to the heterogeneity of the different primary malignancies ($T = 2.4 \pm 2.6$). In 19 of the 21 patients with metastases, lesions were hypovascular (Fig. 19-4). Two patients with metastatic gastrinoma and carcinoid showed hypervascular masses (Fig. 19-5).

Differences between T and D were significant for the mean values between the metastases and HCCs ($p < 0.05$), but not between the metastases and the CACs. The hypervascular metastases of gastrinoma and carcinoid showed T and D values similar to HCC. All studies were diagnostic. Image quality was excellent in 79 to 88 percent and good in 12 to 21 percent of the angio-CT studies (Table 19-2).

DISCUSSION

The differentiation of benign and malignant liver tumors by their contrast enhancement patterns

TABLE 19-1. *T- and D-Ratios for HCCs, CACs, and Metastases*

HCC ($n = 25$):
  $T = 0.34 \pm 0.3$
  $D = 1.3 \pm 0.3$
CAC ($n = 14$):
  $T = 3.2 \pm 1.7$
  $D = 0.8 \pm 0.2$
Metastases ($n = 21$):
  $T = 2.4 \pm 2.6$
  $D = 0.6 \pm 0.3$

TABLE 19-2. *Image Quality for HCC, CAC, and Metastases*

	Unenhanced CT	Angio-CT	Incremental Dynamic CT
HCC ($n = 25$):			
−	6	0	0
(+)	11	0	8
+	8	3	11
+ +	0	22	6
CAC ($n = 14$):			
−	1	0	0
(+)	3	0	1
+	10	3	7
+ +	0	11	6
Metastases ($n = 21$):			
−	1	0	0
(+)	7	0	0
+	13	3	3
+ +	0	18	18

Note: −: no delineation between lesion(s) and normal liver tissue; (+): poor delineation between lesion(s) and liver; +: good delineation between lesion(s) and liver; and + +: excellent delineation between lesion(s) and liver.

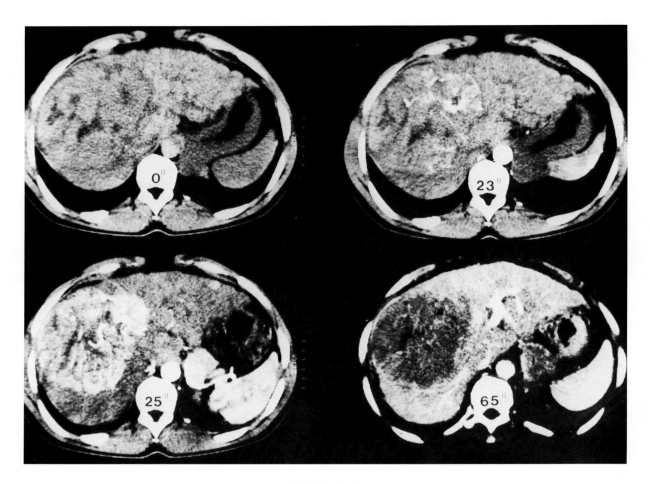

FIGURE 19-1

Hepatocellular carcinoma in liver cirrhosis, angio-CT. 0", unenhanced CT: hypodense mass in the right liver lobe, surrounded by a capsule. Necrotic areas are seen within the tumor. 23" (after the start of the contrast medium injection, start of the scan with 10-s delay), early arterial phase. Tumor appears hyperperfused beginning in the periphery. Tumor vessels are already enhanced. 25", arterial phase. Markedly hyperdense tumor with persistent tumor vessel enhancement. Note satellite in the lateral segment of the left lobe. Tumor and satellite are hyperdense compared with the adjacent liver tissue. 65", portal venous phase. Tumor is hypodense compared with the surrounding liver tissue with persistent peripheral enhancement.

has been studied since abdominal CT was introduced into clinical practice. Among the many different variables studied have been different intravenous contrast material injection techniques, but also more invasive CT modalities, such as CT during hepatic arteriography (CT-HA) and CT during arterial portography (CT-AP) (1–10). In comparison with these more invasive CT procedures, intravenous contrast medium injection by a computer-triggered injector for single-level subsecond dynamic CT (angio-CT) is less invasive (4,9,10). The major advantage of the subsecond CT scanner is that a larger number of scans can be obtained during the arterial phase, using a scanning time of 0.7 s and an interscan delay of less than 1 s. The clinical usefulness of these scanning

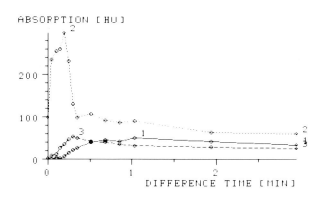

FIGURE 19-2
Time-density curve of the same patient as in Fig. 19-1 with HCC (0: start of the CT scan with 10-s delay p.i.); 1: normal liver; 2: abdominal aorta, 3: tumor.

parameters has been demonstrated for posttransplant evaluation of arterial liver perfusion, especially in patients with suspected arterial anastomotic complications (4,9,10).

Our results point out that there are also diagnostic advantages in analyzing the arterial perfusion of liver tumors when compared with results obtainable with conventional CT scanners. HCCs typically show hyperperfusion, starting in the early arterial phase, with a peak at 25 ± 2 s, lasting up to 40 s after the beginning of the contrast medium injection, whereas they are hypodense during the portal venous phase.

In the early arterial phase, the tumor-supplying arteries also can be visualized by this method in most cases. Our results demonstrate clearly that hypervascular HCCs can be easily differentiated from CACs and hypovascular metastases by time-density curves and calculated T ratios in addition to their morphologic appearance. On the other hand, HCCs cannot be differentiated from hypervascular metastases by the perfusion studies alone. A similar contrast enhancement pattern for HCCs and hypervascular metastases also was reported by Foley (2).

CACs cannot be differentiated from hypovascular metastases. For this differentiation, the patient's history, clinical data, laboratory findings, and morphologic CT criteria must be taken into consideration. There also was a considerable overlap in the T values of metastases and the rare type of small hypovascular HCC. For the differential diagnosis of these two entities, the best imaging procedure seems to be ultrasound, where a typically echoic appearance has been demonstrated by Yoshimatsu et al. (8). As pointed out by several authors (11,12), CT is superior to other

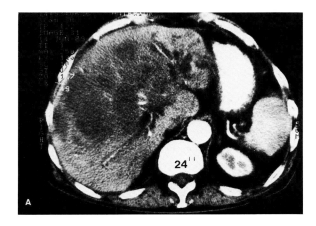 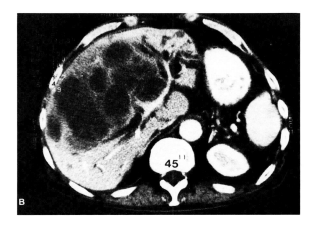

FIGURE 19-3
Infiltrating gallbladder carcinoma with bile duct obstruction and metastases. (A) 24", early arterial phase. Only contrast enhancement of intrahepatic arterial branches is seen. Hypodense tumor is evident. (B) 45", early portal venous phase. Hypodense infiltrating tumor with better delineation of the bile duct obstruction is visible.

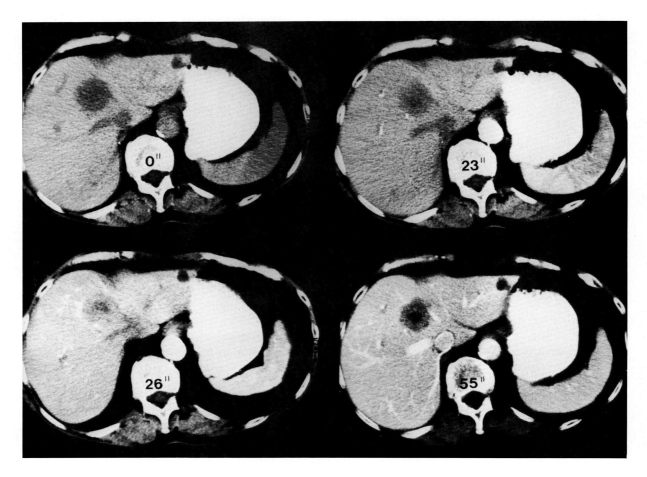

FIGURE 19-4
Metastases of a colonic cancer. 0", unenhanced CT. Multiple hypodense lesions. 23", early arterial phase. No enhancement of the metastases. 26", later arterial phase. Slight peripheral perfusion of the large metastasis adjacent to the falciform ligament. Note better demarcation of the other lesions. 55", early portal venous phase. Metastases remain hypodense in relation to the surrounding liver parenchyma.

imaging modalities, such as MRI or ultrasound, for demonstrating extrahepatic spread of malignant tumors.

CONCLUSIONS

1. Angio-CT is able to distinguish hypervascular HCC from CAC and gallbladder carcinoma and hypovascular metastases.
2. For the differentiation between HCC and hypervascular metastases, and for the differential diagnosis between CAC and hypovascular metastatic lesions, morphologic criteria must be taken into consideration in addition to the perfusion studies.
3. Hypovascular HCC cannot be differentiated from other hepatic malignancies by fast single-level dynamic CT.

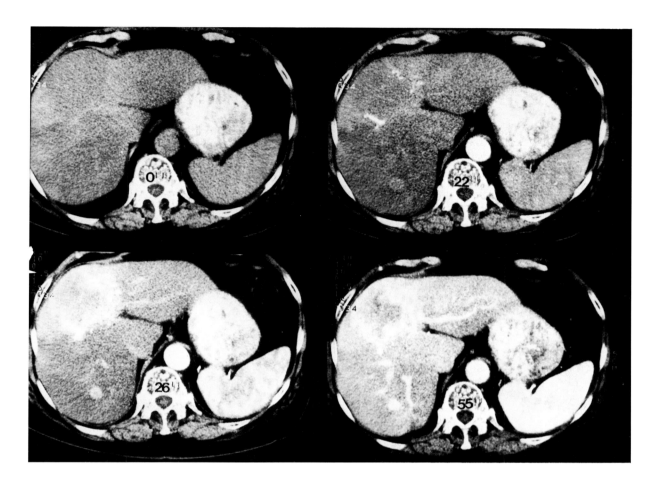

FIGURE 19-5
Hypervascular metastases of a carcinoid. 0″, unenhanced CT. Inhomogeneous liver parenchyma without distinct delineation of individual lesions. 22″, early arterial phase. Peripheral perfusion of the large metastasis adjacent to the falciform ligament. Small metastasis in the posterior right lobe appears homogeneously hyperdense. 26″, later arterial phase. Increasing hyperdensity of both metastases, beginning demarcation of another metastasis in the left lobe. 55″, late arterial/early portal venous phase. Persistent hyperdensity of the metastases and hypodense center of the largest metastasis are apparent.

REFERENCES

1. Claussen C, Lochner B: Dynamische Computertomographie. Berlin, Springer-Verlag, 1983.
2. Foley W: Dynamic hepatic CT. Radiology 170:617, 1989.
3. Freeny PC, Mark WM: Computed tomographic arteriography of the liver. Radiology 148: 193–197, 1983.
4. Langer M, Zwicker C, Langer R, et al: Dynamic CT of the liver and pancreas with a new subsecond scanner and a computerized contrast medium injector. Radiology 173:146, 1989.
5. Miller DL, Simons JT, Chang R, et al: Hepatic metastasis detection: Comparison of three contrast enhancement methods. Radiology 165:785, 1987.
6. Nelson RC, Chezmar JL, Sugarbaker PH, et al: Hepatic tumors: Comparison of CT during arterial portography, delayed CT and MR imaging for preoperative evaluation. Radiology 172:27, 1989.

7. Schild H, Mildenberger P, Schweden F, et al: Leber-CT mit portalvenöser Kontrastmittelgabe. RöFo 147:623, 1987.
8. Yoshimatsu S, Inoue Y, Ibukuro K, et al: Hypovascular hepatocellular carcinoma, undetected at angiography and CT with iodized oil. Radiology 171:343, 1989.
9. Zwicker C, Langer M, Astinet F, et al: Dynamic CT of malignant liver tumors and liver transplants, in Fuchs WA (ed): Advances in CT. Berlin, Springer-Verlag, 1990.
10. Zwicker C, Langer M, Astinet F, et al: Differenzierung maligner Lebertumoren mit schneller dynamischer CT. RöFo 152:293, 1990.
11. Bernardino M: Lesion Detection by MRI and CT. Comparative Studies, Emory experience. Presented at "Liver Imaging," International Symposium, Boston, June 1990.
12. Chezmar JL, Rumancik WM, Megibow AJ, et al: Liver and abdominal screening in patients with cancer: CT versus MR imaging. Radiology 168:43, 1988.

VII. TISSUE CHARACTERIZATION: BENIGN TUMORS

20

Benign Tumors of the Liver

DIDIER MATHIEU and
ELIE SERGE ZAFRANI

The normal liver is composed of various epithelial and mesenchymal cells, and benign tumors may develop from each of these cells. Benign proliferation of the hepatocytes leads to hepatocellular adenoma (HA), whereas bile duct adenoma and biliary cystadenoma result from the neoplastic growth of biliary cells. In focal nodular hyperplasia (FNH), hepatocyte as well as biliary structure proliferation is observed. These epithelial lesions are much rarer than hepatic hemangioma, which develops from endothelial cells and constitutes the most frequent benign tumor of the liver (1,2). Other mesenchymal tumors include leiomyomas, fibromas, and lipomas, which arise from smooth-muscle cells, fibrocytes, and adipocytes, respectively (3,4). Some tumors are comprised of various cell types, e.g., angiolipomas or angiomyolipomas (3,4).

The purpose of this chapter is to focus on the main pathologic and radiologic features of benign epithelial tumors of the liver in adults. These entities raise several questions concerning their pathogenesis and their differential diagnosis from various malignant tumors or pseudotumoral lesions of the liver. Hepatic hemangiomas will be extensively detailed in another chapter of this book, and other mesenchymal tumors will not be further considered because of their extreme rarity (3,4).

FOCAL NODULAR HYPERPLASIA

Focal nodular hyperplasia is a rare benign tumor of the liver that is usually discovered fortuitously during physical examination, abdominal imaging workup, or at laparotomy. This lesion, which has also been referred to as *focal cirrhosis, hepatic hamartoma,* or *mixed adenoma,* should be considered a tumor-like malformation rather than a neoplasm (5). Wanless et al. (5) have indeed suggested that FNH was secondary to an arterial malformation leading to a hyperplastic response of the liver parenchyma due to increased blood flow. This vascular theory is supported by the association of FNH with other vascular abnormalities, such as telangiectases, hereditary hemorrhagic telangiectasia, arteriovenous malformations, and anomalous pulmonary drainage. The association with hepatic hemangioma could represent an additional argument for this theory. In a recent study including 27 patients with HA and 26 patients with FNH, we have demonstrated the presence of hemangioma on the basis of ultrasonography (US), dynamic CT, and pathologic findings in 23 percent of the patients with FNH and in none of the patients with HA (2). The hemangiomas associated with FNH varied in size, ranging from 1.5 to 4 cm, and were located close to or at a distance from the FNH. This association has previously been described in occasional reports and

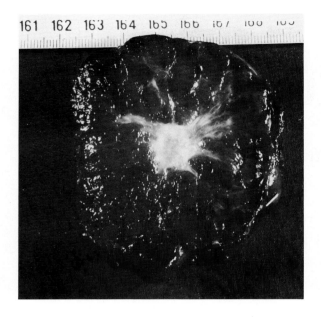

FIGURE 20-1
Focal nodular hyperplasia. Cut section of the tumor shows the characteristic central stellate scar with radiating fibrous septa.

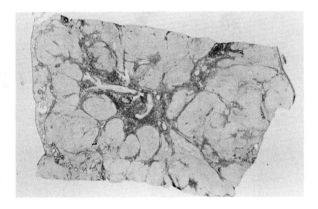

FIGURE 20-2
Focal nodular hyperplasia. Microscopic examination shows that the branches of the central stellate fibrous scar irradiate toward the periphery of the tumor and completely or incompletely delineate hepatocyte nodules. Vascular sections are seen within the central scar.

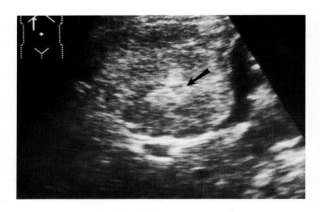

FIGURE 20-3
Focal nodular hyperplasia. Sonography. Hyperechoic structure within the mass corresponding to the central scar (arrow).

incidentally noted in an autopsy study in which single or multiple small cavernous hemangiomas were observed in 7 of 34 cases (21 percent) of FNH (6). It is noteworthy that the prevalence of hemangioma found in our series was very similar to that observed in this autopsy study and markedly higher than the prevalence of 0.7 to 7 percent noted in the general population (7).

Focal nodular hyperplasia occurs in both sexes and at all ages (3,8,9), but most of the cases have been reported in 20- to 50-year-old adults (3,8). In addition, females outnumber males by two or more to one (3,8). Although the responsibility of estroprogestatives in the occurrence of the lesion has not been demonstrated, it is very probable that these agents or endogenous estrogens play a role in its enlargement and complications (8,10,11).

In 80 percent of the cases, FNH is a solitary nodule and its macroscopic appearance is highly characteristic (Fig. 20-1). The mass is usually globular, lobulated, and well circumscribed, although unencapsulated. Its color is lighter than the surrounding normal liver. The pathognomonic gross feature is the presence, on cut sections, of a central stellate scar with radiating fibrous septa dividing the lesion into nodules (Fig. 20-1). The tumor is usually small. Among 130 patients with FNH, 110 (84 percent) had a single nodule measuring less than 5 cm in diameter, 16 (13 percent) had a tumor between 5 and 10 cm, and only 4 (3 percent) had a lesion greater than 10 cm (8).

Microscopic examination shows the central stellate fibrous scar irradiating toward the periphery of the tumor and dividing the hyperplastic

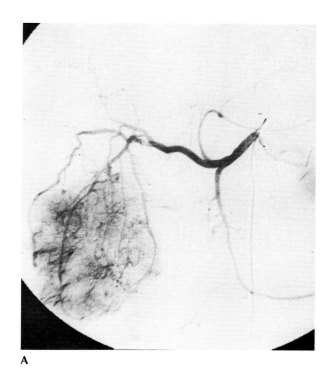 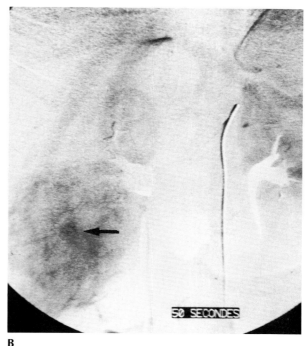

FIGURE 20-4
Focal nodular hyperplasia. (A) Angiography, at the arterial phase. Hypervascular mass of the right lobe. (B) Angiography, at the venous phase. The parenchymal staining shows the opacification of the central scar (arrow), with large hepatic veins draining the tumor.

hepatocyte nodules into smaller units (Fig. 20-2). Marked proliferation of biliary structures surrounded by inflammatory cells is observed within the fibrous septa. Various vascular abnormalities, such as intimal and medial fibromuscular hyperplasia of large vessels in the fibrous scar, sinusoidal dilatation, and hemorrhagic foci, are frequently observed in FNH and are aggravated by the administration of estroprogestatives (10,11). Intake of such agents might favor clinical recognition of the tumor by facilitating its growth and its hemorrhagic complications (2,11). This could well explain the higher prevalence of reported cases in women than in men.

To the best of our knowledge, malignant transformation of FNH has never been reported. However, it must be emphasized that histologic examination of the resection specimen is necessary, since the gross appearance of FNH may mimic that of the fibrolamellar variant of hepatocellular carcinoma (3,12).

Despite the use of different imaging modalities, FNH is often difficult to differentiate from other hepatic lesions. Sonography is nonspecific for FNH characterization, since various echo patterns have been reported. In a series of 23 patients with FNH, we have observed 8 hypoechoic, 8 hyperechoic, 4 isoechoic, and 3 mixed lesions (13). This concurs with the findings of Rogers et al. (14) and Welch et al. (15). The value of ultrasonography (US) is its sensitivity for the detection of lesions by revealing the particular echostructure, the displacement of vascular structures, or the deformation of hepatic contours in the case of isoechoic lesions. In some cases, different authors have described a central hyperechoic band corresponding to the stellate scar (Fig. 20-3).

Angiography appears nonspecific for FNH characterization, demonstrating a hypo- or hypervascular mass with parenchymal staining that reveals septations corresponding to the bands of radiating fibrous tissue (Fig. 20-4). In the majority of cases, the vascular supply appears to arise centrally and to radiate peripherally in a spoke-wheel pattern. However, in some cases, the vessels appear to enter the tumor from its periphery. Initially, a peripheral vascular supply was believed to be more typical of HA. Both types have been described in FNH, but with a predominance of the central supply pattern.

Dynamic CT is of particular value because of its ability to characterize tumor vascularity and to analyze intratumoral elements. As pointed out by different authors, FNH is often slightly hypodense prior to the injection of contrast medium (13). In some cases, the tumor is isodense, and bolus injection must be performed in the plane of the lesion demonstrated by US. After contrast medium injection, the lesion exhibits a considerable enhancement at the arterial phase and becomes rapidly isodense in the portal phase and on late scans (Fig. 20-5). A central scar may be a relatively specific CT feature, but it is noted in only 14 to 43 percent of the cases in recent series (13–16). The scar can be hypodense on the first series of scans after bolus injection, within the hypervascular tumor, and frequently hyperdense in comparison with the isodense or hypodense tumor on delayed scans. This hyperdensity can be explained by the presence of abnormal vessels inside the scar or by the excretion of the iodinated contrast material in the biliary structures existing within the scar. Recently, Kier and Rosenfield (17) demonstrated that FNH, unlike other focal hepatic lesions, may be hyperdense to normal liver parenchyma on delayed contrast-enhanced CT performed 4 h after bolus injection. Since normal hepatocytes secrete 1 to 2 percent of the injected iodine load into the biliary system, the presence of functioning hepatocytes within FNH can explain this hyperdensity on delayed enhanced scans (17).

Scintigraphy has been used to try to differentiate FNH from HA, since areas of normal or increased ^{99m}Tc-sulfur colloid uptake can be identified in 50 to 65 percent of cases of FNH (14,15). This uptake is explained by the presence of Kupffer cells and has been considered diagnostic of FNH (Fig. 20-6). However, Goodman et al. (18) recently demonstrated the presence of Kupffer cells in HA as well. Lubbers et al. (19) also showed an uptake of colloid by HA in 3 of 13 cases. ^{99m}Tc-IDA is concentrated by the hepatocytes but

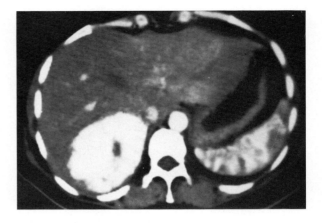

FIGURE 20-5
Focal nodular hyperplasia. Dynamic CT scan, at the arterial phase. Hypervascular tumor with hypodense central scar.

is associated with a prolonged washout owing to the presence of poorly formed biliary structures (20). On ^{99m}Tc-labeled erythrocytes, the lesion exhibits a normal or increased first-pass perfusion and blood pool activity (20).

Magnetic resonance imaging (MRI) allows differential diagnosis of hepatic tumors on the basis of signal-intensity characteristics and/or morphologic features. As reported by three previous studies, FNH can be visualized on unenhanced MRI as an isointense lesion on all pulse sequences (21–23). The isointensity can be explained by the presence of normal hepatocytes and Kupffer cells in the tumor (Fig. 20-7). However, at low field or on unenhanced turbo flash sequences, the lesion is frequently hypointense on the heavily T1-weighted images (24) (Fig. 20-7E). On T2-weighted images, FNH appears frequently isointense or slightly hyperintense (21–23). In addition, MRI appears to be more sensitive than other imaging techniques for the detection of the central scar, which is visualized as a dark area on the T1-weighted images and as a bright region on the T2-weighted images (21–23) (Fig. 20-7B to D). This may be due to the presence of abundant tortuous and abnormal vascular channels with slowly flowing blood in the dense or loose fibrous tissue. On dynamic MRI using fast techniques such as flash and turbo flash, the lesion exhibits, as on dynamic CT, a peak of enhancement at the arterial phase after bolus injection of a paramagnetic

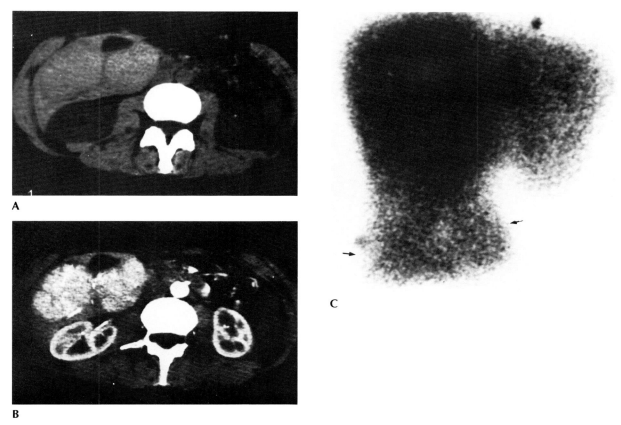

FIGURE 20-6
Focal nodular hyperplasia (A) On precontrast CT scan, presence of two lesions isodense to the surrounding liver, displacing the gallbladder anteriorly. (B) At the arterial phase, a significant enhancement is noticed in the two homogeneous lesions. No stellate central scar is present. (C) Uptake on ^{99m}Tc-sulfur colloid is demonstrated in these two tumors of the right lobe (arrows).

contrast agent (Fig. 20-7F). Then the lesion becomes isointense to the surrounding parenchyma. The superior soft-tissue contrast of paramagnetic-enhanced MRI enables constant visualization of the contrast material within the scar on the postcontrast MRI images, particularly on T1-weighted images (25) (Fig. 20-7G).

HEPATOCELLULAR ADENOMA

Hepatocellular adenoma is a benign proliferation of the hepatocytes within an otherwise normal liver. Although it has been occasionally described in association with type I glycogen storage disease, diabetes mellitus, and iron overload secondary to beta-thalassemia (3), it is now well established that this uncommon tumor occurs, in most of the cases, in women using oral contraceptives (OCs) (8,26,27). The incidence is estimated to be 3 to 4 per year per 100,000 long-term OC users, but only 1 per million in nonusers or women who have used OCs for less than 2 years (3,27). Furthermore, the risk of developing HA increases with the duration of OC use and with the potency of the preparations (3,27).

Patients with HA seek medical attention for several reasons. In approximately 5 to 10 percent of the cases, HA is found incidentally (3). Twenty-five to 35 percent of the patients have an abdominal mass, 20 to 25 percent have chronic or mild episodic abdominal pain, and 30 to 40 percent present with acute abdominal pain due to hemorrhage (3).

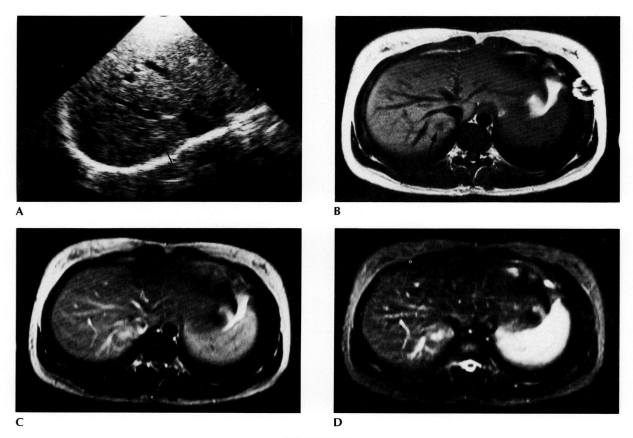

FIGURE 20-7
Focal nodular hyperplasia. (A) Sonography. Isoechoic lesion, with internal echoes (arrow), displacing the right hepatic vein and the inferior vena cava. (B) MRI, T1-weighted SE image, 400/15. The lesion is isointense relative to the surrounding parenchyma, displacing the veins, with a hypointense central scar (arrow). (C) MRI, proton-density image, 2200/40. The lesion is always isointense to the surrounding parenchyma. The central scar appears as an area of increased signal intensity. (D) MRI, heavily T2-weighted SE image, 2200/100. The lesion is slightly hyperintense, and the central scar exhibits a high signal intensity. (E) MRI, turbo flash sequence 7/4, alpha 10 degrees, acquisition time 600 ms. The lesion is now hypointense in comparison with T1-weighted image (part B) due to a pulse of inversion recovery. (F) MRI, turbo flash sequence 7/4, alpha 10 degrees, acquisition time 600 ms. After bolus injection of paramagnetic contrast agent (Gd-DOTA), the tumor exhibits a peak of enhancement, at the arterial phase. (G) MRI, contrast-enhanced T1-weighted image. Persistence of paramagnetic contrast agent in the central scar.

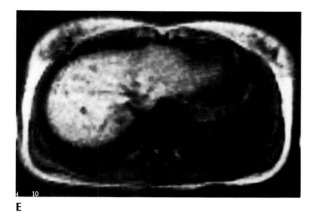
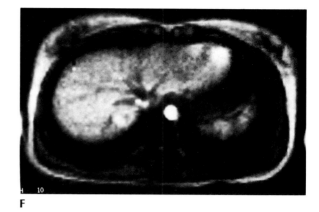
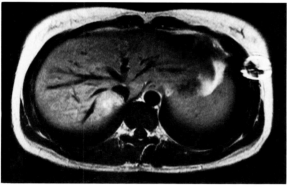

FIGURE 20-7 *(continued)*

Hepatocellular adenoma is usually a solitary nodule, and most reports of multiple adenomas or adenomatosis of the liver (28) should actually be considered examples of nodular regenerative hyperplasia of the liver (3,29). The tumoral nodule, which may be pedunculated, is spherical, with a diameter that may reach 30 cm (3). On cut sections, the tumor is well demarcated from the surrounding liver, but a capsule is usually absent (Fig. 20-8). Areas of necrosis and/or hemorrhage (Fig. 20-9) leading to fibrosis are frequently found. Large blood vessels often run on the surface of the tumor mass, which appears to be vascularized from its periphery (8).

Histologic examination shows a proliferation of benign hepatocytes (Fig. 20-10) that may have an increased content of fat. Vascular abnormalities, similar to those observed in FNH, are frequently noted in HA and are also aggravated by the administration of estroprogestatives (10,11). These vascular lesions are probably responsible for tumor necrosis and occurrence of the life-threatening complications (e.g., intratumoral, subcapsular, or intraperitoneal hemorrhage) of this otherwise benign tumor (11). After withdrawal of estroprogestatives, the tumor may either regress or enlarge, and rare cases of transformation of HA to carcinoma have been reported (3). Therefore, surgical resection is usually proposed, when possible, in order to prove the benign nature of the tumor and to prevent the risk of rupture or hemorrhage.

Sonography is nonspecific for HA characterization, since all echostructural patterns are observed. In a series of 29 patients with HA, we have observed 11 hypoechoic, 8 hyperechoic, 6 isoechoic and 2 mixed lesions (13). In two patients, the lesion was anechoic because of the presence

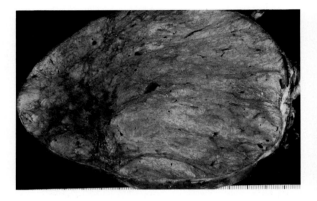

FIGURE 20-8
Hepatocellular adenoma. This large tumor nodule is homogeneous and well-limited. No fibrous scar is observed.

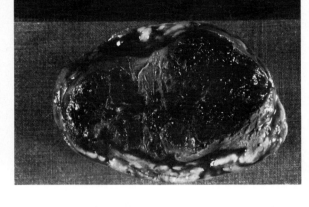

FIGURE 20-9
Hepatocellular adenoma. Most of the tumor nodule is replaced by dark areas of hemorrhage.

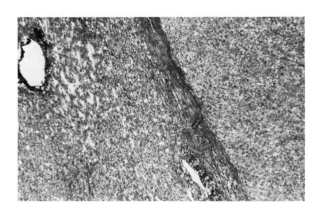

FIGURE 20-10
Hepatocellular adenoma. Microscopic examination shows that the tumor (right) is made by sheets of normal-appearing proliferating hepatocytes. Normal liver (left) is well-separated from the tumor by a capsule.

of hemorrhage (Fig. 20-11A). As in the case of FNH, the value of US is its sensitivity for lesion detection (13).

Angiography appears nonspecific for HA characterization. Hepatocellular adenoma may be either hypovascular with displacement and draping of hepatic arteries or hypervascular with tortuous vessels coursing through the lesion (30) (Fig. 20-12B). Whether or not the feeding vessels enter from the center or from the periphery of the lesion has no bearing on the differentiation between FNH and HA (30).

Plain CT scans are essential for the detection of intratumoral hemorrhage (see Fig. 20-11B) and determination of the best plane for dynamic CT scanning. Discovery of hemorrhage within a lesion strongly suggests the diagnosis of HA in a young patient using OCs (13). The 15 percent incidence of hemorrhage in our series is similar to that reported by Kerlin et al. (31). On dynamic CT scan, the hyperdense HA shows significant enhancement at the arterial phase and a decrease during the portal phase, becoming isodense or even hypodense with respect to the parenchyma 1 min after bolus injection. In the majority of the cases, lesions smaller than 4 cm appear homogeneous (13). In large tumors, hypodense areas are frequently observed before and after contrast material injection corresponding to bands of necrosis of varied widths that may show fibrous transformation. These hypodense areas also might correspond to the fatty changes that can be observed in tumoral hepatocytes (13,32).

Hepatocellular adenomas are usually visualized as defects on ^{99m}Tc-sulfur colloid scans, a fact that has been attributed to the absence of phagocytic Kupffer cells. As already mentioned, Goodman et al. (18) demonstrated that all HA contain Kupffer cells. In addition, Lubbers et al. (19) observed, in 3 of 13 cases of HA, an uptake on ^{99m}Tc-sulfur colloid scan by the tumor. However,

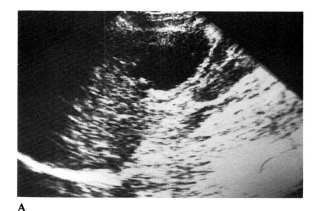
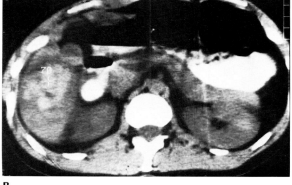
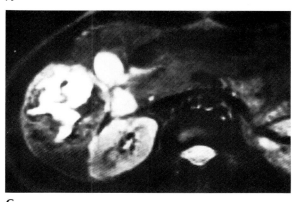

FIGURE 20-11
Hepatocellular adenoma. Subacute hemorrhage. (A) Sonography. Anechoic lesion of the right lobe. (B) Precontrast CT scan shows hemorrhage marked by spontaneous hyperdensity. (C) MRI, T2-weighted SE image 2200/90. Hyperintensity within the tumor corresponding to the subacute hemorrhage.

in the majority of the cases, HA is generally photon deficient relative to normal liver. Several factors might be responsible for this diminished uptake: (1) a decreased number of Kupffer cells in some tumors, (2) an altered blood flow, and (3) an abnormal phagocytic activity of the Kupffer cells. Intratumoral hemorrhage and necrosis also could contribute to this photon-deficient appearance. The presence of proliferating normal hepatocytes and the absence of biliary structures promote the uptake of ^{99m}Tc-IDA without drainage.

At MRI, hepatocellular adenoma can show mild increase in T1 and T2 similar to the relaxation times observed in FNH (33,34). The tumor often appears isointense on T1-weighted images and slightly hyperintense or hyperintense on T2-weighted images (see Figs. 20-11C and 20-12C to E). However, the MRI tissue characteristics vary widely, and HA with long T1 and long T2 relaxation times can be indistinguishable from malignant liver tumors. T1-weighted images may rarely show a low-intensity pseudocapsule, similar to the finding commonly seen in hepatocellular carcinoma (33). The long T2 central scar that is usually observed in FNH has not yet been described in HA. Although HA may undergo necrosis and calcification, the lesion is heterogeneous in relation to these bands of necrosis, appearing as a dark signal on T2-weighted images. As a result of these morphologic variations and the wide range of T1 and T2, a tissue-specific diagnosis of HA is not possible by MRI.

BILIARY CYSTADENOMA

Biliary cystadenoma of the liver is rare and bears a pathologic resemblance to the mucinous cystadenoma arising in the pancreas. Less than 100 cases have been reported in the literature, and over 85 percent of patients are females more than 30 years of age (3). This tumor is slow-growing, and clinical findings (i.e., pain, abdominal enlargement,

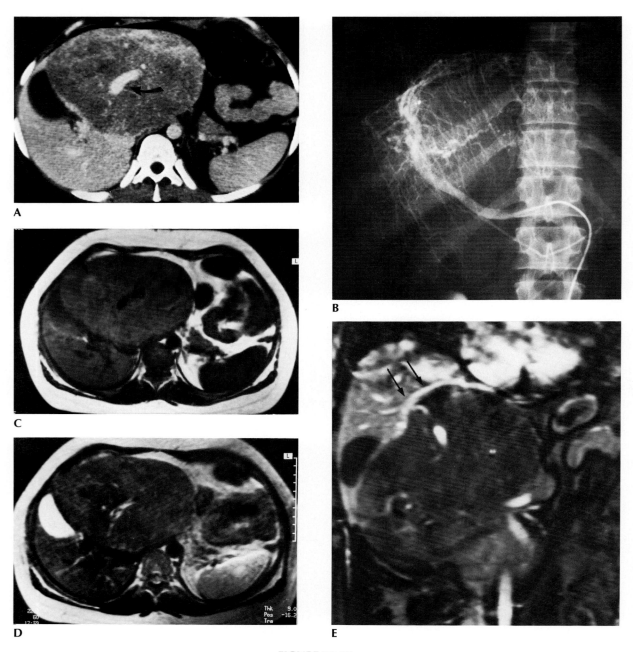

FIGURE 20-12

Hepatocellular adenoma. (A) *Contrast-enhanced CT scan. Large hepatic mass of the left lobe, involving the caudate lobe, with central vein* (arrow). (B) *Selective hepatic arteriogram. Large hepatic artery with abnormal vessels draping the mass.* (C) *MRI, T1-weighted SE image 400/20, shows the large mass that appears heterogeneous by the presence of slightly hyperintense areas* (arrow). (D) *MRI, T2-weighted SE image 2200/50. Persistence of heterogeneous areas within the lesion. Presence of a large and central vessel.* (E) *MRI, flash image 23/12, alpha 30 degrees. After injection of paramagnetic contrast agent, the large lesion appears hypointense with hepatic veins identified in the lesion. The middle hepatic vein is displaced by the tumor* (arrows).

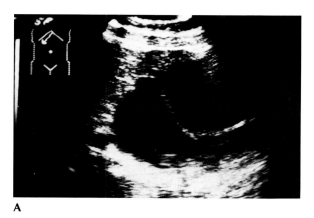 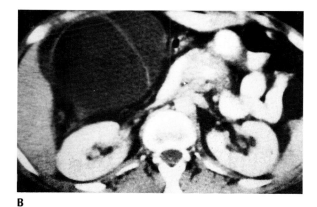

FIGURE 20-13
Biliary cystadenoma. (A) Sonography. Large cystic lesion with thin internal septa. (B) Enhanced CT scan. The large cystic lesion with internal septa is clearly demonstrated displacing the gallbladder.

jaundice, nausea, or vomiting) depend on size (2.5 to 25 cm in diameter) and location (3,35).

The main pathologic feature of biliary cystadenoma is its multilocularity. The locules have various sizes, usually contain a mucinous or gelatinous fluid, and their lining is smooth and thin (35–37). The cystadenoma is globular in shape and has a smooth external surface. Under light microscopy, the locules are lined by a single layer of normal mucin-producing epithelial cells resting on connective tissue. Small polypoid or papillary projections may occasionally be observed in the lumen of the locules. The septa between the cavities can be ulcerated and often contain pigmented or foamy macrophages, cholesterol clefts, calcifications, and various amounts of polymorphous inflammatory cells. Careful examination of the entire tumor is necessary, since foci of adenocarcinoma may arise in an otherwise benign-appearing cystadenoma (35–37). It has been suggested that so-called cystadenomas with mesenchymal stroma could constitute a distinctive subgroup within biliary cystadenomas (36,37). This clinicopathologic entity could be characterized by its exclusive occurrence in women and by the possible malignant transformation of either the epithelial layer or the mesenchymal component in carcinoma or sarcoma, respectively (37). This formal distinction with the other forms of cystadenoma should, however, be confirmed by other studies.

On sonography and CT, the majority of these large lesions are single, multilocular, and cystic (Figs. 20-13 and 20-14). Papillary excrescences, nodular thickening of internal septa, and mural nodules are often observed, and these features appear better demonstrated on sonography than on CT (38,39). A connection with the intrahepatic bile ducts has been showed in three cases by Choi et al. (38). The differential diagnosis of this cystic hepatic neoplasm essentially includes complicated congenital cysts, hematoma, and cystic metastases (38,39). Guided percutaneous aspiration and biopsy of the cystic wall are helpful for the diagnosis of this rare lesion (38). If a cystadenoma is suspected after these procedures, surgery must nevertheless be performed, since biliary cystadenoma and cystadenocarcinoma cannot be reliably differentiated only on the basis of radiologic findings.

BILE DUCT ADENOMA

Bile duct adenoma, also termed *benign cholangioma* or *cholangioadenoma*, is a rare benign lesion of the liver consisting of the proliferation of noncystic biliary structures within a dense fibrous stroma (3,40). The small size, the absence of symptoms, and the indolent behavior of this tumor explain why it is relatively unknown by radiologists. Indeed, it is usually discovered during surgery or at autopsy (40). Its only clinical significance lies in

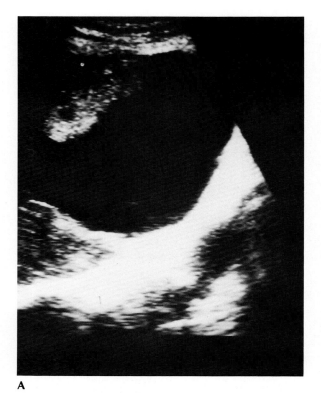

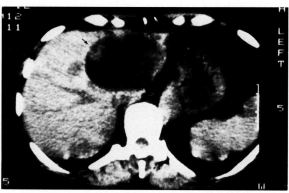

FIGURE 20-14
Biliary cystadenocarcinoma. (A) Sonography. Large mural nodule at the anterior part of the cystic mass. (B) Plain CT scan. The large cystic lesion is located in the left lobe. The mural nodule is clearly demonstrated (arrow).

the possible confusion with a well-differentiated adenocarcinoma or with the Von Meyenburg complex, which is a developmental anomaly of small intrahepatic bile ducts (3). All the 152 cases of bile duct adenoma recently reported by Allaire et al. (40) were asymptomatic nodules. They were observed at all ages, and there was a slight male predominance. The nodules were usually pale, subcapsular, unencapsulated, and solitary in most of the cases (83 percent). Their size ranged from 1 to 20 mm in diameter, with 90 percent of the nodules being less than 10 mm. Follow-up of 38 of the surgically treated patients confirmed the benign behavior of this lesion. The main practical problem raised by this tumor is for the pathologist, since its possible discovery during surgery for carcinoma of another organ (e.g., colon or stomach) leads the surgeon to perform a biopsy for frozen-section diagnosis. The pathologist who is unaware of this rare entity may be puzzled and tempted to call the lesion metastatic adenocarcinoma. No relationship between bile duct adenoma and cholangiocarcinoma has been shown.

REFERENCES

1. Zafrani ES: Update on vascular tumours of the liver. J Hepatol 8:125, 1989.
2. Mathieu D, Zafrani ES, Anglade MC, Dhumeaux D: Association of focal nodular hyperplasia and hepatic hemangioma. Gastroenterology 97:154, 1989.
3. Goodman ZD: Benign tumors of the liver, in Okuda K, Ishak KG (eds): Neoplasms of the Liver. Tokyo, Springer-Verlag, 1987, pp 105–125.
4. Ishak KG: Mesenchymal tumors of the liver, in Okuda K, Peters RL (eds): Hepatocellular carcinoma. New York, Wiley, 1976, pp 247–307.
5. Wanless IR, Mawdsley C, Adams R: On the pathogenesis of focal nodular hyperplasia. Hepatology 5:1194, 1985.
6. Benz EJ, Baggenstoss AH: Focal cirrhosis of the liver: Its relation to the so-called hamartoma (adenoma, benign hepatoma). Cancer 6:743, 1953.
7. Feldman M: Hemangioma of the liver: Special reference to its association with cysts of the liver and pancreas. Am J Clin Pathol 29:160, 1958.
8. Ishak KG: Hepatic neoplasms associated with contraceptive and anabolic steroids, in Lingeman CH (ed): Recent results in cancer research. Berlin, Springer-Verlag, 1979, pp 73–128.
9. Stocker JT, Ishak KG: Focal nodular hyperplasia of the liver: A study of 21 pediatric cases. Cancer 48:336, 1981.

10. Nime F, Pickren JW, Vana J, et al: The histology of liver tumors in oral contraceptive users observed during a national survey by the American College of Surgeons Commission on Cancer. Cancer 44:1481, 1979.
11. Zafrani ES, Pinaudeau Y, Dhumeaux D: Drug-induced vascular lesions of the liver. Arch Intern Med 143:495, 1983.
12. Vecchio FM, Fabiano A, Ghirlanda G, et al: Fibrolamellar carcinoma of the liver: The malignant counterpart of focal nodular hyperplasia with oncocytic change. Am J Clin Pathol 81:521, 1984.
13. Mathieu D, Bruneton JN, Drouillard J, et al: Hepatic adenomas and focal nodular hyperplasia: Dynamic CT study. Radiology 160:53, 1986.
14. Rogers JV, Mack LA, Freeny PC, et al: Hepatic focal nodular hyperplasia: Angiography, CT, sonography, and scintigraphy. AJR 137:983, 1981.
15. Welch TJ, Sheedy PF II, Johnson CM, et al: Focal nodular hyperplasia and hepatic adenoma: Comparison of angiography, CT, US, and scintigraphy. Radiology 156:593, 1985.
16. Fishman EK, Farmlett E, Kadir S, Siegelman SS: Computed tomography of benign hepatic tumors. J Comput Assist Tomogr 6:472, 1982.
17. Kier R, Rosenfeld AT: Focal nodular hyperplasia of the liver on delayed enhanced CT. AJR 153:885, 1989.
18. Goodman ZD, Mikel UV, Lubbers PR, et al: Kupffer cells in hepatocellular adenomas. Am J Surg Pathol 11:191, 1987.
19. Lubbers PR, Ros PR, Goodman ZD, Ishak KG: Accumulation of technetium-99m sulfur colloid by hepatocellular adenoma: Scintigraphic-pathologic correlation. AJR 148:1105, 1987.
20. Tanasescu D, Brachman M, Rigby J, et al: Scintigraphic triad in focal nodular hyperplasia. Am J Gastroenterol 79:61, 1984.
21. Butch RJ, Stark DD, Malt RA: MR imaging of hepatic focal nodular hyperplasia. J Comput Assist Tomogr 10:874, 1986.
22. Mattison GR, Glazer GM, Quint LE, et al: MR imaging of hepatic focal nodular hyperplasia: Characterization and distinction from primary malignant hepatic tumors. AJR 148:711, 1987.
23. Rummeny E, Weissleder R, Sironi S, et al: Central scars in primary liver tumors: MR features, specificity, and pathologic correlation. Radiology 171:323, 1989.
24. Rahman M, Li K, Ros PR: Hepatic focal nodular hyperplasia: New MR findings. Magn Reson Med 7:687, 1989.
25. Tham RT, Holscher HC, Falke TH, et al: Focal nodular hyperplasia of the liver: Features on Gd-DTPA–enhanced MR. AJR 153:884, 1989.
26. Edmondson HA, Henderson B, Benton B: Liver-cell adenomas associated with use of oral contraceptives. N Engl J Med 294:470, 1976.
27. Rooks JB, Ory HW, Ishak KG, et al: The cooperative liver tumor study group. Epidemiology of hepatocellular adenoma: The role of oral contraceptive use. JAMA 242:644, 1979.
28. Flejou JF, Barge J, Menu Y, et al: Liver adenomatosis: An entity distinct from liver adenoma? Gastroenterology 89:1132, 1985.
29. Stromeyer FW, Ishak KG: Nodular transformation (nodular "regenerative" hyperplasia) of the liver: A clinicopathologic study of 30 cases. Hum Pathol 12:60, 1981.
30. Casarella WJ, Knowles DM, Wolff M, Johnson PM: Focal nodular hyperplasia and liver cell adenoma: Radiologic and pathologic differentiation. AJR 131:393, 1978.
31. Kerlin P, Davis GL, McGill DB, et al: Hepatic adenoma and focal nodular hyperplasia: Clinical, pathologic and radiologic features. Gastroenterology 84:994, 1983.
32. Angres G, Carter JB, Velasco JM: Unusual ring in liver cell adenoma. AJR 135:172, 1980.
33. Ferrucci JT: MR imaging of the liver. AJR 147:1103, 1986.
34. Rummeny E, Saini S, Wittenberg J, et al: MR imaging of liver neoplasms: Pictorial essay. AJR 152:493, 1989.
35. Ishak KG, Willis GW, Cummins SD, Bullock AA: Biliary cystadenoma and cystadenocarcinoma: Report of 14 cases and review of the literature. Cancer 38:322, 1977.
36. Wheeler DA, Edmondson HA: Cystadenoma with mesenchymal stroma (CMS) in the liver and bile ducts: A clinicopathologic study of 17 cases, 4 with malignant changes. Cancer 56:1434, 1985.
37. Akwari OE, Tucker A, Seigler HF, Itani KMF: Hepatobiliary cystadenoma with mesenchymal stroma. Ann Surg 211:18, 1990.
38. Choi BI, Lim JH, Han MC, et al: Biliary cystadenoma and cystadenocarcinoma: CT and sonographic findings. Radiology 171:57, 1989.
39. Korobkin M, Stephens DH, Lee JKT, et al: Biliary cystadenoma and cystadenocarcinoma: CT and sonographic findings. AJR 153:507, 1989.
40. Allaire GS, Rabin L, Ishak KG, Sesterhenn IA: Bile duct adenoma. A study of 152 cases. Am J Surg Pathol 12:708, 1988.

21

CT and MRI of Hepatic Cavernous Hemangiomas

SANJAY SAINI

Cavernous hemangioma is one of the most common benign liver tumors (1). Its prevalence in the adult population has been reported to range between 0.4 and 7 percent (2,3). However, it now appears that these figures vastly underestimate the true prevalence of these benign liver tumors. Recent autopsy studies in which the liver was sectioned in 1- to 2-cm-thick slices have revealed that the prevalence of hepatic hemangiomas in adult males is over 20 percent, with multiple tumors being present in 50 percent of these individuals (4). Since hemangiomas are known to occur more frequently in women than in men, their prevalence in females is probably even higher. Although no comparable imaging studies have been performed, the prevailing opinion among experienced liver imagers appears to confirm these data. Advances in cross-sectional imaging techniques, particularly CT and MRI, have heightened an awareness for the high prevalence of benign liver tumors in the general population. In patients evaluated for suspected liver metastases, benign liver tumors are being recognized with increasing frequency, and not infrequently, benign and malignant liver tumors have been found to coexist (Fig 21-1).

In the diagnostic evaluation of the liver, it has long been axiomatic that a cavernous hemangioma must be considered in the differential diagnosis of a solitary liver mass, even in a patient with cancer history. However, it now appears that one can no longer assume a diagnosis of malignant cancer even in a patient with multiple liver masses. Thus the need to define imaging characteristics of benign and malignant liver tumors has achieved even greater importance. This need will only increase with the anticipated ability to rapidly image (with CT and/or MRI) the entire liver in thin (3- to 5-mm) sections that will detect smaller (benign and malignant) liver tumors with even greater frequency. In this chapter I shall examine the appearance of cavernous hemangiomas at CT and MRI, and establish criteria that will permit their differentiation from malignant liver tumors, most notably secondary metastases. The role of other imaging tests such as sonography and nuclear scintigraphy will not be mentioned here but will be addressed in other chapters.

PATHOLOGY

Cavernous hemangiomas are of mesodermal origin and are composed of blood-filled cavernous (or rarely capillary) vascular channels that are divided by thin fibrous septa. Their vascular spaces are lined with a single layer of flat endothelium. Blood flow in hemangiomas is slow and nondirectional, predisposing to thrombosis. With rupture of a vascular space, hemorrhage into the interstitium also can occur. Organization of thrombi and hemorrhages produces scars. These fibrocollagenous scars are most commonly seen in the larger (>2 cm) cavernous hemangiomas (5). Although no data are available on the growth potential of these tumors, cavernous hemangiomas are exceedingly rare in childhood but can ultimately enlarge to over 20 cm.

COMPUTED TOMOGRAPHY (CT)

The diagnosis of cavernous hemangiomas at CT requires exploitation of their vascular hemodynamics. Radiopharmaceutical studies have demonstrated that owing to retarded blood flow in their dilated vascular spaces, hepatic cavernous hemangiomas display slow fill-in and delayed washout of blood-pool agents (6,7). Iodinated x-ray contrast media, while suboptimal blood-pool agents, can be used to display this perfusion profile. Owing to the short intravascular lifetime of these contrast agents, fast imaging techniques are necessary to provide temporal resolution of the tumor's enhancing characteristics. Following bolus infusion of the contrast agent [150 to 180 ml of 60% contrast media at 5 cc/s for 10 s and then at 2 cc/s with a 45-s scanning delay (8)], hemangiomas typically demonstrate peripheral enhancement during the dynamic/vascular phase (0 to 30 s) of the infusion (Fig 21-2A). Initially, the peripheral enhancement may not encircle the entire tumor but may begin at one or more "mural nodules" (9). These nodules are best seen with fast scanning techniques in which dynamic images are obtained in the arterial phase (10 to 30 s after bolus infusion with no scan delay) of contrast infusion. While the pathologic correlate of these mural nodules has not yet been established, fill-in of cavernous hemangiomas often appears to proceed from these foci. It is possible that these mural nodules represent the feeding vascular nidus of cavernous hemangiomas. These nodules are being recognized with increasing frequency as the speeds of cross-sectional imaging techniques have decreased to subsecond times. Indeed, these nodules also have been observed at color flow Doppler sonography and Gd-DTPA dimeglumine-enhanced MRI. At delayed imaging (up to 60 min), the hemangiomas enhance completely from the periphery toward the center, and this fill-in process renders the lesion that was low-attenuation on the noncontrast images isodense to normal liver on the delayed images (Fig. 21-2B).

In a prospective analysis of liver hemangiomas (Fig. 21-3), Freeny and Marks (10) noted that the "typical" features (precontrast: low attenuation; dynamic phase: peripheral enhancement; delayed scan: complete isodense fill-in) are present in only about 54 percent of hemangiomas. The remaining 46 percent hemangiomas display "atypical" enhancement patterns consisting of mixed (central and peripheral) enhancement in the dynamic phase and incomplete fill-in on delayed images. In comparison, only rarely (about

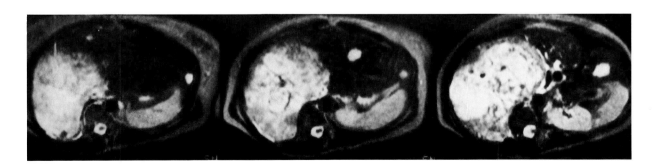

FIGURE 21-1
Coexisting benign and malignant liver tumors. T2-weighted pulse-sequence SE 2350/180. A large hepatic sarcoma replacing the right hepatic lobe and four benign cavernous hemangiomas in the left lobe. The hemangiomas were initially thought to represent atypical metastases but were shown to be hemangiomas following wedge hepatic resection.

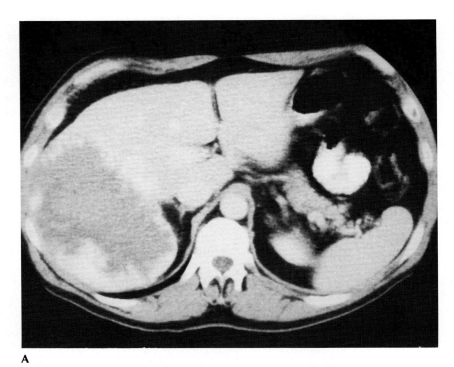

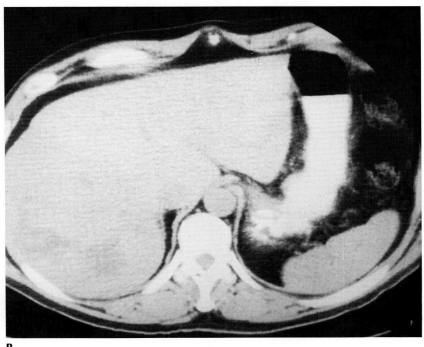

FIGURE 21-2
Typical CT enhancing characteristics of cavernous hemangioma. (A) Dynamic phase. The hypodense tumor demonstrates irregular peripheral enhancement. (B) Delayed phase (25 minutes after infusion). The tumor is nearly uniformly isodense with normal liver.

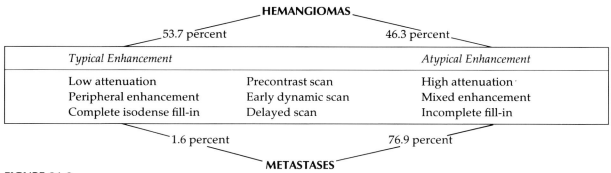

FIGURE 21-3

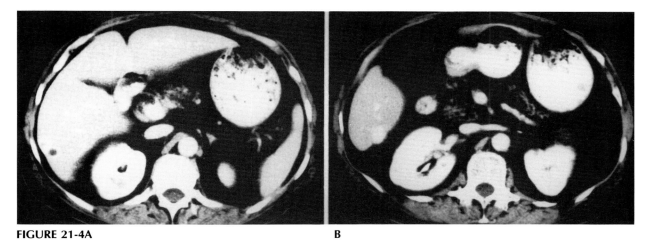

FIGURE 21-3
Typical and atypical features of hemangiomas versus metastases. (From Freeny PC, Marks WM: Hepatic hemangioma: Dynamic bolus CT. AJR 147:711, 1986. Copyright © by American Roentgen Ray Society. Reprinted by permission.)

FIGURE 21-4
Typical and atypical CT enhancing characteristics of cavernous hemangioma. Dynamic phase images. (A) Two lesions demonstrate intense peripheral enhancement typical of cavernous hemangiomas. (B) A similar-sized lesion shows complete intense enhancement, which is atypical of hemangiomas.

1.6 percent) do metastases possess the typical enhancement characteristics. Thus, when present, the typical CT features are a very reliable indicator of the presence of a cavernous hemangioma. However, the atypical characteristics are less reliable, since many (over 76 percent) liver metastases also demonstrate the atypical enhancement features, rendering considerable overlap in this subgroup between benign and malignant liver tumors. Of course, if less rigid CT criteria are utilized, CT can characterize up to 90 percent of cavernous hemangiomas (11).

As the size of hemangiomas decreases, their enhancing characteristics become more atypical. Their peripheral enhancement may be difficult to separate from the enhanced adjacent liver (Fig. 21-4A), or they may enhance completely in the dynamic/arterial phase and can appear uniformly hyperdense (Fig. 21-4B). Furthermore owing to the difficulty in reproducing scan plane because of variations in inspiratory excursion, CT is of extremely limited value in characterizing liver tumors that are less than 1 to 2 cm in diameter.

MAGNETIC RESONANCE IMAGING (MRI)

Relaxation times of hepatic cavernous hemangiomas are considerably greater than those of normal liver, liver metastases and hepatocellular carcinomas (12,13). Thus hemangiomas appear hypointense on T1-weighted images and hyperintense on T2-weighted images (Fig. 21-5). Despite the presence of flowing blood within cavernous hemangiomas, at MRI these tumors have characteristics of a fluid-filled structure. Differentiation from solid liver tumors requires imaging with heavily T2-weighted pulse sequences (12). On multiecho T2-weighted pulse sequences, signal intensity of normal liver and solid liver tumors (e.g., metastases), both having relatively shorter T2 times, fades (Fig. 21-6), while hemangiomas retain signal and become progressively more hyperintense (Fig. 21-7). Thus hemangiomas have what has often been called a "lightbulb" appearance on heavily T2-weighted images (14) (Figs. 21-5B and 21-7C). This high signal intensity is similar to other watery tissues, such as cerebrospinal fluid in the spinal canal or the gallbladder, which can therefore be used as internal reference standards.

Additional features attributed to cavernous hemangiomas include a relatively homogeneous signal intensity and a smooth outer border with a sharp interface with normal liver (14) (Figs. 21-5B and 21-7C). This spectrum of findings is also seen with simple hepatic cysts, which are therefore indistinguishable from hemangiomas on MRI. However, less than 10 percent of solid liver tumors also show these characteristics (13,14). Tumors that may mimic the T2-weighted MRI appearance of hemangiomas are those with a watery matrix, and common examples include cystic tumors, sarcomas, and hypervascular metastases. More commonly, metastases are characterized by a more heterogeneous/amorphous appearance (Fig. 21-7), an indistinct/unsharp outer margin (Fig. 21-8), ringed morphology (Fig. 21-9), or the presence of peritumoral edema (Fig. 21-10) (14). This last characteristic makes metastases appear larger on T2-weighted images when compared with T1-weighted images (blooming) (Fig. 21-8) or may manifest as a peripheral wedge-shaped region of hyperintensity surrounding the metastases (Fig. 21-10).

The concept of homogeneity of tumor signal intensity requires some comment. It is generally thought that hemangiomas appear homogeneous on T2-weighted MRI images, although larger ones can display heterogeneous features as a result of thrombus and scar formation (Fig. 21-11). It appears likely that these features probably occur in smaller lesions as well but are obscured by the window display settings that are invariably selected to portray the lightbulb appearance of hemangiomas (5).

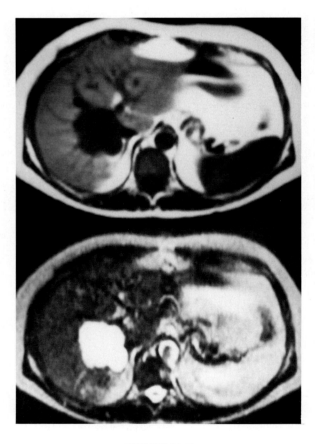

FIGURE 21-5
MRI appearance of hepatic cavernous hemangioma. Images obtained at 0.6 Tesla. (Top) On the T1-weighted image (SE 275/14), hemangiomas are hypointense to normal liver. Liver metastases have a similar appearance on T1-weighted images. (Bottom) On the T2-weighted image (SE 2350/180), hemangiomas are markedly hyperintense (lightbulb), of homogeneous signal intensity, and have a sharp interface with normal liver. Liver metastases rarely possess all three of these features.

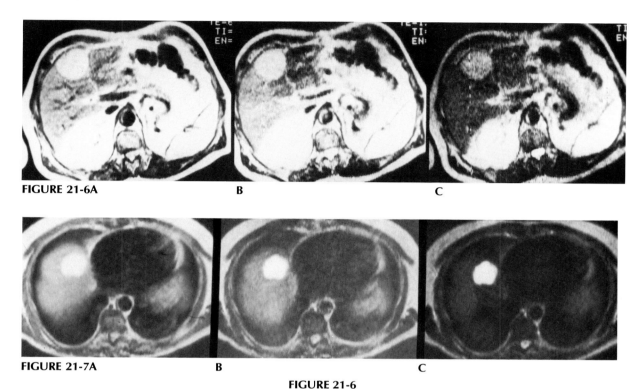

FIGURE 21-6
MRI appearance of solid liver tumor. Multiecho T2-weighted images SE 2350/60 (A)/120 (B)/180 (C) obtained at 0.6 Tesla. Solid liver tumors (benign and malignant) are hyperintense relative to normal liver. However, they are of heterogeneous signal intensities, and their signal intensity diminishes on heavily T2-weighted images (TE 180).

FIGURE 21-7
MRI appearance of cavernous hemangioma. Multiecho T2-weighted images SE 2350/60 (A)/120 (B)/180 (C) obtained at 0.6 Tesla. Cavernous hemangiomas are also hyperintense relative to normal liver. However, they are of homogeneous signal intensity, and they retain this signal intensity on progressively more T2-weighted images (TE 180), which makes them markedly hyperintense (lightbulb-like) on heavily T2-weighted images.

The critical parameter required to confidently make the diagnosis of hemangioma at MRI is the selection of pulse-sequence timing parameters that provide maximal T2 weighting. At midfield this has been shown to be on long TR/long TE pulse sequences with TE times of 180 ms (12). Although no comparable studies have been performed at high field, preliminary results show that at 1.5 Tesla, TEs of 140 ms provide better differentiation than TE times of under 100 ms.

To eliminate subjective analysis of liver tumors, quantitative criteria have been developed to distinguish liver tumors from hemangiomas. This was first done in Japan in an attempt to discriminate hemangiomas from hepatocellular carcinomas. Several Japanese studies have shown that for this differentiation, calculated T2 values obtained with a two-point fit are of some use. Using a cutoff value of 80 ms, Ohtomo et al. (13) were able to correctly classify 92 percent (57 of 62) of hepatocellular carcinomas and hemangiomas at 1.5 Teslas. Several morphologic features unique to hepatocellular carcinomas also assist in differentiating them from hemangiomas. These include an isointense signal intensity to normal liver on T1-weighted images (secondary to T1 time shortening from fatty change) and to tumor capsule (15) (Fig. 21-12). Recently, Egglin et al.

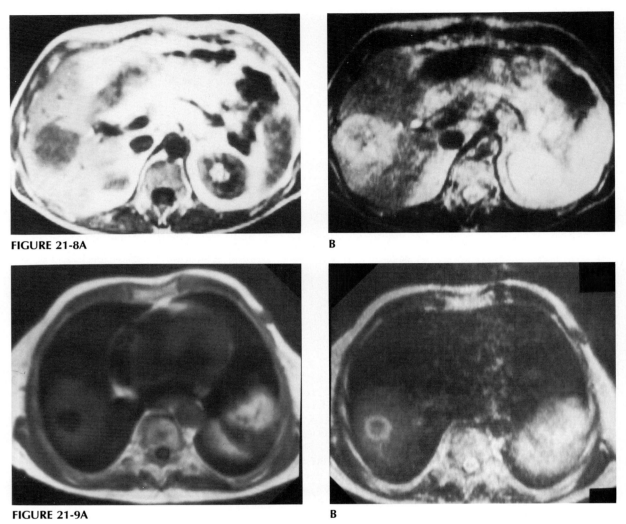

FIGURE 21-8
MRI appearance of malignant liver cancer. The colon metastasis appears hypointense on the T1-weighted image (A: SE 275/14). On the T2-weighted image (B: SE 2350/180), the tumor demonstrates heterogeneous tumor signal intensities and an indistinct outer margin. Also note that owing to peritumoral edema, the lesion appears larger (blooming) on the T2-weighted image.

FIGURE 21-9
MRI appearance of malignant liver cancer. The liver sarcoma appears hypointense on the T1-weighted image (A: SE 275/14). On the T2-weighted image (B: SE 2350/180), the tumor possesses a hyperintense rim (ringed morphology) presumably also due to peritumoral edema.

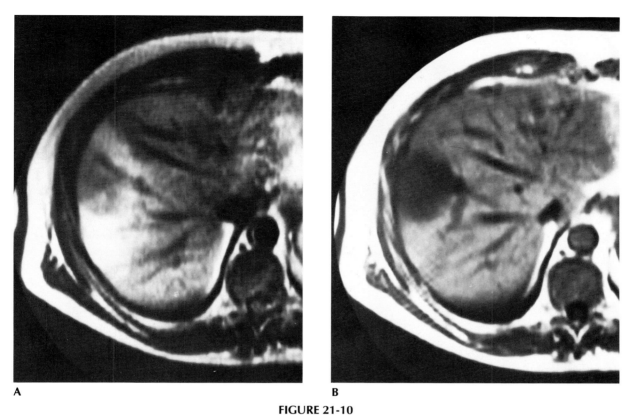

FIGURE 21-10
MRI appearance of malignant liver cancer. On the mildly T2-weighted image (A: SE 2350/60), the colon metastasis is surrounded by a wedge-shaped hyperintense region presumably representing peritumoral edema. Compare with the T1-weighted (B: SE 275/14) image demonstrating the more typical spherical tumor morphology.

(12) developed quantitative criteria at midfield (0.6 Tesla) and reported that a cutoff value for lesion/liver signal-intensity ratio (SIR) of 3.5 rendered a sensitivity of 89 percent and a specificity of 93 percent in discriminating hemangiomas from metastases. Refining these criteria further, Itoh et al. reported that these criteria have size-specific applications and that for the characterization of subcentimeter and 1 to 2-cm lesions, more strict size-specific criteria are required. Indeed, with these quantitative criteria, Itoh et al. were able to characterize a significant proportion of subcentimeter lesions as well. With the availability of echo-planar imaging techniques (17) in the near future, the use of T2 calculations may achieve greater importance. These techniques provide T2-weighted images with no T1 relaxation time contamination, and by obtaining a series of images with varying TEs, a multipoint fit, highly accurate T2 calculation can be performed. Initial studies have shown that there is little overlap in the calculated T2 times of solid liver tumors and metastases (18).

MRI contrast agents also have been utilized to improve the ability of MRI to differentiate hemangiomas from metastases. Gd-DTPA dimeglumine enhances hemangiomas in a fashion that is similar to the effect of iodinated contrast media at CT (19) (Fig. 21-13). However, in addition, owing to the relatively greater effect of Gd-DTPA dimeglumine on MRI signal intensity than of iodinated diatrozoates on CT attenuation values, the slow washout of the

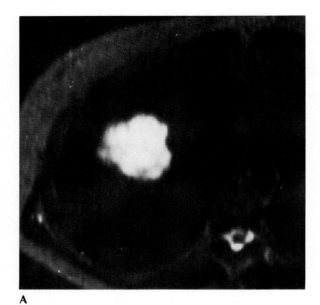

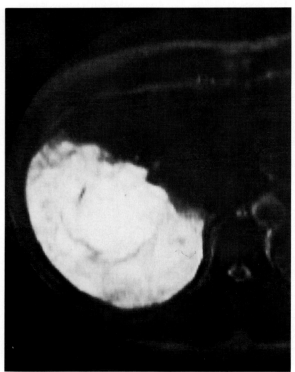

contrast media from hemangiomas renders them hyperintense on delayed MRI images (as opposed to isodense on delayed CT scans). Gd-DTPA dimeglumine thus has been considered a useful adjunct to T2-weighted images for evaluation of atypical hemangiomas and metastases. Using a similar approach, the effect of superparamagnetic iron oxides on hemangiomas and metastases also has been evaluated. During the vascular phase of the contrast agent (AMI-25 blood $t_{1/2}$ 15 min), hemangiomas demonstrate a diminution of signal intensity that is not matched by hypervascular or hypovascular metastases (20). The optimal contrast agent for characterization of liver tumors has as yet not been developed. However, it seems likely that a blood-pool type of agent (21) may be most useful for demonstrating the hemodynamic physiology of hemangiomas and to thereby distinguish them from metastases and primary liver tumors.

Finally, the use of MRI spectroscopy also has received some attention for providing differential diagnostic information. In preliminary studies, Glazer et al. (22) utilized image-localized P-31 MRI spectroscopy and noted that hemangiomas have spectra that differ from those of malignant tumors. The difference was most notable for signal-to-noise ratios (SNRs) using the β-ATP resonance where hemangiomas exhibit lower SNRs than metastases and hepatomas. This difference, however, was difficult to separate from normal liver when hemangiomas occupied less than 50 percent of the CSI section.

CT VERSUS MRI

Both CT and MRI can be utilized to tissue characterize liver tumors. However, at this time, it appears that MRI has considerable advantages over CT. Most important is the much smaller overlap

FIGURE 21-11
MRI appearance of atypical cavernous hemangioma. T2-weighted images: SE 2350/180. Although markedly hyperintense on the heavily T2-weighted images, both hemangiomas are of heterogeneous signal intensities with lobulated but sharp outer margins. These changes are common in hemangiomas over 5 cm and presumably reflect changes in scar formation. Note: Figures 21-2 (CT) and 21-10B (MR) are of the same lesion.

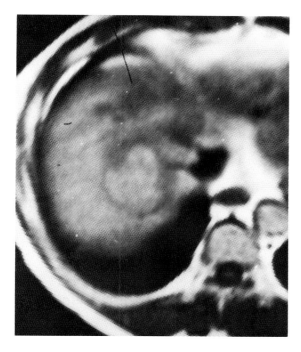

FIGURE 21-12
MRI appearance of hepatocellular carcinoma. T1-weighted: SE 275/14. Often, owing to fatty change, hepatomas are isointense to liver on T1-weighted images, and the presence of hypointense tumor capsule allows its detection.

in the MRI signal-intensity characteristics of malignant liver tumors and metastases. Difficulty in intravenous access and the use of iodinated contrast media and its attendant risks notwithstanding, an important limitation in utilizing CT to characterize liver tumors lies in the fact that CT scanning must be performed on a single anatomic plane so that temporal perfusion information can be obtained. Thus, in patients with multiple liver lesions, it is feasible to examine only those lesions which can be imaged in a single scanning plane. While this is also a limitation in patients undergoing contrast enhanced MRI evaluation, MRI offers the additional advantage that the imaging plane can be varied to portray one or more lesions in a single plane or that multiple slices can be obtained in a single breath-hold (<15 s) scanning period.

A more significant limitation of CT is that a "liver screening" and "lesion characterization" examinations are performed with different scanning protocols. While the latter require single-level imaging over several minutes, screening liver CT examinations (designed to detect liver tumors) require an incremental dynamic protocol so that the entire liver is scanned within 2 to 3 minutes of contrast media infusion. As a result, with CT it is not possible to perform a screening examination and a tissue-characterizing examination at a single sitting and with a single contrast material infusion. This is

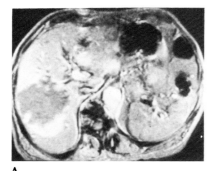 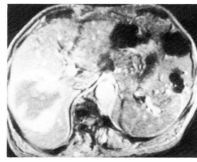 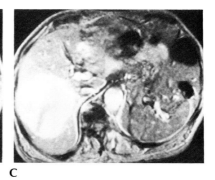

A B C

FIGURE 21-13
Gd-DTPA enhancement characteristics of cavernous hemangiomas. Dynamic imaging GE 110/5/80°. As with contrast-enhanced CT, with dynamic imaging after bolus infusion of Gd-DTPA (0.1 mmol/kg), hemangiomas show peripheral enhancement in the early phase (A), outside-to-center fill-in phenomenon (B: 5 min), and hyperintensity due to delayed washout of the contrast agent on delayed images (C: 20 min). (Courtesy of Dr. Bernd Hamm, Berlin, Germany.)

specially true in the case of CT portography (contrast material infusion into the superior mesenteric artery so that the liver is enhanced by means of the portal vein), which is now considered to be the most sensitive test for detecting focal liver masses (23). Although the superiority of CT portography over contrast-enhanced thin-section MRI has not been confirmed, CT portography is unable to provide any differential diagnostic information on lesions detected.

CONCLUSIONS

Liver tumor imaging requires the optimization of two concurrent goals: tumor detection and lesion characterization. Although the former is of primary importance, its results are of limited value if the latter issue is inadequately addressed. Presently, it appears that CT and MRI offer complementary roles. While, currently, CT portography is the best single test for lesion detection, MRI is the best single test for lesion characterization. Thus both imaging tests are often required to provide complete diagnostic information. Whether in the future a single imaging test can developed to provide the necessary diagnostic information remains to be determined.

REFERENCES

1. Malt RA: Surgery for hepatic neoplasms. N Engl J Med 313:1591, 1985.
2. Edmonson HA: Tumors of the liver and intrahepatic bile ducts, in Atlas of Tumor Pathology, sec 7, fasc 25. Washington, Armed Forces Institute of Pathology, 1958, pp 113–115.
3. Goodman ZD: Benign tumors of the liver, in Okuda K, Ishak KG (eds): Neoplasms of the Liver. New York, Springer-Verlag, 1987, p 114.
4. Karhunen PJ: Benign hepatic tumors and tumor like conditions in men. J Clin Pathol 39:183, 1986.
5. Ros PR, Lubbers PR, Olmstead WW, Morillo G: Hemangioma of the liver: Heterogeneous appearance on T2-weighted images. AJR 149:1167, 1987.
6. Rabinowitz SA, McKusick KA, Strauss HW: ^{99m}Tc red blood cell scintigraphy in evaluating focal liver disease. AJR 143:63, 1984.
7. Tumeh SS, Benson C, Nagel JS, et al: Cavernous hemangioma of the liver: Detection with single-photon emission computed tomography. Radiology 164:353, 1987.
8. Foley WD: Dynamic hepatic CT. Radiology 170:617, 1989.
9. Gaa J, Saini S: Chapter 24 in this textbook.
10. Freeny PC, Marks WM: Hepatic hemangioma: Dynamic bolus CT. AJR 147:711, 1986.
11. Ashida C, Fishman EK, Zerhouni EA, et al: Computed tomography of hepatic cavernous hemangioma. J Comput Assist Tomogr 11:455, 1987.
12. Egglin TK, Rummney E, Wittenberg J, et al: Quantitative tissue characterization by MRI: Hepatic tumors. Radiology 1976:107, 1990.
13. Ohtomo K, Itai Y, Yoshida H, et al: MR differentiation of hepatocellular carcinoma from cavernous hemangioma: Complementary roles of flash and T2 values. AJR 152:505, 1989.
14. Wittenberg J, Stark DD, Forman BH, et al: Differentiation of hepatic metastases from hepatic hemangiomas and cysts by using MR imaging. AJR 151:79, 1988.
15. Itai Y, Ohtomo K, Furui S, et al: MR imaging of hepatocellular carcinoma. J Comput Assist Tomogr 10:963, 1986.
16. Itoh K, Saini S, Hahn PF, et al. MR characterization of small cavernous hemangiomas using quantitative criteria. AJR 155:61, 1990.
17. Saini S, Stark DD, Rzedzian RR, et al: Ultrafast MR imaging of the abdomen at 2.0 T. Radiology 173:111, 1989.
18. Saini S, Stark DD, Pykett IL, et al: Millisecond abdominal MR imaging at 2.0 T, in Abstracts of the Society of Magnetic Resonance Imaging, 1988.
19. Hamm B, Fischer E, Taupitz M. Differentiation of hepatic hemangiomas from hepatic metastases by dynamic contrast enhanced MR imaging. J Comput Assist Tomogr 14:205, 1990.
20. Hahn PF, Stark DD, Weissleder R, et al: Clinical application of superparamagnetic iron oxide to MR imaging of tissue perfusion in vascular liver tumors. Radiology 174:361, 1990.
21. Schmiedl U, Ogan MD, Paajanen H, et al: Albumin labeled with Gd-DPTA as an intravascular, blood pool enhancing agent for MR imaging: Biodistribution and imaging studies. Radiology 162:205, 1987.
22. Glazer GM, Collomb LG, Francis IR, et al: P-31 spectroscopy of hepatic cavernous hemangiomas, in Abstracts of the Society of Magnetic Resonance Imaging, 1989, p 569.
23. Nelson RC, Chezmar JL, Sugarbaker PH, Bernadino ME. Hepatic tumors: Comparison of CT during arterial portography, delayed CT, and MR imaging for preoperative evaluation. Radiology 172:27, 1989.

22

Hepatic Hemangiomas: A Comparison of ^{99m}Tc-Labeled Red Blood Cell SPECT and MRI for Definitive Diagnosis

BERNARD A. BIRNBAUM and JEFFREY C. WEINREB

Hemangioma is the most common benign neoplasm of the liver, with an estimated prevalence of approximately 7.3 percent of the population based on autopsy data (1). It is the second most common hepatic tumor, exceeded only by metastases. Focal masses highly suspicious for hemangiomas are often serendipitously discovered on CT and/or ultrasound (US) examinations. Once a suspected hemangioma is detected, however, further imaging may be necessary to specifically characterize this mass, particularly in a patient with a history of neoplasia or focal hepatic disease. Because the specific CT or US criteria of hemangioma cannot be reliably demonstrated in every case (2–6), additional noninvasive methods have been advocated to specifically and definitively diagnose these lesions. While recent studies have claimed that both MRI and ^{99m}Tc-labeled red blood cell (RBC) single-photon-emission computed tomography (SPECT) are accurate modalities for the definitive diagnosis of hepatic hemangiomas (7–13), it has only recently been demonstrated which examination is most appropriate for an individual case (14). The goal of this report is to help define the appropriate utilization of both MRI and labeled RBC SPECT scanning in this clinical setting.

^{99m}Tc-LABELED RBC SPECT IMAGING
SPECT Technique

At our institution, RBC labeling is performed using a modified in vitro technique with 30 mCi (1110 MBq) of ^{99m}technetium pertechnetate (15). A large-field-of-view tomographic gamma camera fitted with a high-resolution low-energy collimator is used. Once the patient is positioned to optimize visualization of the largest known liver lesion, a dynamic arterial flow phase is acquired at a rate of 3 seconds per frame over a 90-s time interval as the patient's blood is reinjected. Immediately thereafter and without moving the camera or the patient, a 256 × 256 pixel static image is acquired for 2 million counts. Following an interval of approximately 90 to 120 min, a SPECT scan of the liver is obtained (360-degree camera rotation, 64 view angles, approximately 25 to 30 s per projection). Once correction for camera nonuniformity and center-of-rotation deviation is performed, the projections are reconstructed using commercially available filtered-back projection and Chang's method of attenuation correction into 6-mm-thick transaxial slices (16). Coronal and sagittal slices are resorted from these transaxial slices and ultimately are merged pairwise to yield 1.2-cm-thick contiguous axial, coronal, and sagittal slices (64 × 64 pixel matrix). Nuclear image

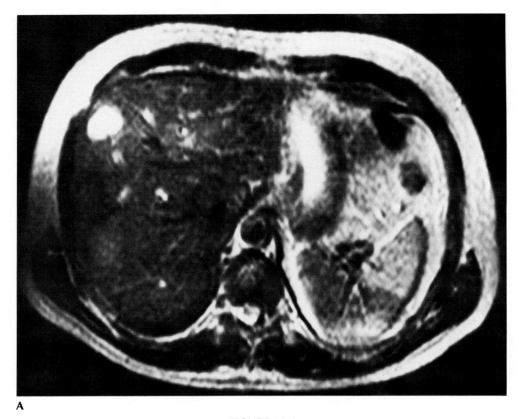

FIGURE 22-1
Typical hemangioma. (A) *T2-weighted (SE 2000/100) MRI image demonstrates homogeneous hyperintense lesion of right hepatic lobe with signal intensity equal to that of CSF.* (B) *Delayed axial SPECT images reveal characteristic uptake of blood pool activity within lesion* (arrows). *Dynamic perfusion phase was normal (not shown).*

acquisition time typically takes approximately 50 min over a total 2.0 to 2.5-hour time interval.

Labeled RBC SPECT Imaging
Numerous studies have demonstrated that ^{99m}Tc-labeled RBC scanning is an accurate method for diagnosing hepatic hemangioma, with the sensitivity of this technique significantly improved with the addition of SPECT imaging (11–13,17–20). Uncomplicated hemangiomas greater than 3.0 cm in size, and occasionally lesions as small as 2.0 cm, may be diagnosed by planar labeled RBC scintigraphy when the patient is optimally positioned to image the suspected region of interest (18,19). SPECT imaging allows improved contrast enhancement, as well as improved size/shape definition afforded by the tomographic removal of superimposed structures, permitting lesion activity on delayed images to be separated from that of overlying liver tissue (11,12). This added capability enables labeled RBC SPECT imaging to routinely detect hemangiomas greater than 2.0 cm in size, and often to identify hemangiomas as small as 1.0 cm when located at the hepatic periphery (11–14,20) (Fig. 22-1). In order to maintain a high degree of diagnostic accuracy, however, it is important that SPECT interpretation involve direct correlation with the referral study (CT/US), especially when evaluating centrally located hemangiomas that may be near major intrahepatic vessels.

The specificity and positive predictive value of labeled RBC SPECT scanning approaches 100 percent (13), with only four documented false-positive results described in the literature. These consisted of three cases of hepatocellular carcinoma (HCC)

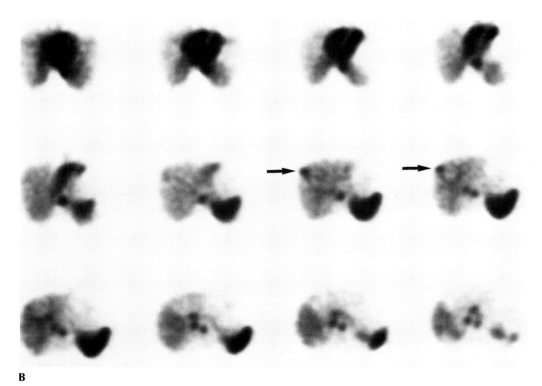

B
FIGURE 22-1 *(continued)*

(18,21) and a single case of hemangiosarcoma (22). Nevertheless, in a recent investigation that evaluated labeled RBC SPECT's ability to distinguish hemangioma from HCC, none of 45 HCCs ranging in size from 1.4 to 5.0 cm displayed delayed blood-pool activity (13). Because hemangiosarcoma is morphologically similar to hemangioma, it is understandable that delayed blood-pool activity may be identified. However, this neoplasm is rare, and unless there is a history of hemochromatosis or chronic exposure to thorium dioxide (Thorotrast), vinyl chloride, arsenicals, or radium, it is generally not a differential diagnostic consideration (13,23).

The importance of the dynamic perfusion phase of labeled RBC scanning in differentiating hemangiomas from other lesions remains controversial (11–13,17–19). Theoretically, it is possible for a primary hepatocellular carcinoma or vascular metastasis to manifest delayed blood-pool activity; however, such lesions should also demonstrate increased arterial perfusion. In order to accurately diagnose hemangioma and exclude such hypervascular lesions, we attempt to identify the presence of perfusion–blood-pool mismatch, i.e. perfusion observed within the lesion equal to or less than that of surrounding normal liver during the arterial phase, associated with delayed blood-pool uptake. Using such diagnostic criteria will maintain a high degree of specificity at the expense of sensitivity, because hemangiomas may occasionally display hyperperfusion relative to normal liver (11,13,14,17,18,24). Hemangioma hyperperfusion is more easily displayed when studying large lesions (>3.0 cm in size), because planar blood-flow imaging may not be sensitive enough to demonstrate the vascular characteristics of small hemangiomas. These hypervascular hemangiomas may be considered indeterminate by some and may require additional evaluation to confirm their benign nature.

It is known that false-negative labeled RBC SPECT scans can occur when hemangiomas are complicated by thrombosis or fibrosis (18,19). The activity in such lesions may either remain stable throughout the study or be absent. When only a portion of a hemangioma is thrombosed or fibrotic, heterogeneous uptake of radionuclide will be observed (19).

Because labeled RBC activity persists in the heart and major intrahepatic blood vessels on delayed SPECT blood-pool images, it may be difficult to discriminate activity originating from small hemangiomas (which are also accumulating activity) when they are located adjacent to these structures. In one study, delayed labeled RBC SPECT scanning failed to identify 33 percent of hemangiomas that were present adjacent to major intrahepatic vessels or were located at the hepatic dome near the heart and/or the confluence of the hepatic veins (Fig. 22-2). These hemangiomas primarily measured less than 2.0 cm, with the largest "missed" hemangioma, measuring 2.5 cm, located at the hepatic dome adjacent to the middle hepatic vein (14). Although a similar difficulty has been reported in the region of the right kidney (13), this may be an inconstant problem, since the amount of activity present within the kidneys on delayed images is often dependent on the efficiency of RBC labeling. When renal activity is significant, lesion detectability will be size-dependent, with multiplanar SPECT imaging capable of correctly diagnosing most hemangiomas greater than 2 cm in size in this location (14).

MAGNETIC RESONANCE IMAGING (MRI)

MRI Technique

For the purposes of this study, MRI examinations were performed using spin-echo (SE) pulse sequences on a 0.5-Tesla superconducting magnet. Following acquisition of a coronal scout, SE axial images are obtained through the entire liver using a repetition interval (TR) of 2000 ms, an echo delay (TE) of 50 and 100 ms, a 128 × 128 matrix (reconstructed at 256 × 256), and 2 NEX. Slice thickness is 10 mm, with an interslice gap equal to 2 mm. MRI acquisition time typically takes about 8.5 min, with approximately 15 min total table time.

Once obtained, the T2-weighted (2000/100) images are specifically photographed at settings whereby cerebrospinal fluid (CSF) appears uniformly and markedly hyperintense. This is important because it is easy to change the appearance of these lesions by manipulation of operator-selected window levels and widths and CSF may be used as an internal reference standard on the hard-copy images.

MRI of Hemangiomas

MRI is the most sensitive imaging modality for the detection of hepatic hemangiomas and is considered to be an accurate and effective means of differentiating these lesions from most malignant hepatic neoplasms (7-10, 25-28). Previous studies have attempted to characterize hemangiomas on the basis of calculated T2 relaxation times, lesion/liver intensity ratios, lesion/liver contrast-to-noise ratios, and morphologic inspection (7-10, 25-28). Recent studies suggest a potential role for gadolinium-enhanced studies (29,30). Nevertheless, certain limitations of these methods exist. For instance, while some reports suggest that the mean T2 relaxation times of hemangiomas may differ significantly from those of other focal liver lesions, the large standard deviations in these calculated T2 values may preclude their use in characterizing a lesion in an individual patient (7-9, 25-28). Quantitative analysis based on calculated T2 relaxation times may not be reproducible in different imaging systems, and inherent inaccuracies exist in commonly used two-point fit measurements. Furthermore, comparing the signal intensity of a mass relative to liver may be inaccurate in the setting of fatty infiltration, hemosiderosis, cirrhosis, or other infiltrating hepatic diseases.

Our MRI analysis is based on visual inspection of hard-copy films, a qualitative assessment that simulates the most commonly utilized interpretive clinical approach and which has proved as reliable as available quantitative techniques (10,27). MRI readers diagnose hemangioma when a lesion is found to be either totally or "predominantly" hyperintense or isointense relative to CSF signal intensity. Small regions of heterogeneity, if present, do not preclude characterization of hemangioma. This interpretation is based on the assumption that (1) a prior CT or US study has excluded the diagnosis of hepatic cyst and (2) the patient has no history of a primary neoplasm known to produce necrotic or hypervascular metastases. When MRI is performed as a screening study, and not as a problem-solving characterization study, the finding of a markedly hyperintense mass on a 2000/100 (TR/TE) pulse sequence may be consistent with either hemangioma, cyst, or hypervascular metastasis.

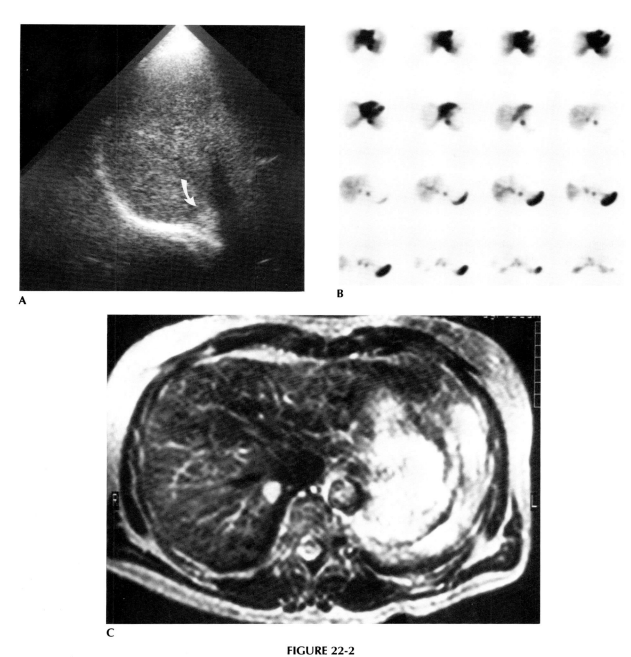

FIGURE 22-2

SPECT-negative hemangioma. (A) Transverse US scan depicts an echogenic mass (arrow) at dome adjacent to right hepatic vein. (B) Delayed axial SPECT scans fail to identify lesion. (C) T2-weighted (SE 2000/100) MRI image clearly demonstrates hemangioma at confluence of right hepatic vein and inferior vena cava. (From Birnbaum BA, Weinreb JC, Megibow AJ, et al: Definitive diagnosis of hepatic hemangiomas: MRI versus ^{99m}Tc-labeled red blood cell SPECT, Radiology *(in press). Reprinted by permission of the publisher.)*

It has been suggested that improved hemangioma/metastasis discrimination may be possible by using SE pulse sequences with TEs ranging up to 120 to 180 ms (8,10). In our experience, this is occasionally helpful; nevertheless, the use of such techniques may still not ensure that all hemangiomas can be differentiated from hypervascular or necrotic neoplasms. We routinely use a TE of 100 ms for practical considerations, since this parameter allows us to study the entire liver in a reasonable amount of time, while providing optimal signal to noise on our system and enabling sufficient T2 weighting for confident characterization.

Hemangiomas typically demonstrate a homogeneous high-signal-intensity appearance on T2-weighted images (10) (Fig. 22-1). Varying degrees of heterogeneity reflecting components of thrombosis, fibrosis, hemorrhage, liquefaction, and calcification may be present, particularly in larger lesions (31,32). These observations agree with those of Ros et al., who found hemangiomas to be frequently heterogeneous on both gross anatomic sections and T2-weighted MRI images (31). In a recent report, 16 of 64 hemangiomas (25 percent) characterized by MRI displayed variable amounts of low-signal-intensity foci (14). Lesions that appeared to be "predominantly" of high signal intensity were further subdivided by appearance into "segmentally heterogeneous" if they contained nonlinear focal regions of low signal intensity, "diffusely heterogeneous" if they contained scattered regions of low signal intensity, or "septated and/or stranded." Strands were defined as linear appearing regions of low signal intensity traversing the lesion. Despite the presence of these low-signal-intensity regions, the MRI readers had no equivocation in characterizing the given lesions as hemangiomas, because the predominant signal was equal to or greater than an internal reference standard, CSF (14). This underscores the importance of interpreting images at standard settings, since the appearance of hemangiomas may be considerably altered depending on the window levels and widths selected.

While the characterization of hemangiomas may be relatively simple when a suspected lesion is homogeneously hyperintense, the diagnosis may become problematic as the degree of heterogeneity present increases. Simply stated, at what point does the diagnosis of a hyperintense mass containing low-signal-intensity foci change from hemangioma with partial thrombosis and/or fibrosis to a metastasis complicated by considerable necrosis? This question will ultimately need to be addressed, because the diagnostic sensitivity of MRI will decrease if only homogeneous "lightbulb" lesions are considered acceptable to be characterized as hemangiomas.

Prior reports have described a homogeneous high-signal-intensity appearance secondary to metastatic carcinoid, islet-cell tumor, pheochromocytoma, and various "sarcomas" (unspecified), as well as with adenocarcinoma of the pancreas, uterus, and lung (10,14,27). Therefore, even when one uses the stringent criteria of a homogeneous hyperintense lesion, MRI is seen to lack the specificity and near 100 percent positive predictive value of a positive SPECT RBC scan (13).

COMPARISON OF LABELED RBC SPECT AND MRI

We retrospectively analyzed the MRI and the ^{99m}technetium-labeled RBC SPECT findings of 37 patients with 69 suspected hemangiomas initially found by CT (peripherally enhanced lesion demonstrated by bolus contrast enhanced sequential dynamic CT) and/or ultrasound (well-circumscribed echogenic mass) (14). Sixty-four "reference" lesions, occurring in 32 patients, were ultimately characterized as hemangiomas. The five remaining lesions that could not be characterized as hemangiomas included two patients with solitary masses of focal nodular hyperplasia, two patients with solitary hepatic metastases (lymphoma and lung cancer), and one patient with a focal normal liver in the setting of fatty infiltration.

Utilizing criteria of perfusion–blood-pool mismatch, SPECT readers correctly diagnosed 50 of 64 hemangiomas and 5 of 5 "nonhemangiomas" (sensitivity 78 percent, accuracy 80 percent) (14). All diagnosed hemangiomas demonstrated either normal or decreased activity during the flow phase and persistent blood-pool accumulation compared with normal liver on delayed SPECT images. Analysis of the 14 false-negative lesions missed by nuclear imaging revealed the following: (1) three lesions greater than 3.0 cm in size were identified on the delayed SPECT images but were interpreted as indeterminate because they displayed increased activity during the arterial flow phase, (2) one hemangioma measuring 2.5

cm located adjacent to the middle hepatic vein was not identified on the SPECT images, and (3) 10 hemangiomas, all less than 2.0 cm, were missed (two located at the hepatic dome or adjacent to vessels, two adjacent to intrahepatic vessels, one at the dome near the heart, two superficial, and three deeply located within hepatic parenchyma).

Qualitative analysis of lesion signal intensity on T2-weighted spin-echo images (TR 2000/TE 100; hemangioma diagnosed when a lesion was found to be either totally or "predominantly" hyperintense or isointense relative to CSF signal intensity) allowed MRI readers to diagnose 58 of 64 hemangiomas and 4 of 5 "nonhemangiomas" (sensitivity 91 percent, accuracy 90 percent) (14). The single MRI false-positive result was a 2.0-cm lesion located at the hepatic dome. This was secondary to metastatic adenocarcinoma of the lung and appeared homogeneously hyperintense with a signal intensity greater than that of CSF. All hemangiomas that were located at the hepatic dome or situated adjacent to major intrahepatic vessels were correctly diagnosed by MRI. Of the six MRI false-negative results, three were located deep within hepatic parenchyma (size range 1.0 to 1.2 cm), while three were superficially located (size range 1.5 to 2.0 cm).

MRI was found to be more accurate than SPECT in characterizing total overall number of lesions. However, when the study data were carefully examined by analyzing lesions according to size and location, the differences between the two techniques were found to be primarily due to two important identifiable trends: (1) MRI was more effective in its ability to detect and diagnose small hemangiomas (<2.0 cm in size), and (2) MRI proved more capable of diagnosing small hemangiomas (≤2.5 cm in size) adjacent to the heart and major intrahepatic vessels (Fig. 22-2). SPECT was seen to compare favorably with MRI for lesions 2.0 cm and greater, where the sensitivity and accuracy of detection were similar for both modalities (14).

A potential limitation of this investigation was that only lesions with features suggestive of hemangioma on CT (peripherally enhanced mass) and/or US (well-circumscribed echogenic mass) were studied. As a result, the resulting inherent selection bias may have artificially increased the accuracies of both MRI and SPECT by excluding those hemangiomas with atypical features which may be difficult to diagnose. In addition, the evaluation of test specificity was limited because only a small number of nonhemangioma lesions were studied. Had more hypervascular or necrotic metastases been included, the results may have been significantly different.

CONCLUSIONS

While the overall accuracy of MRI is slightly greater than that of SPECT for the characterization of hepatic hemangiomas, the differences appear most pronounced in certain specific lesions based on size and location. Labeled RBC SPECT imaging presently has limited sensitivity in routinely detecting hemangiomas less than 2.0 cm, as well as those 2.5 cm or less adjacent to major intrahepatic vessels and the heart. MRI is able to characterize small hemangiomas (1 to 2.0 cm in size), and sensitivity of detection is not limited when hemangiomas are adjacent to regions of vascular activity. MRI characterization of very small lesions (<1.0 cm in size) may be difficult secondary to partial voluming of adjacent hepatic parenchyma. Limitations of MRI include the significant cost and the inability of MRI to categorically differentiate hemangiomas from hypervascular metastases (27).

The decision to utilize labeled RBC SPECT scanning versus MRI as a problem-solving technique for the characterization of hemangiomas should be based on both the size and location of the suspected lesion. Based on the significantly higher cost of MRI and its inability to categorically differentiate hemangiomas from hypervascular metastases, we consider SPECT to be the method of choice for diagnosing hepatic hemangiomas. MRI should be reserved for diagnosing small lesions of less than 2.0 cm, as well as for those 2.5 cm or less when located adjacent to the heart and/or major intrahepatic vessels, where sensitivity of detection is known to be superior to SPECT. MRI may serve as a complimentary technique to SPECT for the noninvasive characterization of those atypical hemangiomas which display increased arterial perfusion on labeled RBC imaging and are considered indeterminate by some. MRI is not advocated for the characterization of hepatic lesions in patients with known primary tumors that may produce hypervascular metastases.

REFERENCES

1. Ishak KG, Rabin L: Benign tumors of the liver. Med Clin North Am 59:995, 1975.
2. Bree RL, Schwab RE, Neiman HL: Solitary echogenic spot in the liver: Is it diagnostic of a hemangioma? AJR 140:41, 1983.
3. Bree RL, Schwab RE, Glazer GM, Fink-Bennett D. The varied appearances of hepatic cavernous hemangiomas with sonography, computed tomography, magnetic resonance imaging and scintigraphy. Radiographics 7(6):1153, 1987.
4. Takayasu K, Moriyama N, Shima Y, et al: Atypical radiographic findings in hepatic cavernous hemangioma: Correlation with histologic features. AJR 146:1149, 1986.
5. Wiener SN, Parulekar SG: Scintigraphy and ultrasonography of hepatic hemangioma. Radiology 132:149, 1979.
6. Freeny PC, Marks WM: Hepatic hemangioma: Dynamic bolus CT. AJR 147:711, 1986.
7. Itai Y, Ohtomo K, Furui S, et al: Noninvasive diagnosis of small cavernous hemangioma of the liver: Advantage of MRI. AJR 145:1195, 1985.
8. Stark DD, Felder RC, Wittenberg J, et al: Magnetic resonance imaging of cavernous hemangioma of the liver: Tissue specific characterization. AJR 145:213, 1985.
9. Ohtomo K, Itai Y, Furui S, et al: Hepatic tumors: Differentiation by transverse relaxation time (T2) of magnetic resonance imaging. Radiology 155:421, 1985.
10. Wittenberg J, Stark DD, Forman BH, et al: Differentiation of hepatic metastases from hepatic hemangiomas and cysts by using MR imaging. AJR 151:79, 1988.
11. Brodsky RI, Friedman AC, Maurer AH, et al: Hepatic cavernous hemangioma: Diagnosis with ^{99m}Tc-labeled red cells and signal photon emission CT. AJR 148:125, 1987.
12. Tumeh SS, Benson C, Nagel JS, et al: Cavernous hemangioma of the liver: Detection with single-photon emission computed tomography. Radiology 164:353, 1987.
13. Kudo M, Ikekubo K, Yamamoto K, et al: Distinction between hemangioma of the liver and hepatocellular carcinoma: Value of labeled RBC SPECT scanning. AJR 152:977, 1989.
14. Birnbaum BA, Weinreb JC, Megibow AJ, et al: Blinded retrospective comparison of MRI and ^{99m}Tc-labeled RBC SPECT for definitive diagnosis of hepatic hemangiomas. Radiology (in press).
15. Front D, Israel O, Groshar O, Weininger J: Tc 99m labeled red blood cell imaging. Semin Nucl Med 14:226, 1984.
16. Chang LT: A method for attenuation correction in radionuclide computed tomography. IEEE Trans Nucl Sci 25:638, 1978.
17. Engel MA, Marks DS, Sandler MA, Shetty P: Differentiation of focal intrahepatic lesions with ^{99m}Tc red blood cell imaging. Radiology 146:777, 1983.
18. Rabinowitz SA, McKusick KA, Strauss HW: ^{99m}Tc red blood cell scintigraphy in evaluating focal liver lesions. AJR 143:63, 1984.
19. Moinuddin M, Allison JR, Montgomery JH, et al: Scintigraphic diagnosis of hepatic hemangioma: Its role in the management of hepatic mass lesions. AJR 145:223, 1985.
20. Malik MH: Blood pool SPECT and planar imaging in hepatic hemangioma. Clin Nucl Med 12:543, 1987.
21. Drum DE: The radiocolloid liver scan in space-occupying disease. Appl Radiol 11:115, 1982.
22. Ginsberg F, Slavin JD Jr, Spencer RP: Hepatic angiosarcoma: Mimicking of angioma on three-phase technetium-99m red blood cell scintigraphy. J Nucl Med 27:1861, 1986.
23. Locker GY, Doroshow JH, Swelling LA, et al: The clinical features of hepatic angiosarcoma: A report of four cases and a review of the English literature. Medicine 58:48, 1979.
24. Larcos G, Farlow DC, Gruenewald SM, Antico VF: Atypical appearance of an hepatic hemangioma with technetium-99m red blood cell scintigraphy. J Nucl Med 30:1885, 1989.
25. Glazer GM, Aisen AM, Francis IR, et al: Hepatic cavernous hemangioma: Magnetic resonance imaging. Radiology 155:417, 1985.
26. Ohtomo K, Itai Y, Yoshikawa K, et al: Hepatocellular carcinoma and cavernous hemangioma: Differentiation with MR imaging. Efficacy of T2 values at 0.35 and 1.5 T. Radiology 168:621, 1988.
27. Li KC, Glazer GM, Quint LE, et al: Distinction of hepatic cavernous hemangioma from hepatic metastases with MR imaging. Radiology 169:409, 1988.
28. Rummeny E, Weissleder R, et al: Primary liver tumors: Diagnosis by MR imaging. AJR 152:63, 1989.
29. Shuman WP, Baron RL, Patten RM, Ekstrom JE: Dynamic gadolinium-enhanced MR imaging of small liver hemangiomas. Radiology 173(P):270, 1989.
30. Van Beers B, Demeure R, Pringot J, et al: Dynamic spin-echo imaging with Gd-DTPA: Value in the differentiation of hepatic tumors. AJR 154:515, 1990.
31. Ros PR, Lubbers PR, Olmsted WW, Morillo G: Hemangioma of the liver: Heterogeneous appearance on T2-weighted images. AJR 149:1167, 1987.
32. Choi BI, Han NC, Park JH, et al: Giant cavernous hemangioma of the liver: CT and MR imaging in 10 cases. AJR 152:1221, 1989.

23

Color Doppler Flow Mapping of Liver Tumors

L. BOLONDI, S. GAIANI, S. LI BASSI,
G. BENZI, G. ZIRONI, V. SANTI,
A. RIGAMONTI, and L. BARBARA

CONVENTIONAL IDENTIFICATION OF FOCAL LIVER LESIONS

The sonographic detection of a solid focal lesion within the liver is quite frequent and often raises a problem of interpretation. The clinical setting is fundamental for an understanding of the ultrasonographic (US) finding and for giving the lesion a probability of being benign or malignant. Every solid nodule found in a cirrhotic liver should in fact be suspected as hepatocellular carcinoma (HCC) until another diagnosis has been proven by guided biopsy or other invasive techniques (angiography). Primary malignant tumors are very rare in healthy livers, where secondary lesions and benign neoplasms are much more common.

Recent experience suggests that some characteristic echo patterns may help in the differential diagnosis: (a) the small (1 to 3 cm) hyperechoic nodules, single or multiple, occasionally found in healthy subjects are generally hemangiomas, (b) the presence of a hypoechoic ring or the appearance of a "target lesion" suggests malignancy, (c) a hyperechoic ring around a hypoechoic lesion suggests the presence of a hemangioma, and (d) an anechoic area seen within a hyperechoic lesion generally corresponds to liquefactive necrosis in the center of a metastatic cancer. There are also other nonneoplastic lesions that sometimes require differentiation from benign and malignant tumors, such as focal fatty infiltration and hydatid cysts, which sometimes display a solid pattern (1).

Computed tomography (CT) may be helpful in identifying large hemangiomas or focal fat. However, in many instances, invasive techniques such as angiography or US-guided biopsy may be required to clarify the nature of a focal mass. When the diagnosis of hemangioma has been excluded, the differential diagnosis of these lesions is usually achieved by US-guided biopsy.

The sensitivity of this technique, performed by fine needle, is very high, varying between 91 and 95.1 percent (2–5), with a specificity of 92.9 to 100 percent. There are, however, some problems of interpretation in cases of small, well-differentiated neoplasms, which can be correctly diagnosed only on the basis of a study of tissue architecture and characteristics by histology (5). It is now accepted that the diagnosis of small, well-differentiated HCC requires a core biopsy, which may be performed with an 18- to 19-gauge cutting needle or with a 22-guage cutting needle passed through a large needle guide inserted to the peritoneum.

PRINCIPLES OF TISSUE CHARACTERIZATION BY THE DOPPLER METHOD

Many investigators have attempted in the past to obtain tissue characterization in a noninvasive way utilizing various acoustic properties of tissues, such as absorption, speed, dispersion, density, compressibility, scattering, and attenuation (6). None of them, however, could be applied in clinical practice. The Doppler technique, therefore, showed great potential for the noninvasive characterization of tumors. This characteristic was originally reported by Wells et al. (1977) in malignant lesions of the breast, where higher signals due to arteriovenous shunts were found at the level of the tumor (7). Several groups (8–10) confirmed the original observation of Wells et al. in breast tumors, and other investigators found characteristic neovascular signals in other lesions (11). Currently, applications of Doppler constitute the best potential for achieving tissue characterization.

The Doppler signal seems to be related to the histologic structure and hemodynamics of the tumor circulation, as has been well documented in histologic and angiographic studies (12–14). It is well accepted that tumor growth depends on the vascular supply. Most of the neoplastic vessels are concentrated in a highly vascularized ring, which constitutes the advancing edge of the tumor. These vessels tend to be thin and lacking in the muscular elements seen in normal vessels. Arteriovenous shunts are also characteristic of some kinds of neoplasms.

In addition, abnormal vascularity includes the presence of vascular tumor lakes, which are thin-walled sinusoids. This morphologic pattern leads to a low-impedance flow, which is represented by a high diastolic flow or even a total lack of systolic/diastolic variation. Another important feature of neovascular flow is high Doppler shift (3 to 10 kHz) depending on large pressure gradients corresponding to arteriovenous communication.

DOPPLER US FEATURES OF LIVER MASSES

A new possibility for the US characterization of HCC and of vascular alterations related to this neoplasm has been recently provided by the application of duplex and color Doppler investigations (15–18). The genesis of the Doppler vascular signals from tumoral masses is quite complex, and several recent studies have attempted to clarify this problem (19). It is well accepted that tumor growth depends on the vascular supply and that most of the neoformed vessels are concentrated in a highly vascularized ring at the periphery of the tumor. These arterioles have a very thin caliber and are impossible to visualize by noninvasive imaging techniques, but Doppler signals may be detected from them. Arteriovenous shunts are characteristic of some HCCs, and they too may show a typical pattern of Doppler spectrum.

According to recent papers (15,17,20), in small HCCs, abnormal signals are characterized by high-peak-velocity Doppler shift frequencies, often over 4 kHz, owing to the large pressure gradient existing in arterioportal shunting. These high-peak signals may be associated with broadening of the spectrum owing to marked turbulence (Fig. 23-1, see color insert). Another pulsed Doppler feature consistent with HCC is the continuous low-impedance signal, probably related to the presence of large intratumoral vascular lakes (Fig. 23-2, see color insert).

In a large series recently published (16), pulsatile or continuous-wave signals have been detected in 87.3 percent of HCC, in 28 percent of metastatic cancers, and in 13.3 percent of hemangiomas. Other Japanese authors (18) found arterial signals within and at the periphery of the tumor in 75.7 percent of small HCC (<3 cm in size) and in 100 percent of HCCs >3 cm.

This method also proved quite sensitive (83.3 percent) in our series of HCCs (17), but its specificity seems to be low, because similar signals can also be found in liver metastasis, in cholangiocarcinomas, and in some benign lesions, such as focal nodular hyperplasia (17).

Color Doppler flow imaging plays an important role in the detection of abnormal tumor signals, allowing a rapid search of the point(s) where flow signals move into or around the tumor (Figs. 23-1, 23-3, and 23-4, see color insert). Otherwise, it should be stressed that color Doppler signals into or around the tumor suggest only the presence of blood flow, without information about the characteristics of flow and its pathologic meaning (Fig. 23-3). Color Doppler should be therefore used as a guide for positioning the sample volume and for obtaining the Doppler trace. A limitation of color Doppler is the relative lower sensitivity in comparison with the Doppler trace, which may give rise to false-negative findings (Fig. 23-4).

Future studies addressed to the development of an ultrasound contrast agent suitable for humans will substantially increase the echogenicity of the neovascular bed of tumors, thus improving the capability of the machines to obtain Doppler signals from small vessels. Another important field of investigation involves the pathologic meaning of the neovascular Doppler signals. It has not yet been established if the presence and the pattern of these vascular signals are related to the growth speed or a particular tendency to vascular invasion. Longitudinal studies correlating the clinical and pathologic outcomes with the Doppler features of tumors are needed. Finally, a promising clinical application of Doppler US is represented by the attempt to evaluate the efficacy of some therapeutic approaches, such as arterial chemoembolization or alcohol injection in case of HCC, based on the disappearing of pathologic signals as a sign of therapeutic success.

REFERENCES

1. Lewall DB, McCorkell SJ: Hepatic echinococcal cyst: Sonographic appearance and classification. Radiology 155:775, 1985.
2. Montali G, Solbiati L, Croce F, et al: Fine-needle aspiration biopsy of liver focal lesions ultrasonically guided with a real time probe: Report on 126 cases. Br J Radiol 55:717, 1982.
3. Schwerk WB, Durr HK, Schmitz-Moormann P: Ultrasound-guided fine-needle biopsies in pancreatic and hepatic neoplasm. Gastrointest Radiol 8:219, 1983.
4. Fornari F, Cavanna L, Civardi G, et al: Ultrasonically guided fine-needle aspiration biopsy: First-stage invasive procedure in the diagnosis of focal lesion of the liver. Ital J Gastroenterol 17:246, 1985.
5. Limberg B, Hopker WW, Kommerell B: Histologic differential diagnosis of focal liver lesions by ultrasonically guided fine-needle biopsy. Gut 28:237, 1987.
6. Taylor KJW, Wells PNT: Tissue characterization. Ultrasound Med Biol 15:421, 1989.
7. Wells PNT, Halliwell M, Skidmore R, et al: Tumor detection by ultrasonic Doppler blood flow signals. Ultrasonics 15:231, 1977.
8. Jellins J: B-mode and Doppler assessment of breast disease, in Jellins J, Kossoff G, Croll J (eds): Proceedings of the Fourth International Congress on the Ultrasonic Examination of the Breast. Sidney 1985. p 215.
9. Schoenberger SG, Sutherland CM, Robinson A: Breast neoplasms: Duplex sonographic imaging as an adjunct in diagnosis. Radiology 168:665, 1988.
10. Scoutt L, Ramos I, Taylor KJW, et al: CW Doppler examination of breast masses. Radiology 169:21, 1988.
11. Ramos I, Taylor KJW, Kier R, et al: Tumor vascular signals in renal masses: Detection with Doppler US. Radiology 168:633, 1988.
12. Ney FG, Feinst JN, Altemus LR, Ordinario VR: Characteristic angiographic criteria of malignancy. Radiology 104:567, 1972.
13. Gammill SL, Shipkey RB, Himmelfarb EH, et al: Roentgenology-pathology correlative study of neovascularity. AJR 126:376, 1976.
14. Okuda K, Obata H, Jinnouchi S, et al: Angiographic assessment of gross anatomy of hepatocellular carcinoma: Comparison of celiac arteriograms and liver pathology in 100 cases. Radiology 123:21, 1977.
15. Taylor KJW, Ramos I, Morse SS, et al: Focal liver masses: Differential diagnosis with pulsed Doppler US. Radiology 164:643, 1987.
16. Yasuhara K, Kimura K, Ohto M, et al: Pulsed Doppler in the diagnosis of small liver tumors. Br J Radiol 61:898, 1988.
17. Bolondi L, Gaiani S, Li Bassi S, et al: Colour Doppler and duplex investigation of vascular signals arising from hepatocellular carcinoma (HCC). Gastroenterol Int 2:30, 1989.
18. Ohnishi K, Nomura F: Ultrasonic Doppler studies of hepatocellular carcinoma and comparison with other hepatic focal lesions. Gastroenterology 97:1489, 1989.
19. Taylor KJW, Ramos I, Carter D, et al: Correlation of Doppler US tumor signals with neovascular morphologic features. Radiology 166:57, 1988.
20. Taylor CR, Taylor KJW: Diagnostic imaging of hepatocellular carcinoma: Progress in noninvasive tissue characterization. J Clin Gastroenterol 10:452, 1988.

24

Hepatic Cavernous Hemangioma: Diagnosis by Means of Rapid Dynamic Nonincremental CT

JOCHEN GAA and
SANJAY SAINI

Cavernous hemangioma, with an incidence of 0.4 to 20 percent, is the most frequent benign tumor of the liver (1). They are often detected during abdominal sonography and usually can be diagnosed by their typical echogenic pattern. However, some cases do not show classic ultrasound features, and in patients with known primary cancer, the differential diagnosis from metastasis is often difficult. Dynamic computed tomography (CT) plays an important role in differentiation and assessing the characteristics of intrahepatic masses (2–5). Modern scanners with continuously rotating measurement systems provide improved spatial resolution and image quality. Additionally, very short scan times permit even more rapid scan rates and thereby a better evaluation of the perfusion features of a lesion. We report our initial experience in diagnosing liver hemangiomas with rapid dynamic CT.

PATIENTS AND METHODS

Thirty-three patients demonstrating 38 liver hemangiomas were examined prospectively using rapid dynamic nonincremental CT. The mean age of the 23 women and 10 men was 52.6 years (range 37 to 80 years). The diameter of lesions ranged from 0.7 to 13 cm (average 3.1 cm). Thirty patients demonstrated single lesions, two patients had two and one patient had four masses. Nine patients had a known underlying malignant disease—four mammary carcinomas, two uterine carcinomas, one lung carcinoma, one non-Hodgkin lymphoma, and one hypernephroma. The diagnosis of hemangioma was verified by fine-needle biopsy ($n = 14$), typical features at angiography ($n = 11$) or nuclear scintigraphy ($n = 10$). Three subcentimeter lesions with a diameter between 7 and 10 mm were presumed to represent hemangiomas because there was no change in size at follow-up imaging at 5, 6, and 8 months. Rapid dynamic CT studies were performed with a CT scanner of the newest generation (Somatom Plus, Siemens AG, Erlangen, FRG). The slice thickness and slice distance of 10 mm each were chosen after precontrast examination of the liver. The plane of focus was established, and a dynamic bolus CT with a scan time of 1 s was performed at this position. All patients were examined in end-expiration in order to retain the selected plane exactly in position. A peripheral, manual bolus injection (1 ml/kg body weight) of 30 percent nonionic contrast medium (Solutrast 300, Byk Gulden, Konstanz, FRG) was administered intravenously within 5 to 7 s by means of an 18-gauge cannula. Fifteen scans were completed in the first 30 s, 10 s after beginning contrast medium administration, at a

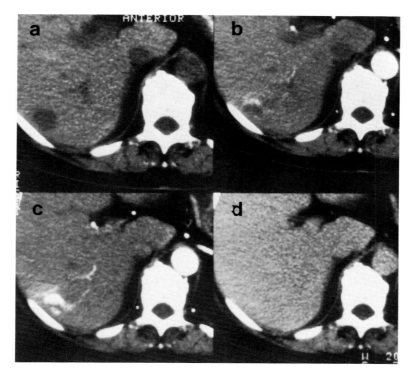

FIGURE 24-1
*Hemangioma (1.5 cm in diameter) located posteriorly in the right liver lobe.
(A) Precontrast view. Evidence of an intense peripheral "nodular" contrast medium
enhancement during the early arterial (B) and arterial (C) phases. (D) The hemangioma
is isodense to the remaining liver parenchyma 90 s after contrast medium administration.*

scan time of 1 s. This was followed by six further scans during the second to fifth minute. Subsequently, one scan per minute was performed until the end of the examination after a maximum of 30 min.

RESULTS

Each of the 38 hemangiomas was seen to be hypodense in the precontrast scan with a mean density value of 44.3 HU (range 38 to 51 HU). Thirty hemangiomas between 1.3 and 13 cm in diameter (average 3.5 cm) demonstrated a characteristic and especially intensive "nodular" enhancement of a focal peripheral vascular space during the arterial phase. This enhancement was of a similarly high density as found in afferent arterial hepatic vessels (Figs. 24-1 and 24-2). The maximum density value (157 HU) in the nodular regions was reached 5.8 s after the highest density in the aorta (380 HU). It was characterized by a persistent contrast medium pooling with only a slow decline in density of 44 HU to an average value of 113 HU after 21 s. A centripetally directed increase in size of the nodular regions was observed simultaneously (Fig. 24-3).

This characteristic pattern was not observed in eight cases; five thrombosed hemangiomas between 1.8 and 4 cm in diameter demonstrated a minimal enhancement in the arterial phase with no evidence of nodular regions. They continued to be hypodense to the surrounding hepatic tissue, even 30 min after contrast medium administration. Three lesions (7, 8, and 10) mm in diameter) demonstrated an intense, homogeneous, hyperdense enhancement in the early arterial phase and were isodense 28 s after contrast medium administration (Fig. 24-4).

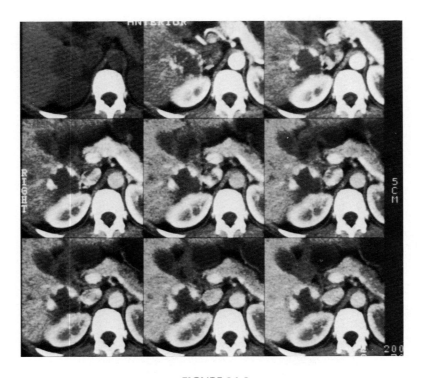

FIGURE 24-2
Rapid dynamic nonincremental CT study demonstrating very intense, sharply outlined "nodular" hyperdensities at the margins of this 3.5-cm hemangioma.

A typical "iris-diaphragm phenomenon" and a total isodensity to the remaining hepatic tissue in delayed scans up to 30 min were found in only 24 hemangiomas.

DISCUSSION

The specificity of conventional CT for the diagnosis of hepatic cavernous hemangioma varies from 55 to 90 percent. This variation reflects both the nature of CT criteria and the quite different examination conditions and system constellations (6,7).

Our dynamic CT criteria depend mainly on early arterial visualization of the vascular spaces of cavernous hemangioma. Earlier papers have described an "iris diaphragm shaped" contrast medium enhancement and a total isodensity compared with the normal liver parenchyma on delayed scans as classic CT signs of hemangioma (4,7). The development of modern CT units makes the performance of even faster scan sequences possible so that the perfusion characteristics of a lesion can be even better evaluated. The following specific criteria are necessary for the diagnosis of hemangioma using rapid dynamic nonincremental CT. They conform to well-known angiographic signs for hemangioma such as the early display of a hypervascularized region and a persistent stasis of contrast medium in the form of mottled contrast medium deposits.

1. In the arterial phase, detection of an intense mural nodular enhancement. The density in the nodular region(s) should have a similar high level to that of the hepatic arteries.
2. A sharp margin of the nodular area(s).
3. An increasing cetripetally oriented spreading of the nodular enhancement for more than 20 s.

Thirty of the 38 hemangiomas (79 percent) could be classified correctly based on these criteria.

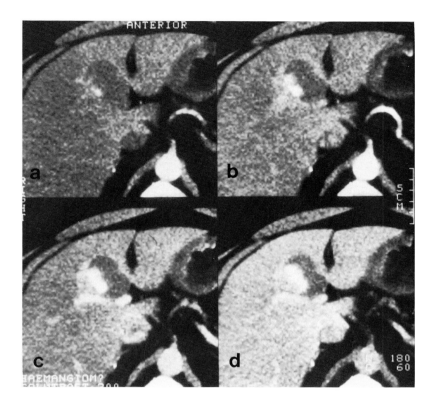

FIGURE 24-3
Hemangioma (4 cm in size) at the level of the portal fissure. An intense peripheral "nodular" density increase is demonstrated during the arterial phase (A, B). A slow, centripetally directed increase in size of the nodular regions with persistent contrast medium pooling is found in the early (C) and late (D) portal phases.

Further signs mentioned in the literature provided no additional diagnostic advantage and were not taken into consideration (e.g., hypodensity of the lesion in the precontrast scan and a complete fill-in in delayed scans). Comparative examinations on 43 patients with liver metastases from colorectal tumors and mammary carcinomas permitted a reliable differentiation to hemangiomas with the use of these criteria (8). Our own results are in accordance with those of Itai and Teraoka (9), who demonstrated only 1 false-positive finding from 110 hemangiomas with the use of similar criteria. This was a very rare angiosarcoma of the liver that could not be differentiated from a hemangioma with CT, angiography, or MRI. The CT diagnosis of thrombosed hemangiomas continues to be a problem because they often demonstrate reduced enhancement. Another problem can be found in foci of 1 cm and less in diameter, since these may show a homogeneous hyperdense enhancement in the arterial phase. Therefore, they cannot be reliably differentiated from hypervascularized metastases of hypernephromas, malignant insulinomas, pheochromocytomas, or carcinoids (10).

In summary, we believe that nonthrombosed hemangiomas larger than 1 cm in diameter demonstrate a nearly pathognomonic CT behavior from the early arterial to the venoportal phase. Therefore, they can be diagnosed reliably based on these specific criteria. An additional advantage is that delayed scans up to 30 min after contrast medium administration are no longer necessary, resulting in a substantial saving of time.

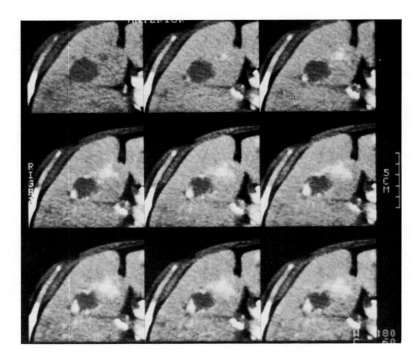

FIGURE 24-4
Two hepatic hemangiomas with a diameter of 2.5 cm and 8 mm. In contrast to the characteristic nodular contrast medium profile of the larger lesion, the smaller hemangioma shows a homogeneous hyperdense enhancement in the arterial phase without evidence of "nodular" regions.

REFERENCES

1. Karhunen PJ: Benign hepatic tumors and tumor-like conditions. J Clin Pathol 39:183, 1986.
2. Araki T, Itai Y, Furui S, Tasaka A: Dynamic CT densitometry of hepatic tumors. AJR 135:1037, 1980.
3. Foley WD: Dynamic hepatic CT. Radiology 170:617, 1989.
4. Freeny PC, Marks WM: Patterns of contrast enhancement of benign and malignant hepatic neoplasms during bolus dynamic and delayed CT. Radiology 160:613, 1986.
5. Itai Y, Araki T, Furui S, Tasaka A: Differential diagnosis of hepatic masses on computed tomography, with particular reference to hepatocellular carcinoma. J Comput Assist Tomogr 5:834, 1981.
6. Ashida C, Fishman EK, Zerhouni EA, et al: Computed tomography of hepatic cavernous hemangioma. J Comput Assist Tomogr 11:455, 1987.
7. Freeny PC, Marks WM: Hepatic hemangioma: Dynamic bolus CT. AJR 147:711, 1986.
8. Gaa J, Deininger HK: Differenzierung benigner und maligner Leberläsionen mit einer schnellen, dynamischen Computertomographie. Radiologe (in press).
9. Itai Y, Teraoka T: Angiosarcoma of the liver mimicking cavernous hemangioma on dynamic CT. J Comput Assist Tomogr 13:910, 1989.
10. Bressler EL, Alpern MB, Glazer GM, et al: Hypervascular hepatic metastases: CT evaluation. Radiology 162:49, 1987.

VIII. STAGING LIVER TUMORS FOR THERAPEUTIC INTERVENTION

25

Principles of Hepatic Surgery

RONALD A. MALT

The late Richard H. Sweet (1901–1962) used to say that thoracic surgery is just an exercise in hemostasis. To the extent that the liver and lungs are plethoric, the aphorism is applicable to both organs; furthermore, certain ductal structures must be controlled during surgery in each of the organs. In the lungs, these are the bronchi; in the liver, the bile ducts.

If hemostasis is perfect and cut bile ducts are closed or are drained into the small bowel, there is no limit to the extent of hepatic surgery, provided only that enough parenchyma is left to synthesize clotting factors, to detoxify and conjugate metabolic products, and to do the myriad other things a liver is expected to do.

While the lung lies passive in the chest, the liver actively helps the surgeon. The liver is an organ with an "expanding" population of long-lived normal cells that can be recruited to undergo mitosis when lost parenchyma must be replaced (1). Although the replacement of parenchymal mass is commonly termed *regeneration*, it is not. *Regeneration* means regrowth of an organ, as in the ability of a newt to produce a new limb from the scar of an amputation stump. The annual sprouting of a stag's antlers is another example. Hepatic regeneration is less complex. It is characterized by hypertrophy and hyperplasia of existing cells, which are mysteriously signaled to begin growth and are equally mysteriously stopped when the demand for new cells is met.

For radiologists, the importance of regeneration is that new parenchyma grows in the area of existing parenchyma. During recovery from a right hepatectomy, the patient's regenerative mass is centered on the remnant left liver, in the epigastrium; after a left hepatectomy, the mass tends to be in the right hypochondrium.

For surgeons, the importance of regeneration is that in it nature provides considerable hepatic reserve if a neoplasm has to be resected. When a potentially resectable neoplasm grows, it displaces normal liver tissue; it does not destroy it. In the unlikely event that parenchyma is actually damaged by the neoplasm, hyperplasia compensates. Thus enormous neoplasms can be removed from the liver with little infringement on its parenchymal mass.

The situation is much different during operations to remedy hepatic trauma. Because there was no occasion for preexisting regeneration, every bit of tissue removed during control of a shattered or otherwise injured liver lessens the hepatic complement. Too generous a resection can, indeed, cause hepatic insufficiency, as can a major elective hepatectomy in which the surgeon underestimates the amount or the vitality of the remnant. If so, the patient will at best be chronically fatigued.

At worst, he or she will be both fatigued and in a state of chronic liver failure.

ANATOMY

In mechanical trauma to the liver, detailed knowledge of anatomy is almost unnecessary because the objectives are only to stop bleeding, to drain bile, and to debride necrotic tissue. Having to repair cut blood vessels or an injured bile duct is uncommon. If bleeding gets out of control, the situation can usually be saved by packing the liver all around with large laparotomy packs, followed by tight closure of the abdominal wall. So effective is packing for control of bleeding in patients with good liver function that their transfer to any medical center in the country is normally feasible if treatment at the first hospital is imprudent.

On the other hand, oncologic surgery and surgery of the intrahepatic bile ducts demand real-time knowledge of the eight anatomic segments of the liver and of the major bile ducts and blood vessels (2,3) (Fig. 25-1). Only this information allows the surgeon, for example, to remove small carcinomas within a cirrhotic liver that is weeping ascites and is likely to trigger a cascade of ominous events if its tenuous homeostasis is disturbed by excessive removal of hepatic tissue. Furthermore, the radiologist must know the segmental anatomy so that he or she can locate a neoplasm precisely for the surgeon, the vascular radiologist, and the radiation therapist and, not least, can hone his or her diagnostic skills.

NOMENCLATURE

Just as the liver has analogies to the lung in terms of its branching ducts and blood vessels, there is a larger similarity: Each organ has two major independent units that become confluent at a carina (2,3). In the lungs, this is the tracheal carina; in the liver, it is the carina at the confluence of the bile ducts. There is a right lung and a left lung. There is a right liver and a left liver. The plane dividing the two livers runs from the gallbladder fossa through the vena cava. (Fig. 25-2).

Removal of the right liver is a right hepatectomy. Removal of the left liver is a left hepatectomy. Because there are no lobes in the liver, except for the portion traditionally called the caudate lobe (segment I), no *lobectomies* are possible. The segmental divisions of the liver imply that eight discrete segmentectomies are feasible. Segment I, the caudate "lobe," is always removed in conjunction with segments II and III, however.

What has historically been called an *extended right hepatectomy* in today's parlance means that segments IV through VIII are removed (everything to the right of the patient's falciform ligament). An *extended left hepatectomy* means that segments

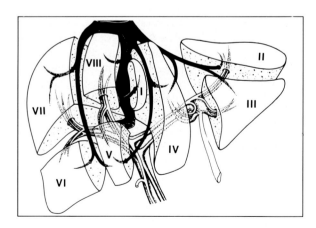

FIGURE 25-1
Couinaud's schema depicting the eight anatomic segments of the liver. (From Bismuth H: Surgical anatomy and anatomical surgery of the liver, World J Surgery 6:3, 1982. Reprinted by permission of Springer-Verlag.)

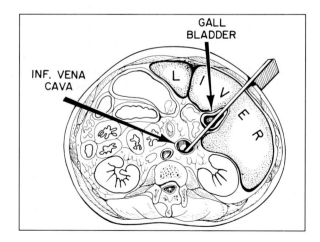

FIGURE 25-2
Plane of division between the right and left livers.

II to IV are certainly removed, plus, on occasion, parts of the remaining segments of the right liver. The introduction into surgical cant of the term *trisegmentectomy* as a replacement for the term *extended hepatectomy* is anatomically wrong. During a right hepatectomy, the gallbladder is nearly always removed. It is also often removed during a left hepatectomy.

DIAGNOSTIC IMAGING

A CT scan enhanced by parenteral injection of a radiopaque contrast substance is normally the only preoperative examination required for elective hepatic surgery. The indication for transhepatic cholangiography is usually the removal of bile ducts that are invaded by cancer or are blocked with stones. MRI is invaluable when resection of cancers metastatic to the liver is being considered, because MRI is the most sensitive means of displaying the number of metastases and of identifying hemangiomas, which might otherwise be confused with malignant neoplasms.

Although angiography was once considered an essential preliminary to hepatectomy, its use now is chiefly limited to circumstances in which a neoplasm seems to involve the inferior vena cava or a renal vein or to surround the extrahepatic transit of the hepatic veins to invade the portal vein (4).

Intraoperative ultrasonography for detection of "minimal" hepatic cancers (<3 to 4 cm in diameter) and delineation of hepatic veins bordering the involved hepatic segment (see below) is valuable in certain instances. The specificity of intraoperative ultrasonography for detection of occult metastases, however, often seems no better than an experienced surgeon's palpation of the liver, except when metastases less than 5 mm in diameter are being sought.

BIOPSY EXAMINATION

Hepatic neoplasms are removed because of what they do, not because of what they are. A 1-cm margin of uninvolved liver around a neoplasm—2 cm at the most—is sufficient (4). Knowing the histologic characteristics of a tumor beforehand does not change the resection that will be done, with one exception: If one were certain that a mass were focal nodular hyperplasia (see below), and if its removal seemed hazardous, the surgeon might argue that this tumor-like condition were better left alone.

Even if a biopsy specimen is indicated, the result might not be definitive because of sampling error. What seems to be benign tissue at the surface of excision or aspiration (needle or trocar) can mask a cancer at the center. Practically the only indications for getting a preoperative tissue specimen are to prove that a neoplasm is too widespread to be resected or to prove that the patient has such bad liver parenchyma as to be unable to withstand an operation.

EXPOSURE FOR SURGERY

Although a right thoracotomy was part of most major hepatectomies a few years ago, retractors fixed to the operating table and capable of lifting the costal margin while distracting the edges of the abdominal wall have made the need for thoracic entry rare. The principal reason to do a thoracotomy nowadays is for exposure of a neoplasm of the vena cava or in the vicinity of the vena cava. Even in these circumstances, however, a median sternotomy generally provides both a more satisfactory view and greater postoperative comfort than does a thoracotomy.

TYPES OF NEOPLASMS

Some tumors should be removed because of their malignant potential and some because their mass causes symptoms. Most should be ignored. The reason is that the vast majority of hepatic neoplasms are benign and innocuous. About 50 percent of the adult population harbors one or more benign hepatic tumors or tumor-like conditions: usually cholangioadenomas, hemangiomas, and focal nodular hyperplasia. The range of size of these benign neoplasms is from a few millimeters to about 2 cm. Generally no treatment is required (5).

Cholangioadenomas

Cholangioadenomas are the firm nodules commonly felt by a surgeon during routine exploration of the abdomen, sometimes leading him or her to wonder if they represent metastatic or primary neoplastic disease from an occult source. If there is no reason to anticipate the presence of metastases in view of the preoperative diagnosis, no attention should be paid to smooth nodules in the liver unless they are exophytic or umbilicated. If they are, taking a biopsy specimen is appropriate.

Hemangiomas

Most people who are referred for excision of a cavernous hemangioma have episodic pain that has nothing to do with the hemangioma. The number of ruptured hemangiomas ever reported is fewer than 50, and all ruptured hemangiomas seem to be over 8 to 10 cm in diameter (6,7). Subcapsular leakage of smaller hemangiomas does occur, however, and causes pain in larger numbers of patients, but the incidence of leakage is so small that hepatic surgeons guard photographs of this event jealously. The reasons that hemangiomas over 20 cm in diameter usually have to be removed is as a result of symptoms provoked by their mass, without the slightest sign of their having bled.

When a hemangioma becomes large enough or painful enough that it has to be removed, the simplest operation should be done. Most hemangiomas can be enucleated rather than being excised in a formal hepatectomy. Control of bleeding from the raw liver bed is easier than might be supposed. A pathologist's subsequent report that hemangioma tissue remains at the resection margin is generally of no importance. Hemangiomas do not regrow, except in rare instances fostered by administration of exogenous estrogens (8).

Hepatoadenoma

Often related to use of birth-control pills or to the administration of steroidal hormones for other reasons, adenomas tend to lie deep in the right liver and to undergo hemorrhagic infarction and rupture—first into the liver and then into the peritoneal cavity (9). An impromptu hepatectomy with a dire outcome often results.

Identification of a hepatoadenoma by imaging studies used to be simple: Since a hepatoadenoma is a neoplasm, it was considered unable to contain Kupffer cells; therefore, it should be unable to concentrate intravenously administered ^{99m}Tc-labeled sulfur colloid. A mass like focal nodular hyperplasia (FNH), which is a tumor-like condition rather than a true neoplasm, should be able to concentrate the colloid because it has Kupffer cells. Theory to the contrary, however, both hepatoadenomas and FNH can take up the labeled colloid.

From a clinical viewpoint, the most important advice for a woman (or a hormone-treated man) thought to have a hepatoadenoma is to withdraw the source of steroidal stimulation. If the mass regresses by 50 percent during the next 3 months, no treatment is likely to be needed. Adenomas that do not regress upon stopping of hormonal therapy should be removed. Because rare adenomas are probably transformed into carcinomas by long-term use of exogenous steroid drugs or by cocarcinogens and promotors (10,11), imaging studies at 3-month intervals for a total of 12 months should be pursued to assess the possibility of malignant growth.

Focal Nodular Hyperplasia (FNH)

This "condition" is not a disease or a neoplasm. It is probably a fibrogenic response to idiopathic ingrowth of blood vessels (12,13). The two reasons to know about FNH are to keep someone from saying that (1) the surgeon who has removed a mass nodular hyperplasia has removed only a whorl of cirrhotic liver and (2) the lesion is a neoplasm, which must be removed. If, because of its central scar and characteristic spherical or oblate shape, the inferential diagnosis of a space-occupying mass is FNH, there is no indication for its removal, absent symptoms. Avid concentration of ^{99m}Tc-labeled sulfur colloid helps in diagnosis.

Cystadenoma

Like FNH, this is a tumor-like condition, not a neoplasm. Cystadenoma probably represents growth of a bud of bile-duct primordia. Fewer than 75 cystadenomas have been reported, the majority of them in women. Although hepatic cystadenomas produce effects of an intrahepatic mass, they do not cause jaundice, unless they happen to be located so as to compress a major bile duct. If symptoms persist, hepatic cystadenomas must be resected for cure and to avoid confusing them with very rare cystadenocarcinomas.

Hepatocellular Carcinoma (HCC)

This is the most common visceral neoplasm in the world, but one that could be virtually eliminated by wide-scale inoculation with hepatitis-B vaccine. In transgeneic mice injected with the virus, progression from intracellular inflammation to carcinoma is unmistakable (14). Alcohol, aflatoxin, and male sex are other putative carcinogens or cocarcinogens.

Because multicentric HCC on the substrate of a liver ravaged by alcoholic cirrhosis is common in the Western world, resection is usually not practical in our civilization, except for the lucky patients who have encapsulated, unicentric cancers. Even if the best 5-year survival rate after resection is only about 35 percent, aggressive surgical removal of a limited HCC is worthwhile, because there is no effective adjunctive or curative chemotherapy.

The fibrolamellar-variant HCC is also reasonable surgical game (15). Encapsulated and growing mostly in women, but sometimes also in steroid-treated men, it can usually be resected, yielding a survival rate that can be as high as 40 percent in 4 years.

Although rare in the United States, "minimal" hepatocellular carcinomas (< 4 cm in maximal diameter) are common in the "hepatic cancer belt" of Africa and Asia as well as in France, as a result of historic referral patterns (16). In the cancer belt, the best screening programs identify these neoplasms as a matter of routine: first, by assaying for abnormally high levels of α-fetoprotein in the blood and, second, if these are high, by sonographic scans. Minimal cancers can be removed, even from abnormal liver parenchyma, without overall compromise of the patient by a bloodless resection of the neoplasm and removal of a few millimeters of apparently normal parenchyma. Either occlusion of portal blood flow from the hepatic segment that is the site of the neoplasm or total occlusion of blood flow to the liver makes a limited hepatectomy possible (17).

Hepatocelluar carcinomas often invade the bile ducts and the hepatic and portal veins, leaving deposits of cancer that produce obstructive jaundice and portal hypertension manifested by bleeding esophageal varices (16,18).

Cystadenocarcinoma

Cystadenocarcinomas are rare, idiopathic, and limited cancers, sometimes curable by resection. By analogy with hepatic cystadenomas, one suspects that cystadenocarcinomas must originate from bile-duct primordia.

Sarcoma

With the exception of angiosarcomas produced by exposure to Thorotrast, testosterone, arsenic, and vinyl chloride (the monomer of polyvinyl chloride plastics), sarcomas are rare (19,20). Although angiosarcoma is incurable, some leiomyosarcomas and embryonal rhabdomyosarcomas are resectable and curable after excision or with therapeutic chemotherapy. Because they might secrete insulin-like growth factors, some fibrosarcomas and leiomyosarcomas first manifest themselves by causing hypoglycemia.

Cholangiocarcinoma

Of speculative etiology, cholangiocarcinomas mimic some of the behavior of hepatocellular carcinomas, in that they may coexist in a parenchymal (or "peripheral") phase and a "central" phase, invading bile ducts widely and producing symptoms of bile-duct obstruction as the chief manifestation of disease (21). Bile ducts can sometimes be freed of cancer, and regions of the biliary system not amenable to "thrombectomy" of the neoplasm can be excised for palliation lasting several years. Unfortunately, the advancement and metastasis of parenchymal multicentricity are inexorable. One of our patients is alive 3 years after resection of all the hepatic segments except I, II, and part of segment V, combined with thrombectomy of the ducts from segments V and VI, which were drained into a roux-en-Y loop.

Metastases

Countless metastases may lodge in the liver. Few of them are worth removing. Nevertheless, huge indolent metastases from exotic sources, such as mesonephric-duct carcinoma, are sometimes resectable with the expectation of cure of or long palliation (22,23). Colorectal primary cancers contribute the greatest number of metastases to the liver. Fortunately, colorectal secondary cancers, too, are often indolent and spare enough parenchyma to be worth resecting. Metastases originating in the right colon tend to be myriad and biologically aggressive, while those from the descending colon and rectum are more likely to be solitary or, at least, enumerable. By removing metastases, the hypothesis is that the patient will be shifted into a group that has a 25 to 35 percent 5-year survival rate rather than one with nil survival. The trouble is that no one knows the natural history of untreated colorectal metastases, but an estimate has been made that only 7 of 1750 patients with untreated hepatic metastases from the colon and rectum have ever survived untreated (24). Metastases are said to have a growth period of 2 to 3 years before they are manifest.

Resection of four or fewer metastases is appropriate, especially if they are satellites around a central neoplasm. Resection of more than four metastases is generally futile. The hope that removal of an enormous mass of metastatic colorectal cancer by a major hepatectomy will relieve pain and discomfort is often unrealized for long. A few highly selected patients with hepatic metastases, and even with an extrahepatic deposit, are potential candidates for orthotopic liver transplantation.

Infusion of 5-FudR, with or without other chemotherapeutic agents, by an implanted pump that delivers only 1 to 2 ml agent daily produces temporary regression in 50 percent of patients with responsive metastases restricted to the liver and a good response in about 20 percent.

REFERENCES

1. Bucher NLR, Malt RA: Regeneration of Liver and Kidney. Boston, Little, Brown, 1971.
2. Couinaud C: Le foie: Études anatomiques et chirurgicales. Paris, Masson, 1957, pp 9–12.
3. Bismuth H: Surgical anatomy and anatomical surgery of the liver. World J Surg 6:3, 1982.
4. Malt RA: Surgery for hepatic neoplasms. N Engl J Med 313:1591, 1985.
5. Karhunen PJ: Benign hepatic tumours and tumour-like conditions in men. J Clin Pathol 39:183, 1986.
6. Trastek VF, vanHeerden JA, Sheedy PF II, Adson MA: Cavernous hemangiomas of the liver: Resect or observe? Am J Surg 145:49, 1983.
7. Takagi H: Diagnosis and management of cavernous hemangioma of the liver. Semin Surg Oncol 1:12, 1985.
8. Conter RL, Longmire WP Jr: Recurrent hepatic hemangiomas: Possible association with estrogen therapy. Ann Surg 207:115, 1988.
9. Mays ET, Christopherson W: Hepatic tumors induced by sex steroids. Semin Liver Dis 4:147, 1984.
10. Forman D, Doll R, Petro R: Trends in mortality from carcinomas of the liver and the use of oral contraceptives. Br J Cancer 48:349, 1983.
11. Palmer JR, Rosenberg L, Kaufman DW, et al: Oral contraceptive use and liver cancer. Am J Epidemiol 130:878, 1989.
12. Stocker JT, Ishak KG: Focal nodular hyperplasia of the liver: A study of 21 pediatric cases. Cancer 48:336, 1981.
13. Wanless IR, Mawdsley C, Adams R: On the pathogenesis of focal nodular hyperplasia of the liver. Hepatology 5:1194, 1985.
14. Chisari FV, Klopchin K, Moriyama T, et al: Molecular pathogenesis of hepatocellular carcinoma in hepatitis B virus transgenic mice. Cell 59:1145, 1989.
15. Nagorney DM, Adson MA, Weiland LH, et al: Fibrolamellar hepatoma. Am J Surg 149:113, 1985.
16. Nagasue N, Yukaya H, Ogawa Y, et al: Hepatic resection in the treatment of hepatocellular carcinoma: Report of 60 cases. Br J Surg 72:292, 1985.
17. Huguet C, Nordlinger B, Galopin JJ, et al: Normothermic hepatic vascular exclusion for extensive hepatectomy. Surg Gynecol Obstet 147:689, 1978.
18. Carella G, Degott C, Benhamou J-P: Invasion of the lumen of bile ducts by hepatocellular carcinoma. Liver 1:251, 1981.
19. Ishak KG, Malt RA: Sarcomas of the liver and spleen, in Raaf JH (ed.): Management of Soft Tissue Sarcomas. Chicago, Year Book Medical Publishers (in press).
20. Malt RA, Galdabini JJ, Jeppsson BW: Abnormal sex-steroid milieu in young adults with hepatocellular carcinoma. World J Surg 7:247, 1983.
21. Kawarada Y, Mizumoto R: Cholangiocellular carcinoma of the liver. Am J Surg 147:354, 1984.
22. Foster JH: Treatment of metastatic disease of the liver: A skeptic's view. Semin Liver Dis 4:170, 1984.
23. Wagner JS, Adson MA, van Heerden HA, et al: The natural history of hepatic metastases from colorectal cancer: A comparison with resective treatment. Ann Surg 199:502, 1984.
24. Steele G, Ravikumar TS: Resection of hepatic metastases from colorectal cancer: Biologic perspectives. Ann Surg 210:127, 1989.

26

Hepatic and Portal Venous Anatomy in Cross-Sectional Imaging for Hepatic Resections

DAVID A. TURNER, TERENCE A.S. MATALON,
ALEXANDER DOOLAS, and BRUCE SILVER

The friability of the liver and the abundance of blood vessels running through it have made hemostatic management of large hepatic wounds seem extremely difficult to surgical pioneers. Successful removal of major portions of the hepatic substance was not reported until the early 1950s (1–3). Thus the development of surgery of the liver has lagged far behind the evolution of the surgery of other abdominal organs. An improved understanding of the internal venous anatomy of the liver and advances in surgical techniques have made major hepatic resection an accepted mode of therapy for selected patients with primary or secondary hepatic neoplasms (4–6) as well as other conditions (7).

Two cardinal rules guide a surgeon in hepatic resections. The first is that a sufficient volume of vascularized liver parenchyma must be left in place to support life (7,8). The exact amount has not been well determined, although removal of more than 65 percent of functioning hepatocytes may increase the risk of postoperative hepatic failure. Survival after removal of up to 80 percent of the volume of the liver has been reported (4); however, most such reports have included tumor with resected hepatic tissue in estimating the percentage of liver removed (8), resulting in an overestimation of the loss of functioning hepatocytes.

Resection of 80 percent of the volume of the liver of a healthy, young person who has sustained massive hepatic trauma would make survival uncertain (4). Patients with diseases characterized by diffuse compromise of hepatocellular function, e.g., cirrhosis, have reduced hepatic reserve and tolerate removal of little, if any, hepatic tissue (7). This has encouraged development of subsegmentectomy techniques to maximize preservation of remaining hepatic tissue.

The second cardinal rule of major hepatic resection is that the vascular supply and the hepatic venous and biliary drainage of liver tissue left in situ must remain intact (5). Adherence to this simple principle is technically demanding. The vascular anatomy of the liver, which is variable, is not readily apparent to the surgeon by inspection of the surface of the liver. Moreover, the distribution of the veins that drain the liver does not parallel its vascular supply, as is the rule in other organs. Finally, there are no significant vascular or biliary anastomoses between hepatic segments (9).

Cross-sectional imaging of the liver with ultrasonography (US), computed tomography (CT),

---

We thank Heidi Hoffer for aid in illustration of this work. We also wish to acknowledge the contribution of John K. Mukai, M.D., whose scientific exhibit and pictorial essays (14,15) served as our starting point in this work.

TABLE 26-1. *Abbreviations Used in Figures 26-4 to 26-7*

Abbreviation	Meaning
CBD	Common bile duct
CL	Caudate lobe
FL	Falciform ligament
FLV	Fissure for ligamentum venosum
GB	Gallbladder
IVC	Inferior vena cava
LHV	Left hepatic vein
LIS	Left lateral segment
LMS	Left medial segment
LPV	Left portal vein
LT	Ligamentum teres hepatis
MHV	Middle hepatic vein
MPV	Main portal vein
RAS	Right anterior segment
RHV	Right hepatic vein
RPV	Right portal vein
RPS	Right posterior segment
SV	Splenic vein

and more recently, magnetic resonance imaging (MRI) provides excellent demonstration of the portal and hepatic veins as well as the lesions to be removed (10–15), allowing planned resections according to sound anatomic principles. As a result, these imaging techniques have come to play a crucial role in the resection of hepatic masses.

The CT, MRI, and US images shown in this chapter, which have been published previously (14,15), were selected to highlight the segmental anatomy of the liver. The CT images are of a patient with fatty liver who also had air in the biliary tree and reflux of oral contrast medium into the gallbladder, the result of a choledochojejunostomy. The sonograms are from a patient who had dilated hepatic veins due to right-sided congestive heart failure. The MRI images are of two patients who had abdominal aortic aneurysms. The abbreviations used in these figures are listed in Table 26-1.

Major hepatic resections cannot be understood without a firm grasp of the anatomy of the liver. Therefore, it is appropriate to begin consideration of the role of cross-sectional imaging in hepatic resections with a discussion of hepatic anatomy.

HEPATIC ANATOMY

Classical descriptions of the gross anatomic divisions of the liver were based solely on surface structures. The traditional right lobe was that portion of the liver to the right of the falciform ligament; the left lobe lay to the left of the falciform ligament and to the left of the fissures for the ligamenta teres and venosum (16). The caudate lobe, bounded by the fissure for the ligamentum venosum and the inferior vena cava (IVC), and the quadrate lobe, bounded by the umbilical fissure, the porta hepatis, and the gallbladder, were considered part of the right lobe (16).

These classical divisions of hepatic anatomy have been of little help to the surgeon and probably contributed to the delay in technical advances. The surface anatomy of the liver poorly reflects the organ's internal vascular structure. It is the relationship of the hepatic parenchyma to the branches of the triad of portal vein, hepatic artery, and bile duct, on the one hand, and the hepatic veins, on the other, that dictates which margins of resection are compatible with maintenance of vascular and biliary drainage and supply of unresected tissue. Consequently, the anatomic divisions of the liver have been redefined in a manner that takes account of the distribution of the branches of the portal vein (9,17).

Two commonly used hepatic segmental nomenclatures based on the branching of the portal triad have been developed. The one usually used in the American and English literature has been outlined by Goldsmith and Woodburne (9). The nomenclature of Couinaud (17) is favored by the French (18). In the discussion that follows, the American/English nomenclature will be described, after which it will be related to Couinaud's system. The anatomy of the portal and hepatic veins will be emphasized. The hepatic arteries and the bile ducts accompany the branches of the portal vein above the porta hepatis. Therefore, the description of the distribution of the portal veins can be considered to apply to the hepatic arteries and bile ducts as well.

The distribution of the portal and hepatic veins is illustrated in Figure 26-1. The liver can be divided into right and left lobes, corresponding, respectively, to the distributions of the right and left branches of the portal vein. This division lies along a plane that passes through the long axis of

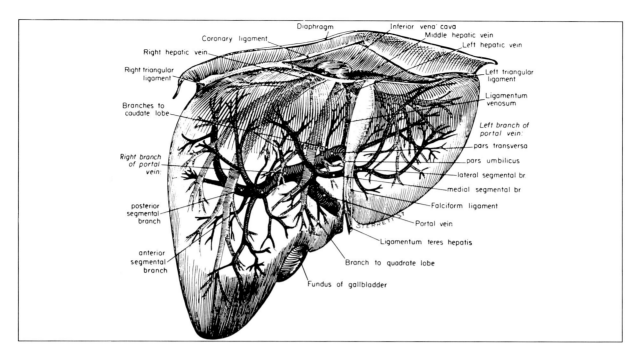

FIGURE 26-1
The liver in transparency to show internal hepatic and portal venous anatomy. (From Goldsmith NA, Woodburne RT: The surgical anatomy pertaining to liver resection. Surg Gynecol Obstet 195:310, 1957. Reprinted by permission.)

the fossa for the gallbladder and through the IVC (9) (plane *B*, Fig. 26-2). As illustrated in Figure 26-2, the middle hepatic vein lies in this plane (9), making it an important landmark of the boundary between the left and right hepatic lobes in transaxial images of the liver. In Figure 26-3 the anatomic levels of Figures 26-4 to 26-7 are indicated respectively by lines *A–D*. As shown in Figures 26-4 to 26-7, the division between the left and right lobes is represented in transaxial images by a line passing through the middle hepatic vein and the IVC (line *B*) or, at more caudal levels, a line passing from the IVC through the center of the gallbladder fossa (14).

At a variable distance (usually 0 to 3 cm) beyond the division of the main portal vein into right and left branches, the right branch of the portal vein divides into anterior and posterior branches (9) (Fig. 26-1). The territories supplied by these two branches are respectively termed (in the American/English nomenclature) the anterior and posterior segments of the right hepatic lobe. As illustrated in Figure 26-2, the plane between these segments (plane *A*) passes through the IVC and contains the right hepatic vein (9). Since the right hepatic vein lies in the intersegmental plane, the vein is an important landmark of the boundary between the anterior and posterior segments of the right hepatic lobe in transaxial images of the liver. As shown in Figures 26-4 to 26-7, the division between the anterior and posterior segments is represented in transaxial images by a line passing through the right hepatic vein and the IVC (line *A*) (14).

The anterior and posterior divisions of the right branch of the portal vein each divide into superior and inferior branches, as shown in Figure 26-1. Thus the anterior and posterior segments of the right lobe each can be divided into superior and inferior subsegments, consisting of the territories supplied, respectively, by the superior and inferior right portal branches (9). The portal and hepatic

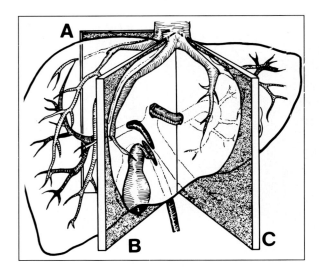

FIGURE 26-2
Hepatic intersegmental boundaries (planes A, B and C) are shown. The right and middle hepatic veins lie, respectively, in planes A and B and thus indicate the position of the planes. Portion of the left hepatic vein close to the IVC lies in plane C. (From Mukai JK, Stack C, Turner DA, et al: Imaging of surgically relevant hepatic vascular and segmental anatomy: I. Normal anatomy. AJR 149:287, 1987. Copyright © by American Roentgen Ray Society. Reprinted by permission.)

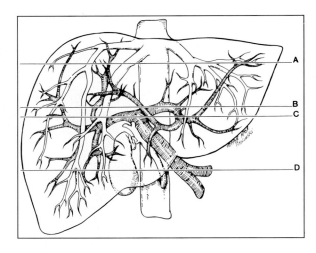

FIGURE 26-3
Lines A through D indicate the anatomic levels of images shown in Figs. 26-4 through 26-7. (Reprinted by permission from same source as Figure 26-2.)

veins interdigitate like the fingers of folded hands. For example, the right hepatic vein can be found bisecting the tissue between the anterior and posterior branches of the right portal vein.

The left lobe of the liver is divided into medial and lateral segments. The boundary between these segments is indicated by the falciform ligament (19) and the umbilical fissure (9). The plane separating the medial and lateral segments is approximated by plane C in Figure 26-2. The main trunk of the left branch of the portal vein consists of two segments (Fig. 26-1), the proximal, or "transverse," part and the distal, or "umbilical," part. The transverse part extends toward the left for approximately 3.5 cm and then curves anteriorly into the umbilical fissure to continue as the umbilical part, ending bluntly in an attachment to the ligamentum teres hepatis (9). Unlike the right branch of the portal vein, which divides into two branches to supply the two segments of the right lobe, the left branch of the portal vein distributes by means of three or four venous radicles into the medial segment of the left lobe and two important branches to the lateral segment (9).

As noted earlier, the falciform ligament and the umbilical fissure denote the boundary between the medial and lateral segments of the left lobe. Since the umbilical part of the left branch of the portal vein and the ligamentum teres hepatis lie within the umbilical fissure, these structures, along with the falciform ligament, serve as important landmarks of the left intersegmental boundary in transaxial images. As shown in Figures 26-5 to 26-7, this boundary is indicated by lines passing from the IVC through the falciform ligament, the umbilical part of the left portal branch, or the ligamentum teres. At levels above the main branches of the portal vein, close to the confluence of the hepatic veins with the IVC, the proximal portion of left hepatic vein marks the left intersegmental boundary (Fig. 26-4). Below this level, the left hepatic vein turns away from the intersegmental boundary and courses within the lateral segment, forming the boundary between the superior and inferior left lateral subsegments (9,19).

The caudate lobe has a vascular drainage that is distinct from the right and left lobes and is

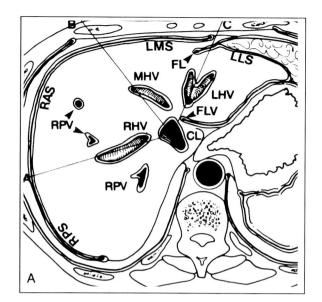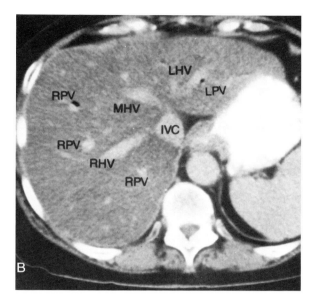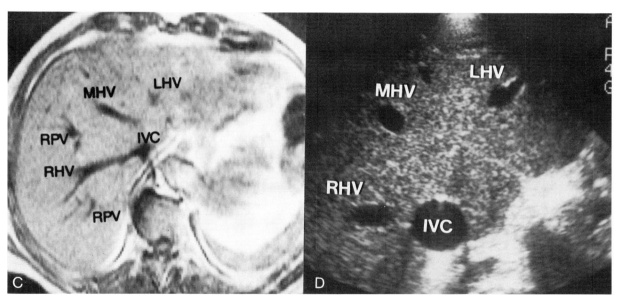

FIGURE 26-4
Transaxial diagram and images at level A of Fig. 26-3. (A) Lines A, B and C indicate intersection of intersegmental planes A, B and C (Fig. 26-3) with the transaxial plane at this level. Note that the lines, which are the boundaries of the hepatic segments, radiate from the inferior vena cava and pass through the hepatic veins. (B) CT image. Air in the distal biliary radicles, within the lateral and anterior segments, is due to choledochojejunostomy. (C) MRI image of another patient shows similar vascular anatomy. (D) Transaxial sonogram at same level. (From Mukai JK, Stack C, Turner DA, et al: Imaging of surgically relevant hepatic vascular and segmental anatomy: I. Normal anatomy. AJR 149:289, 1987. Copyright © by American Roentgen Ray Society. Reprinted by permission.)

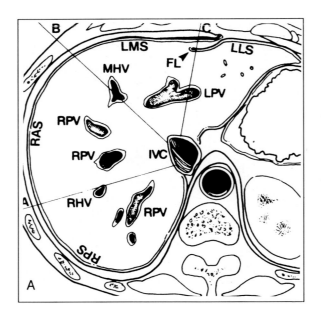

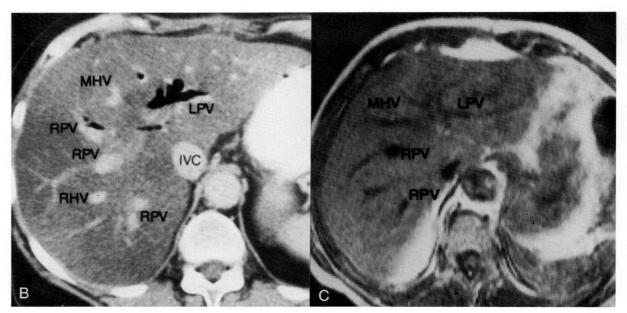

FIGURE 26-5
Transaxial diagram and images at level B of Fig. 26-3. (A) Left hepatic vein not seen at this level. Line from inferior vena cava through falciform ligament (line C) indicates boundary between lateral and medial segments. (B) CT scan, same patient as in Fig. 26-4B. Air in left hepatic duct obscures transverse portion of left portal vein. (C) MRI image, same patient as in Fig. 26-4C, shows anatomy similar to that in B. Biliary system was normal in this patient and therefore is not seen. (From Mukai JK, Stack C, Turner DA, et al: Imaging of surgically relevant hepatic vascular and segmental anatomy: I. Normal anatomy. AJR 149:289, 1987. Copyright © by American Roentgen Ray Society. Reprinted by permission.)

therefore treated as an individual area (9). This pedunculated lobule of tissue lies in direct contact with the IVC. It receives one branch each from the left and right portal veins. The arteries and bile ducts of the caudate lobe are variable in origin. However, the arteries and ducts of the lobe may be derived bilaterally in a manner analogous to the portal veins. The caudate lobe is drained by one to four veins that enter directly into the IVC (19). They are variable in arrangement as well as number.

Caudal to the caval openings of the right, middle, and left hepatic veins are the openings of as few as 3 to as many as 50 "dorsal hepatic veins" that drain into the IVC (19). Most of these are the size of a pinhole. However, the lowest hepatic vein on the right, known as the *inferior right*

FIGURE 26-6
Transaxial diagram and images at level C of Fig. 26-3. (A) Boundary between medial and lateral segments is denoted by line C, which runs from inferior vena cava through umbilical part of left portal vein, ligamentum teres, and falciform ligament. (B) CT scan, same patient as in Fig. 26-4B, shows division of main portal vein into right and left branches, as well as division of right portal vein into anterior and posterior branches. As in Fig. 26-4B, air is seen in biliary system, adjacent to branches of left portal vein. (C) Sonogram, including a small portion of liver at same level as B and C, shows anatomy similar to that seen in A and B. (From Mukai JK, Stack C, Turner DA, et al: Imaging of surgically relevant hepatic vascular and segmental anatomy: I. Normal anatomy. AJR 149:289, 1987. Copyright © by American Roentgen Ray Society. Reprinted by permission.)

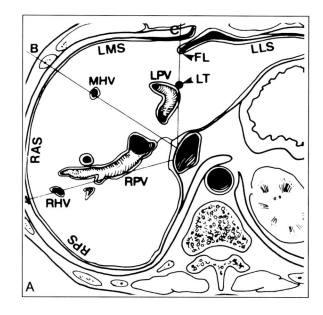

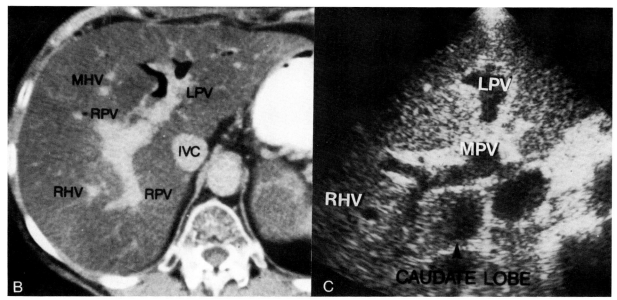

hepatic vein (20) or the *posteroinferior hepatic vein* (19), is quite large and drains much of the posterior segment of the right lobe in 20 percent of cases (9,19,20).

The segmental nomenclature according to Couinaud (17) is also based on the branching of the portal vein, or "portal pedicles" (18), i.e., the branched triad of portal vein, bile duct, and hepatic artery. Couinaud divided the liver into eight segments (Fig. 26-8), which can be related to the American/English nomenclature as described by Goldsmith and Woodburne (9). Segment I is the caudate lobe. Segments II and III are the regions of the lateral segment that are, respectively, posterior and anterior to the left hepatic vein. Segment IV is the quadrate lobe, a part of the medial segment of the left lobe. Segments V and VI are, respectively, the inferior subsegments of the anterior

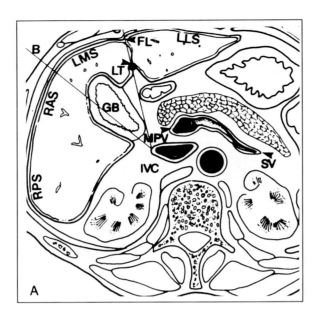

FIGURE 26-7
Transaxial images at level D of Fig. 26-3, at which splenic and superior mesenteric veins join to form the portal vein. (A) Hepatic veins are not readily identified at this level and thus are not used as landmarks for intersegmental boundaries. Line drawn from IVC through gallbladder (line B) approximates boundary between left and right lobes. Line from IVC through ligamentum teres denotes boundary between left medial and left lateral segments. (B) CT scan, same patient as in Fig. 26-4B, shows radiopaque contrast medium in gallbladder due to previous choledochojejunostomy. Left adrenal mass is present. (C) MRI image, same patient as in Fig. 26-4C, shows anatomy similar to that in A and B. (From Mukai JK, Stack C, Turner DA, et al: Imaging of surgically relevant hepatic vascular and segmental anatomy: I. Normal anatomy. AJR 149:289, 1987. Copyright © by American Roentgen Ray Society. Reprinted by permission.)

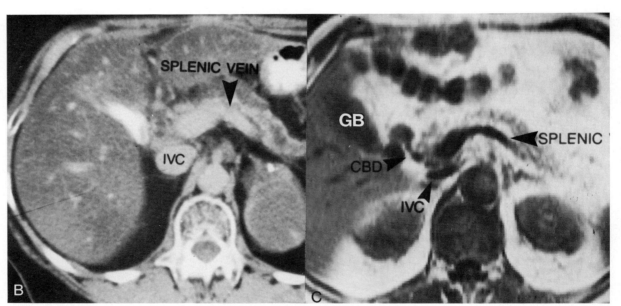

and posterior segments of the right lobe. Segments VII and VIII correspond, respectively, to the superior subsegments of the posterior and anterior segments.

HEPATIC RESECTION

The simplest hepatic resection is the *wedge excision*, which consists of the nonanatomic removal of a small amount of superficial hepatic tissue. The procedure is referred to as *nonanatomic* because the tissue removed does not correspond to a hepatic segment or subsegment. However, as in the case of any hepatic resection, wedge excisions can be performed successfully only if the vascular and biliary structures supplying the remaining hepatic parenchyma are left intact. Thus nonanatomic wedge excisions are

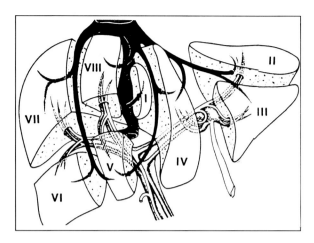

FIGURE 26-8
Segmental anatomy of the liver according to Couinaud's nomenclature. (From Bismuth H: Surgical anatomy and anatomical surgery of the liver. J Surg 6:3, 1982. Reprinted by permission.)

performed only in the hepatic periphery, usually for removing small tumors (21).

In theory, any subsegment (or segment, according to Couinaud's system) can be removed separately (7) by resecting all tissue fed by the corresponding portal venous branch while taking care to leave intact the adjacent intersegmental hepatic veins that drain neighboring segments. In practice, however, single subsegmentectomies have not been widely performed, although Bismuth and associates (7) have reported that selective resection of Couinaud's segments IV through VIII is technically easy. Not all hepatic subsegments can be easily removed; it frequently is technically easier and less hazardous to resect an entire segment or lobe. Adequate exposure of posteriorly located subsegments may be difficult to obtain. For example, removal of the caudate lobe alone might be indicated in some tumors confined to that lobe, but it is usually necessary to remove the medial and lateral segments of the left lobe to gain access to the caudate lobe (7). An important potential source of trouble in resection of subsegments (or larger units of hepatic tissue) is the variability of the venous drainage of the liver, which can make subsegmental boundaries difficult for the surgeon to find. The recent introduction of intraoperative ultrasound (22), by which the internal vascular anatomy of the liver can be readily demonstrated at the operating table, may help overcome this obstacle.

The more commonly performed hepatic resections are procedures in which one, two, or three hepatic segments are removed. For example, the right lobe of the liver is frequently removed in a resection termed a *right lobectomy* (23). As in all major hepatic resections, the success of this procedure depends on adherence to sound anatomic principles. In a right lobectomy, the surgical plane is just to the right of the middle hepatic vein in order to preserve this vessel, which must be left intact because it drains much of the medial segment of the left lobe (9).

The medial segment of the left lobe may be resected along with the right lobe, as described by Starzl in 1975 (23). This procedure is termed a *right trisegmentectomy*, since the posterior, anterior, and medial hepatic segments are removed. The line of resection is just to the right of the falciform ligament. Care must be taken to preserve the umbilical portion of the left portal vein, which runs in the umbilical fissure and supplies the remaining lateral segment.

It is possible to remove the posterior segment of the right hepatic lobe *(posterior segmentectomy)*. However, this procedure, which has been performed by one of us (Doolas), is technically difficult and rarely performed. The right hepatic vein must be preserved in this procedure, since it drains a portion of the anterior segment (9).

The left lateral segment is readily removed in a procedure termed a *lateral segmentectomy* (23). The surgical plane is just to the left of the umbilical fissure so that the umbilical portion of the portal vein, which supplies blood to the medial as well as the lateral segment, will not be injured (9). Much of the left hepatic vein may be taken, since the middle hepatic vein drains all the medial segment (9).

A *left lobectomy* consists of removal of both the medial and lateral segments of the left lobe (23). The caudate lobe may be left in place or removed along with the left lobe (21). The surgical plane in this procedure is just to the the left of the middle hepatic vein; the latter vessel must be preserved because it drains part of the anterior segment of the right lobe (9).

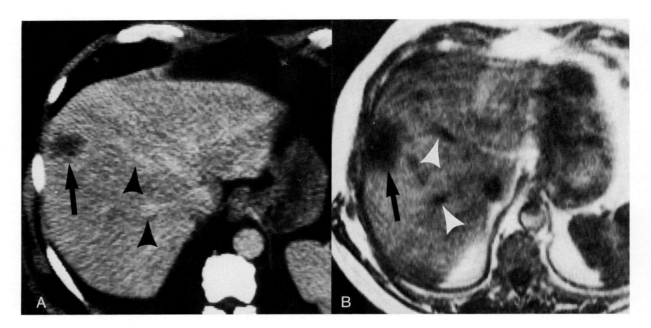

FIGURE 26-9
Resectable metastatic adenocarcinoma of the colon. (A) Contrast-enhanced CT scan reveals lesion in anterior segment of right lobe (arrow), i.e., between right and middle hepatic veins (arrowheads). (B) Inversion spin-echo (inversion recovery with added spin echo) MRI image (inversion, echo, repetition times = 300, 30 and 1400 ms, respectively) shows same lesion as low-intensity (dark) area (arrow). Right and middle hepatic veins, seen as low-intensity, linear structures (arrowheads), are better displayed than by CT. (From Mukai JK, Stack C, Turner DA, et al: Imaging of surgically relevant hepatic vascular and segmental anatomy: II. Extent and resectability of hepatic neoplasms. AJR 149:293, 1987. Copyright © by American Roentgen Ray Society. Reprinted by permission.)

In 1982, Starzl described the *left trisegmentectomy*, in which both segments of the left lobe are resected along with the anterior segment of the right lobe (24). The procedure is technically difficult and rarely performed (21). It is necessary, of course, to preserve the right hepatic vein, since it drains the remaining posterior segment.

THE ROLE OF CROSS-SECTIONAL IMAGING IN HEPATIC RESECTIONS

Preoperative prediction of the resectability of hepatic lesions and rational planning of surgical procedures are based on assessment of the distribution of the lesions and detailed knowledge of internal hepatic vascular anatomy. Cross-sectional imaging with CT, US, and MRI has become the cornerstone of this process, since these imaging modalities provide excellent displays of both the lesions and hepatic and portal venous anatomy (15–19). The relative accuracy of CT and MRI in the detection of hepatic lesions is controversial. We prefer MRI to CT in preoperative planning. In our hands, the two modalities have been equivalent in the demonstration of hepatic lesions. However, the display of vascular anatomy by MRI is generally superior to that afforded by CT (Figs. 26-9 and 26-10).

An example of the impact that cross-sectional imaging can have on hepatic resection is the description by Makuuchi et al. (20) of "four new hepatectomy procedures" in which the right hepatic vein is resected but the infero-posterior subsegment is preserved. These procedures are possible when the infero-posterior subsegment is drained by a large inferior right hepatic vein. In

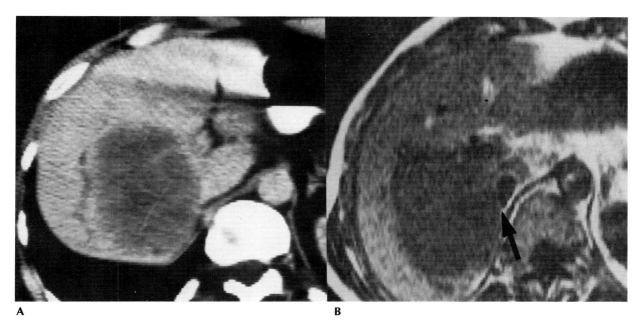

FIGURE 26-10
Metastatic adenocarcinoma of colon with extension to extraluminal margin of inferior vena cava. (A) CT scan of liver immediately after bolus infusion of contrast material. Large lesion is well seen, but inferior vena cava is not. (B) Inversion spin-echo MRI image (inversion, echo, repetition times = 300, 30 and 1800 ms, respectively) shows lesion in the right lobe with intensity lower than normal liver, contiguous with inferior vena cava. Vessel is more easily seen than on CT. One cannot tell from image whether vessel wall has been invaded. Lesion was readily dissected from the IVC at laparotomy. (From Mukai JK, Stack C, Turner DA, et al: Imaging of surgically relevant hepatic vascular and segmental anatomy: II. Extent and resectability of hepatic neoplasms. AJR 149:293, 1987. Copyright © by American Roentgen Ray Society. Reprinted by permission.)

the cases described by Makuuchi et al., the presence of this anatomic variation was demonstrated by preoperative US, enabling the surgeon to plan and execute the tissue-preserving procedures. This illustrates the importance to the surgeon of preoperative recognition of major variations in hepatic venous anatomy.

RESECTABILITY OF LESIONS

Hepatic lesions are resectable (without hepatic transplantation) if it is technically feasible to remove all gross tumor with tumor-free margins, leaving a volume of viable liver parenchyma *in situ* sufficient to support life. In order for the remaining hepatic tissue to be viable, its vascular supply and venous and biliary drainage must remain intact (5).

Lesions in the liver are easily resectable if they spare the porta hepatis, are confined to territory removed by one of the five major heptic resections described earlier, and can be resected with tumor-free margins (Fig. 26-9). Lesions are not resectable if they cannot be removed by these procedures leaving sufficient hepatic tissue to support life (Fig. 26-11). A lesion is generally considered unresectable if it encases or invades the main portal vein, the proper hepatic artery, both intrahepatic bile ducts, or the major branch of these structures contralateral to the hepatic lobe in which the tumor originates (Fig. 26-12).

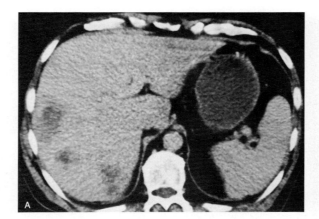 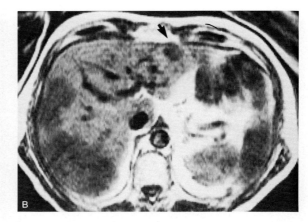

FIGURE 26-11
Adenocarcinoma of the colon, metastatic to the liver, judged unresectable. (A) CT scan demonstrates low-density lesions in the anterior and posterior segments. Left lobe was interpreted as normal. (B) Inversion spin-echo MRI image (inversion, echo, repetition times = 300, 30 and 1400 ms, respectively) shows anterior and posterior segment lesions and an additional lesion in the lateral segment (arrow). Although all lesions theoretically could be removed by a combined right lobectomy and lateral segmentectomy, the volume of tissue in the medial segment that would remain was judged insufficient to ensure a reasonable chance of survival. (From Mukai JK, Stack C, Turner DA, et al: Imaging of surgically relevant hepatic vascular and segmental anatomy: II. Extent and resectability of hepatic neoplasms. AJR 149:293, 1987. Copyright © by American Roentgen Ray Society. Reprinted by permission.)

Resection of a lesion may be possible if there is local, contiguous spread to the margins of the inferior vena cava or the main portal vein, provided that the vessels are not encased or invaded. Since contiguity of tumor with vessel wall does not necessarily mean the vessel has been invaded, the attainability of a tumor-free margin in such a case frequently cannot be predicted by imaging studies (Fig. 26-10).

Spread of tumor to extrahepatic lymph nodes is considered to preclude successful removal of intrahepatic tumors. However, it may be possible to resect tumors that have directly invaded adjacent, nonhepatic structures. For example, one of us (Doolas) has successfully resected a lesion that extended from the liver into the adjacent anterior abdominal wall (Fig. 26-13).

Patients with severe hepatic parenchymal disease are poorly tolerant of major hepatic resections, since they have limited (if any) hepatic reserve. Consequently, hepatic tumors in these patients frequently cannot be resected unless the amount of tissue resected can be minimized (7,20).

CONCLUSION

Hepatic resections are technically demanding procedures that require accurate knowlege of internal hepatic vascular anatomy. Hepatic venous anatomy varies considerably and is poorly reflected by the surface anatomy of the liver, creating difficulties for the surgeon. Cross-sectional imaging with CT, MRI, and US provides excellent preoperative demonstration of the hepatic vasculature as well as the lesions to be removed, allowing surgeons to plan resections according to sound anatomic principles. Consequently, these imaging techniques have come to play a crucial role in the resection of hepatic masses.

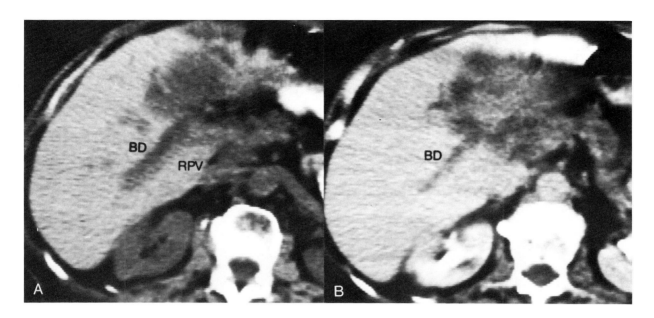

FIGURE 26-12
Adenocarcinoma, primary unknown, metastatic to the liver, unresectable because of involvement of both segments of left lobe, right portal vein, and right hepatic duct. (A) Preinfusion CT shows tumor in left lobe. Dilated right intrahepatic bile duct (BD) is seen anterior to posterior branch of right portal vein (RPV). (B) Postinfusion study shows enhancing tumor, opacification of portal vein, and dilated, low-density right intrahepatic bile duct. Right portal vein obscured by IV contrast medium. (From Mukai JK, Stack C, Turner DA, et al: Imaging of surgically relevant hepatic vascular and segmental anatomy: II. Extent and resectability of hepatic neoplasms. AJR 149:293, 1987. Copyright © by American Roentgen Ray Society. Reprinted by permission.)

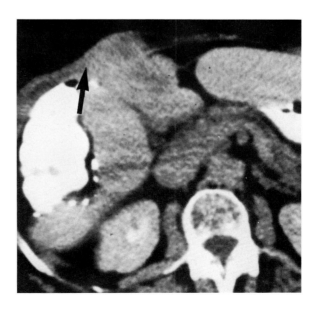

FIGURE 26-13
Local extrahepatic extension of adenocarcinoma of the colon in patient who had previously undergone right hepatic lobectomy. Postinfusion CT study shows lesion extending into anterior abdominal wall (arrow). Lesion was successfully resected (tumor-free margins), but abdominal wall reconstruction was required. (From Turner DA, Doolas A, Silver B, Matalon TAS: Role of cross-sectional imaging in hepatic resections, in Ferrucci JT, Mathieu DG (eds): Advances in hepatobiliary radiology. St. Louis, Mosby, 1990, p 209. Reprinted by permission.)

REFERENCES

1. Lortat-Jacob JL, Robert HG: Hepatectomie droite reglee. Presse Med 60:549, 1952.
2. Quattlebaum JK: Massive resection of the liver. Ann Surg 137:787, 1953.
3. Pack GT, Baker HW: Total right hepatic lobectomy: Report of a case. Ann Surg 138:253, 1953.
4. Malt RA: Surgery for hepatic neoplasms. N Engl J Med 313:1591, 1985.
5. Joishy SK, Balasegaram MB: Hepatic resection for malignant tumors of the liver: Essentials for a unified surgical approach. Am J Surg 139:360, 1980.
6. Tomas-de la Vega JE, Donahue EJ, Doolas A, et al: A ten-year experience with hepatic resection. Surg Gynecol Obstet 159:223, 1984.
7. Bismuth H, Houssin D, Costaing D: Major and minor segmentectomies "reglees" in liver surgery. World J Surg 6:10, 1982.
8. Stone HH, Long WD, Smith RB, Haynes CD: Physiologic considerations in major hepatic resections. Am J Surg 117:78, 1969.
9. Goldsmith NA, Woodburne RT: The surgical anatomy pertaining to liver resection. Surg Gynecol Obstet 195:310, 1957.
10. Pagani JJ: Intrahepatic vascular territories shown by computed tomography (CT). Radiology 147:173, 1983.
11. Sexton CC, Zeman RK: Correlation of computed tomography, sonography, and gross anatomy of the liver. AJR 141:711, 1983.
12. Stark DD, Wittenberg J, Middleton MS, Ferrucci JT Jr: Liver metastases: Detection by phase-contrast MR imaging. Radiology 158:327, 1986.
13. Fisher MR, Wall SD, Hricak H, et al: Hepatic vascular anatomy on magnetic resonance imaging. AJR 144:739, 1985.
14. Mukai JK, Stack C, Turner DA, et al: Imaging of surgically relevant hepatic vascular and segmental anatomy: I. Normal anatomy. AJR 149:287, 1987.
15. Mukai JK, Stack C, Turner DA, et al: Imaging of surgically relevant hepatic vascular and segmental anatomy: II. Extent and resectability of hepatic neoplasms. AJR 149:293, 1987.
16. Lewis WH, Gray H: Anatomy of the Human Body, 21st ed. Philadelphia, Lea and Febiger, 1924, pp 1198–1202.
17. Couinaud C: Le Foie: Etudes Anatomique et Chirurgical. Paris, Masson & Cie, 1957, pp 9–12.
18. Bismuth H: Surgical anatomy and anatomical surgery of the liver. World J Surg 6:3, 1982.
19. Hodgson WJB: Anatomy, in Hodgson WJB (ed): Liver Tumors: Multidisciplinary Management. St. Louis, Warren H. Green, 1988.
20. Makuuchi M, Hasegawa H, Yamazaki S, Takayasu K: Four new hepatectomy procedures for resection of the right hepatic vein and preservation of the inferior right hepatic vein. Surg Gynecol Obstet 164:68, 1987.
21. Hodgson WJB: Hepatic resections, in Hodgson WJB (ed): Liver Tumors: Multidisciplinary Management. St. Louis, Warren H. Green, 1988.
22. Bismuth H, Castaing D: Operative Ultrasound of the Liver and Biliary Ducts. Heidelberg, Springer-Verlag, 1987.
23. Starzl TE, Bell RH, Beart RW, Putnam CW: Hepatic trisegmentectomy and other liver resections. Surg Gynecol Obstet 141:429, 1975.
24. Starzl TE, Iwatsuki S, Shaw BW, et al: Left hepatic trisegmentectomy. Surg Gynecol Obstet 155:21, 1982.

27

Staging Liver Tumors for Therapeutic Intervention: Determination of Resectability by CT-Angiography

RENDON C. NELSON

The liver is second only to lymph nodes as the most frequent site of malignant growth (1). In 1990, there will be an estimated 155,000 new cases of colon and rectal cancer in the United States (2), and of these, approximately 25 percent will have liver metastases at the time of presentation (3). Of patients who die from colorectal cancer, 50 to 70 percent will have liver metastases (4,5). It is estimated that approximately 12 percent of patients with colorectal cancer will have spread limited to the liver alone (6). Patients with liver metastases who do not undergo hepatic resection have a mean 6-month survival of 10 to 35 percent (7). By comparison, patients undergoing resection of hepatic metastases have a 5-year survival rate of 25 to 33 percent (4,8–10). Improvements in long-term survival have been reported not only for large bowel cancer, but also for metastases from endocrine tumors, visceral sarcomas, and occasionally gastric cancer (11).

Candidates for hepatic resection include patients with one to four metastases; without spread to systemic sites such as lung, adrenal glands, or bone; a negative margin of resection for the primary tumor; and without spread to the lymph nodes that drain the liver (12,13). Since progressive liver failure may develop after resecting large portions of hepatic parenchyma, patients with severe liver impairment may be excluded from surgery. It is estimated that at least 30 percent of normal liver parenchyma must remain after resection. This problem is partially resolved by using a parenchymal-sparing segmental surgical approach.

Although patients do survive and can even be disease-free 5 years after hepatic resection (4), 75 percent will develop recurrent cancer within this time period (9). The two most common sites of recurrence are the liver and lungs, involving 43 and 31 percent of patients, respectively. Important determinants of survival after resection include the Dukes' stage of the primary tumor, the number of metastases (if more than three), and the presence of extrahepatic disease (especially hepatic lymph nodes). Factors that are much less important include the number of metastases (one versus two versus three), bilobar versus unilobar disease, the type of surgery (metastasectomy versus major hepatic resection), the preoperative level of carcinoembryonic antigen (CEA), lesion size, the disease-free interval, and the age and sex of the patient (12,14).

Long-term survival is determined not only by the tumors that are detected and subsequently resected, but also by the tumors that are not detected and, therefore, are not resected. As a result, imaging techniques play a critical role in determining the number of lesions, the relationship to the portal and hepatic veins, and an estimate of the tumor-free margin preoperatively. This information is vital in helping the surgeons decide which patients are candidates for resection and the type of resection to perform. Dynamic sequential bolus iodine CT or MRI are, at present, the best techniques for screening the liver for primary or metastatic tumor deposits on a routine basis. In the small group of patients who are potential candidates for hepatic resection, a more invasive, yet more sensitive imaging technique such as CT-angiography is indicated in preparation for surgery.

INTRODUCTION TO CT-ANGIOGRAPHY

The normal liver receives its blood supply from two sources: the hepatic artery and the portal vein. Normal hepatic parenchyma receives 75 percent of its blood from the portal vein, while both primary and metastatic hepatic tumors predominantly receive their blood supply from the hepatic artery (15,16). This difference in the predominant blood supply to normal hepatic parenchyma and hepatic tumors accounts for differential contrast enhancement during CT-angiography. Enhancement of one but not the other vascular system followed by rapid incremental scanning through the liver during the nonequilibrium phase of contrast administration results in very high lesion-to-liver contrast.

TECHNIQUE

CT-angiography can be performed either by means of the hepatic artery directly or by means of the portal vein indirectly. CT during hepatic arteriography (CT-HA) is ideally performed by placing the tip of a no. 5 to 7 French catheter into the proper hepatic artery. Placement into the common hepatic artery or celiac axis is less desirable, since some contrast material flows into the portal system as well. Approximately 300 cc of a 30% iodinated contrast agent is subsequently infused by means of the catheter at a rate of 3 to 5 cc/s (17). Lower infusion rates can result in layering of contrast material along the dependent portion of the artery with differential enhancement of the right and left hepatic lobes. Dynamic incremental CT scanning through the entire liver is subsequently performed immediately following initiation of the contrast material infusion. With CT-HA, focal lesions will demonstrate high contrast enhancement peripherally, while the surrounding normal hepatic parenchyma will be of much lower density (Fig. 27-1).

CT during arterial portography (CT-AP) is ideally performed by placing a no. 5 to 7 French catheter tip in the proximal superior mesenteric artery (SMA). The catheter tip may be alternatively placed in the splenic artery, although layering of contrast material in the main portal vein may be more of a problem. It is important for preliminary angiography to determine if there is a replaced hepatic artery originating from the SMA so that the catheter tip can be appropriately positioned distal to the origin of the anomalous vessel. A total volume of 150 cc of an undiluted 60% iodinated contrast agent is administered by means of the catheter at a rate of 1 to 2 cc/s. Dynamic incremental scanning through the entire liver is initiated 7

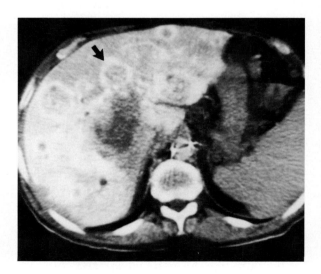

FIGURE 27-1
CT during hepatic arteriography. Lesions demonstrate hyperdense peripheral enhancement (arrow) *surrounded by relatively hypodense hepatic parenchyma. This phenomenon occurs because the predominant blood supply to hepatic tumors is from the hepatic artery.*

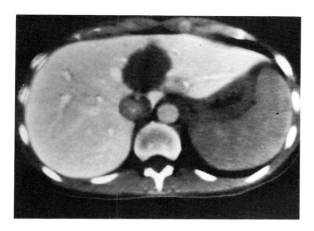

FIGURE 27-2
CT during arterial portography. Focal lesions are hypodense relative to the hyperdense hepatic parenchyma. Note that the IVC is also hypodense owing to mixing with unopacified blood from the lower extremities.

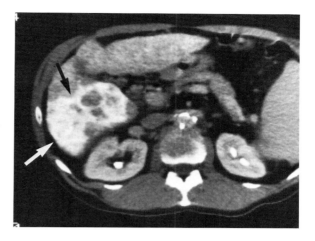

FIGURE 27-3
CT-HA demonstrating a hypodense nodular mass in the right lobe of the liver. The mass has obstructed the right portal vein resulting in arterial-portal shunting and delayed washout. Note that the hepatic parenchyma surrounding the mass is densely stained with contrast material (arrows).

to 10 s after starting the catheter infusion to allow the contrast material to pass through the mesenteric system into the portal vein and opacify both the portal and hepatic venous systems (18). With CT-AP, focal lesions will be of low density, while the surrounding normal hepatic parenchyma will be of very high density (Fig. 27-2).

It is imperative that the volume of contrast material used during preliminary angiography be minimized. These extracellular agents seep into the interstices of tumors and may result in diminished lesion-to-liver contrast on the follow-up CT-angiogram. It must be emphasized that the purpose of the preliminary angiogram is to determine the hepatic arterial anatomy (intraarterial digital subtraction angiography is ideal), to position the catheter tip in the desired vessel for CT-angiography, to administer a test infusion of saline through the catheter to determine the security of the tip within the desired artery, and to estimate the arterial infusion rate for CT-angiography. It is not the purpose of the angiogram to determine the number of focal hepatic lesions, since it has been shown to have a lower sensitivity rate than CT-angiography (19,20).

While CT-HA demonstrates high lesion-to-liver contrast, nontumorous attenuation changes or perfusion abnormalities can be seen in the hepatic parenchyma. Freeny and Marks (21) noted perfusion abnormalities in a total of 17 of 50 patients (34 percent). Most of these abnormalities were due to nonperfusion of a replaced hepatic artery (41 percent), altered hepatic hemodynamics caused by the tumor masses (26 percent) (Fig. 27-3), or cirrhosis and regenerating nodules (11 percent) (Fig. 27-4). Perfusion abnormalities also can be seen with CT-AP, although they are less common and usually are small, subcapsular, and either wedge- or saucer-shaped (18) (Fig. 27-5).

In comparing the two techniques, many imagers prefer CT-AP over CT-HA because the lesions are hypodense relative to normal hepatic parenchyma, similar to that seen routinely on contrast-enhanced CT. Furthermore, in the few studies that have compared CT-HA and CT-AP, performed sequentially in the same patient, it has been shown that if the portal vein is patent, CT-AP is superior to CT-HA for lesion detection (22,23).

COMPARISON WITH OTHER IMAGING MODALITIES

Numerous studies have compared CT-angiography with other imaging techniques to determine if the added sensitivity justifies the risk of this more invasive procedure. In 1985, Matsui

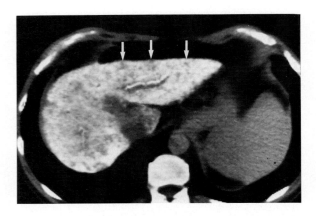

FIGURE 27-4
CT-HA demonstrating multiple, small, hypodense perfusion defects (arrows) *in a patient with cirrhosis and regenerating nodules.*

et al. (19) evaluated 29 small hepatocellular carcinomas (less than 3 cm in diameter, less than three in number) in 19 patients using a number of different imaging techniques. Surgical or autopsy proof was available for 55 percent of the lesions. The sensitivity for detecting focal lesions was as follows: CT-AP, 95 percent; infusion hepatic angiography, 83 percent; real-time ultrasound, 63 percent; contrast-enhanced CT, 58 percent; selective celiac angiography, 58 percent; and ^{99m}Tc-sulfur colloid radionuclide liver scanning, 16 percent.

Later, Matsui et al. (20) used a similar protocol for evaluating 45 liver metastases from colorectal cancer in 22 patients. Surgical proof was available for all lesions. The sensitivity of the various imaging techniques for metastases was similar to that for hepatocellular carcinoma, as follows: CT-AP, 84 percent; contrast-enhanced CT, 63 percent; real-time ultrasound, 58 percent; infusion hepatic angiography, 50 percent; selective celiac angiography, 27 percent; and CT following intraarterial injection of iodized poppyseed oil (Lipiodol), 38 percent. While CT-AP detected 11 of 18 lesions (61 percent) smaller than 15 mm, only one of these small lesions was detected by the other five imaging techniques combined.

In 1989, Heiken et al. (24) evaluated 37 metastatic lesions in 8 patients with MRI and several CT techniques. Surgical proof was available for all lesions. The sensitivity for the various techniques was as follows: CT-AP, 81 percent; MRI at 0.5 Tesla (including T1, T2, and proton density weighted images), 57 percent; delayed iodine CT (4 to 6 h after receiving at least 50 g iodine), 52 percent; and contrast-enhanced CT, 38 percent. The sensitivity for detecting lesions smaller than 1 cm in diameter was 61 percent for CT-AP, 17 percent for MRI, and 0 percent for both delayed iodine CT and contrast-enhanced CT. In the same year, our institution evaluated 143 lesions in 43 patients with similar CT and MRI techniques (18). Surgical proof was available for 60 percent of the lesions, although the sensitivity rates were similar for the surgical and nonsurgical groups of patients. The sensitivity of the two CT techniques was 85 percent for CT-AP and 66 percent for delayed iodine CT (4 to 6 h after 60 g of iodine). The sensitivity of MRI at 0.5 Tesla was 57 percent for T1-weighted inversion recovery (IR), 53 percent for T2-weighted spin echo (SE), and 45 percent for T1-weighted SE. The overall sensitivity for MRI at 0.5 Tesla combining all pulse sequences was 66 percent. The sensitivity of MRI at 1.5 Tesla was 64 percent for T2-weighted SE, 44 percent for T1-weighted IR, and 28 percent for T1-weighted SE. The overall sensitivity at 1.5 Tesla using all pulse sequences combined was 69 percent. Different combinations of imaging techniques yielded the following sensitivities: CT-AP and delayed iodine CT, 85 percent; MRI and delayed iodine CT, 77 percent; and CT-AP and MRI, 96 percent. The major advantage of CT-AP over the other imaging techniques was that of detecting small lesions (Fig. 27-6). CT-AP detected 79 percent of lesions smaller than 1 cm, whereas the technique with the next highest sensitivity (T2-weighted SE at 1.5 Tesla) detected only 47 percent of lesions this size.

In 1990, Merine et al. (25) evaluated 34 hepatocellular carcinomas in 14 patients with CT-AP and CT after intraarterial injection of Lipiodol. Surgical proof was available for all lesions. Overall detection rates for the main tumor were 94 percent for CT-AP and 82 percent for CT-Lipiodol. The detection rates for daughter nodules, however, were considerably lower, at 38 percent for CT-AP and 50 percent for CT-Lipiodol. The authors concluded that many small lesions less than 5 mm in diameter are not detected by either technique.

Not all studies agree, however, that CT-angiography is the best technique for focal hepatic lesion detection prior to surgery. In 1987,

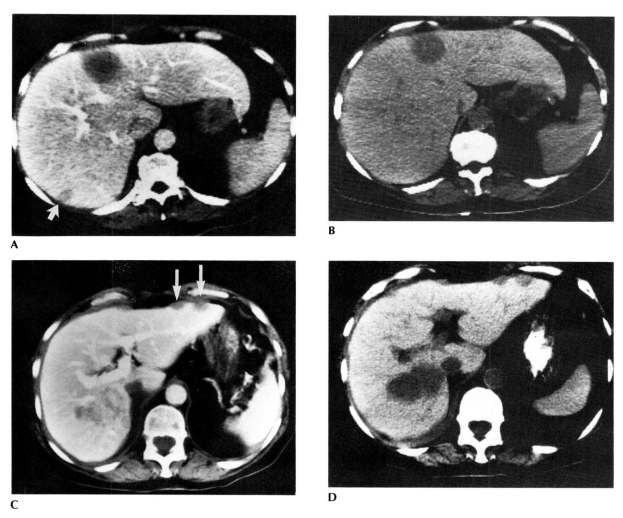

FIGURE 27-5
(A) CT-AP demonstrating a 4.5-cm hypodense mass in the medial segment of the left hepatic lobe and a wedge-shaped hypodense defect in the posterior segment of the right hepatic lobe (arrow). (B) The delayed iodine CT confirms the mass in the left lobe, but the small wedge-shaped mass in the right lobe is no longer seen and is consistent with a perfusion defect. (C) CT-AP in another patient demonstrates an irregular hypodense mass in the right lobe as well as two small subcapsular defects in the lateral segment of the left lobe anteriorly (arrows). (D) The delayed iodine CT also demonstrates the three hypodense lesions and they are therefore tumor deposits not perfusion defects.

Miller et al. (26) evaluated 56 metastases in 15 patients with three CT techniques. Surgical confirmation was obtained for all lesions. The sensitivity of the three CT techniques was 83 percent for delayed iodine CT (3.5 to 5 h after a mean of 79 g iodine), 82 percent for CT after ethiodized oil emulsion (EOE-13), and 77 percent for CT-AP. No significant difference in sensitivity was noted between the three techniques. The false-positive rate for CT-AP, however, was significantly higher than that for either delayed iodine CT or EOE-13 CT. Because of the high false-positive rate, the authors concluded that CT-AP is not clinically useful for detecting hepatic metastases. Why are

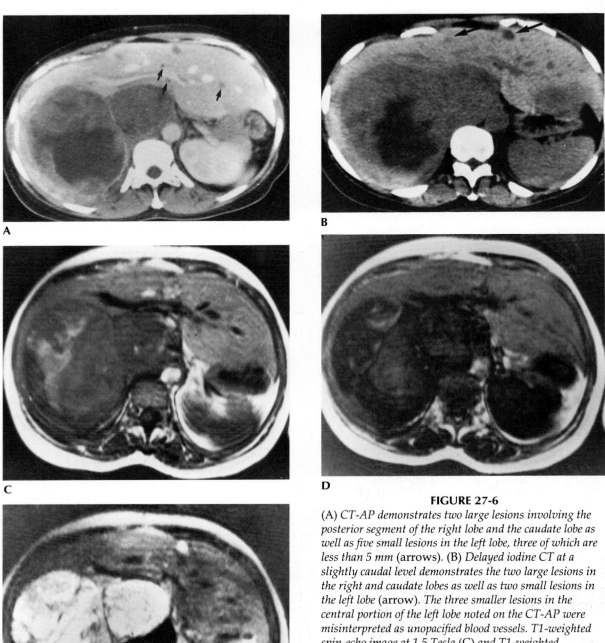

FIGURE 27-6
(A) CT-AP demonstrates two large lesions involving the posterior segment of the right lobe and the caudate lobe as well as five small lesions in the left lobe, three of which are less than 5 mm (arrows). (B) Delayed iodine CT at a slightly caudal level demonstrates the two large lesions in the right and caudate lobes as well as two small lesions in the left lobe (arrow). The three smaller lesions in the central portion of the left lobe noted on the CT-AP were misinterpreted as unopacified blood vessels. T1-weighted spin-echo image at 1.5 Tesla (C) and T1-weighted inversion-recovery sequence at 1.5 Tesla (D) both demonstrate two large hypointense lesions in the right and caudate lobes, but the five small lesions in the left lobe are not detected. (E) T2-weighted spin-echo sequence at 1.5 Tesla demonstrates the two large hyperintense lesions in the right and caudate lobes and one of the five small lesions in the left lobe. (From Nelson RC: Hepatic tumors: Comparison of CT during arterial portography, delayed CT and MR imaging for preoperative evaluation. Radiology, 172:27, 1989. Reprinted by permission.)

the conclusions of this study contrary to the work by the other authors cited? It is not surprising that delayed iodine CT had a comparatively high sensitivity, since very large doses of iodine were administered (mean dose 79 g). Higher doses of iodine in hepatocytes yield a higher hepatic density (27) and, therefore, higher lesion-to-liver contrast. The most likely reason for using larger volumes of contrast material was extensive preliminary angiography. As previously stated, using large amounts of iodine prior to CT-AP results in reduced lesion-to-liver contrast and therefore a lower sensitivity rate. While the high false-positive rate noted by Miller et al. (26) for CT-AP is worrisome, this has not been the experience of other institutions using similar parameters (20). At our institution, we perform delayed iodine CT 4 to 6 h after CT-AP routinely, and most of the false-positive lesions caused by perfusion defects on the CT-AP can be reconciled if they are not present on the follow-up delayed iodine CT (Fig. 27-5). Furthermore, surgeons in general are much less concerned about false-positive lesions that are often subcapsular, superficial in location, and easily investigated intraoperatively. They are much more concerned about false-negative lesions that are located deep within the hepatic parenchyma, are difficult to palpate intraoperatively, but may be important determinants of long-term survival.

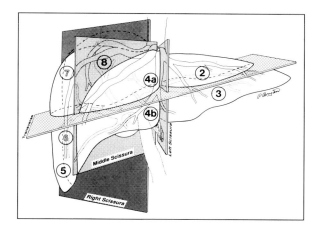

FIGURE 27-7
The liver is divided segmentally by four scissurae, three longitudinal and one transverse. The left longitudinal scissura is parallel to the left hepatic vein and falciform ligament. The middle longitudinal scissura is parallel to the middle hepatic vein and the gallbladder fossa. The right longitudinal scissura is parallel to the right hepatic vein. The transverse scissura is parallel to the right and left portal pedicles (portal vein, hepatic duct, and hepatic artery). Note that the transverse scissura is slightly more cephalad medially and caudad laterally. (From Sugarbaker PH: Surgical decision making for large bowel cancer metastatic to the liver. Radiology, 174:621, 1990. Reprinted by permission.)

SEGMENTAL LOCALIZATION OF FOCAL LESIONS

The liver is divided longitudinally by three scissurae and transversely by one scissura (Fig. 27-7). The longitudinal scissurae are parallel to the right, middle, and left hepatic veins, which along with the gallbladder fossa and falciform ligament are well visualized on CT images. The transverse scissura is parallel to the right and left portal pedicles (portal vein, hepatic duct, hepatic artery). Because it runs nearly parallel to the axial plane, it may be difficult to identify on CT images. In a recent study (28), we evaluated the ability of CT-AP to determine the segmental location of focal hepatic lesions preoperatively. Using the right and left main portal veins as landmarks for the transverse scissura, we found this plane to be consistently located near the middle liver slice of an incremental CT series, with the left portal pedicle slightly cephalad to the right portal pedicle. CT-AP and surgical exploration agreed on the preliminary segmental location in 33 of 36 focal lesions (92 percent) but disagreed on the extent of the tumor in 11 of 36 (31 percent). Upon reanalysis of the CT-AP on these 11 lesions, the extent was felt to have been correctly described at surgery in 6 lesions, correctly described by CT-AP in 4 lesions, and in 1 lesion both surgery and CT-AP correctly described opposite margins of the same tumor. Pitfalls for CT-AP include high lesions under the diaphragm (segment 7 versus 8) and lesions close to a segmental boundary (Fig. 27-8). We concluded that since it may be difficult or impossible to localize deep hepatic lesions intraoperatively by palpation or inspection, CT-AP is an important preoperative tool for determining the segmental location and thereby planning the surgical approach to focal hepatic lesions.

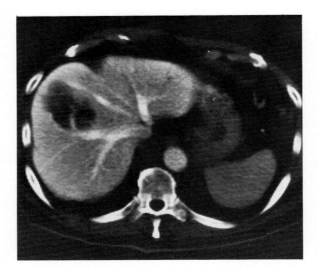

FIGURE 27-8
A 6-cm hypodense mass in the anterior segment of the right hepatic lobe (segment 8) interposed between the middle and right hepatic veins. Even though the CT-AP suggests that the lesion is limited to segment 8, these lesions are often found to extend across segmental boundaries intraoperatively.

PITFALLS OF CT-ANGIOGRAPHY

As previously mentioned, perfusion abnormalities are a major pitfall of CT-angiography. Tyrrel et al. (29) described an additional perfusion abnormality on CT-AP which they called the "straight-line sign." This sign was noted in 16 of 44 patients (36 percent), was associated with a mass at the proximal portion of the defect, and in most patients was not seen on either delayed iodine CT or MRI (Fig. 27-9). Recognition of this sign may indicate to the surgeon that the tumor is inoperable, since it suggests portal venous invasion.

Differential enhancement of the lobes also may result from laminar flow between opacified and unopacified blood in either the hepatic artery or the portal vein. This appears to be uncommon when performing CT-AP; however, in his experience with more than 800 cases, Matsui (30) noted this finding in approximately 5 percent. It is believed that this phenomenon occurs more often when the catheter tip is wedged or directed into a branch of the SMA.

Another pitfall of CT-angiography is the poor sensitivity to porta hepatis lymphadenopathy. Not infrequently we have been told by our liver surgeons that during exploration, adenopathy is

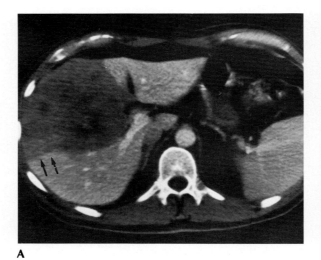
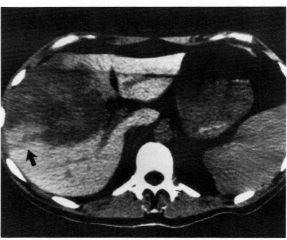

FIGURE 27-9
(A) CT-AP demonstrating a large hypodense mass involving the central portion of the liver and a "straight line" of contrast enhancement extending from the mass to the periphery (arrows). (B) Delayed iodine CT does not demonstrate a "straight line" but rather uptake of contrast material by normally functioning hepatocytes in this nontumorous portion of the liver (arrow). This finding implies obstruction of a branch of the right portal vein.

present in the porta hepatis that was not appreciated on the CT-angiogram and which renders the patient unresectable. This is not surprising, since the contrast technique for CT-AP is optimized for focal hepatic lesion detection, not lymph node detection. Dynamic CT is better suited for this purpose.

CONCLUSIONS

CT-angiography is a highly sensitive cross-sectional imaging technique that should be used routinely in the small group of patients who are candidates for hepatic tumor resection. The major advantage of this technique over other imaging modalities, such as contrast-enhanced CT, delayed iodine CT, and MRI, is the detection of small lesions between 5 and 10 mm in diameter. Many lesions smaller than 5 mm will not be detected reliably by any technique. Accurate detection of lesions prior to surgery will hopefully result in an even better long-term survival rate. We prefer CT-AP over CT-HA because of higher lesion-to-liver contrast and presumably higher lesion-detection rates. CT-AP also has been shown to be helpful for localizing lesions to specific hepatic segments preoperatively. While perfusion abnormalities are an important pitfall, many of these can be clarified by performing follow-up delayed iodine CT routinely.

REFERENCES

1. Bengmark S: Progress in the treatment of liver cancer. World J Surg 6:1, 1982.
2. Silverberg E, Boring CC, Squires TS: Cancer statistics, 1990. CA 40:9, 1990.
3. Wood CB, Gillis CR, Blumgart LH: A retrospective study of the natural history of patients with metastases from colorectal cancer. Clin Oncol 2:285, 1976.
4. Hughes KS, Rosenstein RB, Songhorabodi S, et al: Resection of the liver for colorectal cancer metastases: A multi-institutional study of long-term survivors. Dis Colon Rectum 31:1, 1988.
5. Willis RA: The Spread of Tumors in the Human Body, 3d ed. London, Butterworth, 1973, p 175.
6. August DA, Ottow RT, Sugarbaker PH: Clinical prospective of human colorectal cancer metastases. Cancer Metastasis Rev 3:303, 1984.
7. Bengmark S, Hafstrom L: The natural history of primary and secondary malignant tumors of the liver: I. The prognosis for patients with hepatic metastases from colonic and rectal carcinoma by laparotomy. Cancer 23:198, 1969.
8. Wagner JS, Adson MA, Van Heerden JA, et al: The natural history of hepatic metastases from colorectal cancer: A comparison with resective treatment. Ann Surg 199:502, 1984.
9. Hughes KS, Simon R, Songhorabodi S, et al: Resection of the liver for colorectal cancer metastases: A multi-institutional study of patterns of recurrence. Surgery 100:278, 1986.
10. Adson MA: Hepatic metastases in prospective. AJR 140:695, 1983.
11. Sugarbaker PH, Kemeny NM: Management of metastatic cancer to the liver. Adv Surg 22:1, 1989.
12. Sugarbaker PH: Surgical decision making for large bowel cancer metastatic to the liver. Radiology 174:621, 1990.
13. Joishy SK, Balasegaram M: Hepatic resection for malignant tumors of the liver: Essentials for a unified surgical approach. Am J Surg 139:360, 1980.
14. Hughes KS, Simon RM, Songhorabodi S, et al: Resection of the liver for colorectal carcinoma metastases: A multi-institutional study of indications for resection. Surgery 103:278, 1987.
15. Greenway CV, Stark RD: Hepatic vascular bed. Physiol Rev 51:23, 1971.
16. Ackerman NB, Lin WM, Conde ES, Silverman NA: The blood supply of experimental liver metastases: I. Distribution of hepatic artery and portal vein blood to "small" and "large" tumors. Surgery 66:1067, 1969.
17. Prando A, Wallace S, Bernardino ME, Lindell MM Jr: Computed tomographic arteriography of the liver. Radiology 130:697, 1979.
18. Nelson RC, Chezmar JL, Sugarbaker PH, Bernardino ME: Hepatic tumors: Comparison of CT during arterial portography, delayed CT and MR imaging for preoperative evaluation. Radiology 172:27, 1989.
19. Matsui O, Takashima T, Kadoya M, et al: Dynamic computed tomography during arterial portography: A most sensitive examination for small hepatocellular carcinomas. J Comput Assist Tomogr 9:19, 1985.
20. Matsui O, Takashima T, Kadoya M, et al: Liver metastases from colorectal cancer: Detection with CT during arterial portography. Radiology 165:65, 1987.
21. Freeny PC, Marks WM: Hepatic perfusion abnormalities during CT angiography: Detection and interpretation. Radiology 159:685, 1986.
22. Lundstedt C, Dotberg S, Lunderquist A, et al: Computed tomographic angiography of the liver via the coeliac axis. Acta Radiol Diagn 27:285, 1986.
23. Nakao N, Miura K, Takayasu Y, et al: CT angiography in hepatocellular carcinoma. J Comput Assist Tomogr 7:780, 1983.

24. Heiken JP, Weyman PJ, Lee JKT, et al: Detection of focal hepatic masses: Prospective evaluation with CT, delayed CT, CT during arterial portography and MRI. Radiology 171:47, 1989.
25. Merine D, Takayasu K, Wakao F: Detection of hepatocellular carcinoma: Comparison of CT during arterial portography with CT after intra-arterial injection of iodized oil. Radiology 175:701, 1990.
26. Miller DL, Simmons JT, Chang R, et al: Hepatic metastases detection: Comparison of three CT contrast enhancement methods. Radiology 165:785, 1987.
27. Perkerson RB Jr, Erwin BC, Baumgartner BR, et al: CT density in delayed iodine hepatic scanning. Radiology 155:445, 1985.
28. Nelson RC, Chezmar JL, Sugarbaker PH, et al: Preoperative localization of focal liver lesions to specific liver segments: Utility of CT during arterial portography. Radiology 176:89, 1990.
29. Tyrrel RT, Kaufman SL, Bernardino ME: Straight-line sign: Appearance and significance during CT portography. Radiology 173:635, 1989.
30. Matsui O: Letter to the Editor. Radiology 168:283, 1988.

28

Intraoperative Ultrasonography of Liver

JOSEPH F. SIMEONE

The use of intraoperative ultrasonography (IUS) was first reported in the 1960s, but it was not until the early 1980s that refinements in equipment were adequate enough to make IUS a useful adjunct to routine hepatic surgery (1–8). Intraoperative ultrasound was first used in neurosurgical procedures but is now used in many hepati, biliary, and pancreatic procedures as well.

Intraoperative ultrasound can be used as both a diagnostic and a therapeutic tool. Within the liver, IUS provides the following information:

1. Visualization of normal vascular anatomy and its relationship to pathologic masses.
2. Identification of small (1 to 5 cm), nonpalpable parenchymal liver lesions not detected by preoperative imaging studies.
3. Differentiation of certain benign lesions such as liver cysts or hemangiomas from tumors.
4. Visualization of larger (5 to 10 cm) tumors deep in the liver parenchyma that may not be palpable to the operating surgeon.

Intraoperative ultrasound also displays specific anatomic relationships, which allows precise surgical resection of intrahepatic lesions.

EQUIPMENT

Several manufacturers produce equipment that may be used in the operating room. Individual transducers cost approximately $7500. In general, the ultrasound unit on which a transducer is attached costs approximately $200,000. The equipment, therefore, is moderately expensive. Generally, a superficially focused 5-, 6-, 7.5-, or 10-mHz linear array transducer is preferred. These transducers generally are side-firing so that the transducer may lay flat on the liver surface (Fig. 28-1) and are small enough to fit under the rib cage and above the dome. The transducers generally are no more than 5 cm in length and 1 to 2 cm in width and are easily held within the hand or can be guided by a finger. Other available transducer configurations are the I-shape and T-shape. Transducers require gas sterilization after each use. The particular transducer in use in our institution is a side-firing 5-mHz transducer that may be interposed under the liver, between the ribs and the liver, or the dome (Fig. 28-2).

Intraoperative transducers must be used on machines that are portable from the radiology department to the operating theater. In our institution, a machine is located within the ultrasound unit in radiology and is moved in a portable manner as needed to the operating room. However, a

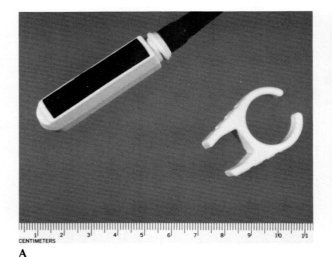
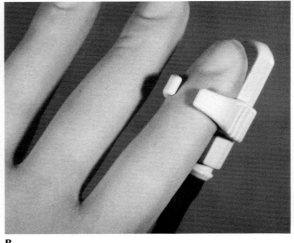
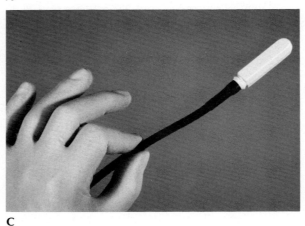

FIGURE 28-1
(A) *En-face view of a 7.5-mHz IUS transducer with attachable finger clip.* (B) *The assembled transducer and finger clip can be used for palpation and precise scanning over the liver surface.* (C) *The transducer can be extended to the most distal portion of the liver by holding the stiff cord at a distance away from the scan head.*

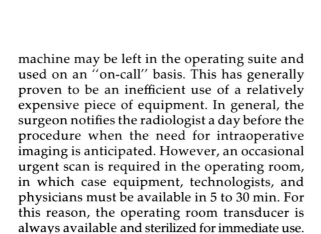

machine may be left in the operating suite and used on an "on-call" basis. This has generally proven to be an inefficient use of a relatively expensive piece of equipment. In general, the surgeon notifies the radiologist a day before the procedure when the need for intraoperative imaging is anticipated. However, an occasional urgent scan is required in the operating room, in which case equipment, technologists, and physicians must be available in 5 to 30 min. For this reason, the operating room transducer is always available and sterilized for immediate use. This is quite feasible in the case of these special transducers because they are limited in use to the operating room.

TECHNICAL CONSIDERATIONS

When in the operating room, the radiologist scrubs and gowns in the usual fashion, positions himself or herself beside the patient, and performs the scan while observing the monitor with the surgeon. Because intraoperative scanning is quite different from routine daily scanning, a radiologist with much IUS experience is needed for these cases. Similarly, one technologist, very familiar with operating room personnel, equipment, and the varying needs of IU scanning is needed for this procedure. The designated US technologist accompanies the radiologist to obtain hard copy and videotape, optimize scan quality, and maximize efficiency. Because most operating room suites have unique electrical outlets that prevent sparks or fire, a special adapter is required for the US unit to be powered in the operating room. We carry this adapter on the US unit at all times. A sterile gel is not needed within the operating room. Contact between the transducer and liver surface is maintained by sterile saline or ambient peritoneal fluid.

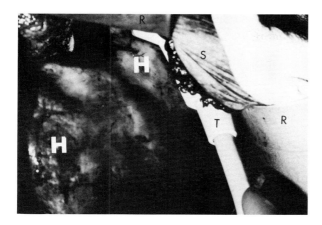

FIGURE 28-2
Demonstration of placement of a different IUS transducer between the anterior ribs and liver parenchyma. The transducer may be placed under the liver, along the side of the liver, or in any of the perihepatic spaces (H = liver; R = retractor; S = skin; T = transducer).

In the operating room, the US scan generally adds 10 to 15 min to the operative procedure. The total time required for the radiologist is approximately 1 h to leave and return to the radiology department. This includes change of clothes, transportation of equipment to the operating room, operative hand cleaning, and scanning itself.

Scanning of the entire liver (especially the left and right lobes) does not require mobilization of the liver or further extension of the skin incision.

ULTRASONOGRAPHIC LIVER ANATOMY

With high-frequency intraoperative transducers, the liver parenchyma is seen as a uniform homogeneous echogenic structure with a recognizable echo pattern (Fig. 28-3) and anatomic landmarks (Fig. 28-4). The intrahepatic vascular structures are easily identified (Fig. 28-5). The hepatic veins course obliquely toward the vena cava, and their walls have little or no echogenicity. Blood flow within these and portal veins is easily seen by real-time imaging as tiny moving echoes that travel within the veins themselves. Portal veins are identified by their echogenic walls and the blood flow occurring within them (see Fig. 28-3).

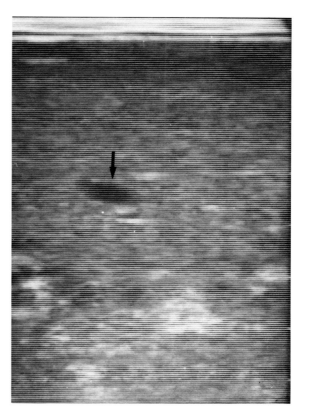

FIGURE 28-3
Appearance of normal hepatic parenchyma. The normal homogeneous echo pattern is recognized throughout the liver. A cross section of a hepatic vein is seen (arrow).

The bile duct can frequently be seen directly anterior or posterior to the portal vein in the left and right lobes and in its expected anterolateral location within the porta itself (Figs. 28-4 and 28-6).

The gallbladder also may be examined at the time of intraoperative sonography (Fig. 28-7). The gallbladder wall and the clear echo-free bile are well seen. Gallstones have a typical appearance as an echogenic focus and posterior acoustical shadowing.

Identification of Liver Tumors
Tumors within the liver have the same appearance intraoperatively as by routine transabdominal scanning. Hemangiomas appear as well-defined echogenic masses. Cysts show no

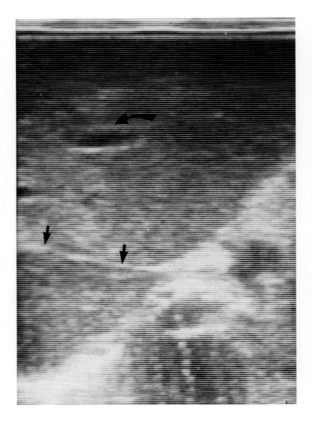 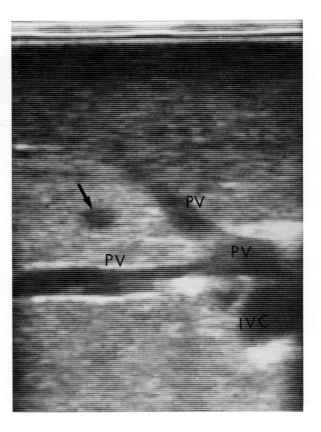

FIGURE 28-4
Left lobe of the liver. The portal vein (curved arrow) in the left lobe is identified by its echogenic wall (straight arrow). The fissure of the ligamentum venosum is seen separating the left lobe of the liver from the caudate lobe.

FIGURE 28-5
Identification of intrahepatic vascular structures. Branching of the portal vein (PV) is clearly demonstrated. The hepatic vein (arrow) seen in cross section between branches of the portal vein (IVC = inferior vena cava).

internal echoes, well-defined walls, and through transmission of sound. Liver tumors, either primary or metastatic, generally appear as hypoechoic, irregularly marginated, solid masses (Figs. 28-8 and 28-9). They are easily recognizable when compared to the normal echogenicity of the liver. While the appearance of malignant disease may be nonspecific, a sure sign of malignancy is vascular invasion, which may occasionally be seen untrasonographically. Proximity of tumor to the vascular structures will usually determine the viability of segmental versus lobar resection of the liver. Intraoperative US can provide precise information about the distance of a tumor from the hepatic vein (Figs. 28-10, 28-11, and 28-12) and therefore determine which surgical resection is best.

DISCUSSION

Routine use of IUS is reported to alter the planned surgical approach in a significant number of patients. Rifkin et al. (1) performed IUS on 49 patients evaluated because of known or suspected disease of the liver. In 55 percent of these patients, no new information was obtained. In 19 percent, new information was gathered that changed the surgical approach. In 14 percent, new information was obtained, but it was such that no change in the therapeutic approach was needed, and in 12 percent, although no new information was gathered, a change in the surgical approach was still possible because of IUS. Bismuth et al. (2) performed a similar study in primary liver tumors. They found that in 79 surgical interventions, IUS provided additional information to that obtained

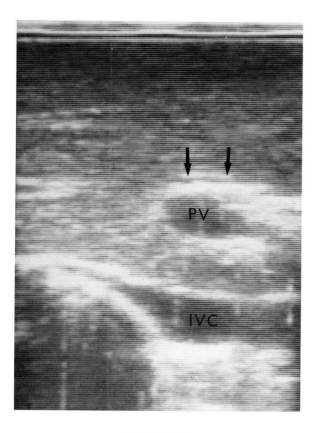

FIGURE 28-6
The intrahepatic bile duct (arrow) *is seen as a tiny submillimeter tubular structure anterior to a portal venous branch within the right lobe of the liver* (PV = *portal vein;* IVC = *inferior vena cava*).

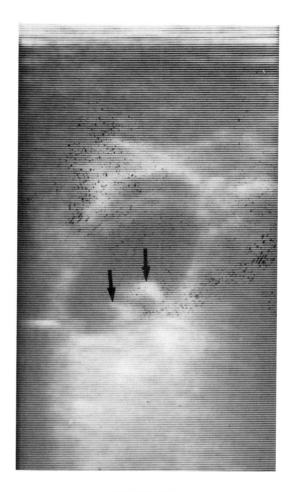

FIGURE 28-7
Appearance of gallstones. The gallbladder is identified in its usual location and in its usual shape. Gallstones (arrows) *are manifested as two echogenic structures within the anechoic bile.*

on preoperative investigations in 33 percent of patients. This information modified the intended surgical procedure in 21 patients, and in 10 patients subsegmental resection was facilitated by ultrasonically guided cannulation of the portal venous branch.

Parker et al. (7) have described similar results. In 42 patients who underwent 45 operations, IUS found 98 percent of lesions compared with 77 percent for preoperative CT. IUS affected operative management in 22 of 45 operations (49 percent). Most helpful findings by IUS were extrahepatic disease (5), more nodules in the liver (4), unsuspected hepatic and portal vein involvement (4), and veins free of tumor (4) when CT demonstrated masses, thereby permitting resection.

Machi and Sigel (8) reviewed their results of IUS in 334 hepatic operations. IUS was determined to be useful in 96 percent of the procedures. IUS provided acquisition of new information in 252 (75 percent), guidance of operation in 77 (23 percent), and confirmation of completion of operation in 29 (9 percent).

Clarke et al. (5) have recently reported on the extraordinary accuracy of IUS in finding liver tumors. In approximately 150 tumors found by IUS, preoperative US found 76 percent, CT found 61 percent, and angiography found 52 percent. Fully 40 percent of the lesions found by IUS were not

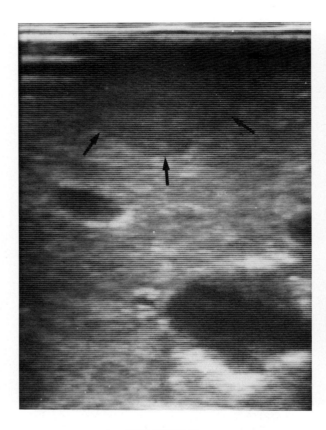 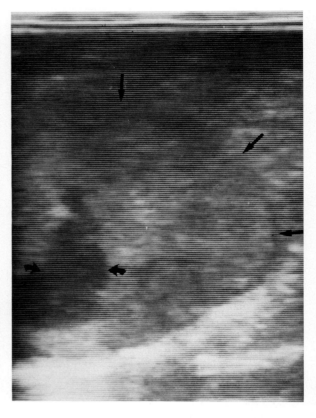

FIGURE 28-8
Appearance of a superficially located hypoechoic liver tumor metastatic from colon. Clear separation is seen between the normal, more echogenic hepatic parenchyma and the round, hypoechoic hepatic tumor (arrows).

FIGURE 28-9
Degenerated cystic area within a large metastatic liver tumor. A hypoechoic capsule (arrows) separates the liver tumor from the normal hepatic parenchyma. A centrally located, irregularly shaped cystic area (curved arrow) of liquefactive degeneration is demonstrated within this liver tumor.

visible or palpable at the time of surgery. IUS was the most accurate of all the imaging techniques in displaying small intrahepatic tumors. This group also was able to perform numerous cryotherapy procedures on liver tumors after identifying and localizing these tumors with IUS. The accuracy of IUS was particularly noticeable in lesions less than 2 cm in size that were located in the lateral segment of the left lobe.

Makuuchi et al. (4) used IUS as an aid in liver resection in patients with hepatocellular carcinoma. In comparing IUS with preoperative US angiography, and CT, IUS was 99 percent sensitive in finding 198 of 203 small HCCs. This compared with sensitivities in the 85 to 95 percent range for the preoperative studies. IUS also revealed 70 percent of the tumor thrombi, while US and angiography disclosed only 21 percent. In the Makuuchi et al. study of HCC associated with liver cirrhosis, 65 percent of patients had invisible or nonpalpable tumors. Therapeutically, IUS also was very helpful in this group of patients. It led to development of new liver-sparing hepatectomy procedures, including systemic subsegmentectomy and hepatectomies that preserved the inferior right hepatic vein. This had led to increased survival at 3 to 5 years.

This author's experience does not equal that of others either in the number of cases performed or in detecting new masses or altering the planned

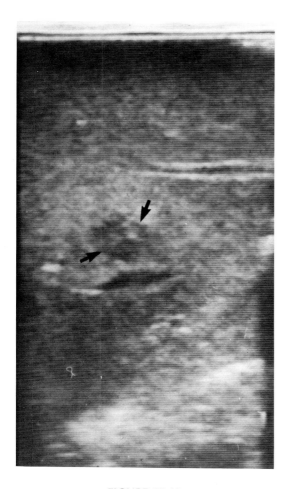

FIGURE 28-10
Nonpalpable small hepatic tumor within the left lobe. Preoperative imaging indicated a left lobe free of tumor. A 1.0-cm hypoechoic, well-defined hypoechoic mass (arrow) is seen anterior to hepatic venous branches.

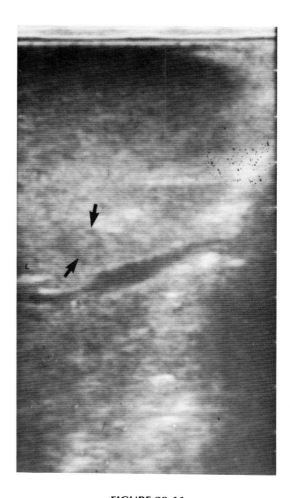

FIGURE 28-11
A second example of a nonpalpable liver tumor within the left lobe. A hypoechoic mass (arrow) is seen just anterior to a portal venous structure. This lesion was not detected by preoperative imaging and was not palpated at the time of surgery. Note the close apposition but absence of invasion of the vascular structure.

surgical procedures. Current techniques for preoperative liver tumor imaging routinely use MRI, CT-AP, and CT with bolus intravenous contrast injection (9). This approach maximizes preoperative liver lesion detection and, therefore, it is unusual for the operating surgeon or the radiologist to be surprised by previously undetected liver lesions. Similarly, detailed examination of the detected liver lesions and their relationship to the hepatic vessels and classic hepatic segmental anatomy makes alteration of the planned surgical approach rare.

The author's major contribution to hepatic surgery in our institution has come in the localization of deeply seated hepatic abscesses (Fig. 28-13) usually found in transplanted livers that have been detected by preoperative imaging studies but cannot be found in the scarred, fibrotic, bloody surgical field at the time of reoperation. On numerous occasions, IUS has been used to find the abscess or abscesses, guide the surgeon during complete evacuation of the infected material, and confirm the absence of other collections.

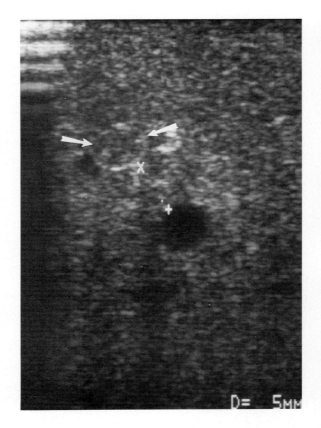

FIGURE 28-12
The distance (X−+) between the hypoechoic hepatic vein and a colonic liver metastasis (arrows) is clearly demonstrated and displayed on the screen (5 min).

CONCLUSION

Intraoperative ultrasound (IUS) of the liver can have the following important uses:

1. To detect previously undetectable and nonpalpable liver lesions within liver parenchyma.
2. To aid in surgery of primary liver tumors by precisely defining the topography of the tumor and liver and the vascular anatomy.
3. For use in planning management of patients at the time of the operation when new disease in the liver is found and disease-free segments of the liver remain.
4. Use for guidance for intraoperative biopsy of nonpalpable lesions.

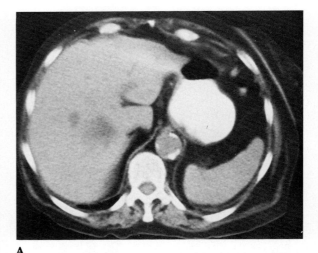

A

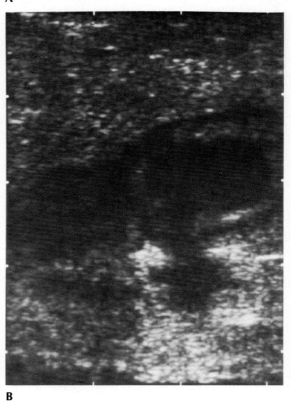

B

FIGURE 28-13
(A) CT scan demonstrates a deeply seated hepatic abscess that was not palpable at the time of surgery. (B) IUS clearly shows the abscess and was used to guide the surgeon to the collection.

Numerous studies have now demonstrated that in 20 to 35 percent of patients who undergo IUS, new information will be provided and a change in surgical technique will be necessary based on the information provided.

However, the author agrees with Sugarbaker regarding the use of IUS in hepatic surgery: "The most valuable aspect of intraoperative ultrasound is that it requires the surgeon, radiologist, x-ray exams, and target organ (liver) to be together in one place. The information exchanged is nearly always beneficial to the physicians and most of all to the patient. Rarely does the intraoperative ultrasound exam impel a definitive change in management" (10).

REFERENCES

1. Rifkin MD, Rosato RE, Branch HM, et al: Intraoperative ultrasound of the liver. Ann Surg 205:466, 1987.
2. Bismuth H, Castaing D, Graden OJ: The use of operative ultrasound in surgery of primary liver tumors. World J Surg 11:610, 1987.
3. Gozzetti G, Angelini L: The use of intraoperative ultrasonography in hepatic surgery, Rifkin M (ed): Intraoperative and Endoscopic Ultrasonography, New York, Churchill-Livingstone, 1987, pp 81–103.
4. Makuuchi M, Hasegawa H, Yamazaki S, et al: The use of operative ultrasound as an aid to liver resection in patients with hepatocellular carcinoma. World J Surg 11:615, 1987.
5. Clarke MP, Kane RA, Steele D: Prospective comparison of preoperative imaging and intraoperative ultrasonography in the detection of liver tumors. Surgery 106:849, 1989.
6. Machi J, Isomoto H, Yamashita Y, et al: Intraoperative ultrasonography in screening for liver metastases from colorectal cancer: Comparative accuracy with traditional procedures. Surgery 678, 1987.
7. Parker GA, Lawrence W, Horsely S, et al: Intraoperative ultrasound of the liver affects operation decision making. Ann Surg 209:569, 1989.
8. Machi J, Sigel B: Overview of benefits of operative sonography during a ten year period. J Ultrasound Med 8:647, 1989.
9. Nelson RC, Chezmar JL, Sugarbaker PH, Bernardino M: Hepatic tumors: Comparison of CT-AP, delayed CT, and MR imaging for preoperative evaluation. Radiology 172:27, 1989.
10. Sugarbaker PH: Surgical decision making for large bowel cancer metastatic to the liver. Radiology 174:621, 1990.

29

Application of a Three-Dimensional Workstation to Liver Tumor Volumetrics

MARK A. GOLDBERG, PETER F. HAHN,
DAVID D. STARK, and JOSEPH T. FERRUCCI

Quantitation of liver tumor burden remains a difficult problem for oncologists, who require this information to plan therapy and assess treatment response. Traditionally, the information provided by the radiologist has been limited to a qualitative impression based on comparison with the patient's prior studies. To provide a more objective assessment, a semiautomated method of quantitating liver tumor burden using a three-dimensional (3-D) workstation has been developed. Three-dimensional technology lends itself to this problem because volume calculations are inherent to the reconstruction process. In addition, the workstation allows for interactive analysis of the three-dimensional object using display features such as rotation, transparency, and cut planes. The interactive display provides the user with a unique spatial representation that can only be conceptualized with cross-sectional imaging techniques. This spatial information is also of potential value in planning radiation therapy or surgery.

MATERIALS AND METHODS

Three-dimensional reconstructions of the liver have been performed on an independent three-dimensional workstation (ISG Technologies, Inc., Toronto) using standard contrast-enhanced CT scans (10 × 10 mm). Performing a reconstruction of the liver involves two steps. The first step is to demarcate the boundaries of the liver using regions of interest (ROI). The second step is to segment the liver, i.e., to discriminate between normal and abnormal pixels within the liver based on their CT density. A range of CT densities is selected to specify which pixels within the indicated region of interest are to be included in the reconstructed object.

The segmentation process is straightforward for skeletal applications because of the significant density difference between the bony structures of interest and the surrounding soft tissues. As a result, a variety of skeletal applications for three-dimensional imaging have been described in the literature, including trauma, orthopaedic surgery planning, and prosthesis design (1–7). The problem is more complex for solid organ imaging, however, because the difference in density between normal and abnormal parenchyma is less distinct. To solve this problem, pixel histogram analysis of the liver is needed. The utility of histogram analysis of the liver was first suggested by Moss et al.(8). A pixel histogram of a normal liver is shown in Figure 29-1. The Gaussian shape of

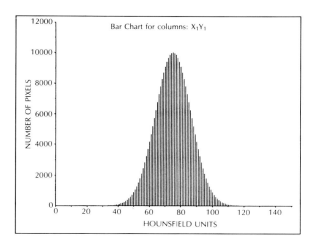

FIGURE 29-1
Pixel histogram of normal liver that has a Gaussian distribution.

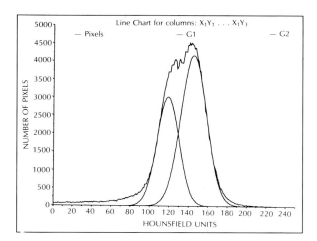

FIGURE 29-3
Pixel histogram from Fig. 29-2 (see color insert) with Gaussian curve fits.

the density distribution arises from randomness introduced by the natural heterogeneity of hepatic parenchyma and by uncertainties in the CT imaging process related to variation in photon flux (8).

As shown by Yang et al. (9), the diseased liver may be accurately and reproducibly modeled as a sum of Gaussian curves. Statistical analysis of the pixel histogram employing a computerized curve-fitting algorithm generates the best-fitting curves from the family of Gaussians.

RESULTS

Three-dimensional reconstructions were performed in 20 patients with known hepatic lesions. The examples that follow serve to illustrate the technique. A CT image from a patient with focal nodular hyperplasia (FNH) is shown in Figure 29-2 (see color insert). Figure 29-3 demonstrates the original histogram and the Gaussian curves which, when added together, model the original curve with a high degree of statistical accuracy. The Gaussian curve with the lower density distribution corresponds to tumor, whereas the curve with the higher mean value represents normal liver parenchyma. In complex cases, such as tumors with solid and necrotic components, three Gaussians may be required to obtain a satisfactory curve fit.

One may calculate the likelihood of tumor involvement for a pixel of any CT density by computing the relative heights of the Gaussian curves for that density. In this manner, a graph demonstrating probability of tumor involvement versus CT density may be constructed, as shown in Figure 29-4. This graph is then referenced to select a probability threshold to determine the segmentation level. All pixels below the threshold are considered to be abnormal, whereas those above are assumed to be normal. The selection of a probability threshold is arbitrary, but the threshold provides a reproducible method of segmenting the liver on follow-up studies. We have found a 60 percent threshold most satisfactory, which means that all pixels with a 60 percent or greater probability of being abnormal are reconstructed as tumor. This threshold was chosen because the pixels identified as abnormal using this level corresponded best to areas interpreted as abnormal by experienced observers.

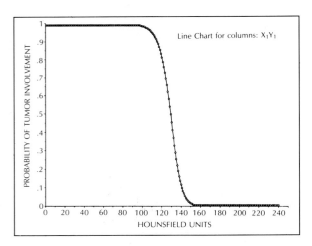

FIGURE 29-4
Plot of probability of tumor involvement versus CT density derived from Fig. 29-3.

Figure 29-5 (see color insert) demonstrates the three-dimensional reconstruction of the liver from the patient with focal nodular hyperplasia shown in the anteroposterior projection. The tumor has been reconstructed in red, and a wedge of normal hepatic parenchyma has been removed by the computer to demonstrate the area of abnormality to better advantage. The calculated tumor volume was 478 cc. In this case, the lesion was surgically resected and the volume of the specimen as measured by water displacement was within 2 percent of the calculated value. However, the calculated value would have varied if a different threshold had been chosen.

One application being investigated at our institution is the follow-up of patients being treated with hepatic arterial chemotherapy infusion. CT images from one such patient are shown in Figure 29-6 (see color insert). Figure 29-6A was obtained initially, and Figure 29-6B was acquired 7 months later. The corresponding pixel histograms are shown in Figure 29-7, demonstrating considerable interval improvement in the tumor component of the curve, as would be predicted from the accompanying CT images. The three-dimensional reconstructions shown in Figure 29-8 (see color insert) demonstrate a 90 percent reduction in tumor burden and a 30 percent reduction in the total volume of the liver.

DISCUSSION

The thresholding technique described above is designed to provide reproducibility on follow-up studies rather than absolute accuracy. Since all pixels below the threshold are included in the reconstruction of abnormal tissue, some normal structures such as bile ducts or fat in fissures will be included in the tumor segment. However, this does not compromise the technique as long as these structures do not change from study to study. On the other hand, development of fatty infiltration or biliary obstruction during the follow-up interval could render the technique misleading. In our experience, this has not been a major impediment.

To date we have been using standard, contrast-enhanced studies with 10×10 mm sections. Studies in the literature employing 10-mm slices and less sophisticated volumetric techniques, such as tracing and summation, report error rates in the 5 to 10 percent range for organ volumes (10–14). Ettinger et al. (15) reported a 6.4 percent error in calculated volumes of two surgically resected primary liver tumors using a manual contouring technique (15). Volumetric error increases with small lesions, and thinner slices may be required to maintain accuracy. The available evidence suggests that 5 to 10 percent error can be obtained using 1-cm slices for lesions as small as 35 to 40 cc (10). This volume corresponds to spherical lesions with a diameter of approximately 2.2 cm.

The use of iodinated contrast may affect reproducibility if the timing of the dynamic bolus is different from study to study. Noncontrast studies eliminate this problem at the expense of lesion contrast. We are investigating delayed imaging following contrast injection as a possible solution.

Three-dimensional reconstructions of the liver from MRI data have been performed and utilized to calculate organ volumes (16). New fast-scanning techniques may allow three-dimensional acquisitions of the liver which can then be reconstructed for display as three-dimensional objects. Data sets obtained in this manner would provide improved anatomic detail.

We believe that three-dimensional volumetrics of the liver is a promising technique for use in planning therapy and assessing treatment response. Additional clinical trials are underway.

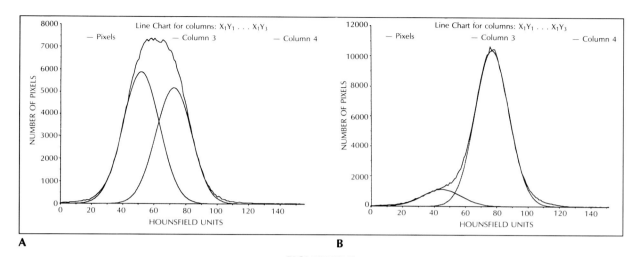

FIGURE 29-7
Pixel histograms, including curve fits, corresponding to the CT scans depicted in Fig. 29-6 (see color insert). The decrease in the tumor component of the curves reflects the demonstrated interval improvement.

REFERENCES

1. Burk DL Jr, Mears DC, Kennedy WH: Three-dimensional computed tomography of acetabular fractures. Radiology 155:183, 1985.
2. Robertson DD, Walker PS, Granholm JW, et al: Design of custom hip stem prostheses using three-dimensional CT modeling. J Comput Assist Tomogr 11:804, 1987.
3. Wojcik WG, Edeiken-Monroe BS, Harris JH Jr: Three-dimensional computed tomography in acute cervical spine trauma: A preliminary report. Skeletal Radiol 16:261, 1987.
4. Mayer JS, Wainwright DJ, Yeakley JW, et al: The role of three-dimensional computed tomography in the management of maxillofacial trauma. J Trauma 28:1043, 1988.
5. Magid D, Fishman EK, Sponseller PD: 2D and 3D computed tomography of the pediatric hip. Radiographics 8:901, 1988.
6. Magid D, Fishman EK: Imaging of musculoskeletal trauma in three dimensions: An integrated two-dimensional/three-dimensional approach with computed tomography. Radiol Clin North Am 27:945, 1989.
7. Kuhlman JE, Fishman EK, Ney DR, et al: Two- and three-dimensional imaging of the painful shoulder. Orthop Rev 18:1201, 1989.
8. Moss AA, Cann CE, Friedman MA, et al: Volumetric CT analysis of hepatic tumors. J Comput Assist Tomogr 5:714, 1981.
9. Yang N, Leichner PK, Fishman EK, et al: CT volumetrics of primary liver cancers. J Comput Assist Tomogr 10:621, 1986.
10. Breiman RS, Beck JW, Korobkin M, et al: Volume determinations using computed tomography. AJR 138:329, 1982.
11. Heymsfield SB, Fulenwider T, Nordlinger B, et al: Accurate measurement of liver, kidney, and spleen volume and mass by computerized axial tomography. Ann Intern Med 90:185, 1979.
12. Moss AA, Friedman MA, Brito AC: Determination of liver, kidney, and spleen volumes by computed tomography: An experimental study in dogs. J Comput Assist Tomogr 5:12, 1981.
13. Brenner DE, Whitley NO, Houk TL, et al: Volume determinations in computed tomography. JAMA 247:1299, 1982.
14. Albright RE, Fram, EK: Microcomputer-based technique for 3-D reconstruction and volume measurement of computed tomographic images. Invest Radiol 23:881, 1988.
15. Ettinger DS, Leichner PK, Siegelman SS, et al: Computed tomography assisted volumetric analysis of primary liver tumor as a measure of response to therapy. Am J Clin Oncol 8:413, 1985.
16. McNeal GR, Maynard WH, Branch RA, et al: Liver volume measurements and three-dimensional display from MR images. Radiology 169:851, 1988.

IX. HEPATIC VASCULAR DISEASES

30

Imaging of the Budd-Chiari Syndrome

PETER F. HAHN and
E. KENT YUCEL

CLINICAL FEATURES

Budd-Chiari syndrome is a clinical entity consisting of ascites, abdominal pain, hepatomegaly, and jaundice arising as a consequence of hepatic vein obstruction. Symptomatic hepatic vein occlusion has been found in 0.05 percent of autopsies (1). Obstruction can occur in the small veins, in the major hepatic veins, or in the suprahepatic inferior vena cava (IVC). The eponym *Budd-Chiari syndrome* is usually reserved for obstruction at the level of the three large hepatic veins or the IVC.

Obstruction of the large hepatic veins can arise from primary thrombus formation, from tumor thrombus or compression, or from obstructed outflow of the hepatic veins into the suprahepatic segment of the IVC. When obstruction is secondary to thrombosis, a hypercoagulable state is usually present. A tumor is responsible in 20 percent of cases. Cancer chemotherapy and hepatic transplantation also contribute some cases. Although older literature suggests that the condition is idiopathic in up to a third of cases, there is recent evidence that an occult myeloproliferative disorder is present in many of these (2).

Obstruction of the IVC can result in thrombosis that extends into the major hepatic veins. Alternatively, the hepatic veins may remain patent, but with outflow restricted because of thrombus, intraluminal tumor, compression, or an obstructing membrane affecting the IVC itself. Obstructing membranes, much more common in the Orient and in South Africa than in the Occident, accounted for one-third of a large Japanese series of Budd-Chiari syndrome (3).

Hepatic venocclusive disease is the term used to denote obstruction of hepatic outflow from obliteration of the small sublobular veins. In developing countries, hepatic venocclusive disease is often mediated by toxins, especially pyrrolizidine alkaloids found in Jamaican bush tea. In the United States, hepatic venocclusive disease is more often a consequence of chemotherapy and hepatic irradiation, especially when used in combination for bone marrow transplantation, as well as in immunodeficiency disorders and in hypercoagulable states such as arise from systemic lupus erythematosus and the use of oral contraceptives (4). At least in the early stages of venocclusive disease, the large veins visible on imaging studies are patent. Liver biopsy documents occlusion of the terminal hepatic venules and sublobular veins, with centrolobular necrosis.

A clinically distinct but related entity is impaired hepatic venous outflow occurring when right-sided heart failure or constrictive pericarditis raises pressure in the IVC. Histologically, centrilobular congestion caused by heart failure also mimicks the appearance of Budd-Chiari syndrome in liver biopsies.

Patients with Budd-Chiari syndrome may present acutely or with an insidious illness resulting in liver failure. The acute presentation may actually be a variant of the chronic form, resulting from occlusion of the last patent hepatic vein. With acute onset of hepatic vein occlusion, the liver is tender and swollen, and there is greater liver cell injury and more marked elevation in transaminase levels than in chronic Budd-Chiari syndrome. When Budd-Chiari syndrome is associated with IVC obstruction, additional findings may include severe edema and cutaneous ulceration of the lower extremities, proteinuria, and clinically visible collateral circulation over the back and abdomen.

IMAGING

Imaging plays a crucial role in the evaluation of patients suspected of having hepatic venous outflow obstruction. Imaging evidence of Budd-Chiari syndrome may be direct or indirect. Direct evidence comes from demonstrating the hepatic veins and IVC and confirming their patency or, conversely, documenting thrombus or obstruction of the lumen. Indirect evidence includes abnormalities in the appearance of the liver parenchyma, morphologic changes in liver contour, ascites, or a tumor such as hepatocellular carcinoma with a predilection for venous extension. Although the surgical literature contains a series of over 100 patients treated for Budd-Chiari syndrome, published imaging studies have been small, retrospective, and usually limited to one imaging modality at a time. Therefore, current knowledge about the sensitivity and specificity of cross-sectional imaging technologies for Budd-Chiari syndrome is limited.

Ultrasound

Ultrasound with pulsed and color flow Doppler provides both direct and indirect evaluation of the liver and venous system. Because sonography offers a rapid and portable assessment of the right upper quadrant, this modality is usually the first examination performed when Budd-Chiari syndrome is suspected. For the most reliable sonographic evaluations, color flow Doppler is required. Insufficient sonographic windows may

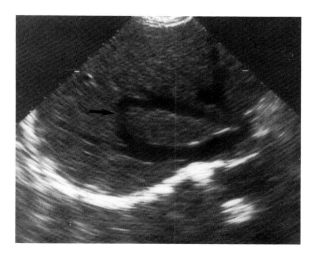

FIGURE 30-1
Diagnostic ultrasound finding in Budd-Chiari syndrome. Real-time sonogram shows large collateral vein (arrow) between the middle and right hepatic veins. (From Mathieu D, Kracht M, Zafrani ES, et al: Budd-Chiari syndrome, in Ferrucci J, Mathieu D (eds): Advances in Hepatobiliary Radiology. St. Louis, Mosby, 1990, pp. 3–28. Reprinted by permission.)

prevent complete evaluation of all three hepatic veins, especially in patients with shrunken livers and copious ascites.

Indirect features that may suggest Budd-Chiari syndrome by sonography include ascites and morphologic changes in the liver, particularly enlargement of the caudate lobe. In acute presentations, the liver is enlarged, but when cirrhosis supervenes, the liver becomes small. There may be echogenic or hypoechoic zones of hepatic hemorrhage, necrosis, and fibrosis. More specific features include tumors in the liver or vena cava, thrombosis or stenosis of the hepatic veins, or a caval web. However, ultrasound has been found to underestimate obstruction of the vena cava in Budd-Chiari syndrome (5), a critical issue in planning surgical therapy. Intraluminal thrombi, mural thickening, stenosis, irregularity, proximal dilatation, and intrahepatic collaterals should be sought. Demonstration of comma-shaped intrahepatic varices or intrahepatic venous collaterals (Fig. 30-1), either between major veins or through capsular pathways, has been considered a pathognomonic ultrasound sign of Budd-Chiari

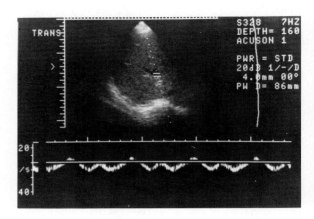

FIGURE 30-2
Normal triphasic Doppler ultrasound pattern in hepatic vein.

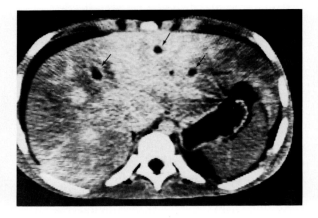

FIGURE 30-3
Diagnostic CT finding in acute Budd-Chiari syndrome. One minute after intravenous injection of iodinated contrast, mural enhancement is visible around the low-attenuation lumens of thrombosed hepatic veins (arrows). (From Mathieu D, Vasile N, Menu Y, et al: Budd-Chiari syndrome: Dynamic CT. Radiology 165:409, 1987. Reprinted by permission.)

syndrome (5,6); however, intrahepatic portosystemic venous shunts can occur and mimic the collaterals of Budd-Chiari syndrome even in the absence of cirrhosis (7). Because acute thrombosis of a single hepatic vein can produce right upper quadrant pain simulating acute cholecystitis, this rare diagnosis should be considered when the gallbladder is sonographically and surgically normal (2).

Doppler flow evaluation is an important part of the evaluation of patients suspected of hepatic vein occlusion. Failure to demonstrate one or more main hepatic veins by static ultrasound does not prove that these veins are occluded (8). Hepatic veins may be compressed when the liver is acutely swollen. In advanced cirrhosis, the veins are attenuated and tortuous and may be invisible with conventional sonography. With color Doppler, flow can be demonstrated in the hepatic veins even when they are not visible by conventional sonography. In a small series, the inability to demonstrate hepatic veins by color flow Doppler was sensitive for Budd-Chiari syndrome (8), but neither the sensitivity nor specificity of this finding has been determined prospectively.

Pulsed Doppler offers important indirect information in patients with Budd-Chiari syndrome. The normal IVC has phasic flow toward the heart. With obstruction there may be absence or reversal of flow, velocity reduction, loss of pulsatility, or turbulence in the IVC. Diminished or hepatofugal flow in the portal vein or extrahepatic collaterals may be found. Flow in the major hepatic veins, which is normally triphasic (Fig. 30-2), will be absent or abnormal in Budd-Chiari patients, but a reliable Doppler signal may be difficult to elicit in these patients.

In hepatic venocclusive disease, anatomic findings are lacking unless thrombosis has propagated from the sublobular veins into the large hepatic veins. Doppler sonography can give evidence to support the diagnosis of venocclusive disease. In a bone marrow recipient, development of venocclusive disease was associated with overnight reversal of flow in the portal vein with progressive thickening of the gallbladder wall (9). Paradoxical acceleration of flow in normal-appearing hepatic veins also has been reported (10).

Computed Tomography (CT)
The CT appearance of Budd-Chiari syndrome varies according to whether or not presentation is acute. In acute Budd-Chiari syndrome, unenhanced CT shows a swollen, low-attenuation liver, usually with ascites. There may be some heterogeneity in the liver from hemorrhage or infarction. Intermediate- or high-attenuation thrombus in the major hepatic veins or in the IVC may be

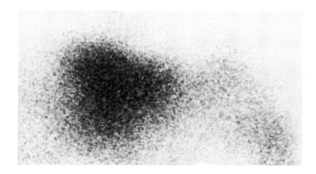

FIGURE 30-4
^{99m}Tc-sulfur colloid scintiscan in chronic Budd-Chiari syndrome. There is marked hypertrophy of the caudate lobe, with reduced tracer uptake in the periphery of the liver. (Courtesy of Dr. M. Clouse, Boston.)

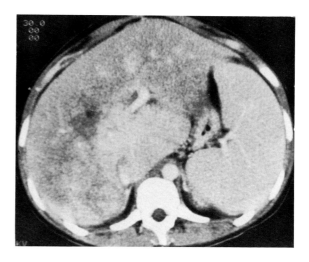

FIGURE 30-5
CT appearance of chronic Budd-Chiari syndrome. Bolus contrast scan shows enhancement of the periportal liver tissue with hypertrophy of the caudate lobe. Enhancement of the periphery of the liver is delayed.

detected; attenuation values fall to isointensity 3 to 5 weeks after an acute presentation (11). However, the most characteristic findings are exhibited after intravenous bolus enhancement with iodinated contrast material.

In acute presentations of Budd-Chiari syndrome there is patchy perihilar enhancement with diminished opacification of peripheral areas. Because the vasa vasora of the occluded hepatic veins opacify, the veins appear as low-intensity structures with enhancing rims (2) (Fig. 30-3).

In nonacute Budd-Chiari syndrome auxiliary hepatic veins come into play. Most important and constant of these is the vein from the caudate lobe into the intrahepatic segment of the IVC. These veins exert a moderating influence on the damaging effects of main hepatic vein obstruction, resulting in hypertrophy of those liver segments having auxiliary venous outflow (12). The caudate lobe is hypertrophied in about 80 percent of cases, giving rise to the classic scintigraphic appearance (Fig. 30-4). Right or left lobe hypertrophy has been found in 40 percent.

Dynamic CT in chronic Budd-Chiari syndrome shows enhancement of the enlarged caudate lobe and periportal area (Fig. 30-5), often with fan-shaped zones of peripheral increased attenuation (13). Peripheral areas tend to fill in with contrast on equilibrium-phase images, and there may be a reversal of the earlier pattern. Thrombosis in the portal circulation occurs in association with Budd-Chiari syndrome and can be demonstrated as low-attenuation filling defects in the portal, splenic, or mesenteric veins (14). The hepatic veins are not visible (13). However, poor timing of the contrast bolus relative to imaging also can obscure the hepatic veins so that CT is predominantly a modality for imaging the secondary signs of Budd-Chiari syndrome.

Severe right-sided heart failure can produce a pattern of patchy hepatic contrast enhancement similar in appearance to that reported in Budd-Chiari syndrome (15). In 85 percent of these cases, elevated filling pressure in the right atrium causes reflux of contrast material into the hepatic veins, in contrast to the absent visualization of hepatic veins seen in most cases of Budd-Chiari syndrome. However, in 15 percent, hepatic vein reflux is not seen. Histologically, centrilobular congestion caused by heart failure also mimics the appearance of Budd-Chiari syndrome in interpretation of liver biopsies. Therefore, clinical evidence must be taken into account before a CT diagnosis of Budd-Chiari syndrome is accepted. Ultrasound helps in this setting by demonstrating enlarged patent hepatic veins with a v-wave from tricuspid regurgitation in severe right-sided heart failure.

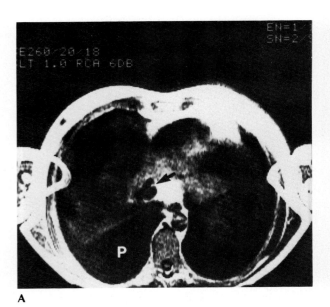 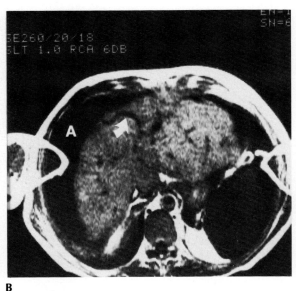

FIGURE 30-6
*Chronic, untreated Budd-Chiari syndrome secondary to an IVC membranous web.
(A) Axial T1-weighted image near the inferior vena cava–right atrial junction shows a web (arrow) separating two channels of flowing blood. Note ascites (A) and right pleural effusion (P). (B) Caudal to (A), the inferior vena cava is compressed and the hepatic veins are absent. Liver is shrunken and irregular because of cirrhosis secondary to the longstanding venous obstruction. Note comma-shaped intrahepatic venous collateral (curved arrow). (From Stark DD, Hahn PF, Trey C, et al: MRI of Budd-Chiari syndrome. AJR 146:1141, 1986. Copyright © by American Roentgen Ray Society. Reprinted by permission.)*

Magnetic Resonance Imaging (MRI)
MRI contributes both anatomic findings and information about blood flow in evaluating Budd-Chiari syndrome. In acute Budd-Chiari syndrome, short T1 thrombus can sometimes be demonstrated in the hepatic veins (16). Since the hepatic venous flow void contrasts with the signal from hepatic parenchyma, absence of hepatic veins on good-quality images is strong evidence in favor of Budd-Chiari syndrome (17). However, low-signal-intensity hepatic veins can sometimes be demonstrated in acute Budd-Chiari syndrome (2).

In chronic Budd-Chiari syndrome, intrahepatic venous collaterals develop to decompress segments with particularly poor drainage. Demonstration of these characteristic comma-shaped varices confirms the diagnosis (Fig. 30-6). Good-quality MRI images also are capable of demonstrating a web in the IVC (17). MRI is very sensitive to the presence of hepatocellular carcinomas; coronal images show tumor thrombus extending into the IVC and right atrium (Fig. 30-7). Hepatic congestion prolongs the T2 of tissue in the right and left lobes; the caudate lobe is usually spared (17,18).

Since MRI images are sensitive to flow, MRI can assess the status of the IVC and hepatic veins directly. A flow void on spin-echo images has been used to confirm vascular patency. However, artifactual intraluminal signal resulting from flow artifacts such as entry slice enhancement and even echo rephasing may be confusing. Techniques specifically designed to image flow include phase images and gradient-echo images. Phase images provide a map of blood flow as white or dark areas on gray background and can be used to quantitate blood flow (Fig. 30-7). Gradient-echo images take advantage of entry slice phenomena and motion compensating techniques to demonstrate

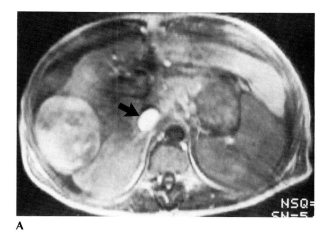
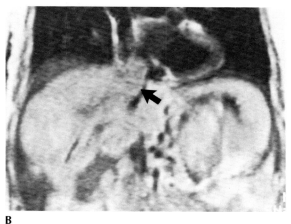
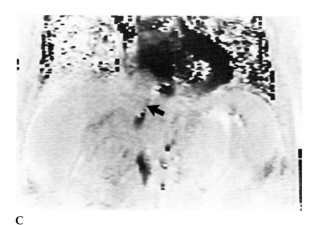

FIGURE 30-7
Hepatocellular carcinoma with venous extension. (A) Axial GE 120/11/120-degree (T1-weighted) image shows fatty, encapsulated tumor in the right lobe. High signal intensity arises in the IVC (arrow) from entry slice effect, confirming patency at this level. (B) Coronal SE 260/14 image shows tumor thrombus extending into the IVC and right atrium (arrow). (C) Coronal phase reconstruction of the data set also used to reconstruct part B. Loss of signal from moving blood in intrahepatic segment of IVC and right atrium contrasts with stationary spins from tumor (arrow).

flowing blood as bright signal on a dark background. The positive signal associated with gradient-echo images is a more reliable indicator of vascular patency than conventional images (19).

The dome of the liver is a difficult and noisy area to image, and seriously ill patients may not be able to lie still with quiet respirations, resulting in nondiagnostic MRI images. As techniques for motion suppression and MRI angiography improve, MRI may become a first-line diagnostic technique in evaluating patients suspected of having hepatic venous obstruction.

Angiography
Angiography is the "gold standard" in studying patients suspected of having this condition. In most centers, angiographic evaluation is pursued even when there is strong histologic and noninvasive imaging evidence of Budd-Chiari syndrome. Vena cavography definitively evaluates the IVC, accurately distinguishing intrinsic obstruction from extrinsic compression. Direct cannulation of the major hepatic veins is performed to establish patency; a wedge venogram showing a "spider web" pattern of collaterals is pathognomonic of Budd-Chiari syndrome (Fig. 30-8). Transhepatic antegrade hepatic venography is an alternative, but more invasive method to demonstrate the hepatic veins and to obtain pressure measurements.

IMAGING IN THE THERAPY OF BUDD-CHIARI SYNDROME

Therapy of Budd-Chiari syndrome involves anticoagulation and diuresis, shunting, and transplantation. Anticoagulation is instituted in patients in whom hepatic vein thrombosis is associated with a hypercoagulable state. However, anticoagulation has not been shown to prolong survival (20). For patients with severe liver damage, hepatic transplantation has been recommended. Anticoagulation is continued after transplantation. Surgical shunting may provide symptomatic relief for patients with Budd-Chiari syndrome. The type of shunt depends on the level of obstruction. Mesocaval and portacaval shunts are used when the IVC is not obstructed; mesoatrial shunts are used to decompress the portal system and systemic circulation through portosystemic collaterals when the IVC is occluded or compressed by hepatic congestion. Mesoatrial shunts are constructed from GorTex or Dacron and are interposed between the superior mesenteric vein and the right atrium. IVC webs can be treated by membranotomy or surgical resection.

Imaging is a mainstay in the assessment of shunt patency. Mesoatrial shunts are particularly prone to occlusion because of their length and slow flow (21) and therefore require frequent assessment. Hepatofugal flow in the portal vein by Doppler ultrasound suggests shunt patency if flow was hepatopedal preoperatively. Since the graft material transmits sound poorly, MRI has been advocated for evaluating mesoatrial shunts (21) (Fig. 30-9). Sometimes a mesoatrial shunt

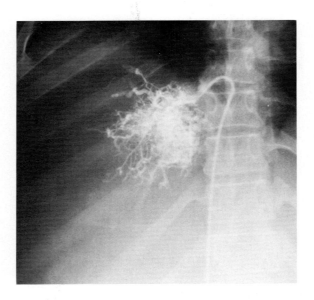

FIGURE 30-8
Hepatic venogram in Budd-Chiari syndrome showing characteristic "spiderweb" pattern of small venous collaterals. Because partial hepatic vein occlusions can occur, all three major hepatic veins must be demonstrated before a hepatic venogram is considered normal.

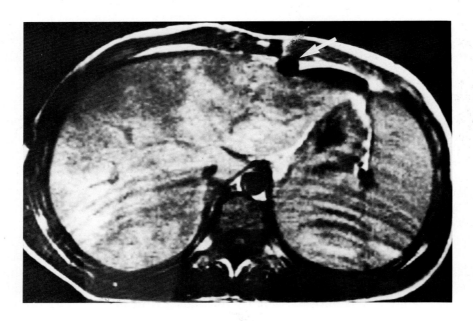

FIGURE 30-9
MRI of mesoatrial shunt for Budd-Chiari syndrome. On this SE 500/25 axial image, flow void in shunt (arrow) indicates shunt patency. Synthetic shunt material transmits ultrasound poorly. (From Mathieu D, Kracht M, Zafrani ES, et al: Budd-Chiari syndrome, in Ferrucci J, Mathieu D (eds): Advances in Hepatobiliary Radiology. St. Louis, Mosby, 1990, pp. 3–28. Reprinted by permission.)

provides sufficient relief of IVC compression that by the time shunt failure occurs, the patient has become a candidate for a portacaval shunt.

For portosystemic venous shunts, color Doppler ultrasound may permit shunt visualization and assessment of shunt patency. In the absence of shunt visualization, hepatofugal portal flow provides indirect evidence of patency. MRI also has been used to investigate shunt patency but remains a secondary technique, since ultrasound is faster and more convenient. Angiography remains the gold standard; pressure measurements above and below the shunt are particularly helpful in assessing the hemodynamic significance of a stenosis.

Image-guided interventional techniques have been applied to selected patients with Budd-Chiari syndrome. Percutaneous transluminal disruption of IVC webs has been used in a small number of patients. Initial success is the rule, but recurrent stenosis is common. Repeat angioplasty may be performed with similar results (22). There have also been reports of angiographic recanalization of hepatic veins after thrombosis (23). Percutaneous balloon dilatation of strictured shunts may restore function. However, stenoses tend to recur, requiring careful follow-up and repeated interventions (22).

SUMMARY

Budd-Chiari syndrome is an uncommon entity, varied in presentation, etiology, and therapy. Ultrasound is the principal imaging modality used initially in the differential diagnosis and follow-up. Angiography remains the gold standard. However, because the clinical diagnosis is difficult, patients with Budd-Chiari syndrome may enter the imaging system through other studies, including CT, MRI, and scintigraphy, each of which may help to establish the diagnosis.

REFERENCES

1. Gall EA, Mostofi FK (eds): The Liver (International Academy of Pathology Monograph No. 13). Baltimore, Williams & Wilkins, 1973, pp 406–430.
2. Mathieu D, Kracht M, Zafrani ES, et al: Budd-Chiari syndrome, in Ferrucci JT, Mathieu D (eds): Advances in Hepatobiliary Radiology. St. Louis, Mosby, 1990, pp 3–28.
3. Hirooka M, Kimura C: Membranous obstruction of the hepatic portion of the inferior vena cava. Arch Surg 100:656, 1970.
4. Pappas SC, Malone DG, Rabin L, et al: Hepatic veno-occlusive disease in a patient with systemic lupus erythematosus. Arthritis Rheum 27:104, 1984.
5. Menu Y, Alison D, Lorphelin J-M, et al: Budd-Chiari syndrome: US evaluation. Radiology 157:761, 1985.
6. Baert AL, Fevery J, Marchal G, et al: Early diagnosis of Budd-Chiari syndrome by computed tomography and ultrasonography: Report of five cases. Gastroenterology 84:587, 1983.
7. Mori H, Hayashi K, Fukuda T, et al: Intrahepatic portosystemic venous shunt: Occurrence in patients with and without liver cirrhosis. AJR 149:711, 1987.
8. Grant EG, Perrella R, Tessler FN, et al: Budd-Chiari syndrome: The results of duplex and color Doppler imaging. AJR 152:377, 1989.
9. Kriegshauser JS, Charboneau JW, Letendre L: Hepatic venocclusive disease after bone-marrow transplantation: Diagnosis with duplex sonography. AJR 150:289, 1988.
10. Hosoki T, Kuroda C, Tokunaga K, et al: Hepatic venous outflow obstruction: Evaluation with pulsed duplex sonography. Radiology 170:733, 1989.
11. Mori H, Maeda H, Fukuda T, et al: Acute thrombosis of the inferior vena cava and hepatic veins in patients with Budd-Chiari syndrome: CT demonstration. AJR 153:987, 1989.
12. Picard M, Carrier L, Chartrand R, et al: Budd-Chiari syndrome: Typical and atypical scintigraphic aspects. J Nucl Med 28:803, 1987.
13. Mathieu D, Vasile N, Menu Y, et al: Budd-Chiari syndrome: Dynamic CT. Radiology 165:409, 1987.
14. Vogelzang RL, Anschutz SL, Gore RM: Budd-Chiari syndrome: CT observations. Radiology 163:h329, 1987.
15. Holley HC, Koslin DB, Berland LL, Stanley RJ: Inhomogeneous enhancement of liver parenchyma secondary to passive congestion: Contrast-enhanced CT. Radiology 170:795, 1989.
16. Murphy FB, Steinberg HV, Shires GT III, et al: The Budd-Chiari syndrome: A review. AJR 147:9, 1986.
17. Stark DD, Hahn PF, Trey C, et al: MRI of the Budd-Chiari syndrome. AJR 146:1141, 1986.
18. Friedman AC, Ramchandani P, Black M, et al: Magnetic resonance imaging diagnosis of the Budd-Chiari syndrome. Gastroenterology 91:1289, 1986.
19. von Schulthess GK, Augustiny N: Calculation of T2 values versus phase imaging for the distinction between flow and thrombus in MR imaging. Radiology 164:549, 1987.

20. Boyer TD: Major sequelae of cirrhosis, in Wyngaarden JB, Smith LH (eds): Cecil's Textbook of Medicine, 18th ed. Philadelphia, Saunders, 1988, pp 847–852.
21. Chezmar JL, Bernardino ME: Mesoatrial shunt for the treatment of Budd-Chiari syndrome: Radiologic evaluation in eight patients. AJR 149:707, 1987.
22. Martin LG, Henderson JM, Millikan WJ Jr, et al: Angioplasty for long-term treatment of patients with Budd-Chiari syndrome. AJR 154:1007, 1990.
23. Lois JF, Harzman S, McGlade CT, et al: Budd-Chiari syndrome: Treatment with percutaneous transhepatic recanalization and dilation. Radiology 170:791, 1989.

31

Portal Hypertension: Doppler US Flow Imaging

L. BARBARA, L. BOLONDI, S. GAIANI,
S. LI BASSI, G. ZIRONI, and G. BENZI

The hemodynamic data provided by Doppler US can be classified as *qualitative, semiquantitative,* and *quantitative*. Qualitative data include the assessment of (a) the presence, (b) the direction, and (c) the characteristics of blood flow and its disturbances. The assessment of flow disturbances from the waveform of the Doppler trace may include some semiquantitative measurements, such as an assessment of vascular impedance by means of the pulsatility and resistance indexes of the arterial bed. Finally, quantitative data include calculation of the maximal and mean velocity of blood flow as well as of flow volume in the major abdominal vessels. On the basis of these many possibilities, numerous clinical papers have been published dealing with the use of this technique in patients with portal hypertension. However, if qualitative information about flow pattern is no longer in question, the availability of quantitative measurements, particularly in small arterial vessels and in collateral pathways, is still questioned. Areas where this new method is able to provide useful and reliable data have been defined recently at a consensus conference held in Bologna, Italy (1).

QUALITATIVE DOPPLER FINDINGS IN PORTAL HYPERTENSION

Thrombosis of the Portal Venous System
The presence of blood flow moving within the portal vein is the simplest Doppler finding to ascertain. Color Doppler further facilitates the evaluation of vascular hemodynamics, directly visualizing flow moving within the vessels and easily distinguishing vascular from other channel structures (Fig. 31-1, see color insert).

In cases of chronic portal vein thrombosis, when the portal vein is small and echogenic at real-time examination, Doppler investigation of the porta hepatis will reveal no evidence of blood flow. When cavernous transformation has occurred, turbulent flow can be demonstrated by color Doppler within the small tortuous vessels (Fig. 31-2, see color insert). Because of the arterialization of hepatic blood supply in portal thrombosis, the presence of high-frequency arterial signals at the porta hepatis and within the liver may be considered an indirect sign of the occlusion.

The diagnosis of portal vein obstruction is sometimes uncertain at real-time US imaging, especially in cases of recent thrombosis, when the echo pattern of the thrombus is markedly hypoechoic and may be missed, so that the lumen appears to be patent. In these cases, the absence of the Doppler signal from the portal vein confirms the diagnosis (Fig. 31-3, see color insert). Color Doppler also facilitates visualization of mural thrombosis (see Fig. 31-1), which may escape real-time imaging and may not produce any alteration of the Doppler signal.

The sensitivity of Doppler US in diagnosing portal vein thrombosis has been reported to be similar to that of dynamic CT (2). Others (3) found Doppler US less sensitive in cases of nonocclusive thrombosis or occlusion of portal branches. In some instances, Doppler US may be even more accurate than arterioportography, which can erroneously suggest portal thrombosis in cases of complete diversion of the contrast medium into large portosystemic collaterals (4). Doppler US may therefore be considered extremely sensitive in the diagnosis of portal thrombosis (5). The extensive application of Doppler US flowmetry in nonselected patients affected by liver cirrhosis will contribute to clarification of the actual prevalence of portal thrombosis. In our experience, based on the investigation of 228 consecutive cirrhotic patients, we found a prevalence of partial and total thrombosis of the portal vein, unrelated to hepatocellular carcinoma, respectively, of 1.8 and 4.4 percent (6).

Reversal of Flow in the Portal Venous System
This is another unequivocal qualitative finding provided by Doppler US (Fig. 31-4). Its importance in the investigation of hepatic hemodynamics is striking. The actual prevalence of a reversed flow in the portal venous system in an unselected cirrhotic population is still undefined. L'Hermine (7) reported reversed intrahepatic portal flow (demonstrated by arterioportography) in about 5 percent of his patients. One-third of these patients had a completely hepatofugal portal flow. Therefore, this hemodynamic abnormality is not so uncommon, but it is unclear if it is related to a poor prognosis. However, the rate of reversed flow detected by arterioportography may not exactly reflect the actual prevalence of this abnormality in a nonselected population of cirrhotics, because only patients with complicated portal hypertension and/or candidates for surgery undergo this invasive procedure.

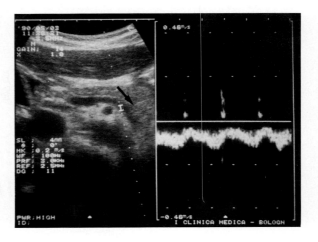

FIGURE 31-4
Hepatofugal flow in the splenic vein. The Doppler trace below the zero line indicates a flow running toward the spleen (arrow). Transverse scan at the epigastrium.

Kawasaki et al. (8) report a prevalence of spontaneous hepatofugal flow of 6.1 percent in cirrhotic patients and of 5.3 percent in patients with hepatocellular carcinoma. In our experience (6), the overall prevalence of hepatofugal flow in liver cirrhosis (without hepatocellular carcinoma) was 8.3 percent (19 of 228). Reversal portal flow was associated with a significantly reduced caliber of the portal vein. We found (6) that this event is more frequently found in Child B and C patients in comparison with Child A patients. We also tried to assess in a prospective case-control study the predictive value of this finding on the risk of bleeding, and we found that patients with hepatofugal flow present a significantly lower incidence of bleeding episodes. Finally, hepatofugal flow in the splenic vein has proved to be closely correlated with hepatic encephalopathy (9), in relation to the drainage of large amounts of blood into large splenorenal collaterals.

Color Doppler easily demonstrates reversals of flow, even in small peripheral portal branches, which show an opposite color in comparison with the arterial branches. The actual prevalence of this finding and its diagnostic importance are still unknown.

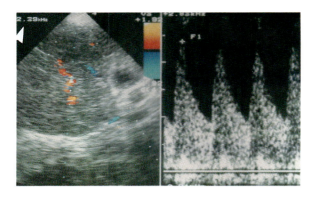

FIGURE 23-1
Hepatocellular carcinoma. Color flow mapping indicates the presence of flow into the mass (in orange-red). The Doppler waveform is characterized by a high-frequency signal (2.39 kHz) (arrowhead) with broadened spectrum.

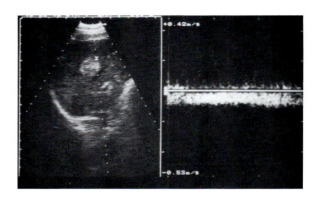

FIGURE 23-2
Small hyperechoic hepatocellular carcinoma. The Doppler feature is characterized by a low impedance and continuous signal, similar to that occurring in normal intrahepatic branches.

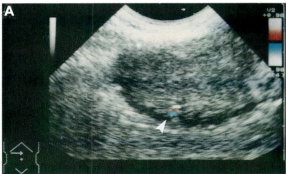

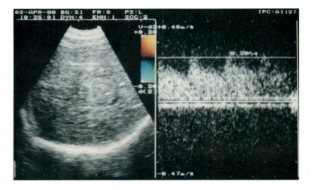

FIGURE 23-4
In this case, the color flow mapping is negative, while the Doppler trace demonstrates a moderately high signal with marked broadening of the spectrum.

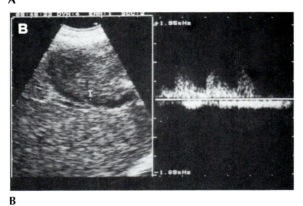

FIGURE 23-3
(A) In the peripheral part of the tumor, color Doppler shows the presence of red and blue signals (arrowhead). (B) Doppler waveform suggests that they correspond to arterial and venous signals (above and below zero line, respectively). The opposite direction of flow is probably related to an arteriovenous shunt, which reverses venous flow.

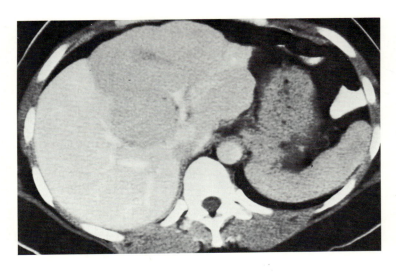

FIGURE 29-2
CT image from a patient with a large mass due to focal nodular hyperplasia replacing the left hepatic lobe.

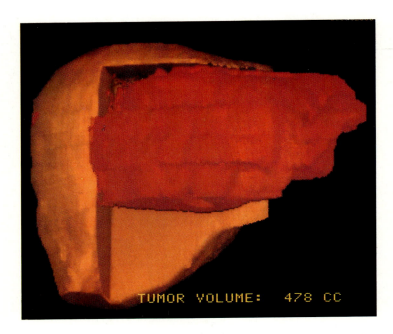

FIGURE 29-5
Image from patient with FNH shown in Figs. 29-2 to 29-4. Tumor is reconstructed in red, and a wedge of normal liver has been removed (using cut planes) to demonstrate the lesion to better advantage. The calculated tumor volume was 478 cc.

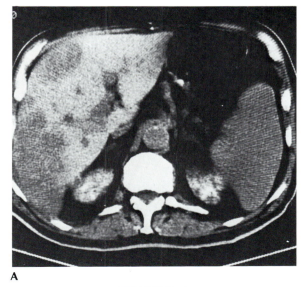
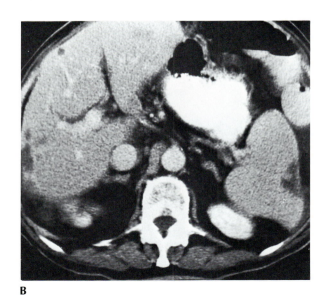

FIGURE 29-6
Initial (A) and 7-month follow-up (B) CT scans in patient with colonic metastases on hepatic arterial chemotherapy. There has been considerable interval decrease in tumor burden.

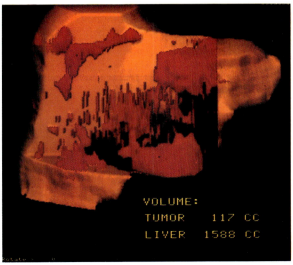

FIGURE 29-8
Reconstructions of the CT scans shown in Figs. 29-6A and 29-6B using cut planes to better demonstrate the areas of abnormality and improvement on therapy.

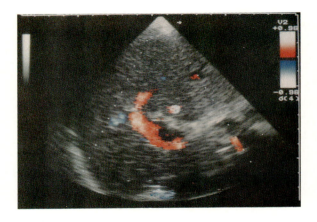

FIGURE 31-1
Color flow mapping of the portal vein clearly shows blood flowing into the liver (in red). Color is lacking in a part of the vessel due to a mural thrombosis, missed at ultrasound examination. Right intercostal scan.

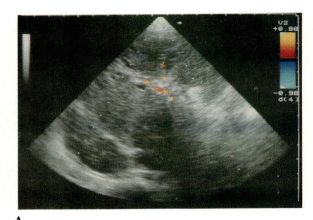
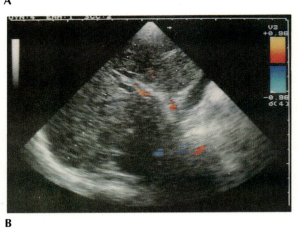

FIGURE 31-2
Cavernous transformation of the portal vein. The portal vein is replaced by an echogenic structure with thin channels, in which color Doppler demonstrates the presence of flow direct toward the liver (in red). Right intercostal scans.

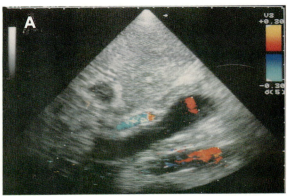
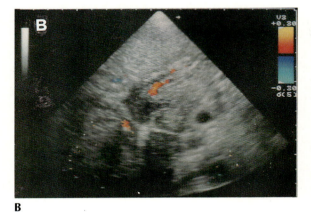

FIGURE 31-3
(A) Recent thrombosis of the portal vein. Color Doppler failed to demonstrate any signal in the vein; meanwhile there is signal (light blue) in the hepatic artery. Longitudinal right scan. (B) Thrombosis of the left portal vein, which appears slightly echogenic. Orange indicates high flow into the branches of the hepatic artery. Transverse scan at the epigastrium.

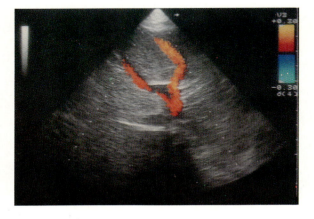

FIGURE 31-5
Color flow mapping of dilated paraumbilical vein in portal hypertension. In this case, there are two paraumbilical vessels, one in the ligamentum teres and another in the surrounding liver parenchyma. Right subcostal scan.

Collateral Pathways
Only some of the collateral vessels are accessible to Doppler investigation, and they usually are the paraumbilical veins (Fig. 31-5, see color insert), the splenorenal veins, and the left gastric vein with the gastroesophageal collaterals. The contribution of Doppler US is essentially to provide a rough idea of their hemodynamic importance. It must be stressed that flow in collateral vessels cannot be measured with the exception of paraumbilical veins, which are often of a quite large caliber and run straight toward the umbilicus near the skin surface, and sometimes the left gastric vein. In all other instances, Doppler analysis may only indicate the heopatofugal direction of blood flow.

Characteristics of Blood Flow and Its Disturbances
One of the most meaningful features of Doppler signal analysis is that the characteristics of the waveform and spectral distribution of frequencies are direct consequences of hemodynamic factors and location of the vessel. Therefore, the pattern of Doppler signal (and its acoustic characteristics) often permits recognition of its origin, even in circumstances in which the image is equivocal. It can be said that any vessel has its own "signature," from which it can be recognized (10).

Investigation of the hepatic veins also may provide interesting data. The hepatic veins in healthy humans display a triphasic waveform depending on cardiac cycles and particularly the fluctuating right atrial pressure. These phasic variations in flow may be completely lost in about 25 percent of cases of liver cirrhosis with portal hypertension and greatly reduced in another 25 percent (11) (Fig. 31-6). The pathophysiology of this alteration is still unclear, even though we found a correlation between these changes and the severity of the disease.

The portal vein also shows, in normal conditions, a Doppler trace with wild oscillations. These oscillations tend to be completely lost in cases of portal hypertension, where slow and turbulent flow is often found. The assessment of flow disturbances from waveform data also can provide semiquantitative methods based on an analysis of the velocity profile and calculation of the interrelationships between maximum, minimum,

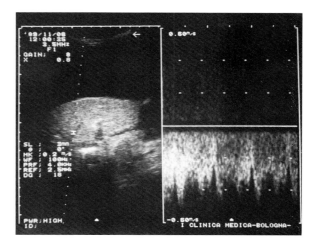

FIGURE 31-6
Doppler US of the hepatic vein in a patient with decompensated liver cirrhosis. The Doppler waveform is turbulent, with reduced phasicity. Right intercostal scan.

and mean frequencies of the spectrum. Numerous indices have been proposed to describe waveforms of arterial flow. One of the most commonly used is the *pulsatility index (PI)*, defined as

$$PI = \frac{A - B}{\text{mean}}$$

where A is the maximum value over the cardiac cycle, B the minimum, and mean is the average value.

Resistance index (RI) is defined as

$$RI = \frac{A - B}{A}$$

Because it is not necessary to know the angle of incidence of the ultrasonic beam when calculating one of these indices, they can be assessed in vessels that are too small or tortuous to be imaged (e.g., the intrahepatic arteries). Since pulsatility of an arterial vessel is influenced by the impedance of the distal vascular bed, the investigation of this parameter could be useful in liver diseases.

An example is provided by study of the superior mesenteric artery. One of the most striking characteristics of cirrhotic patients is the hyperdynamic circulation associated with a fall in arterial resistance (12). This phenomenon has been studied utilizing the Doppler method by a French group (13), who found that the *PI* of the superior mesenteric artery is significantly decreased in patients affected by liver cirrhosis and acute hepatitis, but not in cases of portal vein thrombosis unrelated to liver cirrhosis. Changes in the waveform of hepatic and splenic arteries in the course of portal hypertension has received little prior attention. These vessels normally have a well-represented diastolic component owing to a low-resistance peripheral bed, and therefore, their waveform significantly differs from that of the superior mesenteric artery (10).

QUANTITATIVE MEASUREMENT OF BLOOD FLOW

While several invasive methods have been recently developed and are currently used to measure portal and hepatic venous pressure (14,15), measurement of flow volume has always proved much more difficult. Noninvasive measurement using Doppler US has attracted a great deal of attention in recent years. This measurement is based on the principle of the uniform isonation method, by which the entire volume of blood in a cross section of the vessel is exposed to a uniform ultrasonic beam. The instantaneous mean velocity Vm calculated from the mean Doppler shift is multiplied by the cross-sectional area A of the vessel, thus giving the volume flow Q: $Q = Vm \cdot A$. Sources of errors, however, are measurement of the beam-vessel angle (necessary to transform the frequencies of the Doppler shift into velocities) and of the cross-sectional area of the vessel. Errors increase rapidly with increasing angles of approach (16).

Measurement of the cross-sectional area of the vessel presents even greater problems because most vessels, especially veins, are not circular in section (26). For these reasons, flow velocity and volume calculations taken at angles over 60 degrees or in small and tortuous vessels show a low reproducibility and are unacceptable in clinical practice.

One additional critical point is the calculation of mean velocity Vm. Its determination from the maximal velocity by a fixed coefficient (18,19) may be inaccurate because the velocity profile in the portal vein is different from patient to patient. It is therefore necessary to calculate Vm directly on the Doppler spectrum, and this can be achieved by the software of recent instrumentation.

As far as the portal vein is concerned, it must be said that its 3- to 4-cm straight course, its quite large caliber, and its oblique position with respect to the abdominal wall are favorable factors for Doppler investigation. Measurements of Vm are made in Doppler traces of 4 to 6 s in order to avoid flow-velocity fluctuations, which are also reduced by examining patients during suspended respiration. Errors in measuring the cross-sectional area also may affect the calculation of flow volume in the portal vein. However, it is accepted that repeated measurement of the diameter reduces the error of flow calculation to within 10 percent (20).

The accuracy of Doppler flowmetry for measuring flow volume in the portal vein has been validated by showing a good correlation with the results of Lipiodol droplet cineangiography (18) and electromagnetic flowmetry (19,21). Dauzat and Pomier Layrargues (21) found, however, that the coefficient of variation was higher for Doppler measurements than for electromagnetic measurements (10.9 versus 5.9 percent).

In a recent study (22), the intra- and interobserver variability of Doppler US measurements was assessed in normal volunteers. Intraobserver variability was found to be low in repeated examinations on the same day, with a tendency to increase in consecutive days (which could be related to physiologic changes in the portal flow, however).

The interobserver agreement was always poor. Instrumentation variability (23) has also been noted, thus suggesting that follow-up examinations must be carried out on the same equipment with the same transducer.

On the basis of these data, at present it is reasonable to affirm that the Doppler spectrum reflects the actual blood flow in the portal vein, even though the absolute values expressed in milliliters per minute may not correspond to the real flow volumes. Changes of Vm and flow volume assessed by Doppler flowmetry in the same subject under different conditions are more acceptable, since possible sources of error in measuring the absolute values are expected to affect different measurements in the same way. The method seems to be suitable, therefore, for in vivo monitoring of acute hemodynamic changes in the portal vein, such as those induced by meals, hormones, and drugs (1,21,24). The latter possibility opens large perspectives for the evaluation of the effect of vasoactive drugs. By means of evaluation of different Doppler parameters in a selected group of patients, we demonstrated the action of propranolol on venous collateral resistance (25). Numerous papers dealing with quantitative measurements of flow in the portal vein have been published in recent years (1,8,24,26–29), and they agree that velocity is reduced, to a greater or lesser degree, in cirrhotic patients in comparison with healthy subjects (Fig. 31-7). The variability of values reported for portal vein flow velocity is partly dependent on the limits of the method and partly on the variability of the hemodynamic patterns in relation to the stage and etiology of the cirrhosis. Data about portal flow volumes in liver cirrhosis are even more variable because the development of collateral pathways, which are different from case to case and greatly influence portal flow volume. A patent and dilated paraumbilical vein may explain high velocity and volume of portal flow, while large splenorenal collaterals may reduce portal flow and even cause it to reverse. One important point for the clinician, and in particular for the hepatologist, is to utilize the diagnostic information in a prospective way to better assess the prognosis. Thus we tried to assess the relationship of Doppler information to some clinical variables. Regarding the etiology of liver cirrhosis, we found a significant decrease in flow velocity in cases of alcoholic and virus-related cirrhosis, but not in primary biliary cirrhosis (30). We also found that patients with previous bleeding have a significantly lower velocity in the portal vein in comparison with nonbleeders (31).

Flow volume in the splenic and superior mesenteric veins has been reported in several studies, showing the different contribution of these vessels to the postprandial increase in portal flow (29) and in the attempt to draw new insights in the pathophysiology of portal hypertension (32,33). In our opinion, however, the parallel course of the superior mesenteric vein with respect to the abdominal wall sometimes makes it difficult to find a beam-vessel angle of less than 60 degrees, and the curved course of the splenic

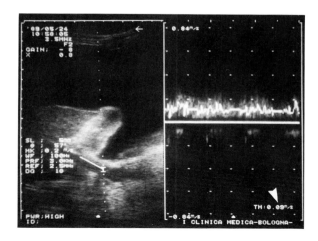

FIGURE 31-7
Doppler US of the portal vein in a patient with liver cirrhosis and gross ascites. The mean velocity of flow is markedly reduced (9 cm/s) (arrowhead).

vein, making the measurement of the angle uncertain, greatly reduces the reliability of Doppler US quantitative flowmetry of this vessel. In a very recent study investigating the feasibility of Doppler flow measurements in splanchnic vessels in a nonselected patient population and in cirrhotics (34), the splenic and superior mesenteric veins showed adequate visibility in only 53 to 69 percent of patients.

EVALUATION OF PORTOSYSTEMIC SURGICAL SHUNTS

Experience in recent years with Doppler US has shown this method to be extremely useful in both the preoperative evaluation of patients and in postoperative follow-up. Preoperatively, Doppler flowmetry can be of great help in guiding the choice of surgery. Thrombosis or reversal of portal flow generally argues against selective shunts. In the postoperative period, Doppler flowmetry is the investigation of choice to assess shunt patency and the hemodynamic consequences of the procedure. Within certain limits, it is possible to quantify flow through the shunt and to assess the amount of portal flow perfusing the liver.

With regard to the direct assessment of flow through the anastomosis, series published in the

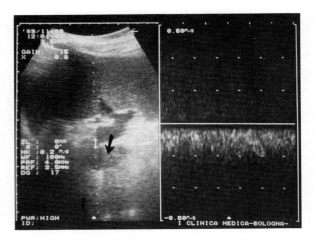

FIGURE 31-8
Distal splenorenal shunt (Warren). Doppler study shows continuous flow directed from the splenic to the left renal vein (arrow). *Left longitudinal scan.*

literature show considerable variations of sensitivity ranging from 55 to 87 percent (35–39). Turbulent high-speed flow can be detected within the shunt itself directed toward the systemic circulation (Fig. 31-8). In some cases, this flow may show a phasic profile on account of the variations in caval pressure.

In practically all patients, indirect signs of patency can be found on the basis of the direction of flow in the portal vein or characteristics of the flow directed toward the shunt. When a *side-to-side portocaval shunt* cannot be visualized at conventional real-time US, the presence of hepatofugal flow in the intrahepatic portal branches is considered a reliable indicator of patency of the shunt (37). However, it must be remembered that the hemodynamic situation changes only gradually, and thus in the immediate postoperative period, a slow hepatopetal portal flow may still be detected despite a patent shunt. On the contrary, hepatopetal portal flow detected on a late postoperative control should make one suspect a thrombosis of the shunt, especially if on a previous study flow was hepatofugal.

Proof of patency of the *conventional splenorenal shunt* is the reversal of flow in the splenic vein and even in the portal vein. In *distal splenorenal shunts*, visualization at real-time US is not always feasible (53.5 percent in our group of patients) (39). When visualization is not possible, useful information can be obtained from the flow pattern in the splenic vein, which displays a typical phasic profile in synchrony with caval pulsatility. The goal of this kind of shunt is to selectively decompress gastroesophageal varices while maintaining a hepatopetal flow in the mesoportal venous bed in order to reduce the incidence of encephalopathy. By means of Doppler flowmetry, we found (39) that in 77 percent of patients a low-velocity hepatopetal flow was maintained at 12 months after the operation. The incidence of late reversal flow in our series was lower than that reported by other authors (40) using other techniques.

CONCLUSIONS

On the basis of present experience and following the statements of the Consensus Conference of Bologna, current clinical applications of Doppler US can be summarized as follows:

1. Doppler US can provide useful information for assessment of portal hypertension from a diagnostic point of view.
2. It has not yet been determined if Doppler US contributes to a better assessment of the bleeding risk. Many Doppler-derived indices need to be evaluated for their prognostic significance and compared with portal pressure and endoscopic scores, as well as with the clinical occurrence of bleeding.
3. Doppler US may contribute to an understanding of the mechanism of action of vasoactive drugs and to the evaluation of treatment efficacy.
4. Doppler US should be used routinely as a follow-up method on patients submitted to portosystemic surgical shunts.

REFERENCES

1. The value of Doppler US in the study of hepatic hemodynamics. Consensus Conference, Bologna, Italy, September 12, 1989. J Hepatol 10:553, 1990.
2. Miller VE, Berland LL: Pulsed Doppler duplex sonography and CT of portal vein thrombosis. AJR 145:73, 1985.

3. Alpern MB, Rubin JM, Williams DM, Cape KP: Porta hepatic: Duplex Doppler US with angiographic correlation. Radiology 162:53, 1987.
4. Burchell AR, Moreno AH, Panke WF, Rousselot LM: Some limitations of splenic portography: I. Incidence, hemodynamic and surgical implications of the nonvisualized portal vein. Ann Surg 162:981, 1965.
5. Scoutt LM, Zawin ML, Taylor KJW: Doppler US: II. Clinical applications. Radiology 174:309, 1990.
6. Gaiani S, Bolondi L, Li Bassi S, et al: Prevalence of spontaneous hepatofugal portal flow in liver cirrhosis: Clinical and endoscopic correlation in 228 patients. Gastroenterology (in press).
7. L'Hermine C: Radiology of Liver Circulation. Dordrecht, Martinus Nijhoff, 1985.
8. Kawasaki T, Moriyasu F, Nishida O, et al: Analysis of hepatofugal flow in portal venous system using ultrasonic Doppler duplex system. Am J Gastroenterol 84:937, 1989.
9. Ohnishi K, Saito M, Sato S, et al: Direction of splenic venous flow assessed by pulsed Doppler flowmetry in patients with a large splenorenal shunt: Relation to spontaneous hepatic encephalopathy. Gastroenterology 89:180, 1985.
10. Taylor KJW, Burns PN, Woodcock JP, et al: Blood flow in deep abdominal and pelvic vessels: Ultrasonic pulsed Doppler analysis. Radiology 154: 487, 1985.
11. Bolondi L, Gaiani S, Li Bassi S, et al: Changes in the hepatic vein waveform detected by Doppler US in liver cirrhosis. J Hepatol 9:S117, 1989.
12. Benoit JN, Granger N: Splanchnic hemodynamics in chronic portal venous hypertension. Semin Liver Dis 6:287, 1986.
13. Darnault P, Bretagne JF, Raoul J, et al: Assessment of the role of portal hypertension and liver failure in lowering splanchnic vascular resistance. Gastroenterology 96:A590, 1989.
14. Paton A, Reynolds TB, Sherlock S: Assessment of portal venous hypertension by catheterization of hepatic vein. Lancet 1:918, 1953.
15. Groszmann RJ, Glickmann M, Blei A, et al: Wedget and free hepatic venous pressure measured with a balloon catheter. Gastroenterology 76:253, 1978.
16. Burns PN: Interpretation and analysis of Doppler signals, in Taylor KJW, Burns PN, Wells PNT (eds): Clinical Applications of Doppler Ultrasound. New York, Raven Press, 1988.
17. Niederau C, Sonnen A, Muller JE, et al: Sonographic measurements of the normal liver, spleen, pancreas and portal vein. Radiology 149:537, 1983.
18. Ohnishi K, Saito M, Nakayama T, et al: Portal venous hemodynamic in chronic liver disease: Effects of posture change and exercise. Radiology 155:757, 1985.
19. Moriyasu F, Ban N, Nishida O, et al: "Congestion index" of the portal vein. AJR 146:735, 1985.
20. Eik-Nes SH, Marsal K, Kristoffersen K: Methodology and basic problems related to blood flow studies in the human fetus. Ultrasound Med Biol 10:329, 1984.
21. Dauzat M, Pomier Layrargues G: Portal vein blood flow measurements using pulsed Doppler and electromagnetic flowmetry in dogs: A comparative study. Gastroenterology 96:913, 1989.
22. Sabba C, Weltin G, Cicchetti D, et al: Observer variability in echo-Doppler measurements of portal flow in cirrhotic patients and normal volunteers. Gastroenterology 98:1603, 1990.
23. Kimme-Smith C, Hussain R, Duerinckx A, et al: Reproducibility of Doppler abdominal flow rates: Instrumentation variability. J Ultrasound Med 7:S90, 1988.
24. Brown HS, Halliwell M, Qamar M, et al: Measurement of normal portal venous blood flow by Doppler ultrasound. Gut 30:503, 1989.
25. Gaiani S, Bolondi L, Li Bassi S, et al: Effect of propranolol on splanchnic arteries, portal vein and left gastric vein blood flow in liver cirrhosis. Gastroenterology 98:A21, 1990.
26. Gaiani S, Bolondi L, Li Bassi S, et al: Effect of meal on portal hemodynamics in healthy humans and in patients with chronic liver disease. Hepatology 9:815, 1989.
27. Moriyasu F, Nishida O, Ban N, et al: Measurement of portal vascular resistance in patients with portal hypertension. Gastroenterology 90:710, 1986.
28. Zoli M, Marchesini G, Cordiani MR, et al: Echo-Doppler measurement of splanchnic blood flow in control and in cirrhotic subjects. J Clin Ultrasound 14:429, 1986.
29. Pugliese D, Ohnishi K, Tsunoda T, et al: Portal hemodynamics after meal in normal subjects and in patients with chronic liver disease studied by echo-Doppler flowmeter. Am J Gastroenterol 10:1052, 1987.
30. Bolondi L, Gaiani S, Li Bassi S, et al: Noninvasive Doppler US evaluation of portal flow in posthepatic (HC), alcoholic (AC) and primary biliary cirrhosis (PBC). J Hepatol 9:S117, 1989.
31. Bolondi L, Gaiani S, Zironi G, et al: Doppler US flowmetry of the portal vein in patients with liver cirrhosis: Relation to esophageal varices. Hepatology 10:A579, 1989.
32. Ohnishi K, Saito M, Sato S, et al: Portal hemodynamics in idiopathic portal hypertension (Banti's syndrome). Gastroenterology 92:751, 1987.
33. Darnault P, Bretagne JF, Fournier V, Raoul J: Splanchnic hemodynamics assessment in patients

with liver cirrhosis and hypersplenism. Gastroenterology 96:A589, 1989.
34. Sabbà C, Ferraioli G, Sarin SK, et al: Feasibility for Doppler flow measurements in splanchnic vessels in nonselected patient population and in cirrhotics. Gastroenterology 96:A432, 1989.
35. Forsberg L, Holmin R: Pulsed Doppler and B-mode ultrasound features of interposition mesocaval and portocaval shunts. Acta Radiol 24:353, 1983.
36. Ackroyd N, Gill R, Griffiths K, et al: Duplex scanning of the portal vein and portosystemic shunts. Surgery 99:591, 1986.
37. Lafortune M, Patriquin H, Pomier G, et al: Hemodynamic changes in portal circulation after portosystemic shunts: Use of duplex sonography in 43 patients. AJR 149:701, 1987.
38. Moryiasu F, Nishida O, Ban N, et al: Ultrasonic Doppler duplex study of hemodynamic changes from portosystemic shunt operation. Ann Surg 205:151, 1987.
39. Bolondi L, Gaiani S, Mazziotti A, et al: Morphological and hemodynamic changes in the portal venous system after distal spleno-renal shunt: An ultrasound and pulsed Doppler study. Hepatology 8:652, 1988.
40. Tylen U, Simert G, Vang J: Hemodynamic changes after distal splenorenal shunt studied by sequential angiography. Radiology 121:585, 1986.

32

Magnetic Resonance Angiography (MRA) of the Hepatic Vein and Portal System

YUJI YUASA and
KYOICHI HIRAMATSU

Since its advent, magnetic resonance imaging (MRI) has steadily evolved and its clinical applications have widened considerably. Among other things, magnetic resonance angiography (MRA) has attracted great attention and is being assessed in various parts of the body (1).

MRA techniques can be divided into two major categories, phase-related methods and time-of-flight (TOF) methods, depending on the dominant contrast mechanism (2,3). In the study reported here, we performed two-dimensional TOF MRA in the upper abdominal region to evaluate normal and abnormal portal and hepatic veins.

MATERIALS AND METHODS

A 1.5 Tesla MRI scanner (GE Signa) was used in this study. Two-dimensional gradient-echo (GRASS) images were successively obtained with 5-mm-thick multisections covering the whole liver. A rectangular field of view (FOV) was used to shorten acquisition time, making breath-holding techniques available. The following are the sequence parameters we used: TR, 22 to 42 ms; TE, 12 to 13 ms; flip angle, 30 degrees; NEX, 1; 128 × 256 matrices (rectangular FOV), with or without a presaturation pulse technique.

Presaturation RF pulses were used to obtain selective magnetic resonance portography by eliminating the abdominal aorta and the inferior vena cava. As a postprocessing technique, projection angiograms were reconstructed with the maximum intensity profile algorithm from the original axial-slice data set. Figure 32-1 shows the images of a normal volunteer acquired with the sequence parameters just described. The original GRASS images and the reconstructed TOF images are shown in Figure 32-1A and B, respectively.

Twenty-eight patients with liver diseases (15 with hepatocellular carcinoma, 4 with liver cirrhosis, 3 with nonneoplastic portal vein occlusion, 2 with portovenous fistulas, and 3 with metastatic liver tumors) and seven patients with biliary tract diseases (6 with bile duct carcinoma and 1 with gallbladder carcinoma) were examined with this method. MRA findings were compared with the corresponding conventional angiograms (transarterial portography) in the 28 patients.

RESULTS

Tables 32-1 and 32-2 summarize the MRA findings in each category and their correlation with conventional angiography. Sixteen patients appeared normal with respect to the vascular system. MRA demonstrated occlusive changes in

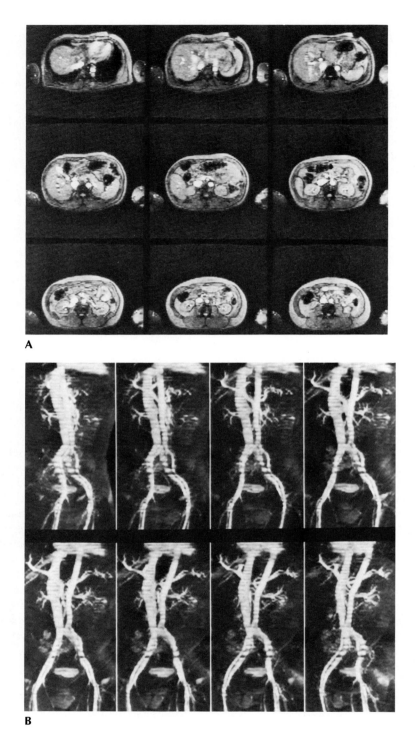

FIGURE 32-1
Normal TOF MRA. (A) Original axial GRASS images. (B) Reconstructed projection images.

TABLE 32-1. MRA Findings

	Normal	Occlusion of Main PV	Occlusion of PV Branch	Narrowing of Main PV	Varix	PV Fistula and PV Aneurysm	No. of Patients
Hepatocellular carcinoma	8	1	4		2(+1)		15
Metastatic liver tumor	3						3
Liver cirrhosis	4			1			5
Other PV abnormalities		3			(+1)	2	5
Bile duct carcinoma	1	1	3	1			6
Gallbladder carcinoma					1		1

TABLE 32-2. MRA versus Conventional Angiography (28 Patients)

Conventional Angiographic Findings	MRA Findings					
	Normal	Occlusion of Main PV	Occlusion of PV Branch	Narrowing of Main PV	Varix	PV fistula and PV Aneurysm
Normal	11					
Occlusion of main PV		3				
Occlusion of PV branch		1	4			
Narrowing of main PV		1	1	1		
Varix	2				3	
PV fistula and PV aneurysm						2

12 patients and stenotic changes in 2 patients within the portal system. Varices of the coronary veins and esophageal veins were detected in 4 patients. A portal vein aneurysm was found in 2 patients with a dilated hepatic vein due to a portovenous fistula.

A good correlation between MRA and conventional angiography was observed, but with MRA there was a tendency to overestimate stenotic lesions in the portal system. The coronary and esophageal varices were poorly visualized by MRA compared with conventional angiography.

CASE REPORTS

Case 1: Metastatic Liver Tumor, 53-Year-Old Man
A solitary metastatic tumor from a colonic carcinoma was found in the posteroinferior segment of the liver with ultrasound (US) and CT. MRI was performed as a preoperative checkup. Figure 32-2A shows a TOF angiogram in coronal projection, and the solitary tumor appears hyperintense after Gd-DTPA injection (arrow). The portal system and hepatic veins appear normal, and an accessory right hepatic vein (arrowhead) is seen just anterior to the tumor. A projection MRA in axial view (Fig. 32-2B) also clearly shows normal intrahepatic vascular structures.

Case 2: Bile Duct Carcinoma, 72-Year-Old Woman
A mass lesion was found at the porta hepatis, and MRA showed a total occlusion of the right portal branch. A short-segment defect also was noted in the left portal branch (Fig. 32-3A). Transarterial portography was performed after the MRA study, and occlusion of the right portal branch was confirmed. The left portal branch showed a severe narrowing corresponding to a small defect seen in MRA (Fig. 32-3B).

Case 3: Portal Aneurysm and Portovenous Fistula, 54-Year-Old Woman
Transarterial portography revealed an intrahepatic portal vein aneurysm in the right portal branch, and fistula formation also was noted (Fig. 32-4A). MRA with presaturation pulses selectively showed the portal system and the hepatic veins.

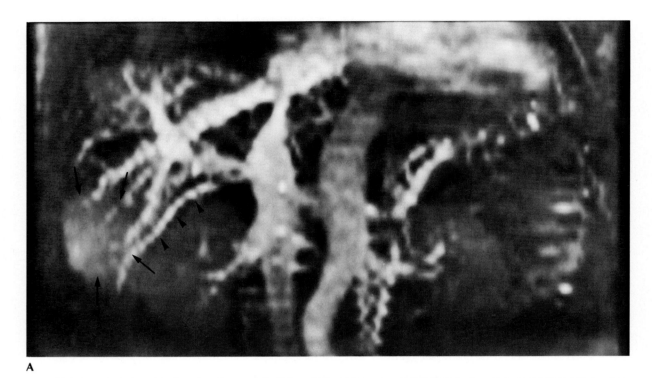

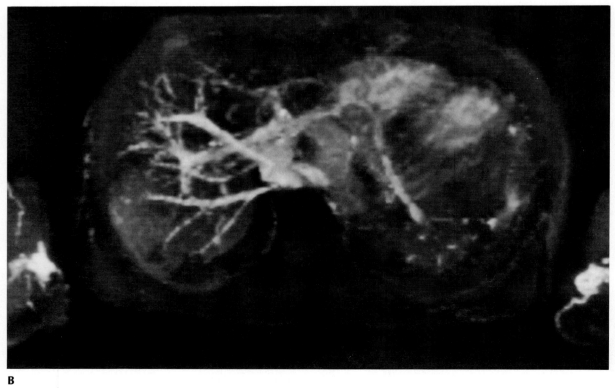

FIGURE 32-2
Metastatic liver tumor. (A) Coronal-projection MRA image. (B) Axial-projection MRA image.

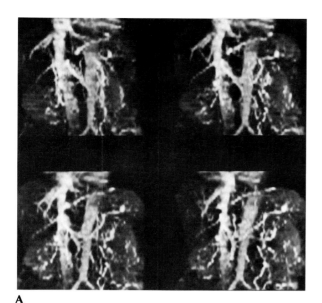

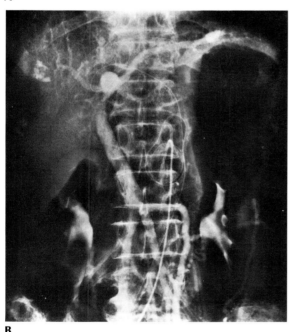

FIGURE 32-3
Bile duct carcinoma. (A) *Coronal-projection MRA images.* (B) *Conventional angiogram (transarterial portography).*

The right portal vein aneurysm is readily identified. The right hepatic vein is markedly dilated, suggesting the presence of portovenous direct communication (Fig. 32-4B). Figure 32-4C is an MRA in axial projection, and the portovenous abnormality is well depicted.

DISCUSSION

A preoperative assessment of the portal and hepatic venous anatomy and abnormality is mandatory for liver surgery, especially in cases of liver segmentectomy. Transarterial portography and selective hepatic venography may be used for this purpose, but these techniques are invasive and are not always successful. MRI has been used to analyze normal and abnormal vascular anatomy, and its usefulness in the liver has been reported (4–7). MRA is a new method to address this clinical demand. Several different approaches have been proposed. Among them, the time-of-flight technique is currently the most popular and robust method in the upper abdominal region (8).

In our study, the hepatic venous structures and portal system were clearly visualized in almost all cases, while the arterial structures were not. As for occlusive portal disease, such as tumor thrombosis of hepatocellular carcinoma, TOF angiography had a tendency to overestimate extent. This is explained by the intravoxel phase dispersion related to turbulent flow at the narrowing point, an effect that is well known in cranial and cervical MRA (9). In the diagnosis of coronary and esophageal varices, MRA was inferior to conventional transarterial portography, probably owing to very slow flow and the small caliber of the vessels. Use of thinner slice thicknesses could be a solution for these problems, thus reducing voxel size and avoiding signal saturation within a slice.

Selective MRA obtained by a presaturation technique further facilitates the assessment of portal anatomy and the diagnosis of abnormalities such as portal obstruction by tumors, collateral venous channels associated with portal vein hypertension, and portovenous shunting. Although this technique has a disadvantage—prolongation of repetition time—the elimination of the great vessels (the abdominal aorta and the inferior vena cava) makes it easier to analyze the portal structures. We strongly recommend use of this technique in upper abdominal TOF MRA.

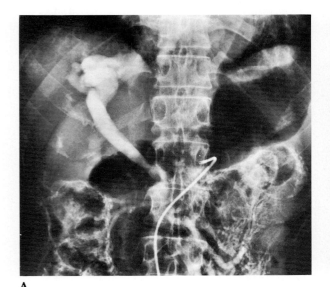

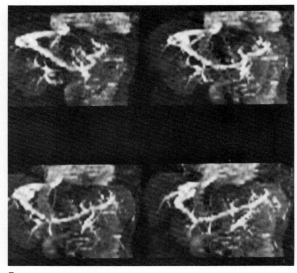

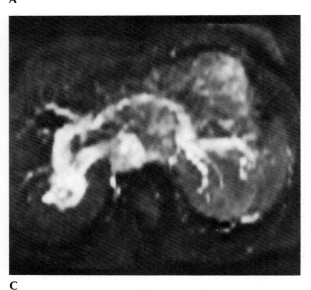

FIGURE 32-4
Portal vein aneurysm and portovenous fistula. (A) Conventional angiogram (transarterial portography). (B) Coronal-projection MRA images. (C) Axial-projection MRA image.

In conclusion, two-dimensional time-of-flight MRA was found to be a good alternative method for the evaluation of hepatic and portal venous structures, and it was particularly of use as a noninvasive preoperative examination.

REFERENCES

1. Alfidi RJ, Masaryk TJ, Haacke EM, et al: MR angiography of peripheral, carotid, and coronary arteries. AJR 149:1097, 1987.
2. Dumoulin CL, Hart HR: Magnetic resonance angiography. Radiology 161:717, 1986.
3. Edelman RR, Wentz KU, Mattle H, et al: Projection arteriography and venography: Initial clinical results using magnetic resonance. Radiology 172:351, 1989.
4. Mukai JK, Stack CM, Turner DA, et al: Imaging of surgically relevant hepatic vascular and segmental anatomy: 1. Normal anatomy. AJR 149:287, 1987.
5. Mukai JK, Stack CM, Turner DA, et al: Imaging of surgically relevant hepatic vascular anatomy: 2. Extent and resectability of hepatic neoplasms. AJR 149:293, 1987.
6. Torres WE, Gaylord GM, Whitmire L, et al: The correlation between MR and angiography in portal hypertension. AJR 148:1109, 1987.
7. Zirinsky K, Markisz JA, Rubenstein WA, et al: MR imaging of portal venous thrombosis: Correlation with CT and sonography. AJR 150:283, 1988.
8. Edelman RR, Zhao B, Liu C, et al: MR angiography and dynamic flow evaluation of the portal venous system. AJR 153:755, 1989.
9. Anderson CM, Saloner D, Tsuruda JS, et al: Artifacts in maximum-intensity-projection display of MR angiograms. AJR 154:623, 1990.

33

Radiology of Liver Transplantation: Complications and Interventions

MICHAEL P. FEDERLE and
WILLIAM L. CAMPBELL

Liver transplantation is now an acceptable treatment for end-stage hepatic disease. A 1-year survival rate of over 70 percent has been achieved in some series as a result of improved immunosuppression medications, advances in surgical techniques, and improved diagnosis and treatment of the causes of postoperative hepatic dysfunction (1–3). A new immunosuppressive drug, FK506, shows great promise in being a further improvement over cyclosporine and may similarly lead to increased enthusiasm and better results for liver transplantation.

Liver transplantation is indicated for irreversible chronic liver disease in which medical or surgical therapy is not effective. Indications are controversial but may include congenital or acquired end-stage cirrhosis, metabolic disorders resulting in liver failure, hepatic-based metabolic defects, Budd-Chiari syndrome, and primary hepatocellular malignancy.

PREOPERATIVE EVALUATION

Radiologic evaluation prior to surgery is performed to detect conditions that may preclude transplantation or require a change in surgical approach (4). Such conditions may include portal vein occlusion, primary malignancy outside the hepatobiliary system or metastatic hepatobiliary malignancy, a focus of infection and sepsis outside the hepatobiliary system, and vascular anomalies of the portal vein or the inferior vena cava, especially in children. Liver volume may be measured to permit an optimal match of donor liver size to the recipient (5).

Real-time sonography with pulsed or color Doppler is the single most useful preoperative imaging study because it permits evaluation of portal vein patency, other vascular anomalies or disease, liver size and echogenicity, masses, and biliary dilation. Computed tomography (CT) is routinely performed as well and is particularly useful in the evaluation of liver masses for size, extent, and possible extrahepatic spread. Liver volume determinations are routinely performed. An upper gastrointestinal barium study is obtained in children to look for intestinal malrotation. Biliary atresia, the most common indication for transplantation in children, may be associated with polysplenia syndrome, which may in turn be associated with intestinal malrotation and anomalies of the portal vein or inferior vena cava. These anomalies may preclude transplantation. Angiography is indicated if malrotation is discovered. Cholangiography is not a routine part of the pretransplantation evaluation but may be necessary if a biliary abnormality is suspected. The possibility of primary sclerosing cholangitis may be an indication for endoscopic retrograde cholangiography or percutaneous transhepatic cholangiography. Involvement of the recipient common bile duct with primary sclerosing cholangitis precludes its anastomosis to the donor common duct and makes biliary anastomosis by choledochojejunostomy mandatory. Magnetic resonance imaging (MRI) may demonstrate hepatic and vascular abnormalities, but it is unclear whether MRI will have significant advantages over CT and ultrasound in the liver transplantation patient.

POSTOPERATIVE CONSIDERATIONS

Anatomy

Orthotopic liver transplantation requires anastomosis of the bile duct, hepatic artery, portal vein, and inferior vena cava.

Bile Duct. In most adult patients with normal bile ducts, an end-to-end anastomosis is performed between the donor and recipient common ducts. The gallbladders are removed. A T-tube is inserted by means of the recipient common duct to stent the anastomosis and monitor bile output. The T-tube usually remains in place for 2 to 3 months. In patients in whom the common duct is abnormal, absent, too short, or too small, biliary reconstruction is accomplished by end-to-side choledochojejunostomy in roux-en-Y with internal biliary stent. Choledochojejunostomy is the most common biliary reconstruction in children.

Hepatic Artery. In most patients, an end-to-end anastomosis is performed between the donor celiac axis and the recipient common hepatic artery. If the donor liver has a dual blood supply (e.g., right hepatic artery from the superior mesenteric artery), a single arterial trunk is created for the anastomosis. In children, direct end-to-end anastomoses are used when possible. Otherwise, the donor thoracic or abdominal aorta with attached celiac axis may be used for arterial revascularization. Because of thrombosis in aortic conduits, graphs of donor iliac artery interposed between the recipient infrarenal aorta and the donor celiac artery have recently gained favor.

Portal Vein. Portal venous revascularization is accomplished by end-to-end anastomosis between the extra hepatic portal veins of the donor and the recipient. If an abnormally small or occluded recipient portal vein is encountered, transplantation is still possible. A venous allograft from the donor inferior vena cava, iliac vein, or pulmonary vein may be interposed between the donor extrahepatic portal vein and the confluence of the recipient superior mesenteric and splenic veins.

Inferior Vena Cava. Reconstruction of the inferior vena cava is accomplished by anastomoses of the infrahepatic and suprahepatic vena cava segments of both donor and recipient.

COMPLICATIONS

Liver transplantation is a major surgical procedure frequently performed in debilitated individuals who must recuperate under the stress of immunosuppression. A greater than 50 percent incidence of significant complications has been reported. The following discussion is limited to those complications with which the radiologist is most frequently and significantly involved.

Biliary Complications

Biliary complications have occurred in approximately 13 percent of liver transplantation patients. Cholangiography, either T-tube, percutaneous transhepatic, or endoscopic retrograde, is the most definitive imaging approach. Ultrasound, CT, and radionuclide scanning with iminodiacetic acid (IDA) analogs may be useful to screen for biliary obstruction or leak but are neither sensitive nor specific.

Biliary complications include obstruction, bile leaks, tube problems, stones, bilomas, and fistulas (Figs. 33-1, and 33-2). Most occur in the first few weeks after transplantation. Complications unique to liver transplantation are related to the choledochocholedochostomy anastomosis and ductal ischemia. Anastomotic strictures or leaks may occur. Strictures in the donor biliary tree, nonanastomotic bile leaks, and bilomas may result from bile duct ischemia and necrosis. Complications related to the small-caliber T-tubes or stents include abnormal location of the proximal limb of the T-tube in the donor cystic duct remnant, tubes outside the common duct, folded

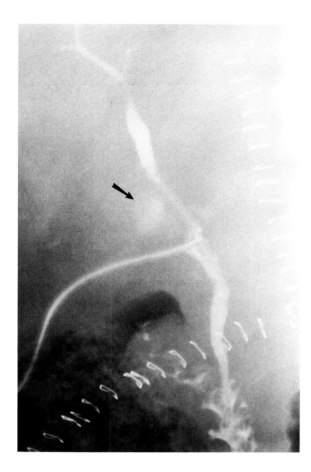

FIGURE 33-1
Bile leak at duct anastomosis. T-tube cholangiogram with tube placed in donor common duct. Mild stricture and bile leak (arrow) *at site of anastomosis.*

tubes, and tube occlusion by sludge and bile encrustation. A T-tube distal limb that crosses the ampulla can result in biliary obstruction.

Vascular Complications

A vascular complication is a primary diagnostic consideration in the liver transplantation patient with fulminant hepatic failure, bile leak, relapsing bacteremia, gastrointestinal or abdominal bleeding, or hemobilia. The most common and serious complication is hepatic artery thrombosis, which has occurred in 12 percent of pediatric and 3 percent of adult transplants.

Hepatic Artery Thrombosis. Hepatic artery thrombosis is a devastating event requiring emergency retransplantation in most cases (6,7). Duplex sonography is currently the optimal screening test. If no hepatic arterial flow is identified by pulsed Doppler imaging, angiography is warranted.

CT and real-time sonography are also predictive of hepatic artery thrombosis. Of transplantation patients with focal inhomogeneity of the liver architecture by CT or sonography, 86 percent have thrombosis. These areas of inhomogeneity represent infarcts (with or without infection) or abscesses. The combination of pulsed Doppler imaging of the hepatic artery and real-time sonography or CT of the liver parenchyma is highly sensitive as a screening test (Fig. 33-3). Hepatic infarcts, abscesses, and bilomas also may be detected on technetium-99m IDA or other radionuclide scans.

Arterial collaterals have been documented angiographically in some children with hepatic artery thrombosis who have survived without retransplantation. Arterial collaterals have not been observed in adults with hepatic artery thrombosis; most such patients have required retransplantation.

Portal Vein Thrombosis. Thrombosis or stenosis occurs much less commonly in the portal vein than in the hepatic artery. Hepatopetal venous collaterals may develop in transplantation patients after portal vein thrombosis. The angiographic appearance is identical to that of cavernous transformation of the portal vein. Occasionally, a bypass shunt is required for control of portal hypertension.

Miscellaneous Vascular Complications. Uncommon vascular complications include anastomotic and donor hepatic artery pseudoaneurysms, hepatic artery dissecting aneurysms, mycotic aneurysms, hepatic artery–portal vein fistulas, biliary-portal vein fistulas, hepatic vein occlusion, and stenosis or thrombosis of the inferior vena cava.

Fluid Collections

CT and real-time sonography are the most useful modalities for the evaluation of possible abdominal abscess or other fluid collections. Fluid collections that may mimic abscesses include loculated

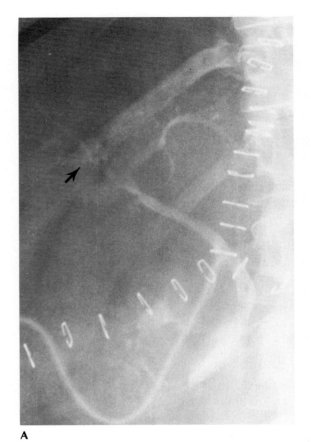 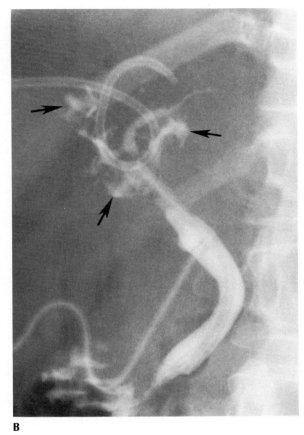

FIGURE 33-2
Bile duct necrosis in hepatic artery thrombosis. (A) T-tube cholangiogram demonstrates poor filling of intrahepatic ducts and an amorphous collection of extravasated bile (arrow). (B) Repeat cholangiogram after placement of a drainage catheter within the biloma (arrows).

ascites and lymphatic fluid, hematomas, and bilomas. Percutaneous aspiration with a 22-gauge needle is safe and diagnostic in most cases. Percutaneous catheter drainage can be performed if an abscess is found.

Rejection
Despite advances in immunosuppression with cyclosporine, rejection is the most common cause of posttransplantation hepatic dysfunction and retransplantation. A recent study documented rejection in at least 37 percent of patients. Without liver biopsy, the diagnosis is often made by exclusion.

Other Complications
Nearly all liver transplantation patients develop pleural effusions, predominantly on the right side. Pulmonary infection, including pneumonia, empyema, and lung abscess, occurs in nearly 20 percent of patients. A variety of organisms are encountered, including bacte-

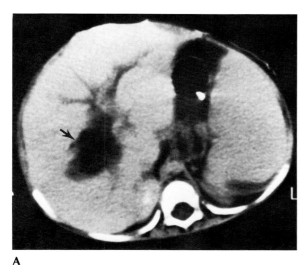 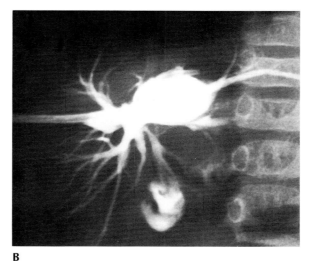

FIGURE 33-3
(A) *Biloma* (arrow) *shown on CT following hepatic artery thrombosis.* (B) *Percutaneous catheter drains biloma.*

rial, viral, and fungal agents as well as *Pneumocystis carinii*. Segmental or lobar atelectasis occurs commonly. Infarction and hemorrhage of the right adrenal gland comprise a common complication owing to ligation of the adrenal veins during transplantation (Fig. 33-4).

INTERVENTIONAL RADIOLOGY

Interventional radiologic techniques are important in treating certain postoperative complications in liver transplantation patients. In many cases, additional surgery can be avoided. Most procedures involve the biliary tree and include percutaneous biliary drainage, balloon dilation of bile duct strictures, replacement of dislodged T-tubes, restoring patency to obstructed T-tubes, and percutaneous removal of internal biliary stents (8).

Procedures outside the biliary tree include percutaneous drainage of postoperative hepatic and abdominal abscesses, bilomas, and other fluid collections. Vascular interventions also are infrequently performed and include angioplasty, embolization, and thrombolytic therapy.

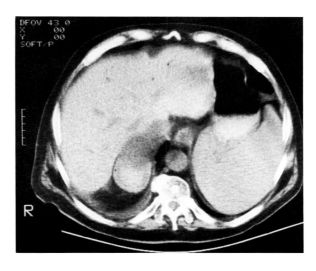

FIGURE 33-4
Adrenal infarction/hemorrhage. High-density hematoma in right adrenal area is due to ligation of adrenal veins during liver transplantation.

REFERENCES

1. Starzl TE, Iwatsuki S, Shaw BW Jr, et al: Immunosuppression and other nonsurgical factors in the improved results of liver transplantation. Semin Liver Dis 5:334, 1985.

2. Busuttil RW, Goldstein LI, Danovitch GM, et al: Liver transplantation today. Ann Intern Med 104:377, 1986.
3. Starzl TE, Iwatsuki S, Shaw BW Jr, et al: Analysis of liver transplantation. Hepatology 4:47S, 1984..
4. Ledesma-Medina J, Dominquez R, Bowen A, et al: Pediatric liver transplantation: 1. Standardization of preoperative diagnostic imaging. Radiology 157:335, 1985.
5. Van Thiel DH, Hagler NG, Schade RR, et al: In vivo hepatic volume determination using sonography and computed tomography: Validation and a comparison of the two techniques. Gastroenterology 88:1812, 1985.
6. Zajko AB, Bron KM, Starzl TE, et al: Angiography of liver transplantation patients. Radiology 157:305, 1985.
7. Wozney P, Zajko AB, Bron KM, et al: Vascular complications after liver transplantation: A 5-year experience. AJR 147:657, 1986.
8. Zajko AB, Campbell WL, Bron KM, et al: Cholangiography and interventional biliary radiology in adult liver transplantation. AJR 144:127, 1985.

X. SPECTROSCOPY

34

Magnetic Resonance Spectroscopy of the Liver: A Review

DIETER J. MEYERHOFF and
MICHAEL W. WEINER

Magnetic resonance spectroscopy (MRS) uses the same basic instrumentation as conventional MRI. Some additional hardware and software allow one to noninvasively measure important metabolites in the living human body (in vivo) that often cannot be measured by other methods. In contrast to MRI, MRS must be performed in a much more homogeneous magnetic field to obtain frequency-selective information, no gradients are desired during data acquisition, and because of the inherently lower sensitivity and concentration of all nuclei compared with protons (^{1}H), the volume size required for MRS is always much larger than that for MRI. (For a more elaborate treatment of the magnetic resonance phenomenon, see, for example, ref. 1).

MRS may be performed on many nuclei. For clinical liver studies, ^{31}P and ^{19}F MRS have been primarily used. Figure 34-1 shows a typical ^{31}P MRS spectrum obtained from a healthy human liver. ^{31}P MRS of the liver detects the high-energy phosphate ATP (giving rise to three resonances owing to the α-, β-, and γ-phosphate groups), inorganic phosphate (P_i), as well as important phosphorus components of phospholipid metabolism (PME and PDE). The intracellular pH of hepatic tissue (for reviews on pH, see ref. 2) can be determined from the P_i chemical shift as derived from the horizontal axis of the spectrum. The chemical shift of the α- and β-ATP resonances can be used to derive the intracellular concentration of free magnesium ions (Mg^{2+}) (3). Precursors of phospholipid synthesis and phospholipid breakdown products are detected in the peaks labeled phosphomonoesters (PME) and phosphodiesters (PDE).

The ^{19}F isotope of fluorine is a highly sensitive, NMR-visible nucleus that is present at 100 percent natural abundance. ^{19}F MRS has potential in clinical studies of 5-fluorouracil (FU) metabolism (for a review, see ref. 4).

The ^{13}C isotope is detectable by MRS, although its natural abundance is only 1.1 percent. Therefore, ^{13}C signals in vivo can only be obtained from highly abundant glycogen and fat (5,6). Despite its high molecular weight, glycogen has been shown to have sufficient molecular mobility to be fully detectable by in vivo MRS (6), opening up the ability of studying glycogen metabolism (7) noninvasively in humans.

^{1}H MRS easily detects water and hepatic lipids. Signals from protons of biochemically interesting compounds of much lower concentrations (millimolar range), such as lactate, N-acetylaspartate, glutamine, glutamate, creatine, and a variety of amino acids (8) that are detected in human brain are obscured by the large lipid signals of liver. Owing to experimental difficulties in suppressing this strong signal, no good ^{1}H MRS spectrum of liver has been published.

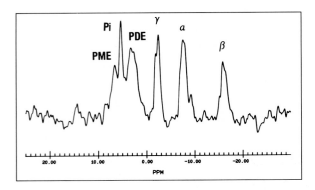

FIGURE 34-1
Typical ^{31}P MRS spectrum of the posterior segment of the right lobe of a healthy liver. The spectrum was obtained with an ISIS localization technique. Peak assignments: PME = phosphomonoesters; P_i = inorganic phosphate; PDE = phosphodiesters; γ, α, β = γ-, α-, and β-phosphates of ATP. Note the absence of a phosphocreatine peak at 0 ppm.

METABOLIC PATHWAYS IN LIVER DETECTED BY MRS

Major energy-producing metabolic pathways occurring in the hepatocyte can be detected by MRS. Cellular energy in the form of ATP is derived from oxidation of food by two pathways: Under anaerobic conditions, glucose is converted to lactate in the glycolytic pathway, directly affecting the acid-base status of the liver and generating relatively small amounts of ATP. In the presence of oxygen, pyruvate and/or fatty acids derived from glucose are oxidized to CO_2 by the citric acid cycle within the mitochondria. This oxidative phosphorylation pathway produces a large amount of ATP, which is transported to the cytoplasm to be used for cellular work. Sodium transport by the enzyme sodium-potassium ATPase uses most of the produced ATP. The reactions of the urea cycle, bile production, gluconeogenesis, lipogenesis, and synthesis of protein and nucleic acids require ATP. In most cases, biological work fueled by the hydrolysis of ATP produces ADP and inorganic phosphate (P_i). These metabolites reenter the mitochondria for resynthesis of ATP if oxygen is available. For some synthetic reactions, ATP is hydrolyzed to AMP and pyrophosphate and further to adenosine, inosine, and ultimately to uric acid. Phosphocreatine (PCr) is not present in the liver because the liver lacks the enzyme creatine kinase.

In summary, MRS is able to measure noninvasively such important hepatic metabolites as ATP, P_i, H^+ (through pH), glycogen, and theoretically, lactate. It proves to be a valuable tool in assessing the energy state and viability of hepatic tissue.

LOCALIZED MRS OF THE HUMAN LIVER

Clinical MRS of the liver became possible with the advent of whole-body magnets with a field strength of 1.5 Tesla or greater. If the RF coil is simply placed on the body wall over the liver (surface coil), a part of the detected RF signal will also be from fat and muscle surrounding the liver, giving rise to signal contribution from phosphocreatine (PCr), which is highly abundant in muscle. To avoid this "contamination," use of a localization technique that acquires signal from a defined volume of interest (VOI) is required (for a short review, see ref. 9). Radda and colleagues (10) employed a "field profiling" technique (11) and "rotating-frame depth selection" (12) to acquire signal only from the liver. MRI-guided three-dimensional ^{31}P MRS (ISIS) uses the three-dimensional information provided by MRI for visualizing and defining the VOI (13). It was used by Segebarth et al. (14) and Meyerhoff et al. (15) to obtain localized MRS spectra from normal and diseased human liver (16). Disadvantages of the ISIS technique are that it is subject to movement artifacts and that the VOIs for each metabolite are slightly spatially displaced from each other as a function of gradient strength and resonance frequency [chemical-shift offset effect (15)]. However, an important advantage of ISIS is the spatial definition of this method, which allows the derivation of absolute molar concentrations of metabolites in the VOI.

Magnetic resonance spectroscopic imaging (*MRSI* or *SI*) (sometimes also termed *chemical shift imaging*) (17,18) uses time-varying magnetic field gradients (phase encoding) after signal excitation to obtain spectra simultaneously from multiple volume elements within the liver. The result can be displayed either as spectra from individual volumes (19) or as coarse images of individual metabolites (20), much as standard ^1H MRS images of water and fat. A determination of the VOI at the time of the examination is not necessary as in all the single-volume localization techniques described above. Several investigators (see refs. 21–23) recently reported encouraging results with ^{31}P SI of the human liver.

CLINICAL LIVER MRS

Previous Clinical Studies

This chapter summarizes clinical liver studies using ^{31}P, ^{13}C, and ^{19}F NMR since 1985. For other reviews on clinical MRS at John Radcliffe and Hammersmith Hospitals, see references 24 and 25. For a short review of studies using animal models of hepatic disease, see reference 26.

Clinical studies were first performed in 1985 on infants with neuroblastoma (27), demonstrating a fall of the hepatic PME/ATP ratio as a function of successful therapeutic intervention. In another ^{31}P MRS study (28), the PME/β-ATP ratio predicted response of an infant neuroblastoma to chemotherapy within 24 hours. ^{31}P MRS spectra were obtained from hepatoblastoma and endometrial adenocarcinoma (29). The adenocarcinoma showed high levels of PME, relatively small amounts of PDE, and some PCr. After embolization of the tumor, the P_i/ATP ratio increased while the intracellular pH fell from 7.15 to 6.8. These early reports on liver tumors suggested that ^{31}P MRS may provide a sensitive and rapid indication of therapeutic response. The liver of a patient with Caroli syndrome (25) showed higher amounts of PME, especially around the porta hepatis, corresponding to the region of thickened bile duct system. Other clinical studies included Budd-Chiari syndrome (25), obstructive jaundice with sclerosing cholangitis (25), and alcoholic hepatitis with jaundice (unpublished results of this laboratory). In all cases, high PME levels were detected, which are probably due to relative high concentrations of phosphoethanolamine (PE) and/or phosphocholine (PC), compounds involved in phospholipid biosynthesis. High PME therefore does not seem to be a specific indicator of hepatic disease, but rather an indicator of structural damage.

In a patient with a glycogen storage disease (glucose-6-phosphatase deficiency) (10), ^{31}P spectra demonstrated relatively strong resonances in the sugar phosphate region of the spectrum (see below) and, consequently, reduced P_i and ATP levels. All these metabolic changes observed in disease were similar to those which are deliberately produced by administration of substances such as fructose, glucose, lactate, or alanine (14,25,30,31). These liver function tests are designed to stress hepatic adenine nucleotide metabolism, which can be monitored by ^{31}P MRS. As has been shown by ^{31}P NMR in animal studies of hepatic disease (for a review, see ref. 26), fructose, for example, is rapidly phosphorylated to fructose-1-phosphate (F-1-P). Since F-1-P is slowly converted to triosephosphate by aldolase B, it accumulates in liver cells and is easily detectable in ^{31}P MRS spectra. The trapping of cytosolic P_i as F-1-P can be followed by serial ^{31}P MRS. Low P_i in turn activates the enzyme AMP deaminase, depleting ATP and leading to increased levels of inosine and uric acid. ^{31}P MRS showed these reversible changes of hepatic phosphorus metabolites (30) in individual heterozygotes for fructose intolerance treated with small amounts of fructose. The chronic accumulation of adenine nucleotide degradation products was suspected to cause gout in these patients.

^{19}F MRS was used without localization to monitor 5-fluorouracil (5-FU) catabolism in the human liver (32) and in liver tumors (33). The kinetics and the time course of the relative concentrations of 5-FU and its main catabolite α-fluoro-β-alanine were measured immediately after drug administration. In contrast to animal livers, the catabolite α-fluoro-β-uridopropionic acid could not be convincingly measured, suggesting a species-dependent 5-FU catabolism (4). The studies show the feasibility of monitoring short-term therapy with ^{19}F MRS.

Studies in This Laboratory: Quantitative Clinical ^{31}P MRS

Results of MRS studies are most commonly presented as ratios of metabolite peak intensities. These ratios, however, are a function of experimental and nuclei-specific parameters, such as RF pulse repetition time of the experiment and relaxation times of the nuclei. Therefore, it is desirable to express MRS results independent of these parameters in absolute terms such as metabolite concentrations (34,35). This allows direct comparison of different and nonrelated patient groups.

This research group has developed a computer-supported method to derive absolute molar concentrations from image-guided localized in vivo spectra (ISIS) (36,37). These calculations assume homogeneous distribution of metabolite concentrations throughout the VOI so that the concentrations obtained indicate mean values over the sample volume and do not indicate cellular concentrations. Calculations also assume relaxation times measured in normal controls for patient studies even though these times may be slightly altered in the patients. Owing to time constraints, it is currently impossible to perform accurate relaxation time measurements on every patient studied. Therefore, inaccurate relaxation times may cause some inaccuracy in calculated concentrations.

Normal Liver. Figure 34-1 shows a typical healthy liver ^{31}P MRS spectrum obtained using the ISIS technique with a surface coil at a magnetic field strength of 1.5 Tesla (15). The spectrum was obtained in 9 min from 150 ml of right lobe liver tissue. The absence of a PCr peak in the spectrum at 0 ppm, characteristic for muscle, confirms good localization within the liver. The peak labeled P_i represents intracellular (primarily cytosolic) and extracellular P_i. The PME peak is composed of overlapping signals from several phosphomonoesters that can be tentatively assigned on the basis of their chemical shifts, human biopsy data, and MRS results from isolated perfused rat liver and rat liver extracts. These results suggest that the major contributors to the PME peak are PC and PE, followed by sugar phosphates such as fructose-1-phosphate and 3-phospho- glycerate (38). The PDE peak is the major resonance in liver spectra obtained at 2 Tesla static magnetic field strength or below. The usually very broad peak consists of several unresolved resonances between 1 and 4 ppm. The PDE peak in rat liver is composed of resonances due to glycero-3-phosphoethanolamine, glycero-3-phosphocholine, and phosphoenol-pyruvate (39,40). It is generally assumed that the same compounds contribute to the PDE region in human liver spectra. From the three ATP resonances, the α-ATP peak has a contribution of approximately 20 percent nicotinamide adenine dinucleotides (NAD/NADH and their phosphates). Resonances from free ADP are not visible in the spectra because of its low concentration and possible line broadening of peaks due to compartmentation in the mitochondria and/or binding to rigid proteins.

The chemical shifts of all major hepatic resonances as determined from spectra of 21 normal subjects relative to α-ATP (set at -7.66 ppm) were 6.76 ± 0.23, 5.28 ± 0.20, 4.5 to 1, -2.41 ± 0.19, and -16.15 ± 0.20 ppm [mean ± standard deviation (SD)] for PME, P_i, PDE, γ-, and β-ATP, respectively. Normal hepatic pH was calculated (2,40) from the chemical shift of P_i to 7.4 ± 0.2 ($n = 21$). Average ^{31}P metabolite relaxation times (T1) measured in healthy human liver at 2 Tesla (15) were 0.4 s for ATP, 1 s for P_i, 0.8 s for PME, and 1.4 s for PDE. Metabolite ratios, derived from ISIS peak integrals and corrected for T1 relaxation times in 8 normal controls were 1.1 for P_i/ATP, 0.4 for PME/ATP, and 2.6 for PDE/ATP. Average metabolite concentrations in millimoles per kilogram wet weight derived from normal liver ISIS spectra corrected for the chemical-shift offset effect are as follows: ATP = 2.0 ± 0.1, $P_i = 2.2 \pm 0.4$, PME = 0.8 ± 0.4, and PDE = 5.3 ± 1.9. The calculated ATP and P_i concentrations were less than those determined by freeze-clamping studies of human liver (42,43). This is so because MRS detects only freely tumbling molecules, and not those which are bound to macromolecules and membranes or those which are localized in the mitochondria (38 and references cited therein). Furthermore, liver biopsy data tend to overestimate P_i content due to hydrolysis prior to freezing.

The result of a ^{31}P study using SI on the liver of a healthy volunteer is shown in Figure 34-2. The figure shows an axial total phosphorus metabolite image on the left and three spectra obtained from different (numbered) regions of the image. The surface coil that was used to acquire the data is not seen on the image, but it is underneath the high-intensity signal area at the right lobe of the liver. The sensitive area of the coil covers approximately 11 × 20 cm, which includes back muscle and spine (low intensity) and most of the posterior part of the right lobe of the liver. Spectra 1 through 3, obtained from approximately 20 ml of tissue, are typical for liver, muscle and liver, and back muscle tissue, respectively. Note the absence of PCr in the liver spectrum, proving proper localization.

Alcoholic Liver Disease. Liver biopsy is the procedure of choice in the diagnosis of hepatic pathology due to alcoholic liver disease. Improved

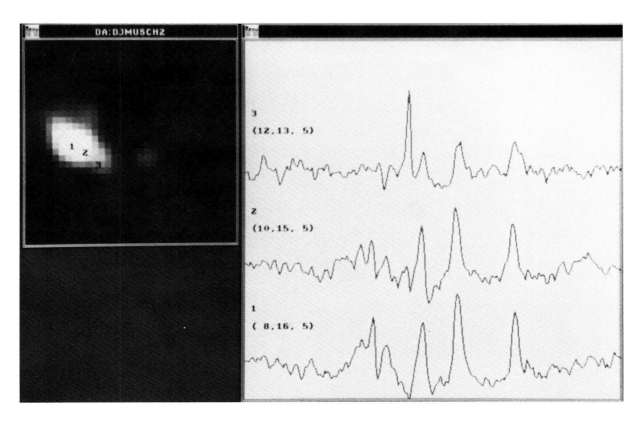

FIGURE 34-2
^{31}P spectroscopic image of the liver and back muscle region of a normal volunteer in supine position. The axial image is composed of the sum of all phosphorus metabolites and corresponds to the region of the body excited by a surface coil underneath the subject's back. Spectra were obtained from approximately 20 ml of liver (1), liver and muscle (2), and back muscle only (3) (unpublished result).

imaging modalities to at least supplement biopsy would be clinically valuable. These spectroscopic findings (16) demonstrate that quantitative ^{31}P MRS provides important information concerning metabolic abnormalities associated with human liver disease not obtained by other methods. Using the ^{31}P ISIS technique, we could show that metabolite *ratios* obtained in normal controls, 10 patients with alcoholic hepatitis, and 9 patients with alcoholic cirrhosis were not statistically different from each other. While preliminary studies of cirrhotic and normal livers by others (44,45) showed similar results, one study (46) showed slightly increased PME/ATP in cirrhotic patients. In our study, alcoholic cirrhosis patients showed a comparatively high contribution of phosphocholine to the PME resonance (based on chemical shift), while alcoholic hepatitis patients showed significant sugar phosphate contribution to the PME peak in 8 of 10 cases.

More important, we noted a significant reduction of absolute signal intensity in all ISIS spectra obtained from patients with alcoholic liver disease. Calculated hepatic phosphorus metabolite concentrations in alcoholic hepatitis patients were significantly decreased by 31 to 46 percent compared with normal controls, whereas the decrease in the alcoholic cirrhosis group was between 18 and 50 percent. Except for PME, all decreases were statistically significant ($p < 0.05$) compared with controls. There was, however, no significant difference between hepatic metabolite concentrations in alcoholic hepatitis and cirrhosis. The most likely reason for such a decrease is loss of hepatocytes due to necrosis and/or diffuse replacement of hepatocytes with fat or collagen. Stereoanalysis of biopsied material indicates that the amount of viable tissue in severely alcohol-damaged livers is significantly reduced compared with normal controls. If hepatitis is chronic and occurs without necrosis (viral hepatitis, see below), metabolite concentrations (except for PME) are normal. Another reason for the reduced metabolite concentrations may be hidden in the assumption made for calculation of molar concentrations that the ^{31}P metabolite relaxation times (T1) are the same in normal volunteers and patients. This may not be correct, especially since longer ^{1}H T1 relaxation times have been found in liver disease (47).

Hepatic intracellular pH as calculated from the chemical shift of the P_i resonance in spectra of normal controls was 7.4. Hepatic pH in alcoholic hepatitis was significantly higher, in alcoholic cirrhosis, significantly lower (7.3). All pH differences were statistically significant ($p < 0.05$). There is some evidence from cell experiments with growth factors that the high pH in alcoholic hepatitis may indicate hepatic cell regeneration (48). Other possible explanations for this increased pH are impaired urea synthesis, leading to an accumulation of HCO_3^- (49), and low rate of glycolysis producing less lactate. The low pH in cirrhotic livers, however, may reflect the loss of capability of a great portion of the liver to regenerate. Acidosis, although it is not very common, is thought to occur with severe hepatic damage, where decreased oxidative metabolism leads to lactic acidosis (50).

Figure 34-3 summarizes the main results of this work on alcoholic liver disease. Calculated hepatic ATP concentrations are plotted versus P_i chemical shift/pH for alcoholic hepatitis, alcoholic cirrhosis, and normal controls. The plot can be divided into the three sectors shown: the upper sector (>1.8 mmol/kg wet weight ATP) contains only measured values for normal controls, the lower left sector (<1.8 mmol/kg wet weight ATP and <5.4 ppm) contains 7 of 8 alcoholic cirrhosis patients, and the lower right sector contains 6 of 7 alcoholic hepatitis patients. The figure demonstrates that molar concentrations of ATP and pH, both determined by ^{31}P MRS, can be used not

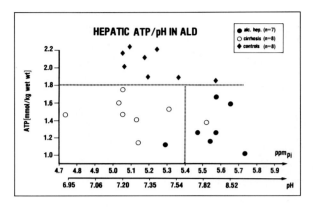

FIGURE 34-3
Calculated ATP concentrations versus chemical shift of inorganic phosphate (in ppm) and intracellular pH for control subjects, alcoholic hepatitis patients, and alcoholic cirrhosis patients. The dashed lines indicate sector limits explained in the text. (From Meyerhoff DJ, Boska MD, Thomas AM, Weiner MW: Alcoholic liver disease: Quantitative image-guided P-31 MR spectroscopy. Radiology 173:393, 1989. Reprinted by permission.)

only to differentiate normal from diseased livers, but also to distinguish non-invasively between alcoholic hepatitis and cirrhosis. However, it should be emphasized that these are early results and that more patient studies and improved methods of quantitation are required to determine the validity of this differentiation.

Viral Hepatitis B. ^{31}P MRS of alcoholic liver disease showed that low ATP and high pH are specific for alcoholic hepatitis. To determine whether this is characteristic for all forms of hepatitis, patients with viral hepatitis B were examined with quantitative ^{31}P ISIS. Metabolite concentrations measured in viral hepatitis B were normal, except for a very high PME (138 percent above normal), most likely due to high concentrations of phosphoethanolamine and/or phosphocholine as determined from the chemical shift of the PME resonance. The study confirms earlier qualitative findings by Radda et al. (24). Intracellular pH was normal, but significantly lower than in alcoholic hepatitis. These results demonstrate that quantitative ^{31}P MRS can be used to distinguish between viral and alcoholic hepatitis.

Liver Metastases. Human tumors often have increased PME and PDE levels compared with their host tissues, indicating an altered phospholipid metabolism (51 and references cited therein). Chemotherapy has been shown to decrease PME/ATP ratios and PME levels (51,52). Embolization and local chemotherapy (chemoembolization) of one lobe of the liver or of the entire liver are being used to treat hepatic metastases and primary cancers of the liver. Therapeutic outcome is usually monitored by serial MRI, CT, and protein measurements, but these methods have not proved very useful. Therefore, we have used serial ^{31}P MRS to directly monitor the effects of chemoembolization on hepatic tumor metabolism (53). High-energy phosphate concentrations derived from ISIS spectra obtained from hepatic tumors before chemoembolization were reduced by 30 to 50 percent, while PME was elevated by 60 to 90 percent. Following chemoembolization, ATP, PME, and PDE levels dropped initially, while P_i levels transiently increased. These findings were consistent with tissue necrosis and/or ischemia in the tumorous region as a direct response to the chemoembolization procedure. MRI and CT failed to show therapeutic responses. During the weeks following the onset of chemoembolization in one patient with a primary liver cancer, the constant increase in ATP concentrations and the constant decrease in the PME/ATP ratio correlated well with clinical recovery.

In conclusion, the clinical use of MRS in the assessment of liver disease is at an early stage. The few studies performed, however, show that many disturbances of hepatic metabolism due to disease or to deliberately produced stress can be detected noninvasively by MRS. ^{31}P MRS at its current stage is especially useful for the evaluation of diffuse liver diseases and large tumors. Even though the total number of examined patients is still small, there is enough evidence to believe that quantitative ^{31}P MRS may be very helpful as a clinical tool in diagnosis of hepatic pathology and in monitoring of cancer therapy. Metabolite concentrations can be obtained from ^{31}P MR spectra in addition to metabolite ratios and provide valuable information at no extra expense to the patient. The authors expect that in the future MRS will have an increasing role in medical investigation, clinical diagnosis, and patient treatment.

REFERENCES

1. Roth K: NMR-Tomography and -Spectroscopy in Medicine; An Introduction. Berlin, Springer-Verlag, 1984.
2. Gadian DG, Radda GK, Dawson MJ, Wilkie DR: pH$_i$ measurements of cardiac and skeletal muscle using ^{31}P-NMR, in Liss AR (ed): Intracellular pH: Its Measurement, Regulation, and Utilization in Cellular Functions. New York, Academic Press, 1982, pp 61–77.
3. Gupta RK, Benovic JL, Rose ZB: The determination of the free magnesium level in the human red blood cell by ^{31}P NMR. J Biol Chem 253:6172, 1978.
4. Evelhoch JL: In vivo ^{19}F nuclear magnetic resonance spectroscopy: A potential monitor of 5-fluorouracil pharmacokinetics and metabolism. Invest New Drugs 7:5, 1989.
5. Sillerud LO, Shulman RG: Structure and metabolism of mammalian liver glycogen monitored by carbon-13 nuclear magnetic resonance. Biochemistry 22:1087, 1983.
6. Jue T, Lohman JAB, Ordidge RJ, Shulman RG: Natural abundance ^{13}C NMR spectrum of glycogen in humans. Magn Reson Med 5:377, 1987.
7. Cohen SM: Application of nuclear magnetic resonance to the study of liver physiology and disease. Hepatology 3:738, 1983.
8. Behar KL, den Hollander JA, Stromski ME, et al: High resolution ^{1}H NMR study of cerebral hypoxia in vivo. Proc Natl Acad Sci USA 80:4954, 1984.
9. Weiner MW: The promise of magnetic resonance spectroscopy for medical diagnosis. Invest Radiol 23:253, 1988.
10. Oberhaensli RD, Galloway GJ, Hilton-Jones D, et al: The study of human organs by phosphorus-31 topical magnetic resonance spectroscopy. Br J Radiol 60:367, 1987.
11. Oberhaensli RD, Galloway GJ, Taylor DJ, et al: First year of experience with P-31 magnetic resonance studies of human liver. Magn Reson Imaging 4:413, 1986.
12. Blackledge MJ, Oberhaensli RD, Styles P, Radda GK: Measurement of in vivo ^{31}P relaxation rates and spectral editing in human organs using rotating-frame depth selection. J Magn Reson 71:331, 1987.
13. Ordidge RJ, Connelly A, Lohman JAB: Image-selected in vivo spectroscopy (ISIS). A new technique for spatially selective NMR spectroscopy. J Magn Reson 66:283, 1986.
14. Segebarth C, Grivegnee A, Luyten PR, Den Hollander JA: ^{1}H image-guided localized ^{31}P MR spectroscopy of the human liver. Magn Reson Med Biol 1:7, 1988.
15. Meyerhoff DJ, Karczmar GS, Matson GB, et al: Non-invasive quantitation of human liver metabolites

using image-guided ^{31}P magnetic resonance spectroscopy. NMR Biomed 3:17, 1990.
16. Meyerhoff DJ, Boska MD, Thomas AM, Weiner MW: Alcoholic liver disease: Quantitative image-guided P-31 MR spectroscopy. Radiology 173:393, 1989.
17. Maudsley AA, Hilal SK, Perman WH, Simon HE: Spatially resolved high resolution spectroscopy by "four-dimensional" NMR. J Magn Reson 51:147, 1983.
18. Brown TR, Kincaid BM, Ugurbil K: NMR chemical shift imaging in three dimensions. Proc Natl Acad Sci USA 79:3252, 1982.
19. Twieg D, Meyerhoff DJ, Hubesch B, et al: Localized phosphorus-31 MRS in humans by spectroscopic imaging. Magn Reson Med 12:291, 1989.
20. Maudsley AA, Twieg DB, Sappey-Marinier DS, et al: Spin echo ^{31}P spectroscopic imaging in the human brain. Magn Reson Med 14:415, 1990.
21. Bailes DR, Bryant DJ, Bydder GM, et al: Localized phosphorus-31 NMR spectroscopy of normal and pathological human organs in vivo using phase-encoding techniques. J Magn Reson 74:158, 1987.
22. Cox IJ, Bryant DJ, Collins AG, et al: Four-dimensional chemical shift MR imaging of phosphorus metabolites of normal and diseased human liver. J Comp Assist Tomogr 12:369, 1988.
23. Meyerhoff DJ, Maudsley AA, Twieg DB, Weiner MW: Phosphorus metabolite mapping of human heart, liver, and kidney by surface coil spectroscopic imaging (abstract). Soc Magn Reson Med 1:140, 1990.
24. Radda G, Oberhaensli RD, Taylor DJ: The biochemistry of human diseases as studied by ^{31}P NMR in man and animal models. Ann NY Acad Sci 508:300, 1987.
25. Ross BD: The current state of clinical magnetic resonance spectroscopy with phosphorus-31: A view from Hammersmith. Magn Reson Med Biol 1:81, 1988.
26. Meyerhoff DJ, Weiner MW: Magnetic resonance spectroscopy of the liver, in Margulis A, Burhenne HJ (eds): Alimentary Tract Radiology, 4th ed. St. Louis, Mosby, 1989.
27. Maris JM, Evans AE, McLaughlin AC, et al: ^{31}P nuclear magnetic resonance spectroscopic investigation of human neuroblastoma in situ. N Engl J Med 312:1500, 1985.
28. Chance B, Northrop J: How MR spectroscopy is deployed depends upon intended goals. Diagn Imaging 11:311, 1986.
29. Oberhaensli RD, Hilton-Jones D, Bore PJ, et al: Biochemical investigation of human tumours in vivo with phosphorus-31 magnetic resonance spectroscopy. Lancet 5:8, 1986.
30. Oberhaensli RD, Rajagopalan B, Taylor DJ, Radda GK: Study of hereditary fructose intolerance by use of ^{31}P magnetic resonance spectroscopy. Lancet 24:931, 1987.
31. Terrier F, Vock P, Cotting J, et al: Effect of intravenous fructose on the P-31 spectrum of the liver: Dose response in healthy volunteers. Radiology 171:557, 1989.
32. Wolf W, Albright MJ, Silver MS, et al: Fluorine-19 NMR spectroscopic studies of the metabolism of 5-fluorouracil in the liver of patients undergoing chemotherapy. Magn Reson Imaging 5:165, 1987.
33. Semmler W, Bachert-Baumann P, Gueckel F, et al: Real-time follow-up of 5-fluorouracil metabolism in the liver of tumor patients by means of F-19 MR spectroscopy. Radiology 174:141, 1990.
34. Thulborn KR, Ackerman JJH: Absolute molar concentrations by NMR in inhomogeneous B_1. J Magn Reson 55:357, 1983.
35. Tofts PS: The noninvasive measurement of metabolite concentrations in vivo using surface coil NMR spectroscopy. J Magn Reson 80:84, 1988.
36. Roth K, Hubesch B, Meyerhoff DJ, et al: Noninvasive quantitation of phosphorous metabolites in human tissue by NMR spectroscopy. J Magn Reson 81:299, 1988.
37. Weiner MW, Hetherington H, Hubesch B, et al: Clinical magnetic resonance spectroscopy of brain, heart, liver, kidney, and cancer: A quantitative approach. NMR Biomed 2:290, 1989.
38. Murphy E, Gabel SA, Funk A, London RE: NMR observability of ATP: Preferential depletion of cytosolic ATP during ischemia in perfused rat liver. Biochemistry 27:526, 1988.
39. Cohen SM, Ogawa S, Rottenberg H, et al: ^{31}P nuclear magnetic resonance studies of isolated rat liver cells. Nature 273:554, 1978.
40. Iles RA, Stevens AN, Griffiths JR, Morris PC: Phosphorylation status of liver by ^{31}P-NMR spectroscopy, and its implications for metabolic control. Biochem J 229:141, 1985.
41. Luyten PR, Brutnik G, Sloff FM, et al: Broadband proton decoupling in human 31P NMR spectroscopy. NMR Biomed 1:177, 1989.
42. Bode JC, Zelder O, Rumpelt, HJ, Wittkamp U: Depletion of liver adenosine phosphates and metabolic effects of intravenous infusion of fructose or sorbitol in man and in the rat. Eur J Clin Invest 3:436, 1973.
43. Hultman E, Nilsson LH, Sahlin K: Adenine nucleotide content of human liver. Normal values and fructose-induced depletion. Scand J Clin Lab Invest 35:245, 1975.

44. Ban N, Moriyasu F, Tamada T, et al: In vivo P-31 MR spectroscopic studies of liver in normal adults and cirrhotic patients (abstract). Radiol Soc North Am 1:340, 1986.
45. Naruse S, Tanaka C, Horikawa Y, et al: Clinical study of the hepatic energy metabolism in cirrhotics using localized ^{31}P MRS (abstract). Soc Magn Reson Med 1:319, 1988.
46. Angus PW, Dixon RM, Rajagopalan B, et al: A study of patients with alcoholic liver disease by ^{31}P nuclear magnetic resonance spectroscopy. Clin Sci 78:33, 1990.
47. The Clinical NMR Group: Magnetic resonance imaging of parenchymal liver disease: a comparison with ultrasound, radionuclide scintigraphy and x-ray computed tomography. Clin Radiol 38:495, 1987.
48. Schuldiner S, Rozengurt E: Na$^+$/H$^+$ antiport in Swiss 3T3 cells: Mitogenic stimulation leads to cytoplasmic alkalinization. Proc Natl Acad Sci USA 79:7778, 1982.
49. Haussinger D, Gerok W, Sies H: The effect of urea synthesis on extracellular pH in isolated perfused rat liver. Biochem J 236:261, 1986.
50. Oster JR, Perez GO: Acid-base disturbances in liver disease. J Hepatol 2:299, 1986.
51. Steen GR: Response of solid tumors to chemotherapy monitored by in vivo ^{31}P nuclear magnetic resonance spectroscopy: A review. Cancer Res 49:4075, 1989.
52. Maris JM, Chance B: Magnetic resonance spectroscopy of neoplasm, in Kressel HJ (ed): Magnetic Resonance Annual. New York, Raven Press, 1986, p 213.
53. Meyerhoff DJ, Karczmar GS, Venook AP, et al: Effects of chemoembolization on human hepatic cancers monitored by ^{31}P ISIS spectroscopy (abstract). Soc Magn Reson Med 1:318, 1990.

35

Metabolic Liver Disease Observed Through MRS: Hepatic Encephalopathy

BRIAN D. ROSS

Biochemistry of the liver, an understanding of which would greatly aid in diagnosis by clinical magnetic resonance spectroscopy (MRS), is diverse and covers many metabolic pathways. The major biosynthetic pathways—glycogen synthesis, gluconeogenesis, and lipid and urea synthesis—require ATP. Each is the target of a number of single enzyme defects in inborn errors of metabolism. Energy metabolism, however, which in the liver involves oxidative phosphorylation, ATP and ADP, but not creatine kinase or phosphocreatine (PCr), is rather well conserved in disease, leaving the concentration of ATP, that is, [ATP], relatively unchanged.

In this chapter, the present contribution of ^{31}P MRS to the understanding of metabolic liver disease will be discussed. Cirrhosis and hepatic encephalopathy (HE) will be discussed in more detail.

TECHNIQUES

MRS of the liver has proved relatively easy to perform (see Chap. 34) (Fig. 35-1). The larger voxels of MRS examinations, characteristically 2 cm^3, appear to make it almost insensitive to respiratory motion artifacts.

Surface coils are generally used, but body coils appear even more effective. T_1 relaxation values for hepatic metabolites are typically 30 percent of those found in other organs, so that the use of short TRs is appropriate.

Quantification and pH Determination

I believe it will be essential to give quantitative information in MRS examinations; the method illustrated in Figure 35-2 yields the desired result. T_1 variations as well as unrecognized changes in the sample (liver cell) volume also should be taken into account. pH cannot be determined by chemical shift of Pi (inorganic phosphate) compared with an internal reference, since PCr is absent from the liver. The external standard MDP

The work discussed here was performed at Hammersmith (RPMS) and Royal Free Hospitals, London, with the participation of Drs. Kathleen Hawley, Marcia Morgan (RFH), Humphrey Hodgson, and David Robinson (RPMS); at the University of California, San Francisco Liver Unit (Drs. John P. Roberts and Nathan Bass); and at Huntington Hospital (Dr. Myron Tong).

Clinical MRS studies were performed with Dr. Ian Young (Picker 1.6-Tesla prototype; RPMS); Drs. James Tropp, Kevin Derby and Christine Hawryszko (2.0-Tesla; formerly Diasonics Corp., San Franciso; now Toshiba Corp.); Drs. Peter Luyten and Jan den Hollander at Philips, Best (1.5-Tesla); and at Huntington Medical Research Institutes (GE Signa, 1.5-Tesla), where we acknowledge the generous support of the L. K. Whittier Foundation.

I am most grateful to my colleagues at HMRI; Dr. Roland Kreis (Boswell Fellow of California Institute of Technology), Neil Farrow, and Dr. Vasanthan Rajanayagam.

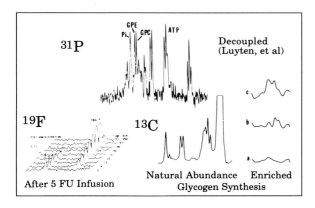

FIGURE 35-1
Multinuclear NMR for human liver studies.

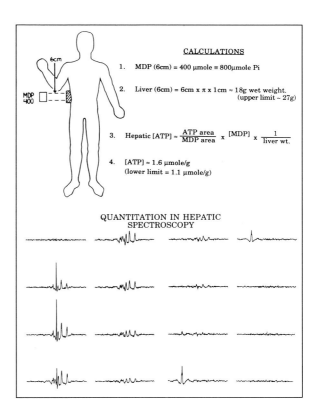

FIGURE 35-2
Quantitation in hepatic spectroscopy.

offers an acceptable alternative to comparison of P_i shift with α- or γ-ATP.

Normal ^{31}P MRS of Human Liver

Metabolite ratios of normal liver vary, with some minor discrepancies between groups and between methods (Table 35-1). Remarkable spectral resolution can be achieved despite the known large accumulation of paramagnetics in the liver. At 1.6 Tesla, 13 or 14 metabolites are resolved in vivo (Fig. 35-3). In addition to three coupled resonances of ATP and inorganic phosphate, ADP and total pyridine nucleotide (NAD + NADH + NADP + NADPH) are partially resolved in the region of the alpha peak. Uridine diphosphoglucose (UDPG), an important reactant in glycogen synthesis and in bilirubin conjugation, can be identified. Intracellular pH is 7.20, indicating intracellular $[HCO_3^-]$ to be less than 20 mM. From the position of the alpha and beta ATP resonances, and the J-coupling observed, intracellular free magnesium, that is, $[Mg^{2+}]$, of liver may be estimated (1).

The phosphomonoester (PME $\approx$ 5 to 6 ppm) region of the spectrum includes many of the intermediates of glycogenolysis, glycolysis, and gluconeogenesis, but it is impossible in this in vivo spectrum to identify them with certainty. Here also are the metabolites of lipid biosynthesis, phosphocholine (PC) and phosphoethanolamine (PE), compounds that assume some significance in hepatic encephalopathy (HE).

TABLE 35-1. *Metabolites of Normal Human Liver*

	Study		
	1 (N = 11)	2[†] (N = 6)	3 (N = 7)
PME/ATP	0.43 ± 0.06	0.7 ± 0.2	0.37 ± 0.07
P_i/ATP	0.72 ± 0.11	0.9 ± 0.1	0.45 ± 0.06
pH	7.24 ± 0.07	—	7.14[‡] ± 0.08
PME/PDE	—	0.6 ± 0.1	—
[ATP]	—	2.0 ± 0.1	—
[PME]	—	1.1 ± 0.2	—
[PDE]	—	5.6 ± 0.9	—
[P_i]	—	2.4 ± 0.2	1.03 ± 0.14

TABLE 35-2. *Metabolic Abnormalities in Liver Disease (^{31}P)*

	[ATP]	PME	[P$_i$]	pH	PDE	Line Width	Reference	Comments
Acute hepatitis	(N)	▲	—	—	—	—	1	Viral or alcoholic
Biliary cirrhosis	(N)	—	—	▲	—	—	1	—
Hemochromatosis	(N)	—	—	—	—	▲	1	MRI better
Cirrhosis	▼	N	▼	—	—	—	2	—
Acute hepatitis	▼	▲	—	—	—	—	2	Alcoholic
Sclerosing cholangitis (1)	—	▲	—	—	—	—	3	—
Caroli syndrome (1)	—	▲	—	—	—	—	3	—
Secondary cancer, medullary (1)	—	N	—	—	▲	—	3	—
Carcinoid syndrome (1)	—	▲	—	—	—	—	4	—
Cirrhosis (7)	(▼)	▲	—	—	—	—	3	PME − ve or PME + ve

In the phosphodiester region are glycerophosphoryl choline and glycerophosphoryl ethanolamine (GPC and GPE), intermediates in lipid metabolism. These important metabolites have been resolved in vivo by decoupling ^{1}H and ^{31}P signals (Fig. 35-1).

What Is the "Free" Intrahepatic ADP Concentration? [ADP] probably regulates the entire electron-transport–related mitochondrial oxidative phosphorylation and, through it, the hepatic [ATP] and ATP-synthesis rate.

With the advent of ^{31}P MRS, we know intrahepatic [ADP] to be only 40 micromolar. How this was achieved represents a study of great ingenuity, carried out in transgeneic mice by Koretsky and colleagues (2). By introducing creatine kinase (and feeding creatine) into a tissue that does not normally possess this enzyme, PCr was formed and assayed, together with ATP and pH, by ^{31}P MRS. From the resultant enzyme equilibria, hepatic free [ADP] can be calculated to be in the same range as that established by ^{31}P MRS for skeletal muscle, heart, and brain (3). This value should probably replace the often quoted hepatic [ADP] of ~2 mM from enzymatic analysis and the even more approximate value of ~0.5 mM from direct ^{31}P MRS on human liver. Unfortunately, this leaves us, for the present, without a means of accurately determining human hepatic [ADP].

Pathology
Despite considerable abnormality in ^{31}P spectra in pathologic conditions (Table 35-2 and Fig. 35-4), there is little evidence of a disease-specific spectrum. Increased PME concentration, the most common abnormality, includes a change in one or more of the three components observed in the best-resolved spectrum (Fig. 35-1) and in any or all of the glycolytic intermediates.

Enhancing the Diagnostic Precision of ^{31}P MRS of the Liver by Metabolic Imaging
A significant improvement derives from the complete spatial localization of metabolism across the liver (spectroscopic imaging) (Fig. 35-5). Elevated PME, a nonspecific finding, is confined to regions of the liver where duct proliferation is occurring or where secondary neoplasms are present. By extension, it may be possible to reclassify cirrhosis as PME + (positive) and PME − (negative) (see Fig. 35-4) if the disease is more localized.

^{31}P MRS of Cirrhosis
   The Origins of Metabolic Alkalosis. Metabolic alkalosis is a feature of cirrhosis with plasma bicarbonate > 29 mM and pH > 7.46. A current view places the liver as a critical player in acid-base homeostasis by virtue of the consumption of HCO_3^- in urea synthesis (4):

$$2NH_4^+ + 2HCO_3^- \rightarrow urea + CO_2 + 3H_2O \qquad (35\text{-}1)$$

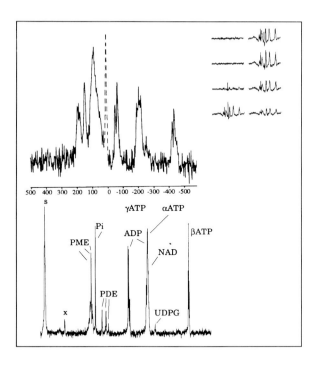

FIGURE 35-3
Resolution in a liver spectrum.

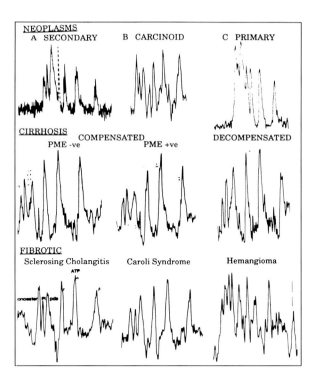

FIGURE 35-4
Pathology of the liver.

Conversely, extracellular and intracellular acidosis markedly inhibit urea synthesis in vitro (5). Thus the determination of intracellular hepatic pH may clarify the mechanism of alkalosis in patients with cirrhosis.

Oberhaensli et al. (6) established the intracellular pH of the cirrhotic liver in vivo, from ^{31}P MRS, to be 7.48 versus 7.24 for normal subjects. However, intracellular pH of the brain in cirrhotics with an alkaline intrahepatic pH is within normal limits, suggesting that the liver events are primary (7).

It appears most likely, therefore, that the systemic alkalosis of cirrhosis is a consequence of the intrinsic loss of urea-synthesis enzymes and may be in part adaptive, an attempt to maximize ammonia detoxification and urea synthesis in the residual liver.

The Failure of Urea Synthesis. Although it is rare to detect hyperammonemia in uncomplicated cirrhosis, urea synthesis is certainly impaired. In a cirrhotic liver biopsy, the urea synthesis rate is reduced as much as 85 percent (4). The urea cycle has a significant requirement for ATP:

$$2NH_3 + CO_2 + 3ATP \rightarrow urea + 2ADP + AMP + PPi + 2Pi \tag{35-2}$$

constituting

(a) $H_2O + CO_2 + NH_3 \xrightarrow{2ATP\ 2ADP + P_i} NH_2-\overset{O}{\underset{\|}{C}}-ONP$
carbamoyl phosphate

(b) Citrulline + aspartate $\xrightarrow{ATP\ AMP + PP_i}$ argininosuccinate

so that it is possible that either reduction in [ATP] or ATP supply from oxidative phosphorylation may contribute to failure of urea synthesis.

^{31}P MRS of the liver in cirrhotic patients from many centers indicates a normal appearance of the ATP/Pi ratio and that PME (which includes AMP) is normal or elevated (Table 35-2). We might assume, therefore, that hepatic energy failure in cirrhosis is unlikely.

This is incorrect. Weiner's group (8) was the first to publish quantitative ^{31}P MRS results of [ATP] in the human liver. A significant reduction in total hepatic [ATP] was detected in the cirrhotic

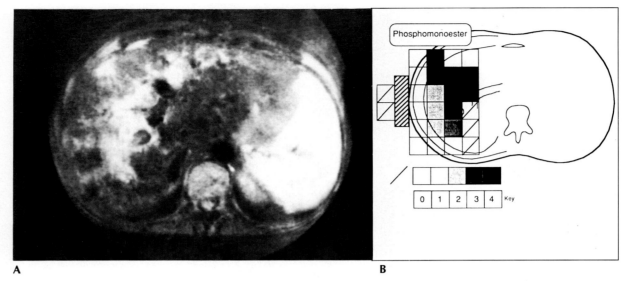

FIGURE 35-5
Imaging of metabolites.

liver (Table 35-2). The K_m of ATP for carbamoyl phosphate synthetase $\approx$ 1mM [in rat liver (9) and personal communication], while the normal [ATP] in healthy human liver lies around 2 mM. As little as a 50 percent reduction in [ATP] could therefore seriously impair urea synthesis and lead to ammonia toxicity.

Control of Intrahepatic [ATP]

[ATP] or the ratio ATP/ADP reflects the redox state of the liver; embolization of a tumor or hemangioma has been shown to reduce [ATP] and increase Pi.

The rate of ATP synthesis might limit the rate of urea synthesis even in the normal human liver. Alanine given IV stimulates urea synthesis. Depending on which pathway (oxidative phosphorylation or the urea cycle) fails first, the infusion of alanine could result in a fall in hepatic [ATP] in the diseased liver. In normal liver (Fig. 35-6), a fall in P_i and a parallel increase in PME is observed, but [ATP] is not markedly reduced.

Hepatic phosphorylation of fructose or sorbitol, administered in the older formulations of parenteral feed solutions, was regularly accompanied by a serious hypophosphatemia. Using ^{31}P MRS, the causative intrahepatic events have been demonstrated in normal volunteers (10).

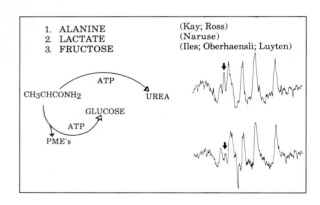

FIGURE 35-6
Metabolic stress tests. Physiologic (alanine/lactate) or pathologic ATP consumption.

Shortly after fructose administration, hepatic [ATP] and P_i fell, and the "missing" phosphate was accounted for almost quantitatively as PME, i.e., fructose-6-phosphate. MR spectroscopists have sometimes advocated fructose loading as a clinical test of liver function. Except in the rare instance of hereditary fructose intolerance and the detection of carriers, fructose-loading is unlikely to be a useful test and might even be risky.

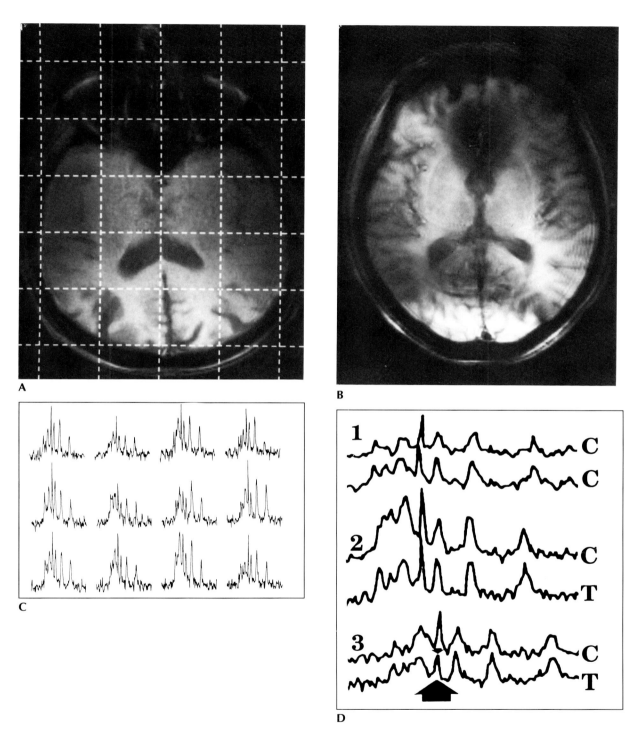

FIGURE 35-7
MRI and ^{31}P spectroscopic imaging of three patients with chronic HE. (A,B) Axial images showing voxel dimensions for ^{31}P images. (C) Complete data set from single slice of ^{31}P chemical shift image. (D) Representative pairs of spectra (C = cortex; T = "thalamus") for three patients. Patient 3 is referred to in the text.

MRI Techniques in Hepatic Encephalopathy
Because there is no completely appropriate animal model of hepatic encephalopathy (HE), the mechanism of this syndrome remains unclear. MRI demonstrates two somewhat surprising features:

1. Cerebral atrophy, quantitated by an increase in the width of sulci and by an increased ventricular width in coronal section, has been sporadically observed (11) and now has been systematically documented by Zeneroli and her colleagues (12).
2. Hyperintensity in the globus pallidus on T_1 weighted images is reported in liver failure in patients with acute (13) or chronic HE (14). The significance of these changes and their temporal association with the development of HE are at present unknown.

Energy Metabolism. Our earliest results in patients with chronic HE by ^{31}P MRS revealed a statistically significant reduction in [P_i] in the frontal cortex, but no consistent change in [ATP] or [PCr] (7). Poor localization may have influenced the results, since, as we now know, the volume of frontal cortex is reduced by cerebral atrophy. No reduction in [PCr] or [ATP] of the parietal cortex was found by den Hollander and colleagues (15). On the other hand, one of three patients with chronic HE requiring liver transplantation studied by Roberts and colleagues (16) using a spectroscopic imaging technique showed a significant reduction in cerebral [PCr] (Fig. 35-7), most marked in the "thalamus." This patient died before transplant could be performed, while the remaining two subjects, with normal cerebral [PCr], survived.

Phospholipid Composition. Ross et al. (7) noted, but could not explain, a shift in the mean resonant frequency of PME in chronic HE from 6.6 to 6.3 ppm. Now with the much improved resolution of cerebral ^{31}P MRS (15), it is clear that this is the result of increased cerebral phosphoryl choline (PC) ($\sigma = 6.3$ ppm), relative to phosphoethanolamine (PE) ($\sigma \approx 6.6$ ppm) (Fig. 35-8).

Neurotransmitter Function. Many neurotransmitters have been implicated in HE. With ^{1}H MRS, glutamine, glutamate, and possibly GABA can be noninvasively assayed (17). [With ^{15}N MRS, we can currently detect all three unequivocally in ex vivo rat brain (18,19).] In patients with

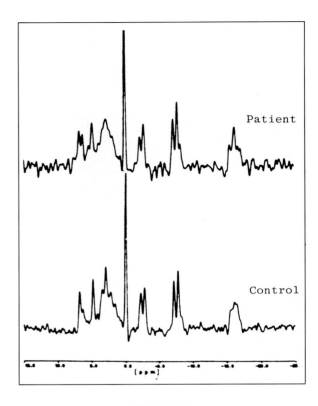

FIGURE 35-8
^{1}H decoupled ^{31}P NMR spectra of a volunteer and of a patient.

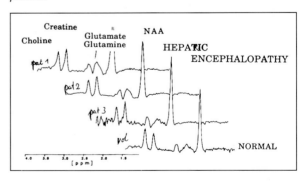

FIGURE 35-9
^{1}H spectra of human brain.

chronic HE, cerebral glutamine concentration was elevated (15) (Fig. 35-9). Using a shorter echo time of 30 ms, we confirmed this observation (20). In addition, these patients ($n = 9$) lacked a resonance at 3.6 ppm. This resonance has been attributed to "phosphoinositols" (17) and may indicate the involvement in chronic HE of yet another family of neurotransmitters, the inositolphosphates.

CONCLUSIONS

1. In cirrhosis, intrahepatic [ATP] is reduced. This may contribute to hyperammonemia and HE by inhibition of urea synthesis.
2. Cerebral energy metabolism is abnormal in chronic HE, but a fall in [PCr] may be a rare, serious sign.
3. Structural changes in the brain, together with abnormalities in phospholipid content are markers of chronic HE.
4. Cerebral neurotransmitter content is abnormal in patients with chronic HE.

Metabolic disorders associated with liver disease invite multiorgan studies with multinuclear MRS.

REFERENCES

1. Malloy C, Cunningham C, Radda G: The metabolic state of the rat liver in vivo measured by ^{31}P NMR spectroscopy. Biochim Biophys Acta 885:1, 1986.
2. Koretsky A, Brosnan M, Chen L, et al: Expression of creatine kinase in the livers of transgenic mice: in vivo detection by ^{31}P NMR (abstract). Magn Reson Med 1:258, 1989.
3. Veech R, Lawson J, Cornell N, Krebs H: Cytosolic phosphorylation potential. J Biol Chem 254:6538, 1979.
4. Häussinger D, Steeb R, Gerok W: Ammonium and bicarbonate homeostasis in chronic liver disease. Klin Wochenschr 68:175, 1990.
5. Oliver J, Bourke E: Adaptations in urea and ammonium excretion in metabolic acidosis in the rat: A reinterpretation. Clin Sci Mol Med 48:515, 1975.
6. Oberhaensli R, Rajagopalan B, Taylor D, Radda G: Assessment of human liver disease by P-31 magnetic resonance spectroscopy (abstract). Clin Sci 73:82P, 1987.
7. Ross B, Morgan M, Cox I, et al: Cerebral energy deficit in patients with chronic hepatic encephalopathy monitoring with ^{31}P MRS. J Cereb Blood Flow Metab 7:5396, 1987.
8. Meyerhoff D, Boska M, Thomas A, Weiner M: Quantitative image-guided ^{31}P magnetic resonance spectroscopy of alcoholic liver disease. Radiology 173:393, 1989.
9. Cohen N, Kyan F, Kyan S, et al: The apparent K_m of ammonia for carbamoyl phosphate synthetase (ammonia) in situ. Biochem J 229:205, 1985.
10. Oberhaensli RD, Galloway GJ, Taylor DJ, Bore PJ, Radda GK: Assessment of human liver metabolism by phosphorus-31 magnetic resonance spectroscopy. Brit J Radiol 59:695, 1986.
11. Ross B, Roberts J, Tropp J, et al: Phosphorus imaging of brain in HE (abstract). Magn Reson Imaging 7:82, 1989.
12. Zeneroli M, Cioni A, Vezzelli C, et al: Prevalence of brain atrophy in liver cirrhosis patients with chronic persistent encephalopathy. J Hepatol 4:283, 1987.
13. McConnell JR, Castaldo P: (abstract), Striatal hyperemia, transient liver failure and chorea after liver transplantation (LTx). J Hepatology 10(1):S 16, 1990.
14. Zeneroli M, Cioni G, Vezzelli C, Crisi G, Ventura E: (abstract), Brain magnetic resonance imaging in liver cirrhosis patients with encephalopathy. J Hepatology 10(1):S 26, 1990.
15. Luyten P, den Hollander J, Bovée W, et al: ^{31}P and ^{1}H NMR spectroscopy of the human brain in chronic hepatic encephalopathy (abstract). Magn Reson Med 1:375, 1989.
16. Ross B, Tropp J, Roberts J, et al: ^{31}P spectroscopic imaging of the brain shows energy deficit of thalamus in chronic hepatic encephalopathy (abstract). Magn Reson Med 1:465, 1989.
17. Frähm J, Michaelis T, Merboldt K-D, et al: Localized NMR spectroscopy in vivo: Progress and problems. NMR Biomed 2:188, 1988.
18. Farrow N, Kanamori K, Ross BD, Parivar F: A 15-N NMR study of cerebral, hepatic and renal nitrogen metabolism in hyperammonemic rats. Biochem J 270:473, 1990.
19. Kanamori K, Ross B, Farrow N, Parivar F: An N-15 NMR study of isolated brain in portacaval shunted rats after acute hyperammonemia. Biochem J (in press).
20. Kreis R, Farrow N, Ross B. Diagnosis of hepatic encephalopathy by cerebral ^{1}H magnetic resonance spectroscopy (letter). Lancet Oct 1990 (in press).

XI. DIFFUSE LIVER DISEASES

36

Hepatitis, Fatty Liver, and Cirrhosis

YUJI ITAI and
KUNI OHTOMO

HEPATITIS

Hepatitis is not a good candidate for liver imaging in most cases. However, severe or fulminant hepatitis and subacute hepatitis may give rise to extensive necrosis, which appears as mottled or localized low-density areas on the plain CT (1,2). The extent of fulminant hepatitis is believed to correlate with the prognosis of the disease. If the patients survive, regenerating nodules of varying size are formed and necrotic areas are changed into scarred zones. Scarred zones may be noted in only one lobe, giving a classic postnecrotic scarred liver appearance, but may also be segmental or masslike (Fig. 36-1), radiating or reticular. CT follow-up may clarify discrepancy between larger size of regenerating nodules and decreased size of the necrotic zone (3). Postnecrotic scar is an example of hyperdense or hypodense hepatic zones not corresponding to mass lesions on CT.

Radiation hepatitis is another example of this entity, but it is easily diagnosed by its geometric distribution as well as history of radiation (4). Affected areas also show hypodensity, which disappears after contrast enhancement.

MRI has a similar sensitivity as CT in the diseases just mentioned and shows hyperintensity on T2-weighted images instead of hypodensity on plain CT (1).

FATTY LIVER

Fatty infiltration of the liver may occur evenly or unevenly in distribution and/or degree. Fat-infiltrated areas appear hyperechoic on US, hypodense on CT, and hyperintense on T1-weighted MRI. Ultrasound is sensitive in detection but essentially nonspecific in characterization. CT is less sensitive but more specific compared with US. MRI using conventional spin-echo technique is less sensitive and nonspecific than CT. However, applying proton spectroscopic imaging, MRI is as sensitive and specific as CT in the detection and characterization of fat (5). Semiquantitative analysis is also possible (6). Short TI inversion recovery is also useful in identifying the presence of fat (7). In classic hepatic steatosis, the whole liver is homogeneously affected. However, the degree of fatty infiltration may differ greatly site by site and may be limited to particular area(s) either anatomically or nonanatomically (8).

Anatomic distribution of fat infiltration may be lobar, segmental, subsegmental, or combined. In these cases of moderate to mild degree, local pa-

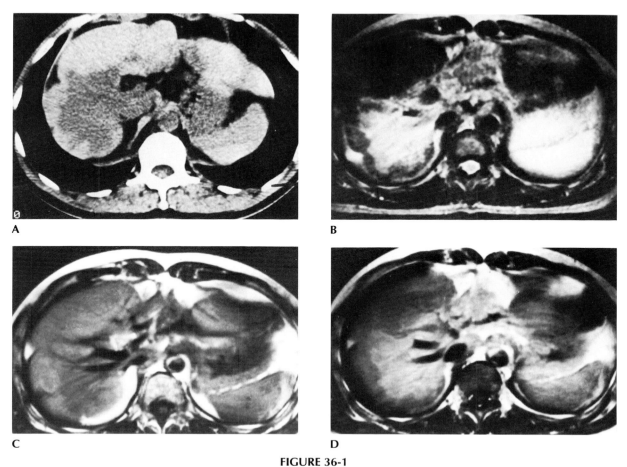

FIGURE 36-1
Postnecrotic scar (subacute hepatitis). (A) *Plain CT reveals a large hypodense area in the right lobe, which disappears after contrast enhancement.* (B) *MRI (T2-weighted image) depicts a hyperdense area. Hypointense area on T1-weighted image* (C) *becomes hyperintense 10 min after injection of Gd-DTPA* (D). *Within the hyperintense area two veins are clearly noted and tumor is excluded.*

renchymal density alterations induced by portal obstruction or cases of hepatic infarction should be distinguished (9,10). Patency of portal veins (absence of tumor thrombus or compression) as well as absence of arterioportal shunts suggest the diagnosis of fatty liver (11).

Nonanatomic distribution of fat may be totally irregular ("irregular" fatty liver) (12), focally noted ("focal" fatty liver; Fig. 36-2) (13,14), or focally lacking in diffuse involvement ("focally spared" fatty liver) (15,16).

In the differentiation of focal fat from hepatic tumor, absence of mass effect and/or normal distribution of intrahepatic vessels is of importance in irregular fatty liver and can be easily demonstrated by incremental dynamic CT, US, and MRI.

However, a focal fatty liver may be too small in size to reveal the findings just mentioned and can simulate hepatic mass(es). The following points are essential clues leading to a correct diagnosis: (1) masslike lesion consisting of abundant fat, (2) vessels noted in the center of the mass by careful observation of US and/or CT enhanced with a large dose of contrast material, (3) the mass not

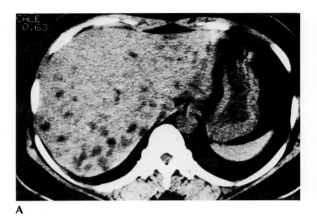
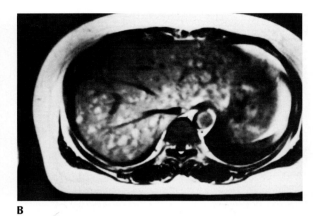

FIGURE 36-2
Focal fatty liver. There are a large number of hypodense masses on CT (A) and hyperintense nodules on T1-weighted MRI (B). (A, courtesy of Tokyo Medical College.)

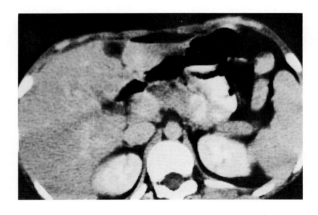

FIGURE 36-3
Focal fatty liver. A hypodense area is noted beneath hepatic surface near the falciform ligament.

being spherical and its contour interdigitating on US, and (4) favorite sites, such as adjacent to the falciform ligament (14) (Fig. 36-3) or near the gallbladder, especially in the presence of a solitary lesion. In focal fatty liver of mild degree, US detects hyperechoic masses, but CT and MRI may fail to detect them.

Focally spared fatty liver also appears as a hepatic mass on cross-sectional imaging (17). The following findings are usually noted, and a correct diagnosis can be suggested: (1) presence of diffuse fatty infiltration, (2) the lesion appears hypoechoic on US and hyperdense on CT, (3) favorite site, such as near the gallbladder or internal side of the lateral segment, and (4) nonspherical appearance on US.

LIVER CIRRHOSIS

Liver cirrhosis is characterized by the presence of regenerating nodules, unbalanced size of individual segments, widened fissures and hepatic hilum attenuated intrahepatic veins, prominent collateral veins, splenomegaly, and ascites. These findings are reflected on US, CT, and MRI to varying degrees.

The presence of regenerating nodules is a direct and confirmative finding for the diagnosis of liver cirrhosis. Regenerating nodules appear as innumerable tiny, hypoechoic, hyperdense, and hypointense nodules on US, CT, and MRI, respectively, when demonstrated.

Using high-frequency US probes, intraoperative or laparoscopic US can reveal regenerating nodules as many hypoechoic nodules with almost the same accuracy as gross specimen study (18). Recently, extracorporal US study has been shown to have an increasing chance of revealing similar findings. However, in most cases, the presence of regenerating nodules is indirectly confirmed by the demonstration of nodularity of the hepatic contour (19). This is possible also with CT,

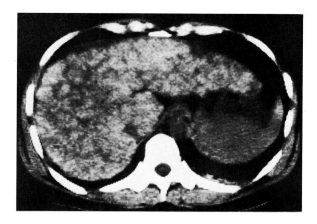

FIGURE 36-4
Regenerating nodules. A large number of hyperdense nodules are shown on plain CT.

but in lesser frequency. Although regenerating nodules are rarely detected by CT, they appear as hyperdense nodules and are more clearly shown on plain CT (Fig. 36-4).

MRI not infrequently demonstrates a large number of tiny nodules in cirrhotic livers (Figs. 36-5 and 36-6). We have suggested such nodules might reflect regenerating nodules (20), since (1) they are detected in patients with liver cirrhosis alone, where US and/or CT often reveal nodularity of the hepatic contour, (2) the size of nodules demonstrated is roughly the same as that of regenerating nodules classified by laparoscopy or surgical specimens, (3) liver tumors appear as hyperintense on T2-weighted images, and (4) liver tumors of such size cannot be detected by MRI. These nodules are well demonstrated on T2-weighted images and/or gradient-echo images, but rarely on T1-weighted images (Fig. 36-7). They can be divided into two groups on the basis of their demonstrability on different pulse sequences (21):

1. Gradient echo detects lesions more clearly in contour and largely in number and size than T2-weighted spin-echo images (Figs. 36-5 and 36-7).
2. T2-weighted spin-echo images are superior in demonstration to gradient-echo images (Fig. 36-6).

Iron-deposits are suggested in group 1 by patterns of MRI imaging: Gamna-Gandy bodies of the spleen (iron-deposit nodules in portal hypertension) have similarly been shown on different pulse sequences (22), and nodules are demonstrated to be larger on gradient echo with longer TEs than on gradient echoes with shorter TEs (23). Histologically, nodules of group 1 have been

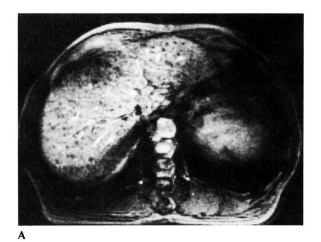
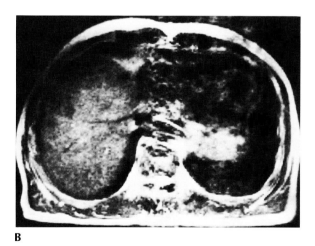

FIGURE 36-5
Regenerating nodules. Gradient-echo image (FLASH 19/12, 90 degrees) reveals a large number of tiny hypointense nodules (A), whereas T-2 weighted spin-echo image does not (B).

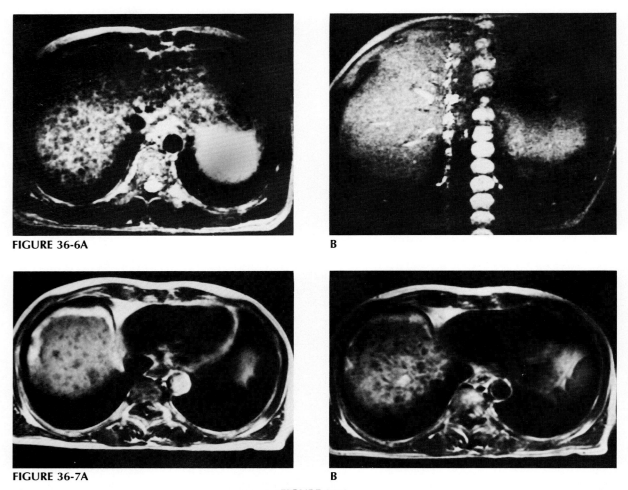

FIGURE 36-6
Regenerating nodules. A large number of hypointense nodules are represented on T-2 weighted spin echo image (A), but a small number of hypointense nodules are equivocally shown on gradient-echo image (B).

FIGURE 36-7
Regenerating nodules. Infrequently, regenerating nodules are clearly shown on T1-weighted spin echo image (A). In such cases, regenerating nodules are more clearly shown on proton-density image (B) and gradient-echo image than T2-weighted image (not shown).

proven to have Prussian-blue-staining iron, and those of group 2 lack iron in pathologic-imaging correlation studies (21). Pathologic states of group 2 have not been clarified as yet. One possibility is the relative hyperintensity of Glisson's sheath on T2-weighted images owing to inflammation, congestion, or hypervascularity therein (21,24) (Fig. 36-8). However, this phenomenon is not necessarily noted in all cases.

It is clinically useful to recall that a small hepatocellular carcinoma, either a primary or a daughter lesion, appears as hyperintense on T2-weighted images, while regenerating nodules are hypointense. Moreover, adenomatous hyperplastic nodules,

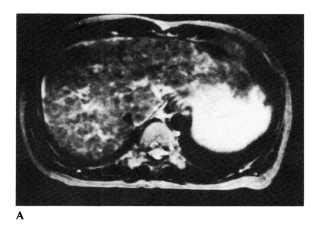
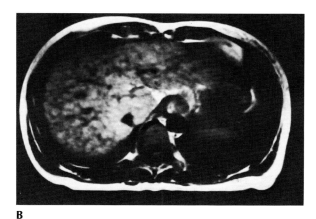

FIGURE 36-8
Regenerating nodules. (A) On T2-weighted image, hypointense nodules are visible partly because of presence of reticular hyperintense shadows. (B) On T1-weighted image, a large number of hyperintense nodules (larger in number and size compared with T2-weighted image) are represented. The same case as in Figure 36-4.

which are solitary or small in number, large in size, and difficult to differentiate from hepatocellular carcinoma, appear as hypointense on T2-weighted images and hyperintense on T1-weighted images (25).

As to other findings of liver cirrhosis, US usually detects the state of the hepatic surface, the edge of the hepatic contour, and the configuration of intrahepatic veins more sensitively, whereas CT depicts unbalance of individual segments and splenomegaly more objectively. Collateral veins developing in liver cirrhosis are well shown by any cross-sectional imaging. Direct angiography is the most accurate in detecting small collaterals. However, cross-sectional imaging compares well with arterial portography in detection and is superior in depicting the exact course and relationship with surrounding organs.

Intrahepatic portosystemic venous shunts are also directly shown in the cross-sectional modalities (26). The paraumbilical vein is one of the most common portosystemic shunts in portal hypertension, and it originates from the umbilical vein recess of the left portal vein. This collateral occasionally runs through the hepatic parenchyma (mostly the medial segment). This course had never been documented by angiography alone owing to its inability to clarify the relationship with the surrounding organs (27) (Fig. 36-9).

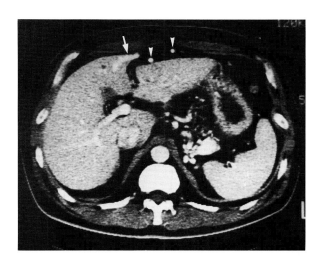

FIGURE 36-9
"Paraumbilical" vein running through the medial segment of the liver. An enhanced vessel (arrow) protrudes from the medial segment and connects with paraumbilical vein (arrowheads). (From Itai Y, Ohtomo K, Kokubo Y, et al: Portosystemic collaterals running through the medial segment of the liver connecting with the paraumbilical vein in portal hypertension. ROEFO 152:357, 1990. Reprinted by permission.)

Applying color Doppler ultrasound, Sugiura et al. found the paraumbilical vein in patients with liver cirrhosis to be more frequently noted than expected previously, and in two-thirds of cases the vein actually traversed the hepatic parenchyma (28). Other rare portosystemic venous shunts are increasingly reported with the advent and wide application of cross-sectional imaging.

REFERENCES

1. Itai Y, Ohtomo K, Kokubo T, et al: CT and MR imaging of postnecrotic liver scars. J Comput Assist Tomogr 12:971, 1988.
2. Ueno E: Magnetic resonance imaging of post massive hepatic necrosis: Comparison with CT and histological findings (abstract in English). Nippon Acta Radiol 48:1406, 1988.
3. Ishikawa N, Nakagawa S, Hirata K, et al: Long-term follow-up of hepatitis using computed tomography. J Computed Assist Tomogr 13:645, 1989.
4. Jefferey RB, Moss A, Quivey J, et al: CT of radiation-induced injury. AJR 135:445, 1980.
5. Heiken JP, Lee JKT, Dixon WA: Fatty infiltration of the liver: Evaluation by proton spectroscopic imaging. Radiology 157:707, 1985.
6. Ohtomo K, Yamada S, Aoyama H, et al.: Semiquantitative analysis of fatty liver using spectroscopic imaging by dephasing amplitude changing (SIDAC). Radiat Med 5:104, 1987.
7. Bydder GM, Steiner RE, Blumgart LH, et al: MR imaging of the liver using short TI inversion recovery sequences. J Comput Assist Tomogr 9:1084, 1985.
8. Halvorsen RA, Korobkin M, Ram PC, et al: CT appearance of focal fatty infiltration of the liver. AJR 139:277, 1982.
9. Nishikawa J, Itai Y, Tasaka A: Lobar attenuation difference of the liver on computed tomography. Radiology 141:725, 1981.
10. Doppman JL, Dwyer A, Vermess M, et al: Segmental hyperlucent defects in the liver. J Comput Assist Tomogr 8:50, 1984.
11. Itai Y, Furui S, Ohtomo K, et al: Dynamic CT features of arterioportal shunt in hepatocellular carcinoma. AJR 146:723, 1986.
12. Scott WW, Sanders RC, Siegelman SS: Irregular fatty infiltration of the liver: Diagnostic dilemmas. AJR 135:67, 1980.
13. Baker ME, Silverman PM: Nodular focal fatty infiltration of the liver: CT appearance. AJR 145:79, 1985.
14. Yoshikawa J, Matsui O, Takashima T, et al: Focal fatty change of the liver adjacent to the falciform ligament: CT and sonographic findings in the surgically confirmed cases. AJR 149:491, 1987.
15. White EM, Simeone JF, Mueller PR, et al: Focal periportal sparing in hepatic fatty infiltration: Cause of hepatic pseudomass on US. Radiology 162:57, 1987.
16. Arai K, Matsui O, Takashima T, et al: Focal spared areas in fatty liver caused by regional decreased portal flow. AJR 151:300, 1988.
17. Yates CK, Streight RA: Focal fatty infiltration of the liver simulating metastatic disease. Radiology 159:83, 1986.
18. Freeman MP, Vick CW, Taylor KJW, et al: Regenerating nodules in cirrhosis: Sonographic appearance with anatomic correlation. AJR 146:533, 1986.
19. DiLelio A, Cestavi C, Lowazzi A, Beretta L: Cirrhosis: Diagnosis with sonographic study of the liver surface. Radiology 172:389, 1989.
20. Itai Y, Ohnishi S, Ohtomo K, et al: Regenerating nodules of liver cirrhosis: MR imaging. Radiology 165:419, 1987.
21. Ohtomo K, Itai Y, Ohtomo Y, et al: Regenerating nodules of liver cirrhosis: MR imaging with pathologic correlation. AJR 154:505, 1990.
22. Minami M, Itai Y, Ohtomo K, et al: Siderotic nodules in the spleen: MR imaging of portal hypertension. Radiology 172:681, 1989.
23. Murakami T, Marukawa T, Kuroda C, et al: Siderotic regenerating nodules in liver cirrhosis: Evaluation by gradient echo (FLASH) imaging 1.5T (abstract in English). Nippon Acta Radiol 49:1427, 1989.
24. Maeda M, Kita K, Nakatani K, et al: MR imaging of liver cirrhosis: Study of image-histology-function relationship. Radiology 173:389, 1989.
25. Matsui O, Kadoya M, Kameyama T, et al: Adenomatous hyperplastic nodules in the cirrhotic liver: Differentiation from hepatocellular carcinoma with MR imaging. Radiology 173:123, 1989.
26. Mori H, Hayashi K, Fukuda T, et al: Intrahepatic portosystemic venous shunt: Occurrence in patients with and without liver cirrhosis. AJR 149:711, 1987.
27. Itai Y, Ohtomo K, Kokubo Y, et al: Portosystemic collaterals running through the medial segment of the liver connecting with the paraumbilical vein in portal hypertension. ROEFO 152:357, 1990.
28. Sugiura N, Karasawa E, Uzawa M, et al: Paraumbilical vein studied by color Doppler (Japanese). Jpn J Gastroenterol 87:645, 1990.

37

Iron Storage Diseases

J. P. KALTWASSER,
U. STRAUBE, and
R. GOTTSCHALK

The term *iron storage disease* describes a group of disorders in which a progressive increase in total-body iron stores results in deposition of iron in the parenchymal cells of the liver, heart, pancreas, and other organs causing tissue damage and functional insufficiency of the organs involved. The increase in total-body iron stores above the normal level results from *inappropriate high intestinal absorption* or *parenteral iron administration* or both.

Different approaches to iron overload as a histopathologic or clinical entity have led to some confusion in terminology. The histopathologic term *hemosiderosis* or *siderosis* is frequently used synonymously with the term *iron overload*. The term *hemochromatosis* is usually reserved for the condition of massive iron overload together with tissue damage (1).

Considering recent knowledge of the pathogenesis of the various iron storage diseases, the term *hereditary* or *genetic hemochromatosis* is used to separate the inherited (formerly called "idiopathic") form of hemochromatosis from the various acquired forms and includes the early preclinical stages of the disease with minor or no increase in body iron stores (2). Hereditary hemochromatosis is caused by an increased iron absorption inappropriate to the body iron stores due to a genetically determined error of iron metabolism, whereas *acquired or secondary hemochromatosis* may be associated with diseases characterized by ineffective erythropoiesis and red cell transfusion requirements or caused by very large amounts of soluble iron in the diet.

IRON STORAGE DISEASE

Hereditary (Genetic) Hemochromatosis

The familial nature of the former "idiopathic" hemochromatosis has been confirmed by the work of Simon and coworkers (3,4), who demonstrated that the iron-loading gene lay close to the HLA locus on the short arm of chromosome 6 and is inherited in an autosomal recessive fashion. The responsible gene(s) has not yet been localized precisely, but there is convincing evidence that the gene is associated with HLA-A3. The hemochromatosis gene is now recognized as probably one of the most common abnormal genes identified in populations of European extraction. For example, the frequency of the hemochromatosis allele has been estimated to be 5 to 7 percent in the United States, which is much higher than previously thought, suggesting that hemochromatosis often remains undiagnosed (5). HLA typing is of

This work was supported by grant G-33-042.2./87 from the German-Israeli Foundation for Scientific Research and Development. The support of the Siemens AG, Erlangen, in providing measurement facilities and assistance in obtaining MRI images is gratefully acknowledged.

no value in population screening because the HLA haplotypes linked to the hemochromatosis gene differ in different families. It may, however, be helpful within a family in which an affected individual has already been identified.

Owing to an inappropriately high food iron absorption and the very limited ability to excrete iron, a chronic progressive accumulation of storage iron resulting in a progressive and predominantly parenchymal cell overload is observed that constitutes the major phenotypic expression of the defective gene. When the iron burden exceeds the body's capacity for safe storage in the form of ferritin and hemosiderin, potentially life-threatening organ damage is the final consequence.

The course of the disease is variable and depends on such factors as sex, dietary iron intake, alcohol consumption, and physiologic (menstrual) blood loss. The disease is latent for many years. Most patients present with symptoms of diabetes, liver disease, hypogonadism, chondrocalcinosis, or heart failure between the ages of 40 and 50 years (1,6,7). Women usually present after menopause. Infrequently, clinical manifestation may occur earlier, in the second or third decades of life, primarily in the form of hypogonadism and cardiomyopathy (8). Once the disease is fully established, the total-body iron content usually has accumulated to 20 to 40 g (360 to 720 mmol). The liver is the first organ to be affected in most cases, and hepatomegaly is present in more than 95 percent of symptomatic patients (6). The major causes of death in patients homozygous for hereditary hemochromatosis are complications of liver cirrhosis and hepatocellular carcinoma. Patients with the greatest risk of death are those with the largest body iron burden (see also "Treatment and Prognosis of Iron Storage Diseases").

Secondary (Acquired) Hemochromatosis
Iron storage diseases due to secondary iron overload form a heterogeneous group of diseases. Iron stores may be increased by the oral intake of large amounts of iron over long periods of time despite a normal regulation of iron uptake, such as in the black population of southern Africa, who formerly ingested large amounts of iron in fermented alcoholic beverages.

Parenteral iron overload is nearly always due to treatment of refractory anemias, such as *thalassemia major*, *sideroblastic anemias*, and *aplastic anemia*. Each unit of blood adds about 225 mg iron to the body's reserve. Some of the refractory anemias (e.g., thalassemia major, sideroblastic anemias) have in common that their erythropoiesis is hypercellular but markedly *ineffective*. These patients tend to accumulate large amounts of iron through excessive food iron absorption.

Massive iron overload may be found in individuals with refractory anemias who have received few or no prior blood transfusions. A rare disorder causing iron overload is *atransferrinemia*, in which inadequate amounts of iron are delivered to the erythroid marrow and iron absorption is increased, presumably as a compensation for the defect in erythropoiesis (9,10). In diseases such as *aplastic anemia* or *pure red cell anemia*, where excess iron has been acquired parenterally by blood transfusion, reticuloendothelial iron excess is dominant and organ damage occurs late after more than 100 units of red cells. In cases where severe iron overload has been observed in association with disorders such as *hereditary spherocytosis* or other *hemolytic anemias*, it is likely that these patients were carriers of the hemochromatosis gene (11).

Iron stores are also often increased in patients with chronic liver disease (12). Hepatic iron concentrations in these patients rarely reach the levels seen in patients with hereditary hemochromatosis. A number of factors have been suggested as possible contributors of increased iron accumulation in patients with liver disease. These include increased oral iron intake (in alcoholic beverages), stimulation of iron absorption by alcohol, pancreatic insufficiency, and folic acid deficiency (13). A modest degree of iron overload (about 5 g) is also seen in patients with *porphyria cutanea tarda* (14). Iron appears to play a key role in this disease, since remission can be induced by venesection therapy (15). With advanced overload, iron deposition in secondary hemochromatosis is found in many organs, and the pattern of accumulation may resemble that seen in hereditary hemochromatosis.

METHODS FOR THE DETECTION OF IRON OVERLOAD

Because of its diffuse topographic distribution, quantitative determination of human iron stores poses significant obstacles. Accurate quantification of the total-body iron burden is possible only by relatively invasive and expensive procedures (Table 37-1). Detailed information on the amount and distribution of tissue iron in iron overload can be obtained from *biopsy specimens* of major iron storage organs such as the liver. Indirect measures such as *serum ferritin, transferrin iron saturation, chelate-induced urinary iron excretion,* or *intestinal iron absorption* may provide useful information on the amount of the body iron reserve. They do, however, all have important limitations in their diagnostic use for evaluating iron overload. Since detection of tissue iron overload at an early stage can help to prevent the detrimental consequences of unphysiologic increases of tissue iron, easily applicable and noninvasive techniques for the repeated direct assessment of total-body iron would be useful.

In the last decade, imaging techniques such as *computed tomography (CT)* and *magnetic resonance imaging (MRI)* as well as *magnetic susceptibility measurements* have been shown to provide noninvasive measures, mainly of hepatic iron content (2, 16–19).

In the following sections, a short description of the more traditional methods for the assessment and location of iron overload will be given, and special emphasis will be placed on recent progress in imaging techniques for the quantitative determination of tissue iron content.

Indirect Measures of Body Iron Stores

Transferrin Saturation. As body iron stores increase, a rise in *serum iron concentration* is observed [normal ranges in men: 100 ± 35 µg/dl (18 ± 6 µmol/liter); in women: 90 ± 40 µg/dl (16 ± 7 µmol/liter)]. *Transferrin,* expressed as *total iron-binding capacity (TIBC),* is low or normal [normal ranges in men: 350 ± 50 µg/dl (63 ± 9 µmol/liter); in women: 380 ± 70 µg/dl (68 ± 13 µmol/liter)] (20). Transferrin iron saturation (percent saturation of TIBC) parallel to the rise in plasma iron increases above the normal range of 20 to 55 percent and may be used as an indirect indicator for iron overload. However, the specificity of this test is reduced by the relatively high frequency of false-positive or false-negative values. Nevertheless, owing to its wide and easy availability in clinical laboratories, transferrin saturation has remained one of the most useful predictors for iron overload (5).

Serum Ferritin. The small concentration of ferritin normally present in the circulating blood (20 to 300 µg/liter) mirrors the size of the body iron store (21–23). This direct relationship of serum ferritin to body iron stores is also seen in hereditary hemochromatosis (24) and in secondary hemochromatosis (25). There are, however, a number of causes of high serum ferritin other than iron overload. Liver diseases, infections, inflammation, and malignant disorders such as leukemias, lymphomas, and certain solid tumors may induce increases in serum ferritin without corresponding increase in storage iron (26,27). Extremely high ferritin levels can be observed in patients with massive hepatic necrosis (concentrations up to more than 30.000 µg/liter). Thus a high serum ferritin concentration does not invariably indicate iron overload.

Calculations derived from the direct correlation of serum ferritin with iron stores in normal healthy subjects as determined by repeated phlebotomy suggest that in normal individuals there

TABLE 37-1. *Methods for the Evaluation of Body Iron Stores*

Indirect measures	Direct measures
Serum ferritin	Liver biopsy
Transferrin iron saturation	Bone marrow biopsy
Chelate-induced urinary iron excretion	Quantitative phlebotomy
Intestinal iron absorption	
Isotope dilution	
Physical methods	
Nuclear resonant scattering of γ-rays (NRS)	
Computed tomography (CT)	
Magnetic susceptibility measurement (by SQUID)	
Magnetic resonance imaging (MRI)	

are 8 to 12 mg storage iron for each microgram per liter of ferritin (1,2). As is shown in Figure 37-1, this ratio of ferritin to storage iron is not constant over the whole range from iron deficiency to heavy iron overload. With increasing iron stores, the ferritin to storage iron decreases, amounting to an average ratio of 15 mg storage iron for each microgram per liter of ferritin at iron stores below 500 mg and decreasing to a ratio of about 6 mg for each microgram per liter of ferritin at storage iron levels about 18 g (Fig. 37-1). For clinical purposes, this variation in the ferritin to storage iron ratio has to be considered when calculating the amount of storage iron from serum ferritin measurements. Nevertheless determination of serum ferritin has its place as a noninvasive screening parameter in detecting iron overload in early stages as well as in the state of advanced iron overload.

Chelator-Induced Urinary Iron Excretion. An estimate of the body iron reserve also can be obtained by determining the quantity of iron excreted in the urine in response to parenteral administration of chelating agents. The agents most frequently used are *desferrioxamine* and *diethylentriamine pentaacetic acid (DTPA)*. Chelator-induced urinary iron excretion exceeding 39 μmol (2.2 mg per 24 h) indicates iron overload (28). Despite being a rather cumbersome and rarely used method, chelator-induced urinary iron excretion has an established place as a reliable method of detecting iron overload, especially in distinguishing the high serum ferritin levels of tissue damage, inflammation, or malignancy from those found in true iron overload (29,30).

Intestinal Iron Absorption. The iron metabolism in normal subjects is regulated by the adaptation of intestinal iron absorption to the body's iron requirements. Intestinal iron absorption, as measured by whole-body counting, is increased in iron deficiency and reduced to subnormal levels in secondary iron overload due to diminished erythropoiesis. In contrast, in patients with hereditary hemochromatosis and patients with iron-loading anemias due to ineffective erythropoiesis, intestinal iron absorption is increased or inappropriate for the amount of storage iron present in the body (2). Thus the determination of intestinal iron absorption may be useful in distinguishing between hereditary hemochromatosis and iron overload secondary to increased iron supply (2).

Direct Measures of Body Iron Stores

Liver Biopsy. Iron stores are located primarily in two tissues, the *hepatic parenchyma* and the *reticuloendothelial system (RES)*. Body iron stores therefore may be assessed most directly by determining nonheme iron concentration in liver or bone marrow biopsies by biochemical methods or histochemical (Prussian blue) tissue staining.

Since increased iron storage with deposition in the parenchymal liver cells is the hallmark of all forms of advanced iron overload, liver biopsy presently is the *definitive* test of assessing both iron distribution and tissue damage (31). The degree of stainable parenchymal iron may be arbitrarily graded from 0 to 4 (32). *Total iron* in biopsy specimens may also be measured by the use of atomic absorption spectrophotometry (33), and *nonheme iron* can be calculated by subtraction of the heme iron measured separately, e.g., using the pyridine hemochromagen technique (34). More applicable for routine use is the direct determination of nonheme iron described by Torrance and Bothwell (30,35). The mean concentration of normal liver iron ranges from 80 to 300 μg/g (1.4 to 5.4 μmol/g) wet weight, equivalant to a total amount of liver iron between 120 and 450 mg (2.2. and 8.1 mmol).

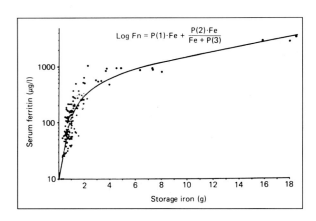

FIGURE 37-1
Correlation of storage iron, mobilized by repeated phlebotomy in 69 healthy male subjects (○) and 71 patients with hereditary hemochromatosis (●) at various clinical stages. The data can be fitted according to the given equation (Fe in mg): P(1) = 3.59 × 10⁻⁵; P(2) = 2.912; P(3) = 432.80. Reprinted, by permission, from Kaltwasser JP, Werner E: Diagnosis and clinical evaluation of iron overload, in Bailliere's Clinical Haematology, vol 2. London, Bailliere Tindall, 1989, pp 363–389.

Bone Marrow Biopsy. Bone marrow aspiration and biopsy provide a direct means of assessing reticuloendothelial iron stores and therefore are particularly useful in iron overload seen in refractory anemias, whereas they are not suitable for the diagnosis of hereditary hemochromatosis, where RES iron stores are normal or only slightly increased. Histologically, the iron stores are usually categorized into four to eight arbitrary grades, ranging from no detectable to massive excess (36). This method is a highly subjective assessment, however, with a substantial variation between and within observers (29).

Quantitative Phlebotomy. Iron mobilization in response to repeated phlebotomy (quantitative phlebotomy) is the only way of quantitatively assessing the total amount of the diffusely distributed body iron reserve in vivo. Subjects are phlebotomized by 500 ml at regular (weekly) intervals until the supply of iron for erythropoiesis has been exhausted (2,37). Quantitative phlebotomy is regarded as a reference method of storage iron measurement in humans. Because of its time-consuming and invasive nature, it is a retrospective measure, applicable only in patients with normal erythropoiesis, e.g., hereditary hemochromatosis.

Physical Methods
In a 10-year-old article on iron methodology, physical methods for measuring storage iron were mentioned in only a few sentences at the end of the appropriate chapter (30). It was stated, however, that none of the traditional methods "permits easy, rapid, and direct determination of body iron stores." During the last decade, physical methods applicable for direct and noninvasive measurement of tissue iron have significantly improved. Radiologic and biomagnetic methods, especially *imaging techniques* such as *computed tomography* (CT) and *magnetic resonance imaging* (MRI), in parallel with their broad clinical application in various diagnostic fields, also became available for the direct and noninvasive determination of tissue iron overload under normal diagnostic conditions.

Nuclear Resonant Scattering (NRS) of γ-Rays. The NRS technique uses gamma rays to raise ^{56}Fe to its first excited state. Subsequent decay back to the ground state by resonant emission produces gamma rays that may be counted by a suitable counter. This technique may be used to quantitate body (or organ) iron content (23). The method is limited by the fact that owing to the short half-life of the source (e.g. [^{56}Mn]Cl$_2$), it can be carried out only in close proximity to a reactor; moreover, a rather high level of radiation exposure is required (38).

Computed Tomography (CT). CT provides a tool for the evaluation of regional distribution of x-ray attenuation within a particular cross section of the body. Since soft tissue is almost exclusively composed of elements of very low atomic number, any increase in iron content results in a significant increase in tissue x-ray attenuation.

Applying the standard *single-energy technique*, where a tissue slice is scanned at one energy level, several groups were able to demonstrate higher densities in liver tissues from patients with iron overload than in those of healthy controls (39–41). CT values of liver density were directly correlated with serum ferritin ($r = 0.72$) but showed a higher predictive value (100 percent) than serum ferritin (24 percent) and transferrin saturation (66 percent) (40). Follow-up of patients undergoing venesection therapy showed a progressive decrease in the liver attenuation coefficient that correlated directly with the amount of mobilized iron ($r = 0.79$) and liver iron concentration ($r = 0.83$) (42).

Using a *dual-energy technique*, where the same tissue slice is scanned at two different energy levels and the difference in CT number is calculated, even better results with respect to accuracy and sensitivity were obtained. A correlation coefficient of $r = 0.99$ between chemically determined liver iron and the CT estimate of liver iron was obtained in patients with hereditary hemochromatosis (17).

CT estimates of tissue iron, especially by applying the dual-energy technique, suggest that CT is a useful method for the evaluation of body iron stores. Since CT involves exposure of the patient to ionizing irradiation, and since manufacturers of CT scanning equipment unfortunately have shown little interest in modifying calibration procedures for their instruments, this potentially quantitative measure currently is not widely used clinically (2,38).

Magnetic Susceptibility Measurements (by SQUID). *Magnetic susceptibility* is the property of a material or tissue responsible for the magnetic response evoked by application of a constant or alternating magnetic field (43). The response varies greatly in different materials, both in magnitude and in orientation of the induced magnetic field. In most human biologic material, this induced field is diametrically opposed to the applied field. Since this *diamagnetic* response is extremely weak (about 10^{-6} of the applied field), its detection requires highly sensitive instrumentation. In contrast, *ferromagnetic* materials, such as the common bar magnet, respond with an induced field as strong as or even stronger than the applied field and in the same direction (38). Intermediate between these two extremes of magnetic response is the *paramagnetic* response of the iron in the iron storage proteins ferritin and hemosiderin. This response is directly proportional to the iron ions present in iron storage compounds and its measurement provides a noninvasive means of determining tissue iron concentration (38,44). Contributions by other paramagnetic materials (hemoglobin or other trace metals) to the magnetic susceptibility are so small, at least in liver tissue, that measurements are highly specific for the content of ferritin and hemosiderin iron. For human liver specimens, a linear relationship was observed in vitro between magnetic susceptibility and tissue iron content (45). The first in vivo measurement applying biomagnetic susceptometry became possible in the 1970s by introduction of the SQUID (*s*uperconducting *q*uantum *i*nterference *d*evice) technology (45). A second-generation SQUID magnetometer with better sensitivity meanwhile has become available (38). Applying the SQUID technique, Brittenham and coworkers (16) at Case Western Reserve University could demonstrate a close correlation ($r = 0.98$) between magnetic susceptibility and liver iron content in biopsy specimens. Values in normal subjects [men: 3.8 ± 1.1 μmol/g (mean ± SD); premenopausal women: 2.5 ± 2.0 μmol/g; iron-deficient subjects: 0.8 ± 1.3 μmol/g] were in good agreement with data in the literature regarding liver biopsies and liver autopsies. In patients with hereditary hemochromatosis, hepatic iron measured by the SQUID technique was greatly increased to 23 to 118 μmol/g wet weight (16). In a more recent summary of data accumulated so far, a close correlation between liver iron and magnetic susceptometry ($r = 0.97$) has been shown up to an iron concentration of about 350 μmol/g liver (38). In 25 patients with beta-thalassemia, significant correlations were observed between hepatic iron as measured by intestinal iron absorption and serum ferritin and magnetic susceptometry (46). Presently, SQUID magnetometers still have to be regarded as investigational devices, available at only very few places in the world. However, the SQUID technique certainly has already been proven to be interesting and promising, owing to its noninvasive properties, and thus it may become more generally available for clinical use in the future.

Magnetic Resonance Imaging (MRI). Iron, when present in sufficient concentration in tissues, causes an enhancement of proton relaxation such that spin-lattice relaxation time (T1) and spin-spin relaxation time (T2) are shortened (18,19,47–52). Liver images from patients with iron overload show abnormally low spin-echo intensities, as is shown in the T2-weighted liver image in Figure 37-2A. The shortening of T1 and T2 relaxation times of protons in iron-loaded liver tissues most probably is caused by the magnetization of iron-containing substances, such as ferritin and hemosiderin, as well as of low-molecular-weight iron ions, when they are placed in a magnetic field (19,53).

Magnetic resonance spectroscopy (MRS) of iron-loaded rat livers in vitro has shown a linear relationship of the relaxation rates 1/T1 and 1/T2 to the hepatic iron levels. The increase in 1/T1 with increasing iron concentrations was, however, only moderate as compared with an extreme increase in 1/T2 (19). The more marked effect of tissue iron on T2 compared with T1 and the physical basis for this disproportionate alteration presently are not well understood (19,53). The difference of the effect of iron on the two relaxation rates 1/T1 and 1/T2, which are in fact different expressions of the same fundamental interactions, may depend on measurement conditions (magnetic field strength, pulse sequence and intensity, repetition rates, delay times, and others) as well as on the fine structure of tissue in a manner that also is incompletely understood (38,54). However, it is most likely that the decrease in spin-echo image intensity in iron overload (Fig. 37-2A) is due mainly to the extreme decrease in T2 relaxation time (19,51).

Since MRI is an entirely noninvasive technique, the effects of tissue iron on spin-echo intensities may be used to detect and quantify tissue iron

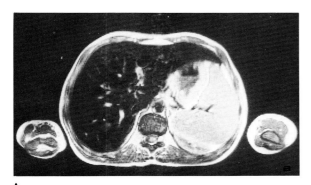

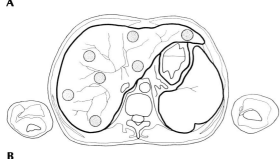

FIGURE 37-2
(A) *T2-weighted image of a section of the liver of a 16-year-old boy with thalassemia major. Serum ferritin amounted to 650 μg/liter. T2 = 11.7 ms.* (B) *Schematic arrangement of the operator-defined regions of interest (ROIs). Each ROI encompasses at least 80 image pixels and was placed in homogeneous areas of the liver away from large vessels and relatively free of artifacts.*

overload. However, using MRI tomographs operating at low field strength (0.15 to 0.35 Tesla), T2 may be so short that MRI signals emitted by the protons cannot be discriminated accurately from the noise level (19,24,48,49,51).

In a recent study using a standard MRI system, we were able to confirm the findings of Stark et al. (19) that in vivo measurements of T1 and T2 using conventional MRI techniques do not allow accurate discrimination between normal iron content and low grade iron overload (15 to 200 μmol/g) in the liver of human subjects (55). It also could be confirmed that T2 is potentially the more sensitive and precise test for determining tissue iron levels.

We therefore concentrated on the measurement of T2 using a Siemens Magnetom 63 (resonance frequency: 63 MHz; homogeneity of the magnetic field: ±5 ppm; CPU: 32 Microvax II and SMI, with array processor; system software: NUMARIS; CPU system software: Micro VMS) operating at 1.5 Tesla. The calculation of very short T2 times such as less than 10 ms was possible applying a minimal of echo-time TE of 10 ms, repetition time TR of 600 ms, and four averages. The circular body coil was generally used, providing a good signal homogeneity across the liver. After an initial localizing measurement, five to seven regions of interest (ROI) were selected in a T2-weighted image that were devoid of liver vessels and displayed homogeneity in the selected slices, as is schematically demonstrated in Figure 37-2B. Within-day variation of T2 measurements amounted to 4.4 percent (range 0.2 to 29 percent) in individuals with various grades of liver iron concentration. T2 results were defined as the arithmetic means of the calculated single T2 values of the ROIs selected.

The clinical applicability of the iron-determination protocol has been tested so far in 35 subjects with various grades of liver iron overload. Serum ferritin was used to estimate the body iron status in healthy volunteers as well as in patients with iron overload due to hereditary and secondary hemochromatosis. In parallel to serum ferritin in 16 patients, liver iron concentration could be determined quantitatively in needle biopsies by the chemical method of Torrance and Bothwell (30,35). In four patients, repeated T2 determinations were carried out during the course of an iron mobilization treatment by phlebotomy or SC desferrioxamine.

Serum ferritin of the study population ranged from 4 to 3140 μg/liter. Liver iron concentration in biopsy specimens ranged from 12 to 1200 μmol/g dry weight. The T2-relaxation rate 1/T2 and serum ferritin (Fig. 37-3) showed a direct but moderate correlation ($r = 0.61$), whereas the 1/T2 to liver iron concentration relationship of the 16 subjects available for liver biopsy exhibited a much closer correlation of $r = 0.92$, as shown in Figure 37-4B. As is shown in Figure 37-4A, the direct correlation between the in vivo measured T2 relaxation time and the chemically measured liver iron over the whole range of iron concentrations observed is not linear, but may be interpreted as a more complicated function, e.g., as two combined linear functions. This can be due to changes in the conformation of the major tissue iron constituents ferritin and hemosiderin at various

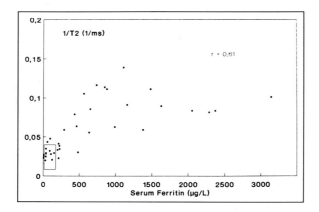

FIGURE 37-3
Relationship between transverse (spin-spin) relaxation rate 1/T2 and serum ferritin concentration in 32 patients with depleted, normal, and increased iron stores, including repeated measurement in 7 patients during iron mobilization treatment. The rectangle encompasses the normal ranges for serum ferritin and 1/T2.

grades of tissue iron overload. The nonlinear relationship between T2 and liver iron does not, however, interfere with an accurate calculation of the iron concentration from T2 measurements in higher grades of iron overload.

In iron-overload syndromes, iron determination in organs other than liver (e.g., heart, spleen, brain, pituitary gland, and synovialis) is of particular clinical interest. Since MRI combines the possibilities of producing high-quality images of various body sections together with the characterization of different tissue constituents (56), MRI also may be a useful measure for the detection and characterization of different organ systems involved in the iron overload process. Besides liver and heart, it is impossible to correlate MRI signals in vivo directly with tissue iron concentration as determined by tissue biopsy. Tissue iron may, however, be estimated approximately by comparing MRI signal intensity with that of tissues with known low iron content, e.g., skeletal muscle or fatty tissues (53,57).

MRI seems also to be superior to CT in differentiating iron deposition from other tissue constituents such as iodine or tissue infiltration by cavernous hemangiomas or tumor metastases (58–61). Not only in the diagnosis but also in the management and monitoring of iron storage diseases, MRI provides a noninvasive method for controlling iron depletion by phlebotomy or chelation therapy as well as of the rate of iron reaccumulation in pretreated patients. As is shown in Figure 37-5, iron mobilization in hereditary as well as in secondary hemochromatosis can be documented by a continuous increase in T2

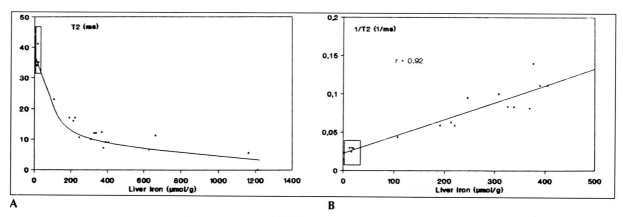

FIGURE 37-4
(A) Relationship between transverse (spin-spin) relaxation time T2 and chemically determined hepatic nonheme iron concentrations of needle biopsies obtained from 19 subjects with various liver iron concentrations. (B) Relationship between transverse (spin-spin) relaxation rate 1/T2 and chemically determined hepatic iron of 16 of the 19 subjects shown in part A. The rectangles encompass the normal ranges of nonheme liver iron concentration and T2 and 1/T2, respectively.

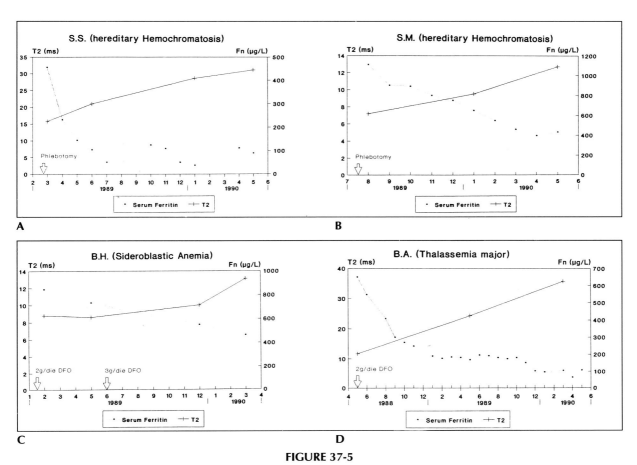

FIGURE 37-5
Follow-up of iron mobilization therapy in patients with iron overload. A and B: Course of T2 time and serum ferritin in 2 patients with hereditary hemochromatosis undergoing phlebotomy treatment. C and D: Course of T2 time and serum ferritin in 2 patients with secondary hemochromatosis due to sideroblastic anemia and thalassemia major during treatment by SC desferrioxamine (DFO) treatment. Note the increase in DFO dosage at 6/89 in patient B.H. and the concomitant increment in the increase in T2 time.

relaxation time, as measured with the above-mentioned MRI protocol. MRI may also be of interest for a population screening for iron overload (2,38). It has to be proved first, however, that T2 measurement can accurately discriminate normal liver iron concentration from minor degrees of iron overload.

As our preliminary data for the T2 to liver iron correlation (Fig. 37-4A, B) indicate, this most probably will be the case. It is necessary, however, to carry out prospective clinical studies, which will be difficult to realize for ethical reasons.

In vivo spectroscopy in combination with MRI probably can add further important information to the diagnostic requirements in iron overload syndromes, e.g., with respect to the discrimination between parenchymal and reticuloendothelial iron deposition (2,18). Improved imager performance is required, however, before all these expectations may become realities.

TREATMENT AND PROGNOSIS OF IRON STORAGE DISEASES

The most effective therapeutic modality in the treatment of hereditary hemochromatosis is the mobilization of surplus iron by repeated phlebotomies (1). In patients in whom phlebotomy is not feasible (e.g., patients with iron-loading anemias or those with hereditary hemochromatosis associated with severe cardiomyopathy or hypoproteinemia), chelation therapy, as described extensively in a recent issue of *Clinical Haematology* (62), provides an effective alternative method for iron removal.

Since early detection and prophylactic treatment can prevent the pathologic complications of all iron-overload syndromes, the primary goal in the handling of this group of diseases is the evaluation of the extent of iron accumulation and organ damage. As has been shown in a carefully controlled study by Niederau et al. (63), life expectancy has greatly improved since, owing to early detection by refined diagnostic procedures and HLA-related identification of affected family members, treatment can be started in hereditary hemochromatosis long before clinical manifestation of the disease. As is shown in Figure 37-6B, noncirrhotic patients in this study have shown an entirely normal life expectancy, whereas survival was significantly reduced in the cirrhotic patients (Fig. 37-6A).

Cumulative survival also has significantly improved during the last 20 years by consequent use of phlebotomy treatment and early detection of the disease, as has been shown in three consecutive series published between 1976 and 1985 (63–65). Causes of death obviously also have changed since introduction of phlebotomy treatment in hereditary hemochromatosis. Primary liver cell carcinoma presently seems to be one of the major causes of death and is not prevented by phlebotomy treatment in patients with advanced disease, whereas this particular risk of the disease seems to be completely absent after treatment in the noncirrhotic stage (66). In secondary hemochromatosis, treatment is more unsatisfactory. Continuous subcutaneous infusion of desferrioxamine can improve survival significantly, but careful long-term management is required and is often hindered by incomplete compliance of the patients (67). This situation may improve when inexpensive, orally active iron chelators become available for routine clinical use (68).

CONCLUSIONS

Early detection of increased iron stores is of particular importance for the course and prognosis of

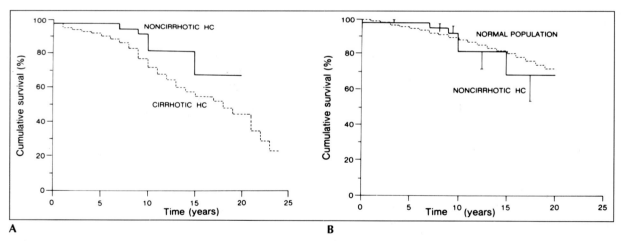

FIGURE 37-6
Survival of patients with hereditary hemochromatosis. (A) Cumulative survival in 112 cirrhotic and 51 noncirrhotic patients. Significance of differences: $p \leq 0.05$ by log-rank test. (B) Cumulative survival in 51 noncirrhotic patients as compared with the expected survival in the normal population; there is no significant difference between both survival curves (Reprinted, by permission, from Strohmeyer G, et al: Survival and cause of death in hemochromatosis: Observations in 163 patients, in Weintraub LR, et al (eds): Hemochromatosis: Proceedings of the First International Conference. Ann NY Acad Sci 526:245, 1988.)

iron storage diseases. In the recent decade, diagnostic procedures as well as therapeutic strategies have significantly improved. Serum ferritin together with transferrin saturation have been proved to be the best indirect methods of screening for iron overload. HLA typing within families of an affected patient is especially useful in the early identification of family members carrying the hemochromatosis gene and in determining the state of inheritance (hetero- or homozygosity) in a particular subject at risk. Liver and bone marrow biopsies still remain the most direct methods that provide detailed information on the amount and distribution of tissue iron as well as on the extent of iron-induced tissue damage.

Three new physical methods presently under investigation offer direct and noninvasive means of assessing tissue iron concentration: Magnetic susceptibility measurements by SQUIDs are promising with respect to accurate quantitation of liver iron concentration. This technique presently is restricted to research purposes only, however, and has the disadvantage of being applicable exclusively to liver iron determination. For clinical use, imaging techniques such as CT and MRI may become of particular interest for a quantitation of tissue iron in various systems simultaneous with the morphologic analysis of the respective body section. Liver biopsy certainly remains the "gold standard" for the quantitative tissue iron determination. Because of its noninvasive nature, the "magnetic biopsy" obtainable from T2-weighted MRI as well as from SQUID measurements may become a substitute of liver needle biopsy for the detection of iron overload and documentation of the response to iron mobilization treatment.

Further improvement is desirable in iron quantitation in tissues other than liver and in the possibility to differentiate noninvasively between parenchymal and reticuloendothelial iron deposition. According to predictions of the European Workshop on NMR in London in 1987, there will be about 3000 MRI imagers in clinical and research use by 1990. This proliferation of equipment together with further improvement in instrumentation should guarantee continuous progress in the further evaluation of the clinical applicability of MRI in the various diagnostic requirements associated with iron storage diseases.

REFERENCES

1. Bothwell TH, Charlton RW, Cook ID, Finch CA: Iron Metabolism in Man. Oxford, Blackwell Scientific, 1979.
2. Kaltwasser JP, Werner E: Assessment of iron overload, in Hershko C (ed): Iron Chelating Therapy: Bailliere's Clinical Haematology, vol 2. London, Bailliere Tindall, 1989, pp 363-389.
3. Simon M, Bourel M, Fauchet R, Genetet B: Association of HLA-A3 and HLA-B14 antigens with idiopathic haemochromatosis. Gut 17:332, 1976.
4. Simon M, Alexanre JL, Bourel M, et al: Heredity of idiopathic haemochromatosis: A study of 106 families. Clin Genet 11:327, 1977.
5. Dadone MM, Kushner JP, Edwards CQ, et al: Hereditary hemochromatosis: Analysis of laboratory expression of the disease genotype in 18 pedigrees. J Clin Pathol 78:196, 1982.
6. Halliday CW, Halliday JW, Powell LW: The clinical manifestation of chronic iron overload, in Hershko C (ed): Iron Chelating Therapy: Bailliere's Clinical Haematology, vol 2. London, Bailliere Tindall, 1989, pp 403-421.
7. Sheldon JH: Haemachromatosis. London, University Press, 1935.
8. Cazzola M, Ascari E, Barosi G, et al: Juvenile idiopathic haemochromatosis: A life-threatening disorder presenting as hypogonadotrophic hypogonadism. Hum Genet 65:149, 1983.
9. Goya N, Miyazaki S, Kodate S, Ushio B: A family of congenital atransferrinemia. Blood 40:239, 1972.
10. Heilmeyer L, Keller W, Vivell D, et al: Kongenitale Atransferrinämie bei einem sieben Jahre alten Kind. Dtsch Wochenschr 86:1745, 1961.
11. Barry M, Scheuer PJ, Sherlock S, et al: Hereditary spherocytosis with secondary haemochromatosis. Lancet 2:481, 1968.
12. Zimmermann HJ, Chomet B, Kulesh HM, McWhorter CA: Hepatic hemosiderin deposits: Incidence in 558 biopsies from patients with and without intrinsic hepatic disease. Arch Intern Med 107:494, 1961.
13. Grace ND, Powell LW: Iron storage disorders of the liver. Gastroenterology 64:1257, 1974.
14. Erickson RP: Haemochromatosis and superoxide metabolism: Free radical influence on iron storage? Lancet 2:743, 1978.
15. Epstein JM, Redeker AG: Porphyra cutanea tarda: A study of the effect of phlebotomy. N Engl J Med 279:1301, 1968.
16. Brittenham GM, Farrell DE, Harris JW, et al: Magnetic-susceptibility measurement of human iron stores. N Engl J Med 307:1671, 1982.

17. Champman RW, Williams G, Bydder G, et al: Computed tomography for determining liver iron content in primary haemochromatosis. Br Med J 280:440, 1980.
18. Stark DD, Bass NM, Moss AA, et al: Nuclear magnetic resonance imaging of experimentally induced liver disease. Radiology 148:743, 1983.
19. Stark DD, Moseley ME, Bacon BR, et al: Magnetic resonance imaging and spectroscopy of hepatic iron overload. Radiology 154:137, 1985.
20. Fielding J: Serum iron and iron binding capacity, in Cook JD (ed): Iron: Methods in Hematology, vol 1, New York, Churchill-Livingstone, 1980, pp 15-43.
21. Kaltwasser JP, Werner E: Quantitative evaluation of body iron stores, in Spittel JA Jr (ed): Clinical Medicine, vol 1, Philadelphia: Harper & Row, 1983, pp 82-103.
22. Walters GO, Miller FM, Worwood M: Serum ferritin concentration and iron stores in normal subjects. J Clin Pathol 26:770, 1973.
23. Worwood M: Serum ferritin, in Cook JD (ed): Iron: Methods in Hematology, vol 1. New York, Churchill-Livingstone, 1980, pp 59-89.
24. Halliday JW, Cowlishaw JL, Russo AM, Powell LM: Serum-ferritin in diagnosis of haemochromatosis. Lancet 2:621, 1977.
25. Letzky EA, Miller F, Worwood M, Flynn DM: Serum ferritin in children with thalassaemia regularly transfused. Clin Pathol 27:652, 1974.
26. Kim HS, Kaltwasser JP, Roth P: Evaluation of serum ferritin in leukaemia by two different ferritin assays. Tumor Diagn Ther 5:166, 1984.
27. Prieto J, Barry M, Sherlock S: Serum ferritin in patients with iron overload and with acute and chronic liver disease. Gastroenterology 68:525, 1975.
28. Balcerzak SP, Westerma MP, Heinle EW, Taylor FH: Measurement of iron stores using desferrioxamine. Ann Intern Med 68:518, 1968.
29. Cavill J: Diagnostic methods, in Clinics in Haematology: Disorders of Iron metabolism, vol 11. Philadelphia, Saunders, 1982, pp 259-273.
30. Torrance JD, Bothwell TJ: Tissue iron stores, in Cook JD (ed): Iron: Methods in Hematology, vol 1. New York, Churchill-Livingstone, 1980, pp 90-115.
31. Powell L, Halliday JW: Idiopathic haemochromatosis, in Jacobs A, Worwood M (eds): Iron in Biochemistry and Medicine, vol 2. London, Academic Press, 1980, pp 461-498.
32. Scheur P, Williams R, Muir AR: Hepatic pathology in relatives of patients with haemochromatosis. Pathol 84:53, 1962.
33. Walker RJ, Miller JPG, Dymock IW, et al: Relationship of hepatic iron concentration to histochemical grading and to total chelatable body iron in conditions associated with iron overload. Gut 12:1011, 1971.
34. Flink EB, Watson GJ: A method for the quantitative determination of haemoglobin and related heme pigments in feces, urine and blood plasma. Radiol Chem 146:171, 1942.
35. Torrance JD, Bothwell TH: A simple technique for measuring storage iron concentrations in formalinised liver samples. S Afr J Med 33:9, 1968.
36. Hausmann K, Kuse R, Sonnenberg AW, et al: Interrelations between iron stores, general factors and intestinal iron absorption. Acta Haematol (Basel) 42:193, 1969.
37. Haskins D, Stevens AR, Finch S, Finch CA: Iron metabolism: Iron stores in man as measured by phlebotomy. J Chem Invest 31:543, 1952.
38. Brittenham GM: Non-invasive methods for the early detection of hereditary hemochromatosis, in Weintraub LR, Edwards CQ, Krikker M (eds): Hemochromatosis: Proceedings of the First International Conference. Ann NY Acad Sci 526:199, 1988.
39. Honang MTW, Arozena X, Skalieka A, et al: Correlation between computed tomographic values and liver iron content in thalassaemia major with iron overload. Lancet 2:1322, 1979.
40. Howard JM, Ghent CN, Carey LS, et al: Diagnostic efficacy of hepatic computed tomography in the detection of body iron overload. Gastroenterology 84:209, 1983.
41. Mills SR, Doppman JL, Nienhuis AW: Computed tomography in diagnosis of disorders of excessive iron storage of the liver. J Comput Assist Tomogr 1:101, 1977.
42. Roudot-Thoraval F, Halpen M, Larde D, et al: Evaluation of liver iron content by computed tomography: Its value in the follow up of treatment in patients with idiopathic hemochromatosis. Hepatology 3:974, 1983.
43. Bastuscheck CM, Brenner D, Williamson SJ, Kaufmann L: Susceptometer for in vivo measurements of iron stored in human tissue, in Erne SN, Hahlbom HD (eds): Biomagnetism. Berlin, W. de Gryter, 1981, pp 519-532.
44. Farrell DE, Tripp JH, Zanzucchi PE, et al: Magnetic measurements of human iron stores. IEEE Trans Magnet 16:818, 1980.
45. Harris JW, Farrell DE, Messer MJ, et al: Assessment of human iron stores by magnetic susceptibility measurements (in vivo and in vitro studies) (abstract). Clin Res 26:504A, 1978.
46. Pootrakul P, Kitcharoen K, Yansukon P, et al: The effect of erythroid hyperplasia on iron balance. Blood F1:1124, 1988.

47. Bernardino ME, Small W, Goldstein J, et al: Multiple NMR T2 relaxation values in human liver tissue. AJR 141:1203, 1983.
48. Brasch RC: Methods of contrast enhancement for NMR imaging and potential applications. Radiology 147:781, 1983.
49. Brown DW, Henkelman RM, Poon PY, Fisher MM: Nuclear magnetic resonance study of iron overload in liver tissue. Magnet Reson Imaging 3:275, 1985.
50. Doyle FH, Pennock JM, Bank LM, et al: Nuclear magnetic resonance imaging of the liver: Inital experience. AJR 138:193, 1982.
51. Leung AW-L, Steiner RE, Young JR: NMR imaging of the liver in two cases of iron overload. Comput Assist Tomogr 8:446, 1984.
52. Runge VM, Clanton JA, Smith FW, et al: Nuclear magnetic resonance of iron and copper disease states. AJR 141:943, 1983.
53. Johnston DL, Rice L, Vick GW, et al: Assessment of tissue iron overload by nuclear magnetic resonance imaging. Am J Med 87:40, 1989.
54. König SH, Brown RD: Determinants of proton relaxation rates in tissue. Magn Reson Med 1:437, 1984.
55. Kaltwasser JP, Gottschalk R, Schalk KP, Hartl W: Non-invasive quantitation of liver iron-overload by magnetic resonance imaging. Br J Haematol 74:360, 1990.
56. Podo F: Tissue characterization by MRI: A multidisciplinary and multi-centre challenge today. Magn Reson Imaging 6:173, 1988.
57. Querfeld U, Dietrich R, Taira RK, et al: Magnetic resonance imaging of iron overload in children treated wih peritoneal dialysis. Nephron 50:220, 1988.
58. Fujisawa J, Morikawa M, Nakano Y, Konishi J: Hemochromatosis of the pituitary gland: MR imaging. Radiology 168:213, 1988.
59. Mirowitz S, Heiken JP, Lee JKT: Potential MR pitfall in relying on lesion liver intensity ratio in presence of hepatic hemochromatosis. J Comput Assist Tomogr 12:323, 1988.
60. Noma S, Konishi J, Morikawa M, Yoshida Y: MR imaging of thyroid hemochromatosis. J Comput Assist Tomogr 12: 623, 1988.
61. Schröder J, Haan J: Extrapyramidales Syndrom bei idiopathischer Hämochromatose (IHC). Bedeutung laborchemischer, neurophysiologischer und bildgebender Verfahren (CT, MRT). Nervenarzt 58:577, 1987.
62. Hershko C (ed): Iron Chelating Therapy: Bailliere's Clinical Haematology, vol 2. London, Bailliere Tindall, 1989.
63. Niederau C, Fischer R, Sonnenberg A, et al: Survival and causes of death in cirrhotic and non-cirrhotic patients with primary hemochromatosis. N Engl J Med 313:1256, 1985.
64. Bomford A, Williams R: Long-term results of venesection therapy in idiopathic hemochromatosis. Q J Med 45:611, 1976.
65. Milder MS, Cook JD, Stray S, Finch CA: Idiopathic hemochromatosis, an interim report. Medicine 59:34, 1980.
66. Strohmeyer G, Niederau C, Stremmel W: Survival and cause of death in hemochromatosis: Observations in 163 patients, in Weintraub LR, Edward SQ, Krikker M (eds): Hemochromatosis: Proceedings of the First International Conference. Ann NY Acad Sci 526:245, 1988.
67. Hoffbrand AV, Wonke B: Results of long-term subcutaneous desferrioxamine therapy, in Hershko C (ed): Iron Chelating Therapy: Baillier's Clinical Haematology, vol 2, London, Bailliere Tindall, 1989, pp 345–362.
68. Kontoghiorghes GH, Hoffbrand AV: Prospects for effective oral chelation in transfusional iron overload, in Hoffbrand AV (ed): Recent Advances in Haematology, vol 5. Edinburg: Churchill-Livingstone, 1988, pp 75–89.
69. Chezmar JL, Nelson RC, Malko JA, Bernardino ME: Hepatic iron overload: Diagnosis and quantification by non-invasive imaging. Gastrointest Radiol 15:27, 1990.
70. Wielopolski L, Ancona RC, Mossey RT, et al: Nuclear resonance scattering measurement of human iron stores. Med Phys 2:401, 1985.

38

Principles for Design of Liver Contrast Agents

DAVID D. STARK

The ability of exogenous pharmaceutical compounds to change MRI signal intensity by altering T1 and/or T2 relaxation times holds great promise for improving the diagnostic information on abdominal MRI images. The rationale for developing MRI contrast agents is to further improve image contrast-to-noise ratios (CNRs), allowing detection of even smaller lesions, simplify the MRI examination, improve patient throughput, and reduce cost. These potential gains must be balanced against the added cost and inconvenience of drug administration and the potential risk of toxicity (1).

Pharmaceutical manipulation of the MRI signal in vivo was first shown by Lauterbur et al. (2) in 1978, when they measured shortened canine myocardial proton relaxation times after administration of a manganese salt. Subsequently, numerous diamagnetic, paramagnetic, superparamagnetic, and ferromagnetic materials have been evaluated as MRI contrast agents (3–7). The general requirements for design of a clinically useful MRI contrast agent are (1) magnetic activity that alters image signal intensity, (2) biodistribution to normal tissue and exclusion by diseased tissue (or the reverse), and (3) low toxicity or a high margin of safety for the effective dose.

MAGNETIC MATERIALS

Magnetic materials are usually classified in terms of their response when placed in an external magnetic field (Fig. 38-1). The ratio (dimensionless) of the magnetization induced in a material to the strength of the applied magnetic field is termed the *magnetic susceptibility* of the substance. The magnetization of a material at a specified field strength can be expressed in terms of electromagnetic units (emu*) per gram of metal. The induced magnetization may be oriented antiparallel (diamagnetic) or parallel (paramagnetic, superparamagnetic, ferrimagnetic, or ferromagnetic) to the external magnetic field (8,9).

Diamagnetic susceptibility is due to motion of spin-paired orbital electrons and therefore contributes to the susceptibility of all materials. However, magnetic susceptibility is very weak, and materials that are exclusively diamagnetic (i.e., most organic and inorganic compounds) are of little interest as contrast agents because they do not have sufficient magnetization to alter nuclear (proton) MRI signals. Diamagnetic materials have been used as MRI contrast agents in situations where they can displace or mix with normal tissue, directly altering the signal of a region on the image. For example, water, fat, perfluorocarbons,

---

*cgs system: 1 emu = 1 erg/gauss = 10^{-3} joules/Tesla: SI system.

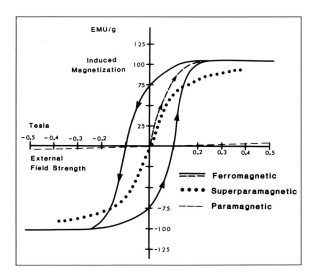

FIGURE 38-1
Magnetic susceptibility. Relationship between applied external field and induced magnetization (emu/g) in various materials. Ferromagnetic materials exhibit residual magnetization after exposure to an external field as described by the histeresis curve (arrowheads). Beginning with a nonmagnetized sample, induced magnetization responds as shown by the dashed line; thereafter, with removal or reversal of the external field, the induced magnetization follows the solid line. Remanence of the induced magnetization, in the absence of an external field (i.e., magnetic memory), allows use as recording material. Superparamagnetic material (dotted line) shows a similarly large induced magnetization but does not show remanence. Generally, superparamagnetic materials approach saturation magnetization (100 emu/g iron in this example) more gradually than do ferromagnetic materials. Paramagnetic materials show weak magnetic susceptibility, develop an induced magnetization in direct proportion to the applied field, and saturate only at extremely high field strengths (not encountered under conditions of MRI imaging). The hysteresis curves for both superparamagnetic and paramagnetic materials pass through the origin, indicating loss of magnetization when the applied field is removed.

and carbon dioxide have been used to displace normal bowel contents and have been proposed as gastrointestinal agents (10–13).

Paramagnetism is characterized by independent action of individual atomic or molecular magnetic moments due to unpaired electron spins. These moments are not aligned in the absence of an external magnetic field. In the presence of a magnetic field, the moments tend (statistically) to align in the field direction, and the net magnetic moment is the sum of individual moments multiplied by a Boltzmann factor (3). Paramagnetism can occur in individual atoms or ions, as well as in collections of atoms or ions in solids such as ferritin, hemosiderin, or the mineral goethite (FeOOH).

Superparamagnetic materials are comprised of crystals of certain materials such as magnetite (Fe_3O_4) and maghemite (Fe_2O_3) large enough to form a solid-phase microscopic volume or "domain" in which atomic unpaired electron spins are aligned by positive exchange forces. A *domain* is a volume of material (5 to 35 nm in size for Fe_3O_4) possessing a uniform magnetization and a specific direction. Superparamagnetic materials are comprised of single-domain crystals with properties intermediate to paramagnetic and ferromagnetic materials. Specifically, the susceptibilities of superparamagnetic materials are very much larger than those of paramagnetic materials, yet are also proportional to 1/T (Curie law; applied in materials science). Unlike ferromagnetic materials, superparamagnetic materials do not exhibit residual magnetism when the external magnetic field is removed. Thermal agitation is sufficient to overcome any net alignment in an ensemble of particles (14).

Ferromagnetic (and ferrimagnetic) particles (8,9) are comprised of multiple magnetic domains. If the domains are randomly aligned, the material is "unmagnetized"; if the domains are aligned with each other, the ferromagnetic material is "magnetized." When placed in an external magnetic field, randomly aligned domains become aligned, and upon removal of the external magnetic field, these materials exhibit residual magnetization described by a hysteresis curve. The property of residual magnetization after removing the magnetic field is called *remanence*, and this allows application as recording media and as structural material for permanent magnets. If the size of a ferromagnetic (or ferrimagnetic) crystal is reduced to that of a single domain, both materials exhibit superparamagnetism. A subset of ferrimagnetic iron oxides having the formula $M^{2+}O \cdot Fe_2^{3+}O_3$ (M^{2+} is a divalent cation) are known as ferrites. The iron oxide particles used in MRI to date (15–19) have not been fully characterized; however, they would all appear to be superparamagnetic, structurally similar to the ferrite magnetite ($Fe^{2+}O \cdot Fe_2^{3+}O_3$).

PROTON RELAXATION ENHANCEMENT
Soluble Agents

In most situations, paramagnetic contrast agents increase both the 1/T1 and 1/T2 relaxation rates. The dose dependency of proton relaxation enhancement is expressed as the ratio of the change in rate to the change in drug concentration, and this measure of drug potency is called *relaxivity*. For example, the efficiency of Gd-DTPA at enhancing longitudinal T1 relaxation in water is expressed as relaxivity R1 = 4.5 $(mM \cdot s)^{-1}$, while the transverse (T2) relaxivity is R2 = 6.0 $(mM \cdot s)^{-1}$ (20–21). The R2/R1 ratio (6.0/4.5) = 1.3) shows slightly greater transverse relaxation enhancement than longitudinal relaxation enhancement for this typical paramagnetic complex. However, in imaging we are primarily interested in tissue relaxation times. In tissues, 1/T2 relaxation rates are normally 10 times faster than 1/T1 relaxation rates, since tissue T1 relaxation times are typically 10 times longer than the T2 relaxation times. For example, if liver T1 is 500 ms and T2 is 50 ms, then the inherent T1 rate of liver is 2.0/s and the T2 rate is 20/s. Since paramagnetic relaxation rates are additive to the inherent tissue relaxation rates, a given dose of Gd-DTPA might then increase the 1/T1 relaxation rate of liver tissue to 2.21/s, while increasing the 1/T2 relaxation rate to 20.6/s. Inverting the rates to express these numbers in terms of tissue relaxation times, we find the enhanced liver T1 to be 408 ms and the enhanced liver T2 to be 49 ms. Therefore, because tissue T1 relaxation is inherently slow compared with T2 relaxation, the predominant effect of paramagnetic contrast agents is on T1. For the hypothetical dose of Gd-DTPA used in this example, the liver T1 decreases 18 percent, while the T2 decreases only 2 percent (22).

Given these changes in T1 and T2, the signal-intensity equation for spin-echo imaging (or any other type of sequence) would predict, and in vivo experimentation confirms, that Gd-DTPA and the entire class of paramagnetic agents behave as "T1 agents" and increase the signal intensity of target tissues. The sensitivity of MRI to paramagnetic contrast enhancement is quite pulse-sequence-dependent (23–25). Short TE T1-weighted SE or IR techniques show the greatest "enhancement," which in the case of paramagnetic contrast agents is manifested as an increase in signal intensity due to shortening of T1. A general advantage of this class of materials is that increased image signal-to-noise ratios (SNRs) may allow faster imaging or reduction of the administered dose.

Paramagnetic enhancement of proton relaxation was first demonstrated in 1946 by Bloch et al. (26), when they added a paramagnetic solvent, ferric nitrate, to water for the convenience of shortening experiments. Studies of water 1H relaxation in solutions of transition metal ions led to a mathematical formulation of paramagnetic-enhanced solvent relaxation first described by Solomon (27) in 1955 and later modified by Bloembergen (28) in 1957. In aqueous solutions or in tissue, the 1/T1 or 1/T2 relaxation rates observed in the presence of a paramagnetic contrast agent are the sum of the proton relaxation rate caused by the electrons of paramagnetic molecules and the proton relaxation rate that would exist without paramagnetic effects:

$$\frac{1}{T_{observed}} = \frac{1}{T_{native}} + \frac{1}{T_{paramagnetic}} \quad (38\text{-}1)$$

The parameter $1/T_{paramagnetic}$ represents many interactions between electrons and hydrogen protons (3). In general, the magnitude of relaxation enhancement is proportional to the magnetic moment of the paramagnetic compound; however, relative effects on T1 and T2 relaxation can be modulated by other factors described in the Solomon-Bloembergen equation. For example, complex interrelationships of various molecular motions are proposed to explain the magnetic field dependence of observed relaxation times (29,30). The structure of paramagnetic molecules is also important, since relaxation enhancement is maximal when water has close access to the paramagnetic center because electron-proton (dipole-dipole) interactions show an r^{-6} dependence.

Particulate Agents

Particles are also capable of interactions with water molecules and can enhance T1 relaxation by mechanisms similar to those described in the

Solomon-Bloembergen equation (31). However, particles differ from small paramagnetic complexes in that most of the unpaired electron spins in particles are not accessible to solvent water protons, therefore limiting the influence of dipole-dipole and scalar relaxation (3). Nevertheless, particles have very large magnetic moments, and significant T1 relaxation enhancement can be observed with either paramagnetic or superparamagnetic materials (31). It is the unique ability of particles to selectively enhance T2 relaxation (R2/R1 $\gg$ 1) that is of greatest interest in MRI (15–22).

Unfortunately, relaxation theory is not sufficiently developed to predict the influence of particle characteristics on longitudinal (R1) and transverse (R2) relaxivity $(mM \cdot s)^{-1}$. While it is agreed that particle size and magnetization are important, five groups working on the theory of proton relaxation by particles have come up with three different explanations of the dependence of relaxation enhancement on fundamental parameters such as particle size and concentration (17, 31–34). For practical purposes, relaxation enhancement by particles having large magnetic moments has been attributed to "magnetic susceptibility effects." This simply means that since particles have a greater magnetic susceptibility than surrounding diamagnetic tissues, the magnetization induced in particles distorts the local magnetic field, creating local magnetic field inhomogeneities.

Inhomogeneities introduced on a microscopic scale by particles have effects similar to other sources of inhomogeneity, such as a poorly shimmed magnet. For example, magnetic field inhomogeneities accelerate the rate of spin dephasing, shortening the apparent transverse relaxation time. Just as magnetic field inhomogeneities caused by imperfections in the magnetic field can be refocused in spin-echo experiments using a 180-degree pulse, static field inhomogeneities caused by particles are also refocused. Gradient-echo experiments that do not use a 180-degree pulse are sensitive to the additional contribution of static field inhomogeneities to transverse relaxation and therefore observe a shorter relaxation time known as T2*.

Magnetic field gradients induced by particles also contribute to the dephasing of protons that move by diffusion from one point to another in the vicinity of a particle. As the field experienced by moving protons changes over time, spin-echo refocusing does not recover this contribution to transverse relaxation. Therefore, the diffusional effects are seen as irreversible T2 decay. The diffusional contribution to T2 relaxation has a well-known dependence on TE2, and therefore, the observed R2 of particulate contrast agents will depend on the circumstances (pulse-sequence timing) used to measure relaxation (32,35). The earliest clinical studies have shown that long TE spin-echo sequences and short TE gradient-echo sequences are both very sensitive to low concentrations of iron oxide particles in tissue (19).

PHARMACOKINETICS AND BIODISTRIBUTION

Contrast agents are most useful when selective accumulation occurs in only one of two tissues being compared (Fig. 38-2). Ideally, a contrast agent would be concentrated in a single target tissue only during the brief period of MRI and would then disappear without subsequent effects on the target tissue or other body organs.

Applications of magnetic contrast agents are largely determined by the physiologic delivery system used. Most agents administered intravenously, such as iodinated radiographic contrast agents or Gd-DTPA, have a nonspecific biodistribution determined by the relative vascular perfusion of different tissues and by capillary permeability, which allows diffusion into the extracellular space (Fig. 38-2B). A functioning blood-brain barrier effectively limits the biodistribution of Gd-DTPA to abnormal tissue in the central nervous system, while free filtration through the renal glomerulus leads to concentration of low-molecular-weight compounds (Gd-DTPA = 590 daltons) in the normal kidney (4–7,20,36–38). The physiology and clinical uses of nonspecific agents are essentially the same for MRI and CT; however, in many applications the enhanced MRI images contain more diagnostic information due to greater image contrast than the corresponding enhanced CT scans.

Vascular contrast agents are retained within the vascular system due to their large size (molecular weight > 30,000), which prevents glomerular filtration or leakage through capillaries (6,39–41). In the absence of accumulation in the extracellular space, vascular contrast agents selectively enhance tissues in proportion to their fractional blood volume and have been used to study perfusion (see below) and ischemia.

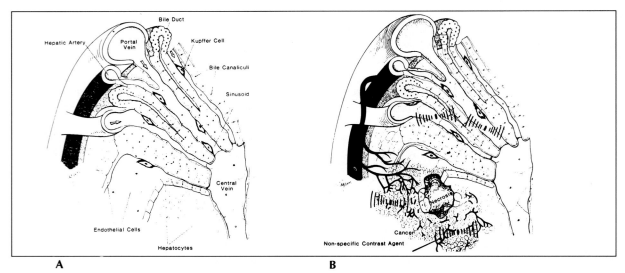
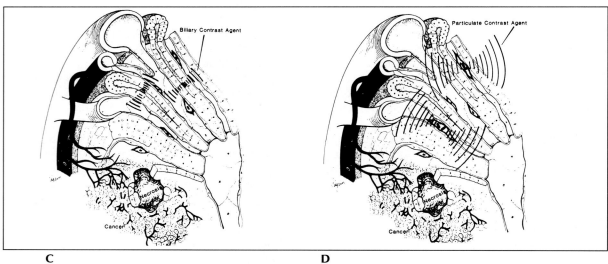

FIGURE 38-2

Contrast agent distribution in liver tissue. (A) Diagram of normal lobular hepatic anatomy showing major structures and cell types. (B) Cancer is shown with peripheral vascular supply and central necrosis. Nonspecific contrast agents delivered by means of the vascular system distribute to both normal liver and perfused cancer tissue. Paramagnetic relaxation enhancement is seen in both tissues. (C) Hepatobiliary contrast agent is taken up by hepatocyte and excreted into bile ducts. Since cancer does not show tissue specific uptake of this material, after the contrast agent has cleared from the bloodstream, selective enhancement is seen in normal liver tissue. (D) Reticuloendothelial (particulate) contrast agents are phagocytosed by Kupffer cells lining the hepatic sinusoids. These cells may ingest more than one particle, and superparamagnetic materials have very large effects on tissue proton relaxation. Since there is no phagocytosis by cancer cells, selective enhancement of liver tissue is seen.

FIGURE 38-3
Schematic diagram of monoclonal antibody targeted to a cancer-specific antigen on the cell surface. M^+ represents a radionuclide for scintigraphy or a magnetic material (paramagnetic or superparamagnetic) for MRI.

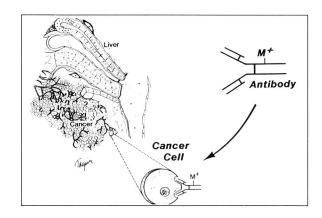

Antibody targeting involves binding magnetic contrast agents to monoclonal antibodies, which would then carry them to cell surface antigens, e.g., carcinoembryonic antigen (CEA) of colon cancer (Fig. 38-3). Unfortunately, the small number of binding sites available on the surface of malignant cells and the limited affinity (low specificity) of available antibodies have thus far prohibited effective contrast enhancement of tumors (42). Scintigraphy offers more ideal circumstances for the initial development of this targeting strategy, since radionuclide concentrations of 10^{-9} M can be detected (3). MRI applications will require much higher drug concentrations ($\sim 10^{-6}$ M), and in many body regions, technical problems further limit the antibody strategy. For example, the liver normally cleans the blood of extraneous proteins, and nonspecific accumulation of antibodies in liver tissue may offset any selective uptake of antibody by tumor.

Receptor targeting has been an effective strategy for selective delivery of paramagnetic contrast agents (Fig. 38-2C). Compounds such as Mn-dipyridoxal diphosphate (Mn-DPDP), an enzymatically active analog of vitamin B_6, show selective uptake by hepatocytes (43) (Fig. 38-4). Compounds similar to the scintigraphic iminodiacetic (IDA) class of agents, targeted to the anionic hepatocyte receptor (potentially competing with bilirubin uptake), have carried paramagnetic iron (Fe-EHPG), manganese, and gadolinium (Gd-BOPTA) to hepatocytes in place of the ^{99m}Tc used in nuclear medicine hepatobiliary imaging (3,44) (Fig. 38-5). The hepatic

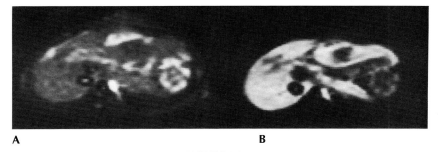

A   B

FIGURE 38-4
Paramagnetic hepatobiliary agent efficacy tested using a rat model of a solitary adenocarcinoma metastasis in the liver. (A) Unenhanced SE 250/18 image. Tumor in the left lobe is barely visible. (B) Thirty minutes following intravenous infusion of Mn-DPDP (50 mol/kg), the 3-mm tumor is obvious. The agent has selectively shortened the T1 of normal liver tissue, increasing the liver signal-to-noise ratio (SNR), increasing anatomic resolution. Conspicuity is increased due to the increased liver/tumor signal difference-to-noise SDN or CNR ratio.

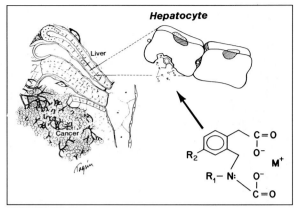

FIGURE 38-5

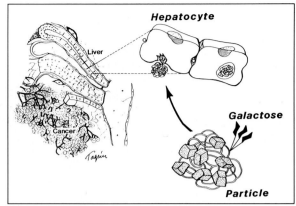

FIGURE 38-6

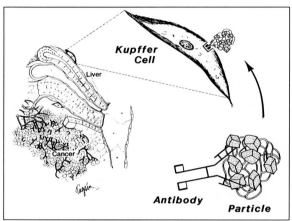

FIGURE 38-7

FIGURE 38-5
Schematic drawing of low-molecular-weight paramagnetic complex targeted to a hepatic cell surface receptor or transport protein. M^+ represents a paramagnetic metal ion (gadolinium, iron, or manganese). The ligand-metal complex shown is schematically representative of Fe-EHPG, Mn-DPDP, and Gd-BOPTA.

FIGURE 38-6
Schematic diagram of a large macromolecule or a small composite particle bearing terminal galactose moieties that are recognized by the hepatic binding protein, also known as the asialoglycoprotein receptor (45–47). In this illustration of a composite iron oxide particle, the gray cubes represent superparamagnetic iron oxide crystals, typically 10 nm in size. Composite particle size is determined by the number of crystals coprecipitated by the macromolecule that forms the composite particle matrix, such as dextran, albumin, or (galactose-bearing) arabinogalactan.

FIGURE 38-7
Model of phagocytosis. A composite particle circulating in the bloodstream is recognized as foreign material and is then coated with antibodies or other opsonins, and the complex is then recognized and internalized by macrophages such as the hepatic Kupffer cells. This process is physiologically distinct from endocytosis of macromolecules and small particles mediated by the hepatic binding protein or internalization of small molecules transporter proteins located in the sinusoidal hepatocyte cell membrane.

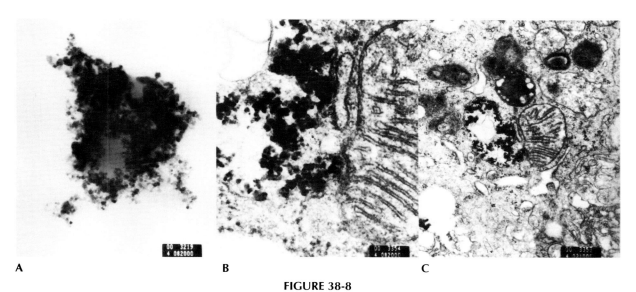

FIGURE 38-8
Transmission electron microscopy. (A) Iron oxide particles were precipitated on Formvar-coated grids. Overall particle size is approximately 1 μm and is composed of individual crystals measuring approximately 10 nm in diameter (original magnification × 82,000). (B) Photomicrograph from a rat that had received 70 μmol Fe/kg IV as particulate iron oxide 24 h before being killed. Particles seen within hepatic Kupffer cells appear similar to the injected material (A). No cellular or organelle abnormalities are seen (original magnification × 82,000). (C) Membrane-bound collection of particles illustrated in (B) is seen within Kupffer cell cytoplasm at lower magnification (original magnification × 21,000).

binding protein (HBP), a tissue-specific hepatocyte receptor for galactose-bearing structures such as asialoglycoprotein, can be targeted with a variety of labeled macromolecules or small iron oxide particles (45–47) (Fig. 38-6).

To the extent that hepatobiliary agents are also distributed by vascular perfusion and less than 100 percent of drug is ultimately taken up by hepatocytes, nonspecific tumor enhancement also occurs, partially offsetting enhancement of normal liver parenchyma. Nevertheless, newer agents with greater than 49 percent hepatobiliary uptake (30 min after injection) significantly improve lesion/liver contrast on MRI images (48). Delayed imaging is appropriate because the vascular-extracellular pool of contrast agent is excreted by the kidneys more rapidly than excretion of the hepatocyte pool. Delayed imaging is also favored because it provides a more flexible time window for clinical throughput.

Phagocytosis is a physiologic strategy traditionally exploited in liver-spleen imaging (Fig. 38-2D). Analogous to the use of ^{99m}Tc-sulfur colloid scintigraphy and the use of iodinated liposomes or ethiodized oil emulsions for CT scanning, several particulate materials have been used in MRI (4,49,50). Particulate materials show the greatest tissue specificity of all contrast agents, since phagocytosis is a highly specialized process by which specific cells (reticuloendothelial macrophages) remove debris from the bloodstream (Fig. 38-7). Lymph nodes and bone marrow also have this capability; however, 80 percent of reticuloendothelial activity resides in the liver and 10 percent in the spleen (63). Targeting of particles can be influenced by the selection of coating materials and composite particle size (Fig. 38-8).

CLINICAL APPLICATIONS

Contrast Agents

Soluble Complexes. Gadolinium-DTPA is initially distributed within the intravascular compartment and rapidly diffuses throughout the interstitial extravascular space, entirely analogous to the patterns seen with CT. As a probe for blood-brain barrier defects, Gd-DTPA has been enormously successful, allowing use of fast T1-weighted imaging techniques with high SNRs per unit time, rather than conventional unenhanced T2-weighted images, which have reduced SNR. However, as a result of nonspecific distribution in other body organs, such as the liver, early trials with Gd-DTPA were disappointing (24,37,51,52). For example, in patients studied 5 to 10 min after infusion of 0.1 mmol/kg Gd-DTPA, images showed tumor nodules to lose contrast and become isointense with surrounding liver. Although precontrast T1-weighted images show tumor nodules as hypointense due to their long T1, tumors have a large extracellular space and increased capillary permeability, which results in greater accumulation of Gd-DTPA in tumor tissue than in surrounding liver. As with contrast-enhanced liver CT, equilibration of drug into the interstitial compartment of the tumor results in a net loss in image contrast (22). Nonequilibrium "dynamic" scanning is a satisfactory solution in some circumstances.

Studies of Gd-DTPA imaging have shown that immediate (1 to 2 min) postinjection scanning maximizes liver/tumor signal-intensity differences, just as with dynamic bolus CT (24,51–56). Later, the tumor "fills in" from the periphery as contrast agent accumulates in the tumor. The rims of hypovascular or necrotic tumors may show increased enhancement due to increased blood flow, and tumors that are inherently hypervascular, such as hepatomas or islet-cell metastases, may show prominent tumor enhancement. In most cases, the enhancement pattern with Gd-DTPA matches that seen with CT.

Cavernous hemangiomas studied with Gd-DTPA show peripheral enhancement during the dynamic phase (53), and most fill in completely during 5 to 30 min, reproducing the well-known contrast-enhanced CT appearance (54–56). The diagnosis of small hemangiomas may benefit from Gd-DTPA–enhanced MRI, since subcentimeter lesions are difficult to characterize by T2-weighted noncontrast techniques. Small lesions are also particularly difficult to characterize using the single-slice, dynamic-bolus CT technique owing to problems with slice misregistration from breath-hold to breath-hold. MRI circumvents this problem because it is a simultaneous multislice technique (22).

Particles. Iron oxide particles show a highly tissue-specific biodistribution and much simpler pharmacokinetics than Gd-DTPA or the hepatobiliary chelates (3,22). Tumors simply lack phagocytic activity and do not take up particles. Therefore, the signal intensity of tumor is unchanged, while surrounding liver shows a reduction in T2 and a loss of signal intensity (Fig. 38-9G). Iron oxide particles have also been used to enhance the detection of focal splenic lesions (57) and also may be useful for imaging of the bone marrow and lymph nodes. Experimental studies have suggested that iron oxide particles are useful in the differential diagnosis of splenomegaly and can detect diffuse splenic lymphoma (58).

Particles also show a blood-pool phase and may have potential development as vascular perfusion agents (64)(Fig. 38-9). Iron oxide particles have a blood half-life of approximately 13 min and then remain intact for several hours, without significant redistribution (19,59). This temporal stability may be desirable for liver/spleen imaging in clinical practice, since careful coordination of drug administration and the time of scanning is not required.

Pulse-sequence selection is simplified because of the potent and selective T2 relaxation enhancement, which essentially eliminates signal from normal liver and spleen tissue. "Balanced" or "mildly T2-weighted" pulse sequences (i.e., with timing parameters in the range of SE 500/30 to SE 2000/60) are similarly effective (60). In clinical practice, use of short TR techniques may be preferred, since they allow ghost artifact reduction by means of signal averaging or shorter scan times and more rapid patient throughput. Recently, we have shown that gradient-echo sequences are maximally sensitive to iron oxide particles, offer high SNRs, and speed and therefore optimize tumor/liver CNR per unit time (19,65).

TOXICITY OF IV MRI CONTRAST MEDIA

Safety is a major issue with all new drugs and is of special concern when particles are administered intravenously. The doses of iron oxide proposed for imaging studies (1 mg Fe/kg) do not significantly increase hepatic iron concentration.

To place this dose in perspective, a 70-kg human taking 325 mg $FeSO_4$ (119 mg Fe) three times a day for 2 days (standard iron replacement therapy) would absorb an equivalent amount of iron (1.02 mg/kg), assuming 10 percent efficiency of intestinal absorption. In toxicity studies, administration of massive iron oxide doses (250 mg iron/kg) causes increased iron concentration in the liver, spleen, and lung macrophages. Even with massive doses, no evidence of lipid peroxidation or enzyme dysfunction can be detected using biochemical indicators known to be sensitive to iron-induced hepatic injury (61). Morphologic and biochemical studies of animals chronically receiving iron oxide particles demonstrate the presence of excess iron in reticuloendothelial cells, without evidence of toxicity. These animal studies are consistent with the clinical finding that selective reticuloendothelial iron deposition (e.g., transfusional iron overload) is less toxic than hepatocellular iron deposition (e.g., hereditary hemochromatosis). Indeed, hepatic iron overload is the experiment of nature that provided the basis for the development of ferrite particles as MRI contrast agents (62).

Degradation of superparamagnetic iron oxide particles has been proven by three independent experiments: (1) histologic examinations show clearance of particles from hepatic Kupffer cells, (2) liver T2 returns to normal, and (3) radiolabeled (^{59}Fe) iron from administered ^{59}Fe-oxide appears in hemoglobin. In fact, superparamagnetic iron oxide has been used to correct iron-deficiency anemia in rats (59). The half-life of iron oxides varies from 2 to 30 days depending on particle size and composition (31,59).

Paramagnetic complexes, while more toxic than iodinated contrast agents on a molar (or weight) basis, are used in much lower doses and therefore have a greater margin of safety. The safety factor, or ratio of LD^{50} per effective dose (in rats), is approximately 10 for iodinated agents, 20 to 100 for paramagnetic agents, and 200 for superparamagnetic iron oxides. However, in addition to the acute LD^{50} in rats, the potential for sensitization and idiosyncratic (allergic) reactions must be considered, especially for macromolecular complexes such as albumin–Gd-DTPA and particulate agents (19,39–41).

GASTROINTESTINAL CONTRAST AGENTS

The major goals of cross-sectional abdominal imaging seldom require examination of the bowel itself. Projective radiographs (barium studies) and endoscopy are far more suitable than sonography, CT, or MRI for detecting mucosal pathology and delineating its effects on the alimentary tube. However, identification of the bowel must be achieved when cross-sectional imaging techniques are used in order to allow discrimination of pathologic masses such as pancreatic and renal tumors for retroperitoneal adenopathy from normal bowel loops. It is expected that an orally administered contrast agent will be required to mark the small bowel lumen on MRI images (10). The stomach and colon are less of a problem owing to their more predictable anatomic relationships and their content of gas, which can be identified as a signal void. Unfortunately, magnetic contrast agents analogous to the radiographic gastrointestinal contrast agents used for CT are not yet available for routine use.

Preliminary attempts to develop gastrointestinal contrast materials for MRI have included use of the full range of magnetic materials, water-soluble and immiscible materials, and materials that either increase or decrease the signal intensity of the intestinal lumen (10–13). The two major goals in the design of gastrointestinal contrast materials are (1) complete and uniform marking of the intestinal lumen and (2) patient acceptance, which requires ease of administration and nonstimulation of peristalsis. Stimulation of peristalsis may have the advantage of increasing the rate at which the contrast is distributed throughout the intestine but results in unacceptable cramping, diarrhea, and MRI image degradation due to increased motion artifacts.

Agents that mix freely with intestinal contents are preferable to immiscible materials, since the latter will by definition "segment" in some bowel loops and leave other loops with unchanged luminal contents. Although it may be equally acceptable for diagnostic purposes to increase or decrease luminal signal intensity, it may be desirable to reduce the luminal signal intensity in order to reduce the intensity of ghost artifacts resulting from bowel motion. Iron oxide particle formulations that are stable in aqueous suspension can reduce luminal signal throughout the stomach, small bowel, and colon.

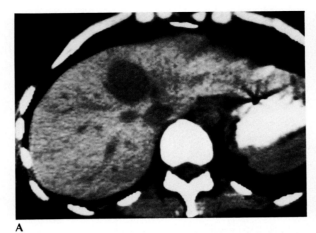
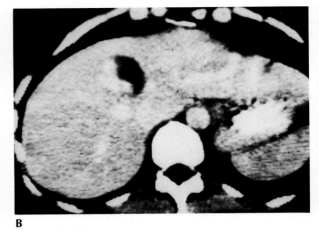
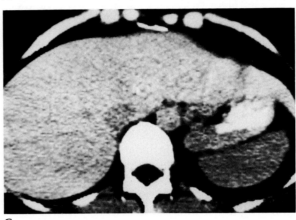

FIGURE 38-9
Perfusion study with superparamagnetic iron oxide. Hepatic cavernous hemangioma shows a tissue-specific perfusion pattern. (A–C) Iodine bolus-enhanced single-slice CT scan shows hypodense baseline (A), with peripheral enhancement of the lesion immediately after injection (B). One hour after injection, (C) the lesion is isodense to liver parenchyma and hyperdense to the blood vessels, reflecting slow flow and retention of iodine within the hemangioma—a pattern that distinguishes this benign tumor from most cancers. (D–G) MRI blood-pool imaging shows the same temporal and spatial pattern after injection of iron oxide. (D) SE 2350/60 baseline precontrast image. (E) Immediately after injection of 20 µmol Fe/kg. One hour after injection; (F) and 24 hours after injection (G) when the contrast

Legend continues on page 337

However, at high concentrations, these highly susceptible materials may sufficiently distort the magnetic field to cause artifacts in regions of hyperconcentration similar to the appearance of magnetic susceptibility artifacts caused by surgical clips. Furthermore, peristaltic motion of the mesenteric fat may continue to limit abdominal MRI image quality, even in the presence of a completely dark intestinal lumen.

Hahn et al. (65) recently reported clinical results using a formulation of superparamagnetic iron oxide that minimizes susceptibility artifact while maximizing T2 relaxivity. Patients ingested 75 ml of a solution containing 175 mg Fe per liter in a low-viscosity osmotic carrier consisting of food-grade materials. Small bowel enhancement (signal loss) improved visualization of retroperitoneal anatomy; however, 33 percent of subjects reported a brief diarrheal episode. Motion-related unsharpness was not affected, and the behavior of ghost artifacts was variable.

Promising approaches for pharmacologic alteration of the intestinal signal intensity include oral administration of paramagnetic agents such as ferric ammonium citrate (Geritol) or solutions of gadolinium-DTPA. The lumen of the stomach and proximal duodenum shows a high signal intensity following administration of paramagnetic materials. Early studies failed to show effects distal to the ligament of Treitz, and this failure was attributed to dilutional effects of gastric, biliary, and pancreatic secretions in the proximal small bowel and complex absorptive processes in the distal small bowel resulting in inappropriate contrast agent concentrations. Recently, oral administration

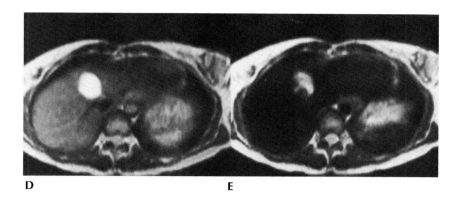

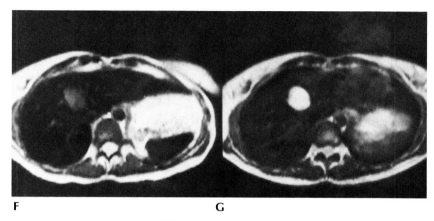

FIGURE 38-9 *(continued)*
agent has cleared the hemangioma as well as the bloodstream. The liver remains enhanced for a longer period of time (3 to 7 days) owing to superparamagnetic iron oxide entrapped in Kupffer cells. (From Hahn PF, Stark DD, Weissleder R, et al: Clinical application of superparamagnetic iron oxide to MR imaging of tissue perfusion in vascular tumors. Radiology 174:361, 1990. Reprinted by permission.)

of 10 ml/kg of a formulation containing 1.0 mM Gd-DTPA solution with 15 g mannitol per liter has successfully marked the distal small bowel within 90 min of administration. However, the mannitol vehicle causes diarrhea in a third of patients, and ghost artifacts may increase—despite the routine use of scopalomine as an antiperistaltic—due to the increased signal intensity of the bowel lumen.

In summary, contrast media under development have shown efficacy in abdominal MRI, and several agents are currently in clinical trials. Considerable work remains with respect to pulse-sequence optimization and suppression of motion artifacts. Ultimately, CT of the abdomen and ultrasound of the pelvis are the standards by which radiologists will judge abdominal MRI.

REFERENCES

1. Wolf GL: Opinion. Safer, more expensive iodinated contrast agents: How should we decide? Radiology 159:557, 1986.
2. Lauterbur PC, Mendoca-Dias MH, Rubin AM: Augmentation of tissue water proton spin lattice relaxation rates by in-vivo addition of paramagnetic ions, in Duttun PL, Leigh JS, Scarpa A. (eds): Frontiers of Biological Energetics. New York, Academic Press, 1983.

3. Engelstad BL, Wolf GL: Contrast agents, in Stark DD, Bradley WG (eds): Magnetic Resonance Imaging. St. Louis, Mosby, 1988, pp 161–181.
4. Wolf GL, Burnett KR, Goldstein EJ, Joseph PM: Contrast agents for magnetic resonance imaging, in Kressel H (ed): in Magnetic Resonance Annual. New York, Raven Press, 1985, pp 231–266.
5. Brasch RC, London DA, Wesbey GE, et al: Work in progress: Nuclear magnetic resonance study of a paramagnetic nitroxide contrast agent for enhancement of renal structures in experimental animals. Radiology 147:773, 1983.
6. Runge VM, Clanton JA, Herzer WA, et al: Intravascular contrast agents suitable for magnetic resonance imaging. Radiology 153:171, 1984.
7. Bousquet JC, Saini S, Stark DD, et al: Gd-DOTA: Characterization of a new paramagnetic complex. Radiology 166:693, 1988.
8. Cullity BD: Introduction to Magnetic Materials. Reading, Mass., Addison-Wesley, 1976.
9. Saini S, Frankel RB, Stark DD, Ferrucci JT: Magnetism: A primer and review, AJR 150:735, 1988.
10. Stark DD: Biliary system, pancreas, spleen, and alimentary tract, in Stark DD, Bradley WG (eds): Magnetic Resonance Imaging. St. Louis, Mosby, 1988, pp 1060–1140.
11. Weinreb JC, Maravilla KR, Redman HC, Nunnally R: Improved MR imaging of the upper abdomen with glucagon and gas. J Comput Assist Tomogr 8:835, 1984.
12. Zerhouni EA, Brennecke CM, Fishman EK, et al: Development of gaseous contrast agent for MRI of the abdomen and pelvis. Proceeding of the 34th Annual Meeting of the Association of University Radiologist, Hartford, Conn., 1986, abstract no 63.
13. Mattrey RF, Hajek PC, Gylys-Morin VM, et al: Perfluorochemicals as gastrointestinal contrast agents for MR imaging: Preliminary studies in rats and humans. AJR 148:1259, 1987.
14. Bean CP, Livingston JD: Superparamagnetism. J Appl Physiol 30:120S, 1959.
15. Mendoca-Dias MH, Lauterbur PC: Ferromagnetic particles as contrast agents for magnetic resonance imaging of the liver and spleen. Magn Reson Med 3:328, 1986.
16. Renshaw PF, Owens CS, MacLaugling AC, et al: Ferromagnetic contrast agents: A new approach. Magn Reson Med 3:217, 1986.
17. Gillis P, Koenig SH: Transverse relaxation of solvent protons induced by magnetized spheres: Application to ferriting, erythrocytes and magnetite. Magn Reson Med 5:323, 1987.
18. Saini S, Stark DD, Hahn PF, et al: Ferrite particles: A superparamagnetic MR contrast agent for the reticuloendothelial system. Radiology 162:211, 1987.
19. Stark DD, Weissleder R, Elizondo G, et al: Superparamagnetic iron oxide: Clinical application as a contrast agent for MR imaging of the liver. Radiology 168:287, 1988.
20. Wolf GL, Fobben ES: Tissue proton T1 and T2 response to gadolinium-DTPA injection in rabbits: A potential contrast agent for MR imaging. Invest Radiol 19:324, 1984.
21. Bousquet JC, Saini S, Stark DD, et al: Gadolinium-DOTA: Characterization of new paramagnetic complex. Radiology 166:693, 1988.
22. Stark DD: MR imaging of the liver, in Stark DD, Bradley WJ Jr (eds): Magnetic Resonance Imaging. St. Louis, Mosby, 1988, pp 934–1059.
23. Greif WL, Buxton RB, Lauffer RB, et al: Pulse sequence optimization for MR imaging using a paramagnetic hepatobiliary contrast agent. Radiology 157:461, 1985.
24. Saini S, Stark DD, Wittenberg J, et al: Dynamic gadolinium-DTPA imaging of liver cancer: Animal investigation. AJR 147:357, 1986.
25. Wolf GL, Joseph PM, Goldstein EJ: Optimal pulsing sequences for MR contrast agents. AJR 147:367, 1986.
26. Bloch F, Hansen WW, Packard P: The nuclear induction experiment. Physiol Rev 70:474, 1946.
27. Solomon I: Relaxation processes in a system of two spins. Physiol Rev 99:559, 1955.
28. Bloembergen N: Proton relaxation times in paramagnetic solutions. J Chem Phys 27:572, 1957.
29. Bloembergen N, Morgan LO: Proton relaxation times in paramagnetic solutions: Effect of electron spin relaxation. J Chem Phys 34:842, 1961.
30. Koenig SH: A novel derivation of the Solomon-Bloembergen-Morgan equations: Application to solvent relaxation by Mn^{2+} protein complexes. J Magn Reson 37:1, 1978.
31. Josephson L, Lewis J, Jacobs P, et al: The effects of iron oxides on proton relaxivity. Magn Reson Imaging 6:647, 1988.
32. Hardy PA, Henkelman RM: Transverse relaxation rate enhancement caused by magnetic particulates. Magn Reson Imaging (submitted).
33. Majumdar S, Zoghbi S, Pope CF, Gore JC: A quantitative study of relaxation rate enhancement produced by ferrite particles in polyacrylamide gels and tissue. Magn Reson Med (submitted).
34. Parrish TB, Haacke EM: The contribution to T2 from local field inhomogeneities in gradient field echo imaging: Predicting the signal loss from ferrite microspheres. Magn Reson Imaging (submitted).
35. Robertson B: Spin-echo decay of spins diffusion in a bounded region. Physiol Rev 151:273, 1966.
36. Brasch RC, Weinmann HJ, Wesbey GE: Contrast-enhanced NMR imaging: Animal studies using gadolinium-DTPA complex. AJR 142:625, 1984.

37. Carr DH, Brown J, Bydder GM, et al: Gadolinium-DTPA as a contrast agent in MRI: Initial clinical experience in 20 patients. AJR 143:215, 1984.
38. Carr DH: The use of proton relaxation enhancers in magnetic resonance imaging. Magn Reson Imaging 3:17, 1985.
39. Schmiedl U, Moseley ME, Ogan MD, et al: Comparison of initial biodistribution patterns of Gd-DTPA and albumin-(Gd-DTPA) using rapid spin echo imaging. J Comput Assist Tomogr 11:306, 1987.
40. Schmiedl U, Ogan MD, Moseley ME, Brasch RC: Comparison of the contrast enhancing properties of albumin-(Gd-DTPA) and Gd-DTPA at 2.0 T: An experimental study in rats. AJR 147:1263, 19.
41. Schmiedl U, Ogan M, Paajanen H, et al: Albumin labeled with Gd-DTPA as an intravascular, blood pool-enhancing agent for MR imaging: Biodistribution and imaging studies. Radiology 162:205, 1987.
42. Renshaw PF, Owen CS, Evans AE, Leigh JS Jr: Ferromagnetic antibody relaxation technique, in SMRM Program, Society of Magnetic Resonance in Medicine, Montreal, August 1986, pp 17–18.
43. Worah D, Rocklage SM, Quay SC, et al: MR hepatobiliary imaging with a paramagnetic manganese chelate derived from pyridoxal-5-phosphate (work in progress), in Abstracts of the Sixth Annual Meeting of the Society of Magnetic Resonance in Medicine, New York, 1987.
44. Lauffer RB, Greif WL, Stark DD, et al: Iron-EHPG as an hepatobiliary MR contrast agent: Initial imaging and biodistribution studies. J Comput Assis Tomogr 9:431, 1985.
45. Vera DR, Krohn KA, Stadalnick RC, Scheibe PO: Tc-99m-galactosyl-neoglycoalbumin: In-vivo characterization of receptor-mediated binding to hepatocytes. Radiology 151:191, 1984.
46. Wu GY, Midford S, Wu CH: A hepatocyte-directed contrast agent for magnetic resonance imaging of hepatic tumors. Hepatology 8:1253, 1988.
47. Menz ET, Rothenberg JM, Groman EV, Josephson L: Receptor-Mediated Endocytosis Type MRI Contrast Agents. International Patent Application No. PCT/US89/03352, publication date 90.02.22.
48. Lauffer RB: Paramagnetic metal complexes as water proton relaxation agents for NMR imaging: Theory and design. Chem Rev 87:901, 1987.
49. Burnett KR, Wolf GL, Schumacher HR, Goldstein EJ: Gadolinium oxide: A prototype agent for contrast enhanced imaging of the liver and spleen with magnetic resonance. Magn Reson Imaging 3:65, 1985.
50. Caride VJ, Sostman HD, Winchell RH, Gore JC: Relaxation enhancement using liposomes carrying paramagnetic species. Magn Reson Imaging 2:107, 1984.
51. Hamm B, Wolf KJ, Felix R.: Conventional and rapid MR imaging of the liver with gadolinium-DTPA in clinical use. Radiology 164:313, 1987.
52. Mano I, Yoshida H, Nakabayasi K, et al: Fast spin-echo imaging with suspended respiration: gadolinium enhanced MR imaging of liver tumors. J Comput Assist Tomogr 11:73, 1987.
53. Ohtomo K, Itai Y, Yoshikawa K, et al: Hepatic tumors: Dynamic MR imaging. Radiology 163:27, 1987.
54. Freeny PC, Marks WM: Patterns of contrast enhancement of benign and malignant hepatic neoplasms during bolus dynamic and delayed CT. Radiology 160:613, 1986.
55. Freeny PC, Marks WM: Hepatic hemangioma: Dynamic bolus CT. AJR 147:711, 1986.
56. Foley WD, Bernland LL, Lawson TL, et al: Contrast enhancement techniques for dynamic hepatic computed tomographic scanning. Radiology 147:797, 1983.
57. Weissleder R, Hahn PF, Stark DD, et al: MR imaging of splenic metastases: Ferrite-enhanced detection in rats. AJR 149:723, 1987.
58. Weissleder R, Stark DD, Rummeny EJ, et al: Splenic lymphoma: Ferrite-enhanced MR imaging in rats. Radiology 166:423, 1988.
59. Stark DD, Groman EV, Saini S, et al: Ferrite: A superparamagnetic contrast agent for MR imaging (abstract), in Society for Magnetic Resonance In Medicine 5th Annual Meeting, Montreal, 1986, pp 15–16.
60. Tsang YM, Stark DD, Chen MC, et al: Hepatic micrometastases in the rat: Ferrite-enhanced MR imaging. Radiology 167:21, 1988.
61. Bacon BR, Stark DD, Park CH, et al: Ferrite particles, a new MRI contrast agent: Lack of acute or chronic hepatotoxicity following intravenous administration. J Lab Clin Med 110:164, 1987.
62. Stark DD, Moseley ME, Bacon BR, et al: Magnetic resonance imaging and spectroscopy of hepatic iron overload. Radiology 154:137, 1985.
63. Weissleder R, Elizondo G, Josephson L, et al: Experimental lymph node metastases: Enhanced detection with MR lymphography. Radiology 171:835, 1989.
64. Fretz CJ, Elizondo G, Weissleder R, et al: Superparamagnetic iron oxide-enhanced MR imaging: Pulse sequence optimization for detection of liver cancer. Radiology 172:393, 1989.
65. Hahn PF, Stark DD, Weissleder R, et al: Clinical application of superparamagnetic iron oxide to MR imaging of tissue perfusion in vascular liver tumors. Radiology 174:361, 1990.

XIII. NONSPECIFIC AGENTS

39

Gadolinium-DTPA: Lesion Detection and Differential Diagnosis

MICHAEL LANIADO, MARTIN SKALEJ,
HILMAR BONGERS, and GERHARD KÖLBEL

In computed tomography (CT) of the liver, iodinated contrast agents are applied in a great percentage of studies. Intravenous bolus injection of contrast material significantly improves diagnostic accuracy (1). Gadopentetate dimeglumine (Gd-DTPA) was the first intravenous contrast agent that became available for clinical magnetic resonance imaging (MRI). The paramagnetic MRI contrast agent enhances both T1 and T2 relaxation rates through short-range dipole-dipole interactions. Gd-DTPA has pharmacokinetic properties entirely analogous to iodinated intravascular contrast media used in excretory urography and contrast-enhanced CT (2). The volume of distribution of Gd-DTPA is the extracellular space (3). After intravenous injection, the complex has rapid plasma clearance ($t_{1/2}$ = 90 min) and is excreted into the urine, with only traces being cleared by means of the bile (2,3).

Gd-DTPA underwent phase I clinical trials in 1983 (4). Since then it has been clinically used in more than 500,000 patients. The initial field of application of Gd-DTPA was MRI of the brain and spinal cord. As a marker of blood-brain barrier disruptions, Gd-DTPA provides excellent visualization of neoplasms, infarctions, and inflammatory processes of the central nervous system (5). MRI of focal liver lesions was one of the first applications of Gd-DTPA outside the central nervous system (6–8).

LESION DETECTION: CONVENTIONAL PULSE SEQUENCES

Normal liver tissue appears relatively bright on plain T1-weighted images. The high signal intensity (SI) is related to the inherent short T1 relaxation time of normal liver parenchyma. The prolonged T1 relaxation time observed in most liver tumors makes these lesions hypointense with liver on T1-weighted images (9). In normal liver tissue, intravenously injected Gd-DTPA is mainly distributed in the large intravascular space provided by the sinusoids. Only a small portion of contrast material is present in the relatively small interstitial compartment. However, liver tumors have leaky capillaries that allow rapid diffusion of Gd-DTPA into the large interstitial space of abnormal tissue. As a result, Gd-DTPA decreases the T1 of normal liver to a moderate degree but usually decreases the T1 of tumors to a greater degree. The net result may be a decrease in the difference between the tumor and normal tissue with conventional T1-weighted sequences (7).

The phenomenon of fading contrast after injection of Gd-DTPA was first described by Carr et al. (7). They studied five patients with liver tumors at 0.15 Tesla (0.1 mmol/kg of Gd-DTPA). Solid liver tumors showed increases of SI to a degree that decreased SI differences versus normal enhancing liver with saturation-recovery, inversion-recovery, and spin-echo (SE) sequences. The same results were reported by Hamm et al. (8). They investigated eight patients with malignant hepatic tumors at 0.5 Tesla. Precontrast MRI included conventional T2, proton-density, and T1-weighted images (SE 200/20; IR 1500/35/400). Following intravenous injection of Gd-DTPA at a dose of 0.1 mmol/kg, T1-weighted SE and IR images showed a decrease of lesion contrast at 5 and 30 min postcontrast. Also, in 15 patients of their study group receiving 0.2 mmol/kg of Gd-DTPA, lesions were less conspicuous on postcontrast images.

In the studies of Carr et al. (7) and Hamm et al. (8), patients were selected on the basis of pathologic findings in preceding imaging studies, and no blinded review of the films was done. Therefore, no reference was given to the sensitivity of Gd-DTPA–enhanced MRI with conventional SE and IR sequences. However, the decrease of lesion contrast on Gd-DTPA–enhanced images precludes improvement of sensitivity compared with plain scans. At our institution, 0.1 mmol/kg of Gd-DTPA was used at 1.5 Tesla. In many cases, focal liver lesions were obscured on postcontrast T1-weighted SE images (Fig. 39-1). In an animal model, Gd-DTPA did not show significant hepatocyte excretion (10). As a result, delayed images (4 to 6 h postcontrast) also failed to provide improved sensitivity.

The data from the literature reported here and our experience were obtained at field strengths ranging from 0.15 to 1.5 Tesla, with Gd-DTPA dosages of 0.1 and 0.2 mmol/kg, and with a variety of conventional T1-weighted imaging techniques including short TR, short TE SE sequences (6–8). However, none of the pulse sequences was suited to match with the rapidity with which Gd-DTPA distributes itself into the extracellular compartment. It is therefore necessary to conclude that Gd-DTPA–enhanced MRI with conventional pulse sequences offers no relevant advantage over plain MRI with regard to lesion detection.

LESION CHARACTERIZATION: CONVENTIONAL PULSE SEQUENCES

MRI has been shown to provide unique information on the characterization of focal liver lesions

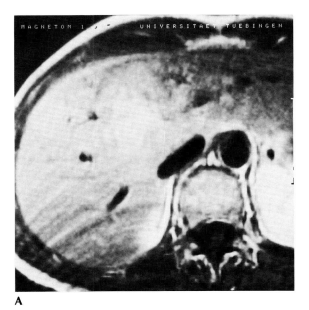
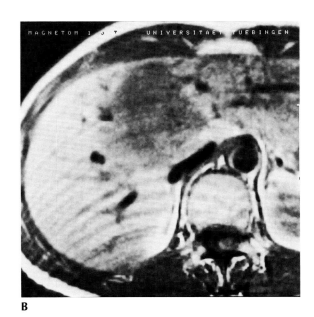

FIGURE 39-1
Hepatic metastasis from colorectal cancer in a 48-year-old woman (SE 500/15). (A) The precontrast image shows a hypointense lesion. (B) After injection of Gd-DTPA (0.1 mmol/kg), isointensity of lesion versus liver obscures the metastasis.

(11). However, equivocal cases remain despite the potential of T1, proton-density, and heavily T2-weighted sequences to predict the nature of a lesion. Therefore, the use of contrast media such as Gd-DTPA is a reasonable approach to further improve tissue characterization.

Tissue characterization with Gd-DTPA–enhanced conventional pulse sequences was the purpose of a study performed by Heintz and Ehrenheim (1.0 Tesla; 0.1 mmol/kg of Gd-DTPA) (12). Sonography and scintigraphy were obtained prior to MRI in all 47 patients. CT was done in some patients. Conventional postcontrast T1-weighted SE images showed marked enhancement in 11 of 13 hemangiomas, lack of contrast enhancement in 8 of 9 instances of focal nodular hyperplasia (FNH), and inhomogeneous enhancement in 11 of 15 hepatocellular carcinomas (HCC). Heintz and Ehrenheim (12) summarize that Gd-DTPA can be of help in partially thrombosed cavernous hemangiomas, that lack of contrast enhancement in FNH 10 min postinjection supports the working diagnosis based on scintigraphy (^{99m}Tc-DISIDA), and that irregular enhancement further narrows differential diagnosis in HCC. However, they fail to discuss whether the pattern of contrast enhancement on conventional T1-weighted images prospectively improved diagnostic efficacy in terms of predicting diagnosis. Considering this limitation of the study (12), and based on our experience, we feel that "static" postcontrast liver MRI alone contributes little to differential diagnosis (Fig. 39-2).

FAST IMAGING: LESION DETECTION AND CHARACTERIZATION

The pharmacologic behavior of Gd-DTPA is identical to that of iodinated contrast media used in CT (2). Thus imaging techniques such as dynamic scanning (13) also may be applicable to MRI. Before gradient-echo sequences became widely available, Saini et al. (14) first described dynamic Gd-DTPA–enhanced MRI of focal liver lesions in an animal model (14). With a heavily T1-weighted SE sequence at 1.4 Tesla (SE 250/15), a nearly threefold increase of liver/tumor contrast was measured 1 min after bolus injection of 0.2 mmol/kg of Gd-DTPA. Tumor/liver signal differences were maximal 1 to 2 min after administration of the contrast agent and gradually diminished thereafter. At approximately 8 min postcontrast, the two tissues became isointense (14). Similar techniques have been applied in humans since then (15–17).

Ohtomo et al. (15,16) and Mano et al. (17) used short TR (100 to 200 ms), short TE (15 to 20 ms) SE sequences at 1.5 and 0.5 Tesla, respectively. In their studies, Gd-DTPA was injected at a dose of 0.05 mmol/kg. Sequential rapid postcontrast MRI with short TR, short TE SE sequences yielded criteria for differentiating hemangioma, HCC, and metastasis, although some overlap of these criteria was reported. For example, five of seven hemangiomas showed peripheral contrast enhancement during the bolus dynamic phase and complete fill-in of high signal intensity on delayed scan images (10 to 15 min postcontrast). In HCC, delayed images displayed no area of high signal intensity in 21 of 28 patients. A peripheral halo with delayed enhancement was noticed in 12 hepatomas (16).

The confinement to single-slice imaging presented a drawback of the studies of Ohtomo et al. (15,16) and Mano et al. (17). For example, small lesions in the target section may be difficult to follow with single-slice imaging owing to differences in the depth of a breath-hold between consecutive images. To overcome this limitation, van Beers et al. (18) performed dynamic MRI using a SE 235/20 sequence that yields three slices in 36 s (1.5 Tesla, 0.1 mmol/kg of Gd-DTPA). They calculated SI ratios in the early phase after Gd-DTPA administration (30 s postcontrast) and at 3 min postcontrast. When a ratio of 1.4 was used as a borderline, correct classification of 28 of 30 focal liver lesions was achieved (hemangioma and benign liver tumor versus malignant liver tumor). Thus dynamic MRI combined with delayed imaging (up to 15 min postcontrast) has the potential to add to the inherent properties of MRI in terms of tissue characterization.

Ohtomo et al. (15,16), Mano et al. (17), and van Beers et al. (18) did not comment on lesion conspicuity and detection. However, even with high lesion contrast during the first 2 min after bolus injection of Gd-DTPA, no improvement of overall sensitivity is to be expected. This is because dynamic imaging of up to three slices at a time precludes detection of additional lesions in adjacent

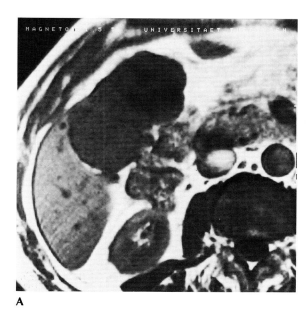
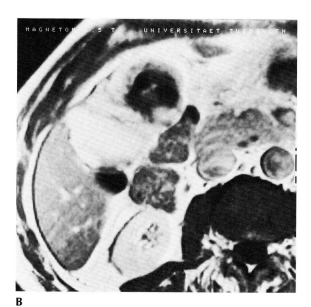
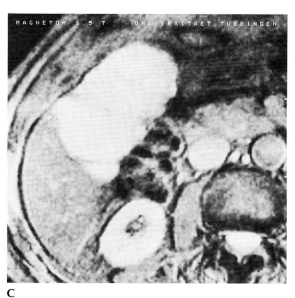

FIGURE 39-2
Hemangioma in the right lobe of the liver in a 70-year-old man. (A) The precontrast T1-weighted image shows the lesion hypointense with liver (SE 600/15). (B) On the postcontrast scan (SE 600/15), the hemangioma is markedly hyperintense relative to enhancing liver parenchyma. Nonenhanced area within hemangioma presumably corresponds to scar tissue. Note also enhancement of the right kidney. (C) The plain T2-weighted gradient-echo image (FLASH 500/15/15 degrees) shows the lesion isointense with CSF. Thus hemangioma was already the most probable diagnosis before Gd-DTPA was injected.

slices. Thus superior lesion conspicuity in a few slices does not translate into overall improved sensitivity.

Dynamic MRI with short TR, short TE SE sequences had confirmed that differences in vascularity and/or extracellular volume between tumor and liver can provide diagnostically relevant signal difference immediately after bolus injection of Gd-DTPA. The advent of gradient-echo sequences brought about a significant improvement in temporal resolution for dynamic MRI. Clinical studies were then initiated to evaluate the potential role of bolus-enhanced dynamic MRI with gradient-echo sequences in characterizing focal liver lesions.

To our knowledge, Hamm et al. (8) were the first to publish results of dynamic MRI of focal liver lesions with gradient-echo sequences (0.5 Tesla). In their series of 19 patients, lesions being hypointense versus liver on precontrast images showed increases of lesion contrast 2 to 3 min postinjection (0.1 and 0.2 mmol/kg of Gd-DTPA). Four tumors with hyperintense SI relative to liver immediately after bolus injection of 0.2 mmol

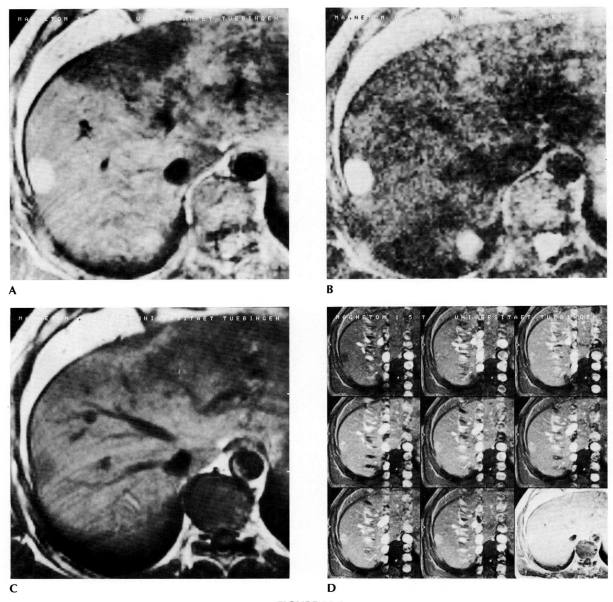

FIGURE 39-3

Hemangioma in right lobe of the liver in a 43-year-old man. (A) The proton-density-weighted image shows a well-delineated lesion with high signal intensity (SE 2300/22). (B) With longer TE, the hemangioma displays the typical "lightbulb" sign (SE 2300/80). A second hemangioma can be identified dorsally. (C) On the T1-weighted image, the lesion is difficult to appreciate due to little contrast versus liver. (D) A bolus-enhanced dynamic study was performed with FLASH 40/10/70 degrees (0.1 mmol/kg of Gd-DTPA). The hemangioma shows peripheral enhancement immediately after injection of Gd-DTPA. With time, filling in can be observed. The scan on the lower right is a conventional T1-weighted delayed image (SE 500/15) obtained 10 min postcontrast (see E). The pattern of contrast enhancement is indicative for hemangioma. (E) Ten minutes after administration of Gd-DTPA, the lesion is homogeneously hyperintense with liver on the T1-weighted SE 500/15 image.

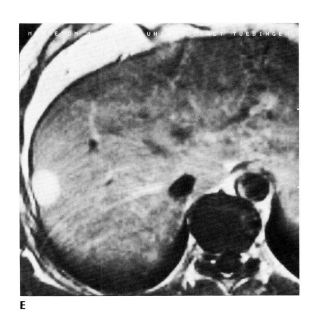

FIGURE 39-3 (continued)

Gd-DTPA per kilogram of body weight demonstrated only slight improvement of lesion contrast 5 min postinjection. Hamm et al. (8) concluded that rapid MRI with intravenous administration of Gd-DTPA improves lesion conspicuity in the first 2 (0.1 mmol/kg of Gd-DTPA) to 3 min (0.2 mmol/kg of Gd-DTPA) after bolus injection. In their pilot study, a single-slice gradient-echo sequence was used. No attempt was made to evaluate sensitivity or diagnostic accuracy in predicting diagnosis. However, Yoshida et al. (19) and Hamm et al. (20), in other studies, investigated tissue characterization by dynamic MRI with gradient-echo sequences.

The study group of Yoshida et al. (19) comprised 22 HCC and 18 hemangiomas all of which were 1 to 3 cm in diameter. A FLASH sequence with a TR of 19 ms, a TE of 12 ms, and a flip angle 90 degrees was used (1.5 Tesla, 0.05 mmol/kg of Gd-DTPA). Yoshida et al. (19) defined criteria of which 17 of 22 HCC and 15 of 18 hemangiomas satisfied 3 or more. Criteria for HCC included hyperintensity prior to administration of contrast material, peak contrast enhancement at 10 s postcontrast, slight to moderate peak contrast enhancement, and absent or minimal delayed contrast enhancement. At morphologic study, HCC often showed a capsule or a nodule-in-nodule appearance. With hemangiomas, they found a hypointense mass precontrast, peak contrast enhancement more than 2 min after injection of Gd-DTPA, marked peak contrast enhancement, moderate to marked delayed enhancement (10 min postcontrast), and at morphological study, filling-in of lesion.

Hamm et al. (20) investigated 29 patients with hepatic hemangiomas ($n = 14$) and hepatic metastases ($n = 15$) by means of Gd-DTPA–enhanced dynamic MRI (0.5 Tesla, 0.2 mmol/kg of Gd-DTPA). Scan variables of the gradient-echo sequence were a TR of 40 ms, a TE of 14 ms, and a flip angle of 40 degrees. Tumor/liver contrast of hemangiomas was higher for all hemangiomas compared with metastases. Furthermore, peripheral enhancement on early postcontrast images and hyperintense fill-in on delayed scans were indicative for hemangiomas.

The studies of Yoshida et al. (19) and Hamm et al. (20) confirm that dynamic MRI with gradient-echo sequences and bolus injection of Gd-DTPA is a useful method to narrow differential diagnosis. It can be recommended as a safe procedure in equivocal cases once a lesion has been detected by other imaging techniques or plain MRI scans. At our institution, this method has been used in many patients, and the results are in keeping with the data from the literature (21) (Figs. 39-3 and 39-4). However, single-slice techniques are not suited for screening purposes; i.e., lesion detection is not improved.

Technical developments of both software and hardware brought about gradient-echo multislice sequences for breath-hold imaging. Edelman et al. (22) used a FLASH sequence with a TR of 110 ms, a TE of 5 ms, a flip angle of 80 degrees and one excitation that yields six contiguous slices within less than 20 s (matrix 256 × 128, 1.5 Tesla). Following bolus injection of 0.1 mmol Gd-DTPA per kilogram of body weight, a first set of images of the entire liver span was obtained in the first 1 to 2 min. Lesion/liver contrast increased immediately postcontrast when compared with plain T1- and T2-weighted images. In this prospective study, the authors detected additional lesions in 2 of 26 patients. To our knowledge, this is the first communication in the literature that reports improvement of sensitivity through Gd-DTPA in focal liver lesions.

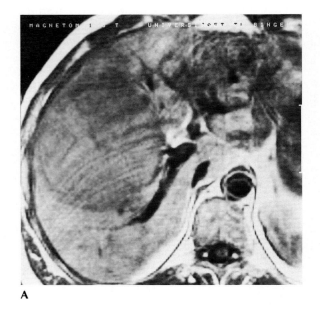

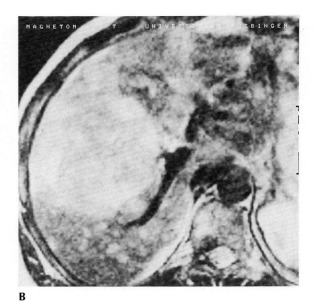

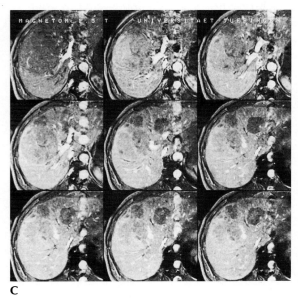

FIGURE 39-4
Hepatocellular carcinoma in a 42-year-old man. (A) The T1-weighted image shows a hypointense mass in the right lobe of the liver that displaces the right portal vein dorsally (SE 500/15). (B) The mass is markedly hyperintense on the T2-weighted scan. There is inhomogeneity of the lesion (SE 1600/80). (C) In the dynamic study after injection of 0.1 mmol Gd-DTPA per kilogram, inhomogeneity of the mass is highlighted (FLASH 50/10/70 degrees). The degree of enhancement is less as compared with the hemangioma in Fig. 39-3.

In Chapter 41, Mirowitz et al. use another approach to multislice dynamic MRI with Gd-DTPA (1.0 Tesla, 0.1 mmol/kg). A short TR (275 ms), short TE (10 ms), one-acquisition T1-weighted SE sequence with half-Fourier sampling (RASE) is applied that yields enough slices to cover the liver within a breath-hold (23 s). Contrast-to-noise ratio (CNR) is highest with Gd-DTPA–enhanced RASE compared with plain T1- and T2-weighted SE scans. As a result, lesion conspicuity is improved, but sensitivity remains unchanged. When compared with the study of Edelman et al. (22), the method of Mirowitz et al. may have the advantage of overall superior image quality because of SE technique but may have the drawback that critically ill patients may not be able to hold their breath for 23 s.

CURRENT CLINICAL ROLE

The review of data from the literature as well as our experience at Tübingen University indicate that Gd-DTPA only contributes to lesion detection when dynamic multislice scanning is performed immediately after bolus injection. However, the inherently high sensitivity of plain

T1- (medium field strength) and T2-weighted images (high field strength), in our view, makes striking improvements of sensitivity through Gd-DTPA unlikely to occur. As regards differential diagnosis of a single lesion or different lesions in the same or adjacent slice, dynamic MRI with a fast imaging sequence that allows simultaneous imaging of at least three slices is a reasonable approach. Dynamic MRI for this purpose should include delayed images 10 to 15 min postcontrast. However, in view of the well-defined MRI criteria for characterization of focal liver lesions (11), only selected patients will need further evaluation by means of dynamic scanning.

FUTURE PROSPECTS

Definition of the value of Gd-DTPA for lesion detection and differential diagnosis is a difficult task. New developments in the field of MRI contrast agents for liver MRI and further improvements in ultrafast-pulse sequences provide a shifting, dynamic background for the evaluation of the ultimate benefits of Gd-DTPA. For example, superparamagnetic iron oxide and hepatobiliary contrast agents both have a specific volume of distribution. Thus both show superior contrast-enhancing properties for liver imaging within a larger time window for postcontrast imaging. However, these agents must exhibit a degree of safety and tolerance comparable with those of Gd-DTPA (23) to ensure that the benefit of improved lesion contrast is not offset by unwanted side effects. Ultrafast-pulse sequences may further change our strategies with contrast-enhanced MRI of focal liver lesions. For example, incremental Gd-DTPA–enhanced snapshot imaging of the liver may be performed rapidly enough to cover the entire liver volume before Gd-DTPA has distributed itself in the extracellular compartment of both liver and tumor tissue.

SUMMARY

Shortening of imaging time from minutes to seconds and from seconds to subseconds has increased the usefulness of Gd-DTPA. Along with the safety of this agent, bolus-enhanced multislice MRI of focal liver lesions is a reasonable method to improve sensitivity. To narrow differential diagnosis in equivocal cases, dynamic MRI with Gd-DTPA can be performed. However, with the imminent clinical availability of other safe contrast agents, the final role of Gd-DTPA in liver MRI will have to be reevaluated.

REFERENCES

1. Freeny PC, Marks WM, Ryan JA, Bolen JW: Colorectal carcinoma evaluation with CT: Preoperative staging and detection of postoperative recurrence. Radiology 158:347, 1986.
2. Weinmann HJ, Brasch RC, Press WR, Wesbey GE: Characteristics of gadolinium-DTPA complex: A potential NMR contrast agent. AJR 142:619, 1984.
3. Weinmann HJ, Laniado M, Mützel W: Pharmacokinetics of Gd-DTPA/dimeglumine after intravenous injection into healthy volunteers. Physiol Chem Med NMR 16:167, 1984.
4. Laniado M, Weinmann HJ, Schörner W, et al: First use of Gd-DTPA/dimeglumine in man. Physiol Chem Phys Med NMR 16:157, 1984.
5. Laniado M, Claussen C, Weinmann HJ, Schörner W: Paramagnetic contrast media in magnetic resonance imaging of the brain, in Taveras J, Ferrucci JT (eds): Radiology: Diagnosis/Imaging/Intervention, vol 3. New York, Lippincott, 1986, chap 59.
6. Hamm B, Römer T, Felix R, Wolf KJ: Magnetische Resonanztomoghraphie fokaler Leberläsionen unter Verwendung des paramagnetischen Kontrastmittels Gadolinium-DTPA. Fortschr Röntgenstr 145:684, 1986.
7. Carr DH, Brown J, Bydder GM, et al: Gadolinium-DTPA as a contrast agent in MRI: Initial clinical experience in 20 patients. AJR 143:215, 1984.
8. Hamm B, Wolf KJ, Felix R: Conventional and rapid MR imaging of the liver with Gd-DTPA. Radiology 164:313, 1987.
9. Moss AA, Goldberg H, Stark DD: Hepatic tumors: Magnetic resonance and CT appearance. Radiology 150:141, 1984.
10. Nelson RC, Umpierrez M, Chezmar JL, Bernardino ME: Delayed magnetic resonance hepatic imaging with gadolinium-DTPA. Invest Radiol 23:509, 1988.
11. Wittenberg J, Stark DD, Forman BH, et al: Differentiation of hepatic metastases from hepatic hemangiomas and cysts by using MR imaging. AJR 151:79, 1988.
12. Heintz P, Ehrenheim C: Differenzierung fokaler Leberläsionen mit der kontratmittelunterstützten KST. Fortschr Röntgenstr 150:297, 1989.
13. Claussen C, Lochner B: Dynamic Computed Tomography. Berlin: Springer, 1985, p 59.

14. Saini S, Stark DD, Brady TJ, et al: Dynamic spin-echo MRI of liver cancer using gadolinium-DTPA: Animal investigation. AJR 147:357, 1986.
15. Ohtomo K, Itai Y, Yoshikawa K, et al: Hepatic hemangioma: Dynamic MRI using gadolinium-DTPA. Eur J Radiol 7:257, 1987.
16. Ohtomo K, Itai Y, Yoshikawa K, et al: Hepatic tumors: Dynamic MR imaging. Radiology 163:27, 1987.
17. Mano I, Yoshida H, Nakabayashi K, et al: Fast spin-echo imaging with suspended respiration: Gadolinium enhanced MR imaging of liver tumors. J Comput Assist Tomogr 11:73, 1987.
18. van Beers B, Demeure R, Pringot J, et al: Dynamic spin-echo imaging with Gd-DTPA: Value in the differentiation of hepatic tumors. AJR 154:515, 1990.
19. Yoshida H, Itai Y, Ohtomo K, et al: Small hepatocellular carcinoma and cavernous hemangioma: Differentiation with dynamic FLASH MR imaging with Gd-DTPA. Radiology 171:339, 1989.
20. Hamm B, Fischer E, Taupitz M: Differentiation of hepatic hemangiomas from metastases by dynamic contrast-enhanced MR imaging. J Comput Assist Tomogr 14:205, 1990.
21. Kölbel G, Schmiedl U, Hess CF, Klose U: Contrast-enhanced MR imaging of focal liver lesions: Application of FLASH and spin-echo sequences (abstract). Radiology 169:221, 1988.
22. Edelman RR, Siegel JB, Singer A, et al: Dynamic MR imaging of the liver with Gd-DTPA: Initial clinical results. AJR 153:1213, 1989.
23. Goldstein HA, Kashanian FK, Blumetti RF, et al: Safety assessment of gadopentetate dimeglumine in U.S. clinical trials. Radiology 174:17, 1990.

40

Gd-DOTA: Chemistry, Toxicity, and Clinical Results

B. BONNEMAIN, A. C. NEISS, D. DOUCET,
S. BEAUTÉ, and D. MEYER

Gd-DOTA meglumine (Dotarem, Laboratoire Guerbet, France) (Fig. 40-1) was first administered in humans in September of 1986 by Professor Caillé (Hôpital Pellegrin, Bordeaux, France). Since that date, many patients have received this contrast agent, and over 6000 patients, including both adults and children, have been evaluated as part of clinical trials or multicenter studies in Europe. The aim of this chapter is to review the main results obtained with Dotarem, the only paramagnetic, macrocyclic chelate marketed so far, with particular emphasis on an indication of paramagnetic complexes that is not very well known, i.e., the investigation of liver diseases. Other indications, such as brain-spine, bone-joint, and soft-tissue diseases, also will be reviewed briefly.

CHARACTERISTICS OF Gd-DOTA MEGLUMINE
Physicochemical Properties

As described by Meyer et al. (1) in 1988, Gd-DOTA meglumine is characterized by the highest thermodynamic stability (Table 40-1) of all gadolinium chelates known to date (2,3) and by extremely slow dissociation kinetics: dissociation $T_{1/2}$ = 21 days at pH 1.15 or 2.10^4 years at pH 7 (4). Another physicochemical property of Gd-DOTA is the rather high affinity of the DOTA ligand for gadolinium. Maegestadt et al. (5) determined that the size of the gadolinium ion perfectly matches that of the cavity of the macrocycle formed by DOTA. These characteristics account for the fact that gadolinium release is most unlikely to occur even in biological media (6) and for the remote capacity of this metal to exchange with endogenous ions when in the form of Gd-DOTA (7).

Gd-DOTA has two other important characteristics: (1) Whereas at 20 MHz its paramagnetic efficacy is comparable to that of Gd-DTPA, it increases at low field strength, a phenomenon probably attributable to the symmetry of the chelate (8); and (2) The osmolality of the Gd-DOTA solution used in clinical practice is less than that of

TABLE 40-1. *Thermodynamic Stability Constants of Gd Chelates*

Chelate	Log K
Gd-DOTA	25.6*
	ND†
Gd-DTPA	22.9*
	19.7†

*Arsenazo III spectrophotometric method.
†Potentiometric method (μ = 0.1 M $(CH_3)_4N^+NO_3^-$ —25°C ± 0.1°C). For Gd-DOTA, determination by this method proves impossible.

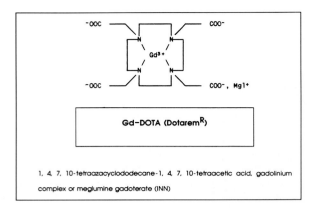

FIGURE 40-1
Gd-DOTA (Dotarem): 1,4,7,10-tetraazacyclododecane-1,4,7,10-tetraacetic acid, gadolinium complex, or meglumine gadoterate (INN).

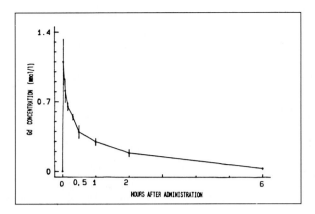

FIGURE 40-2
Plasma concentrations of Gd-DOTA after intravenous injection of 0.1 mmol/kg in six healthy male volunteers (mean and standard deviation).

Gd-DTPA (1300 versus 1900 mOsm/kg H_2O). However, since volumes administered for contrast-enhanced MRI studies are small, the osmolality of gadolinium chelates is not so much a major determinant of clinical safety as it is when using urographic and angiographic iodinated contrast media. Toxicologic, pharmacologic, and efficacy studies performed in animals (9–11) before starting clinical trials in humans have shown the value of these physicochemical properties.

Pharmacokinetic Properties
Pharmacokinetic studies performed in animals (9) and humans (12) demonstrated that Gd-DOTA is a marker of the extracellular space. The plasma half-life of the compound determined after administration in healthy volunteers of a dose of 0.1 mmol/kg (0.2 ml/kg) was approximately 1.3 h, with a steady-state distribution volume of 18 liters. As shown by the plasma disappearance curve, Gd-DOTA is characterized by very rapid distribution kinetics (Fig. 40-2) and is eliminated mainly by the kidney with no metabolization. The affinity of Gd-DOTA for human albumin cannot be measured under usual test conditions because it is too low (10).

CLINICAL EXPERIENCE WITH Gd-DOTA MEGLUMINE

Gd-DOTA was tested in clinical trials according to the usual approach applied to pharmaceuticals at the development stage. In addition to phase I clinical trials in healthy volunteers, phase II and III trials were performed in more than 1500 subjects. More recently, a multicenter study involving nearly 5000 subjects was conducted in more than 100 European hospitals or clinical centers using MR imagers of 0.3 to 1.5 Tesla. The purpose of this trial was to evaluate the advantages and efficacy of Gd-DOTA as well as clinical safety in routine MRI examinations.

Biological Safety of Gd-DOTA
As a result of the increases in serum iron observed in several studies after administration of Gd-DTPA (13), special attention was paid to changes in this parameter between 1 h and 24 h postinjection of Gd-DOTA, both in adults and children. No significant increase in serum iron was found during studies conducted in 178 patients and 6 healthy volunteers given Gd-DOTA (12,14), irrespective of the measuring time (t_0 + 1 h, + 2 h, + 4 h, + 9 h, and + 24 h).

A specific study on the renal tolerability of Gd-DOTA (15) was performed in 12 patients with chronic renal failure (glomerular filtration rates of less than 60 ml/min). Six patients received a dose of 0.1 mmol/kg, and the other six were used as controls. Study findings demonstrated the absence of renal toxicity related to the compound and confirmed preclinical work on the same subject (15).

Overall Safety of Gd-DOTA

The European multicenter clinical trial of Gd-DOTA (16) shows that this agent is remarkably well tolerated in adults and children. Of 4887 patients, only 0.8 percent (i.e., 40 patients) had one or several minor adverse reactions, attributable or not to the contrast agent. These reactions were all observed in adults, except for one. It is also worth noting that no adverse reaction was reported in any of the 228 patients who were administered a dose higher than 0.25 ml/kg and even in the two patients who received a dose higher than or equal to 0.8 ml/kg (i.e., four times the usual clinical dose).

Diagnostic Efficacy

Gd-DOTA, which was first studied in the context of central nervous system (17–23), bone-joint, and soft-tissue (24,25) diseases, as well as liver diseases (26–30), also was evaluated in various pathologic conditions involving the breast (31), pelvis (32–34), ENT, and chest (35–38). On the whole, the diagnostic evaluation made on 4169 patients administered Gd-DOTA as part of the multicenter trial provided the following information (Table 40-2):

1. The purpose of the examination was mainly etiologic diagnosis (32 percent of patients) and frequently tumor staging (28 percent of patients). Another indication for the investigation was recurrence of the disease (13 percent of patients). However, when analyzing study findings organ by organ, the main objective of the examination turns out to be different. The main reasons for using the contrast agent in the investigation of the pelvis and in ENT diseases was tumor staging. In bone-joint and soft-tissue diseases, search for recurrence and postoperative follow-up were the major determinants of the use of the contrast agent.

2. The contribution of Gd-DOTA was fundamental in the majority of examinations. Gd-DOTA–enhanced MRI was found more efficient than plain MRI in more than 60 percent of patients. Nevertheless, this percentage varied depending on the disease explored. It was 62 percent for central nervous system diseases, 71 percent for bone-joint and soft-tissue explorations, and 40 to 50 percent for most of the remaining organs. There are several practical consequences of the diagnostic contribution of Gd-DOTA. In more than 70 percent of patients, the use of the contrast agent had a definite impact on the choice of the initial treatment or on changes in therapy and influenced the decision of whether the initial treatment should be continued or not. In only 26 percent of patients in our series, Gd-DOTA–enhanced MRI did not affect therapeutic decision making. Here again, significant variations can be found depending on the organ explored. Thus, in central nervous system and abdominal diseases, the most important consequence of the contrast-enhanced examination is that it plays a role in the choice of the initial therapy. In contrast, examination of the breast and pelvis with the contrast agent generally had no practical implication on the therapeutic approach in 40 to 60 percent of patients.

TABLE 40-2. *Gd-DOTA Multicenter Trial: Objectives of MRI Examination in Percentage (Several Answers Possible)*

	Etiologic Diagnosis	Tumor Staging	Search for Recurrence	Postoperative Control	Therapeutic Follow-Up	Discovery of New Lesions	Other
Total population ($n = 4169$)	32	28	13	9	5	3	10
Children ($n = 305$)	19	32	21	8	10	4	6
CNS ($n = 3206$)	34	30	12	7	6	4	12
Bone-muscle ($n = 469$)	34	18	34	25	4	2	3
Abdomen ($n = 117$)	37	26	3	1	3	3	8
Breast ($n = 110$)	29	5	4	1	5	4	18
Pelvis ($n = 80$)	19	66	6	4	1	—	—
ENT ($n = 70$)	13	74	13	9	6	1	1
Chest ($n = 27$)	7	26	4	7	7	4	33
Other and missing ($n = 90$)	—	—	—	—	—	—	—

MRI EXAMINATIONS OF THE LIVER: A SPECIAL STUDY ON DIAGNOSTIC EFFICACY

Gadolinium chelates have been evaluated in several studies on the detection of hepatic lesions. Gd-DOTA was tested as part of animal experiments (39–43) and clinical trials in humans involving several hundreds of patients (26–30,44). Four controlled studies were performed in 116 patients. Since the conditions under which these trials were conducted differed from one center to the other (Table 40-3), general conclusions as to the contribution of gadolinium chelates in MRI can hardly be drawn. Parameters modified depending on the study include, among other things, the following:

- *Field strength.* Some studies were performed at 0.5-Tesla field strength, others at 1.5 Tesla. This not only affected both the value of the signal and the effect of the contrast agent, but also the type of sequence practicable.
- *Pulse sequences.* These varied from one MR imager to the other and depended on the center. In some cases, fast imaging and/or dynamic sequences were available.
- *The dose of contrast material and the injection rate.* In most cases, the dose administered was 0.1 mmol/kg (0.2 ml/kg); however, 31 patients received 0.2 mmol/kg so as to evaluate the utility of a higher dose of Gd-DOTA.
- *Diseases explored.* In some trial centers, the majority of patients had liver metastases or hepatocarcinoma. Patient recruitment in other centers was more diverse.

The main objective of these controlled clinical trials was to assess the diagnostic potential of Gd-DOTA using complementary approaches, such as the following:

- Comparison of pre- and postcontrast images obtained with the same sequence
- Comparison of postcontrast images and unenhanced T2-weighted images
- Evaluation of Gd-DOTA–enhanced MRI in comparison with reference diagnostic methods (CT, ultrasound)
- Evaluation of the utility of Gd-DOTA in terms of sensitivity and specificity (assessment of vascularization, characterization of lesions, and so on).

Part of the study published on 4887 patients administered Gd-DOTA (16) relates to patients suffering from a liver disease: 79 patients underwent a Gd-enhanced MRI examination (Table 40-4). The investigations were performed under the usual

TABLE 40-3. *Imaging Techniques in Gd-DOTA Clinical Trials*

	Grellet (Paris, France)	Drouillard (Bordeaux, France)	Bigot (Paris, France)	Marchal (Louvain, Belgium)
Number of patients	39	30	24	23
Field strength	0.5 Tesla	0.5 Tesla	1.5 Tesla	1.5 Tesla
T_2 sequences	SE 2000/60–120–180 ms	SE 2000/50–100–150 ms 2 excitations	GE 33–55/16–19 and 25–24 ms 20 degrees	SE 2200/22–90 ms 4 excitations 8-mm sections Motion compensation
T_1 sequences	SE 350/26 ms GE 200/14 ms GE 35/14 ms Apnea 2 excitations 10 sections every 75 s.	SE 500–700/26 ms 2 excitations SE 260/26 ms 1 excitation 5-section sequence at 1, 3, 5, 10, 15 min	GE 33–55/16–19 ms 80 degrees; Apnea	SE 600/15 ms 4 excitations GE flash 60/10 ms 30 degrees Apnea 10-mm sections
Fast imaging	+	+	+	+
Dynamic mode	+	+	−	+
Dose of Gd-DOTA (mmol/kg)	0.1/0.2	0.1/0.2	0.1 T_2 sequence after Gd-DOTA	0.1

operating conditions of each center, and investigators were free to choose whichever MRI sequence they considered most appropriate.

RESULTS AND DISCUSSION

Role of Administered Dose

Two studies were conducted with the specific objective of evaluating the influence of the Gd-DOTA dose on diagnostic efficacy (30,45). No significant difference in diagnostic efficacy was found between the 0.1 and 0.2 mmol/kg doses in either of the two studies.

Fast versus Conventional Imaging Sequences

This factor is considered essential in the great majority of studies and tests. Fast acquisition sequences taking into account the very rapid pharmacokinetics of Gd-DOTA (29) contribute to a distinct improvement in its diagnostic efficacy, which is consistent with experimental work in the rat (40). Where fast acquisition of MRI data is not possible, the use of gadolinium chelates seems of little interest (46).

Diagnostic Contribution of Gd-DOTA Meglumine

On the whole, as far as plain MRI is concerned, Gd-DOTA injections improve the diagnostic efficacy of MRI in liver diseases in 5 to 75 percent of cases depending on the acquisition method and MRI equipment used (Table 40-5). In comparison with the reference T2 sequence, the contribution of the agent appears to be marginal. In Drouillard's study (47), for instance, lesion count was improved in 67 percent of cases when comparing results obtained with pre- and postcontrast T1 procedures. However, this percentage drops to 16 percent compared with precontrast T2 sequences.

Results from the study by Boudghene et al. (28) appreciably differ from those of other clinical trials. In 30 patients, most of them with metastases (63 percent) or hepatocarcinomas (23 percent), the evaluation of the diagnostic contribution of Gd-DOTA yielded more favorable results (Table 40-6). Indeed, it was shown that Gd-DOTA–enhanced T2 MRI sequences provided better results in 75 percent of patients with respect to T2 reference sequences and in 30 percent of patients compared with CT scanning. Furthermore, the authors noted the following fundamental advantages of Gd-DOTA:

TABLE 40-4. Gd-DOTA Multicenter Trial Liver Investigations (n = 79)

Hepatocarcinoma	27
Metastasis	24
Vascular malformation	15
Adenoma	5
Nodule	2
Not mentioned	6

TABLE 40-5. Summary of Diagnostic Evaluation of Post/Pre Gd-DOTA Sequences

Diagnostic Efficacy	Grellet	Drouillard*	Rolland, Bigot	Marchal	Multicenter Trial	Total
Poorer	41%	25%	5%	17%	4%	16%
Identical	54%	60%	20%	39%	46%	45%
Better	5%	15%	75%	43%	50%	39%
Total	39	20	24	23	79	185

*Calculated on 20 patients with T2-weighted images before Gd-DOTA.

TABLE 40-6. Efficacy of Gd-DOTA MRI in Study by Rolland (29)

Diagnostic Efficacy	MRI T2 Sequence versus CT + Iod. CM (n = 20)	MRI T2 + Gd-DOTA versus CT + Iod. CM (n = 20)	MRI T1 + Gd-DOTA versus MRI T2 Sequence (n = 4)	MRI T2 + Gd-DOTA versus MRI T2 Sequence (n = 24)
Poorer	60%	35%	100%	5%
Identical	20%	35%	—	20%
Better	20%	30%	—	75%

- Better delineation of limits between lesion and necrosis (52 percent of patients)
- Better delineation of normal and diseased tissue (62 percent of patients), which is attributable to an improvement in contrast that is definitely more appreciable in metastases than in hepatocarcinomas (Fig. 40-3)
- Evaluation of other extrahepatic structures (57 percent of patients)
- Detection of other lesions of the liver (25 percent of patients)

Assuming a sensitivity index based on (1) the number of lesions detected, (2) contrast quality, and (3) detectability of lesions less than or equal to 1 cm, the authors conclude that the sensitivity of Gd-DOTA–enhanced T2 sequences was identical to that of CT and definitely superior to plain MRI (Fig. 40-4). Sensitivity is even slightly better than that of CT scanning in the evaluation of metastases (Fig. 40-5). These findings obtained with a small series would be worth confirming in a larger series.

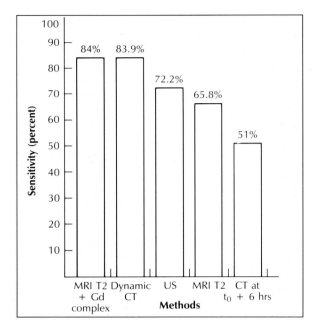

FIGURE 40-4
Sensitivity of the various methods. (From Rolland Y: Détection des Lesions Tumorales Hépatique: Apport du DOTA-Gadolinium en Imagerie Rapide à Haut Champ (1.5 Tesla). Thèse pour le Doctorat en Médecine, Paris, Université René Descartes, 1990. Reprinted by permission.)

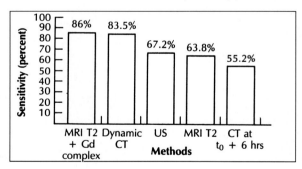

FIGURE 40-5
Sensitivity of the various methods: metastases. (From Rolland Y: Détection des Lesions Tumorales Hépatique: Apport du DOTA-Gadolinium en Imagerie Rapide à Haut Champ (1.5 Tesla). Thèse pour le Doctorat en Médecine, Paris, Université René Descartes, 1990. Reprinted by permission.)

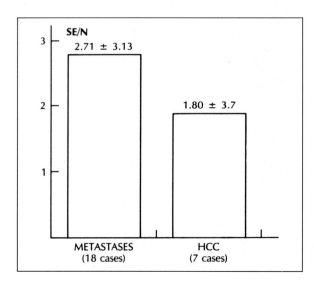

FIGURE 40-3
Mean signal enhancement (SE/N) for metastases and hepatocellular carcinomas. (From Rolland Y: Détection des Lesions Tumorales Hépatique: Apport du DOTA-Gadolinium en Imagerie Rapide à Haut Champ (1.5 Tesla). Thèse pour le Doctorat en Médecine, Paris, Université René Descartes, 1990. Reprinted by permission.)

Injection of Gd-DOTA also permits assessment of the vascularization of lesions. Laurent et al. (26) found different aspects of vascularization depending on the lesion: hemangioma, hepatocarcinoma, or metastases. At 10 and 15 min postinjection of Gd-DOTA, contrast enhancement of hemangiomas is significantly higher than that obtained for other diseases. This is consistent with the findings of Marchal et al. (27) and with CT images of the same lesions after administration of iodinated contrast media.

In the European multicenter clinical trial of Gd-DOTA, in which 79 patients presenting with liver diseases were given the compound, the main indications for the examination were etiologic diagnosis in 44 percent and tumor staging in 27 percent (Table 40-7). Gadolinium was helpful in choosing the initial treatment (35 percent of patients) and even in modifying the ongoing therapy (5 percent of patients). In a third of the patients, the injection of Gd-DOTA had no practical implication on therapeutic decision making (Table 40-8).

TABLE 40-7. *Indications for the Examinations*

	Total Population (n = 4169)	Liver Examinations (n = 79)
Etiologic diagnosis	32%	44%
Tumor staging	28%	27%
Search for recurrence	13%	8%
Postoperative control	9%	—
Therapeutic follow-up	5%	3%
Discovery of new lesions	3%	4%
Other	10%	8%

TABLE 40-8. *Implications of Gd-DOTA–Enhanced Examinations on Therapeutic Decision Making*

	Total Population (n = 4169)	Liver Examinations (n = 79)
No consequence	26%	33%
Choice of initial treatment	29%	35%
Treatment modified	10%	5%
Treatment continued	14%	19%
No treatment	21%	16%

CONCLUSIONS

A large amount of clinical data is available on the first macrocycle injected in humans, Gd-DOTA (Dotarem), which has been shown to be remarkably well tolerated. It is now used in routine clinical practice both in adults and children. Its diagnostic utility has been widely demonstrated in MRI explorations of central nervous system diseases as well as in bone-joint and soft-tissue diseases. Whether gadolinium chelates are useful in liver investigations is hard to evaluate insofar as this is dependent on examination conditions, especially on the type of sequence used and data-acquisition rate. Even though CT scanning remains the standard examination method in liver pathology, Gd-DOTA may under certain conditions contribute to improving diagnosis at MRI. This is most important when CT scans appear to be doubtful or when the patients cannot receive iodinated contrast media. New fast-imaging sequences still have to be evaluated with a view to optimal use of gadolinium chelates in liver imaging and to allow comparison with liver-specific agents such as superparamagnetic iron oxide particles.

REFERENCES

1. Meyer D, Schaefer M, Bonnemain B: Gd-DOTA, a potential MRI contrast agent: Current status of physicochemical knowledge. Invest Radiol 23(Suppl 1): s232, 1988.
2. Loncin MF, Desreux JF, Merciny E: Coordination of lanthanides by two polyamino polycarboxylic macrocycles. Inorg Chem 25:2646, 1986.
3. Sherry AD: Lanthanide chelates as magnetic resonance imaging contrast agents. J Less-Common Metals 149:133, 1989.
4. Merciny E, Desreux JF, Fuger J: Séparation chromatographique des lanthanides en deux groupes basée sur des différences dans la cinétique de décomposition des complexes lanthanides-macrocycles. Anal Chim Acta 189:301, 1986.
5. Knop RH, Franck JA, Dwyer AJ, et al: Gadolinium cryptelates as MR contrast agents. J Comput Assist Tomogr 11:35, 1987.
6. Magerstadt M, Gansow OA, Brechbiel MW, et al: Gd-DOTA: An alternative to Gd-DTPA as a T1,2 relaxation agent for NMR imaging or spectroscopy. Magn Reson Med 3:808, 1986.
7. Tweedle MF, Eaton SM, Eckelman WC, et al: Comparative chemical structure and pharmacokinetics of MRI contrast agents. Invest Radiol 23(Suppl 1): s236, 1988.

8. Muller RN, Maton F, Haverbeke Y: Characterization of MRI contrast media by nuclear magnetic relaxation spectroscopy. Diagn Imag Intern 10:s62, 1988.
9. Doucet D, Meyer D, Bonnemain B: Pharmacological and physicochemical profile of Gd-DOTA, 17e Congrès International de Radiologie, ICR 1989, Paris, 1–8 Juillet 1989, p 122.
10. Doucet D, Meyer D, Bonnemain B, et al: Gd-DOTA, in Runge VM (ed): Enhanced Magnetic Resonance Imaging. St. Louis, Mosby, 1989, pp 87–104.
11. Kien P, Caille JM, Allard M, Bonnemain B: Experimental study of DOTA gadolinium in neuroradiological MRI and in CT, in Fifth Annual Meeting of the Society of Magnetic Resonance in Medicine, Montreal, Canada, August 19–22, 1986, p 1543.
12. Le Mignon MM, Chambon C, Warrington S, Davies R: Gd-DOTA: Pharmacokinetics and tolerability after intravenous injection in healthy volunteers. Invest Radiol 25:933, 1990.
13. Goldstein HA, Kashanian F, Blumetti RF. Safety assessment of gadopentetate dimeglumine in U.S. clinical trials. Radiology 174:17, 1990.
14. Meyer D, Bonnemain B, Schaefer M, Doucet D: Dotarem: The macrocyclic structure of Gd-DOTA and its contribution, in 17e Congrès International de Radiologie, ICR 1989, Paris, 1–8 Juillet, 1989, p 973.
15. Deray G, Bellin MF, Assogba U, et al: Renal tolerance of gadolinium-DOTA and gadolinium-DTPA: A clinical and experimental study, in European Congress of NMR in Medicine and Biology, Book of Abstracts, 301, 1990.
16. Neiss AC, Le Mignon MM, Vitry A: Gd-DOTA: Preliminary results of a multicenter investigation, in European Congress of NMR in Medicine and Biology, Book of Abstracts, 139, 1990.
17. Dietemann JL, Roy C, Tajahmady T, et al: Les produits de contraste en IRM: Essais cliniques d'un nouvel agent paramagnétique le DOTA-gadolinium. J Med Strasbourg 20:93, 1989.
18. Pigeau I, Sigal R, Halimi P, et al: Aspect IRM des craniopharyngiomes à 1.5 Tesla: À propos d'une série de 13 cas. J Neuroradiol 15:276, 1988.
19. Doyon D, Krief O, Halimi P, et al: Contribution of Gd-DOTA in study of medullary tumors and neuromas of petrous part of temporal bone, in Runge VM (ed): Enhanced Magnetic Resonance Imaging. St. Louis, Mosby, 1989, pp 93–96.
20. Caille JM, Gressell JF, Kien P, Allard M: Contribution of Gd-DOTA in assessment of intracranial diseases, in Runge VM (ed): Enhanced Magnetic Resonance Imaging. St. Louis, Mosby, 1989, pp 97–104.
21. Parizel PM, Degryse HR, Gheuens J, et al: Gadolinium-DOTA enhanced MR imaging of intracranial lesions. J Comput Assist Tomogr 13:378, 1989.
22. Lipski S, Baraton J, Taviere V, et al: Gd-DOTA enhanced MRI in neuropediatric patients. Pediatr Radiol 19:267, 1989.
23. Berry I, Manelfe C, Prere J, et al: Le gadolinium-DOTA (Gd-DOTA) dans la pathologie médullaire et rachidienne. Radiologie 9:189, 1989.
24. Vanel D, Coffre C, Contesso G, et al: Apport du gadolinium DOTA dans 20 tumeurs primitives des os et des parties molles. J. Radiol 69:735, 1988.
25. Vanel D, Coffre C, Couanet D, et al: Limites et erreurs dans l'interprétation de l'imagerie par résonance magnétique dans les tumeurs primitives des os et des parties molles. Rev Im Med 2:89, 1990.
26. Laurent F, Drouillard J, Barat JL, et al: Le DOTA-gadolinium en pathologie tumorale hépatique: Evaluation en IRM dynamique à 0.5 T. Rev Im Med 1:61, 1989.
27. Marchal G, Demaerel P, Decrop E, et al: Gadolinium-DOTA enhanced fast imaging of liver tumors at 1.5 T. J Comput Assist Tomogr 14:217, 1990.
28. Boudghene F, Rolland Y, Grange JD, et al: Detection of liver malignancy: T2-weighted rapid MR imaging with DOTA-gadolinium at 1.5 Tesla, in Thirty-Seventh Annual Meeting of the Association of University Radiologists, Seattle, May 19–25, 1989, p s103.
29. Rolland Y: Détection des Lésions Tumorales Hépatiques: Apport du DOTA-Gadolinium en Imagerie Rapide à Haut Champ (1.5 Tesla). Thèse pour le Doctorat en Médecine, Paris, Université René Descartes, Faculté de Médecine, Cochin Port-Royal, 1990.
30. Cuenod CA, Bousquet JC, Duron A, et al: Apport du gadolinium-DOTA dans l'exploration IRM des tumeurs du foie: À propos de 36 Observations, in 17e Congrès International de Radiologie, ICR 1989, Paris, 1–8 Juillet, 1989, p 780.
31. Lamarque JL, Rodiere MJ, Pujol J, et al: Apport des produits de contraste DOTA-gadolinium dans l'exploration du sein, in 10èmes Journées Francophones et 37èmes Journées Françaises de Radiologie, Paris, 7–10 Novembre, 1988, programme scientifique, Société Française de Radiologie Médicale, p 52.
32. Degryse H, Parizel P, De Belder F, et al: Gd-DOTA enhanced MRI of pelvic gynecological tumors, in 17e Congrès International de Radiologie, ICR 1989, Paris, 1–8 Juillet, 1989, p 859.
33. Thurnher S, Hodler J, Marincek B, et al: Contrast enhanced MR imaging of ovarian tumors, in 17e Congrès International de Radiologie, ICR 1989, Paris 1–8 Juillet, 1989, p 859.
34. Gevenois PA, Van Sinoy ML, Stallenberg B, et al: IRM de la prostate: Etude avec gadolinium-DOTA, in 17e Congrès International de Radiologie, ICR 1989, Paris, 1–8 Juillet, 1989, p 495.

35. Bernard P, Jau P, Barth P, Bonnet JL: Magnetic resonance imaging of recent and late myocardial infarction effects of DOTA-gadolinium of contrast enhancement, in 17e Congrès International de Radiologie, ICR 1989, Paris, 1-8 Juillet, 1989, p 731.
36. Kastler B, Germaln P, Dletemann JL, et al: Comparison of multiecho MR images obtained before and after gadolinium injection in myocardial infarction, in 75th Anniversary Scientific Assembly and Annual Meeting, RSNA 1989 Scientific Program, Chicago, November 26-December 1, 1989. Radiology 173P(Suppl 635):481, 1989.
37. Mousseaux E, Guillemin R, Bruneval P, et al: MR imaging with Gd-DOTA for detecting cardiac transplant rejection in humans, in 75th Anniversary Scientific Assembly and Annual Meeting, RSNA 1989 Scientific Program, Chicago, November 26-December 1, 1989. Radiology 173P(Suppl 618):478, 1989.
38. Mousseaux E, Bittoun J, Idy-Peretti I, et al: Contribution of MR imaging to the evaluation of intracardiac and intrapericardial masses diagnosed with echography or CT, in 75th Anniversary Scientific Assembly and Annual Meeting, RSNA 1989 Scientific Program, Chicago, November 26-December 1, 1989. Radiology 173P(Suppl 622):479, 1989.
39. Bousquet JC, Saini S, Stark DD, et al: Gd-DOTA: Characterization of a new paramagnetic complex. Radiology 166:693, 1988.
40. Bousquet JC, Doucet D, Bonnemain B, et al: Hepatic pharmacokinetics of Gd-DOTA in liver MR, in Fifth Annual Meeting of the Society of Magnetic Resonance in Medicine, Book of Abstracts, Montreal, August 19-22, 1986, 1533-1534.
41. Saini S, Weissleder R, Rummeny E, et al: Gd-DOTA: Dose analysis for liver imaging, in Sixth Annual Meeting and Exhibition of the Society of Magnetic Resonance in Medicine, Works in Progress, New York, August 17-21, 1987, p 662.
42. Weissleder R, Stark DD: Magnetic resonance imaging of liver tumors. Semin Ultrasound CT MR 10:63, 1989.
43. Bousquet JC, Doucet D, Saini S, et al: IRM et foie: Etude pharmacodynamique du DOTA-gadolinium, in Second Congrès du GRAMM, Strasbourg, 4-6 Février, 1987, Résumés des Communications Scientifiques, p 157.
44. Bousquet JC, Duron A, Bellin MF, et al: Produit de contraste en IRM hépatique: Aspect respectif du gadolinium et de la ferrite en pathologie tumorale, in 17e Congrès International de Radiologie, ICR 1989, Paris, 1-8 Juillet, 1989, p 123.
45. Laurent F, Drouillard J, Barat JL, et al: IRM et pathologie tumorale hépatique confrontation des séquences sans et avec DOTA-gadolinium, in Troisième Congrès du GRAMM, Bicêtre, 6-8 Avril, 1988, Résumés des Communications Scientifiques, p 64.
46. Hamm B, Wolk KJ, Felix R: Conventional and rapid MR imaging of the liver with Gd-DTPA. Radiology 164:313, 1987.
47. Drouillard J: G 449 06 (DOTA-Gd) en imagerie hépatique par résonance magnétique: Tolérance générale/efficacité diagnostique, Rapport Interne Guerbet, 1988.

41

Dynamic Gadolinium-DTPA–Enhanced MRI of the Liver Using the RASE Technique

SCOTT A. MIROWITZ and
JOSEPH K. T. LEE

The results of several comparative studies indicate that spin-echo MRI has a somewhat higher sensitivity to detection of focal hepatic lesions than does CT (1,2). However, screening examinations of the liver in patients with suspected neoplasia continue to be performed largely with CT. There are several important explanations for the lack of utilization of MRI as a primary screening modality in the liver. Among these are the long imaging times associated with conventional spin-echo pulse sequences, image degradation caused by respiratory motion, and the inability to effectively utilize approved MRI contrast agents in the liver. We have developed a new approach to performing MRI of the liver and other organs called *rapid-acquisition spin-echo (RASE)* (3). This technique successfully addresses many of the impediments that have prevented widespread utilization of MRI for hepatic screening studies. In this chapter we describe the RASE technique and its application for MRI of the liver.

MOTION SUPPRESSION: PRIOR TECHNIQUES

The damaging effects of respiratory motion on abdominal MRI images may be manifested in two ways. Ghost artifacts, which are complete or incomplete replications of moving high-signal-intensity structures (primarily abdominal wall fat), may be observed with periodic motion. Since respiratory motion is essentially periodic in nature, and since the respiratory cycle is short with respect to standard spin-echo imaging sequences, such ghost artifacts are often encountered and may obscure identification of hepatic lesions. The second major effect of respiratory motion is a loss of *anatomic resolution*, which simply refers to the sharpness or definition of structures within the image. Anatomic resolution is to be distinguished from *spatial resolution*, which is a function simply of voxel size and is determined by the slice thickness and imaging matrix. In the liver, the effects of respiratory motion on anatomic resolution may be manifested by a blurring of normally sharp interfaces such as those surrounding hepatic veins, liver margins, or the periphery of hepatic lesions. Such effects also contribute to poor visualization of focal hepatic lesions, particularly those which are small.

A number of methods have been introduced that attempt to reduce the deleterious effects of respiratory motion. These will be briefly reviewed here, although the reader is referred to several excellent discussions of these techniques (4–6). The most widely practiced strategy for reducing respiratory artifacts is that of *multiacquisition imaging*, or *data averaging*. This simply refers to performance of many data sets which are then summated in an effort to "average out" the effects of respiratory motion. This technique is successful in reducing ghost artifacts, with artifact reduction proportional to the square root of the number of data averages performed. Imaging time, however, is directly proportional to the number of data averages, indicating that effective artifact reduction requires significant prolongation of imaging time. Furthermore, the effects of respiratory motion on image blurring are not addressed by this method and may be more pronounced with longer imaging times. Respiratory gating involves acquisition of data during a defined portion of the respiratory cycle—usually during end-expiration. This eliminates the otherwise inconsistent matching of phase encoding with the respiratory cycle and therefore greatly reduces ghost artifacts and image blurring. However, since data acquisition is relatively inefficient with this method, imaging time is markedly prolonged. This renders respiratory gating impractical in most clinical settings, and it is not routinely utilized. In respiratory-ordered phase encoding, imaging takes place throughout the respiratory cycle and is therefore more time-efficient. With this technique, phase-encoding steps are reordered by the computer so as to simulate a single, continuous, slow respiratory cycle. This suppresses but does not eliminate ghost artifacts and does little to improve respiratory-related blurring. Imaging time is essentially unchanged; a bellows device must be positioned on the patient and image reconstruction time may be somewhat prolonged. The effectiveness of respiratory-ordered phase encoding may be severely impaired in patients with erratic respiratory cycles.

It has become apparent that the only means by which respiratory artifacts can be *eliminated*, rather than just *suppressed*, is through breath-hold imaging, as is performed with CT. The difficulty in implementing breath-hold MRI scanning relates, of course, to the prohibitively long imaging times that have been required for spin-echo imaging. However, attention has been recently directed toward reduction of imaging time so as to allow for imaging during suspended respiration. The method that has been most frequently advocated is use of gradient-echo sequences, which utilize a short TR and low flip angle to effect a significant reduction in imaging time. While such sequences can be performed during breath-holding and therefore result in images that are free of respiratory-related artifacts, several important factors must be considered. First, the tissue contrast scale provided by gradient-echo sequences is significantly different from and more complex than that of conventional spin-echo sequences. For example, steady-state gradient-echo sequences such as GRASS and FISP provide tissue contrast that represents a mixture of both T2 and T1 weighting. It is important to remember that the ultimate goal of MRI is to detect lesions, not simply to produce artifact-free images. All the studies referenced at the outset of this chapter were performed with spin-echo pulse sequences. There are presently no studies in the literature that document a lesion detection rate for gradient-echo sequences which is equivalent to that provided by spin-echo MRI. Until such studies become available, it is prudent to consider spin-echo sequences as the "gold standard" for MRI of the liver. Another limitation of gradient-echo sequences is their sensitivity to degradation due to magnetic field inhomogeneities. This arises from the lack of a 180-degree refocusing pulse, such as occurs in spin-echo imaging. As a result, regions of signal void may occur at interfaces of varying magnetic susceptibility such as adjacent to air-containing stomach or bowel or near metallic surgical clips. These artifacts may be reduced with the use of gradient-echo sequences utilizing ultrashort TEs (5 ms), although such sequences are not yet widely available. Finally, since gradient-echo sequences are generally performed with very short TRs (approximately 100 ms), a limited number of imaging slices can be acquired during a single breath-hold (approximately four).

RASE TECHNIQUES: PRINCIPLES

The RASE technique is based on a standard spin-echo pulse sequence performed with short repetition time (TR) and echo delay time (TE). The parameters that we use are a TR of 275 ms and a TE of 10 ms. However, instead of performing multiple data acquisitions in an effort to "average out" the degrading effects of respiratory motion, RASE is performed with a single data acquisition. Because imaging time is directly proportional to the number of data acquisitions (also referred to

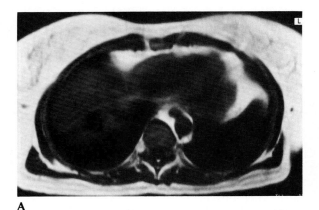
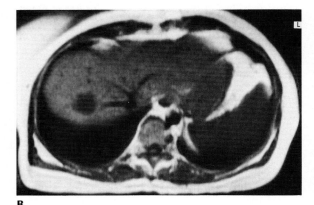
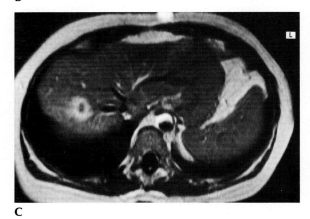

FIGURE 41-1
Metastatic breast carcinoma involving the hepatic dome. (A) Conventional multiacquisition T1-weighted sequence demonstrates the lesion poorly due to blurring and ghost artifacts caused by respiratory motion. The lesion is better visualized using RASE before (B) and after (C) Gd-DTPA administration. A typical halo of contrast enhancement is seen surrounding the metastatic lesion in part C.

as the *number of excitations*, NEX) that are performed, this has the effect of substantially reducing imaging time. However, imaging time continues to exceed the ability of a patient to suspend breathing for the entire acquisition period. In order to bring about a further reduction in imaging time, the half-Fourier data-sampling method is utilized. This indicates that slightly more than one-half the number of phase-encoding steps are performed, with the remaining data generated by computer reconstruction. This is permitted by the inherent symmetry of data provided by the Fourier transform method of image reconstruction. The result is a further reduction in imaging time by approximately 50 percent. Consequently, total imaging time for the RASE sequence is 23 s, which is well within the capacity for most patients to suspend respiration. During this 23 s, 11 imaging slices are obtained. When a slice thickness of 12 mm and interslice gap of 3 mm are utilized, this allows for 16.5 cm of coverage, which is sufficient for imaging of the entire liver in most patients.

RASE provides tissue contrast of a highly T1-weighted spin-echo pulse sequence (hence the name *rapid-acquisition spin-echo*). The strong T1 weighting is advantageous in lesion detection and also renders RASE images highly sensitive to the T1 shortening effects of gadolinium-DTPA (Fig. 41-1). The spin-echo nature of these images indicates that they are relatively less sensitive to susceptibility artifacts than are images acquired with the gradient echo technique. The ability of RASE to image the entire liver during a single breath-hold also has several advantages; the most obvious is in terms of reduced imaging time. When only a portion of the liver can be imaged during a single sequence, time must be allowed for image calculation before the following sequence can be started. Even such apparently minor time delays can be critical if dynamic contrast-enhanced imaging is to be performed effectively. Imaging of the entire liver during a single breath-hold also eliminates one potential source of error that occurs in CT and with performance of interleaved MRI sequences—*misregistration*. This refers to the inability of a patient to precisely replicate the degree of inspiration during repeated breath-holds. This can result in a small portion of the liver not being imaged, and therefore, lesions within that portion could be potentially missed.

The availability of rapid pulse sequences such as RASE presents the opportunity for dynamic contrast-enhanced MRI of the liver. Early experience with gadolinium-DTPA (Gd-DTPA, also referred to as gadopentate dimeglumine DTPA) using conventional spin-echo sequences was disappointing (7). Lesions were often obscured because the long imaging times and slow contrast agent infusion allowed contrast material to equilibrate between lesions and uninvolved liver parenchyma. It is known from experience with CT that for approximately 2 min following rapid intravenous administration of contrast material there is significantly greater contrast enhancement of normal liver parenchyma than liver lesions. As a result, marked improvement in lesion conspicuity can be achieved (8,9) (Fig. 41-2). The biodistribution and pharmacokinetic properties of Gd-DTPA are very similar to those of iodinated contrast material used for CT (10). Therefore, we would expect that "dynamic" contrast-enhanced MRI also may provide improvements in lesion

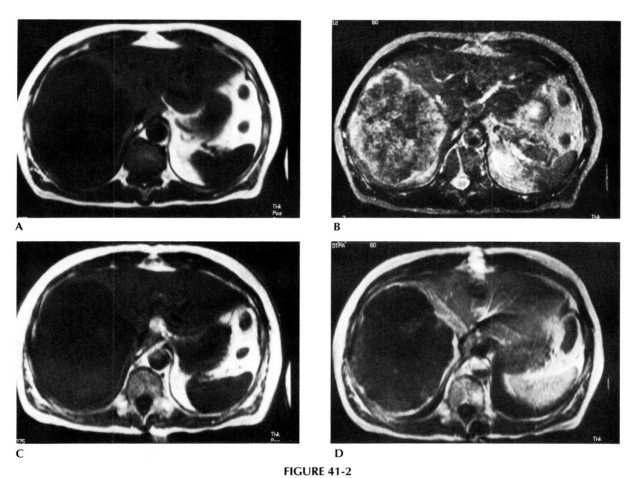

FIGURE 41-2
Metastatic colon carcinoma to the right hepatic lobe. Conventional T1-weighted (A), T2-weighted (B), RASE (C), and dynamic Gd-DTPA enhanced RASE (D) examinations all demonstrate the lesion. However, lesion conspicuity is maximal on dynamic RASE sequence, and a thin rim of enhancement is demonstrated surrounding the lesion (D). Pulsation artifacts from aortic blood flow are pronounced on RASE images due to shorter sampling times and increased blood-pool signal after administration of Gd-DTPA.

conspicuity over nonenhanced MRI. RASE is ideally suited to performance of dynamic MRI liver imaging, since the entire liver can be imaged not only once, but multiple times if desired, during the initial 2 min following bolus contrast material infusion.

LIMITATIONS AND REFINEMENTS

Before discussing the specifics of dynamic liver imaging with RASE, the limitations of this sequence should be addressed. Since imaging time is generally proportional to the square root of the signal-to-noise ratio (SNR), it can be expected that RASE images will have a lower SNR than conventional multiacquisition images of comparable TRs and TEs. The use of half-Fourier data sampling imposes a further reduction in SNR by approximately 40 percent. It can be shown that SNR (defined as signal intensity divided by the standard deviation of noise in the phase-encoding direction) is reduced 2.6 times for a stationary phantom imaged with RASE as compared with a standard 2DFT four-acquisition spin-echo sequence of comparable TR, TE, slice thickness, and field of view (3). When the same comparison is performed in vivo, however, the differences between the sequences become much less significant, with a reduction in SNR of 48 percent for RASE images. This is so because in the conventional sequence noise is increased significantly due to the effects of respiratory motion, resulting in a relative reduction in SNR as compared with phantom measurements. Furthermore, when the mean signal intensity, rather than the square root of signal intensity, of noise is used as an index of relative sequence performance (so-called contrast-to-artifact ratio, CAR), RASE provides a 77 percent improvement in vivo. These statements refer only to RASE images performed without Gd-DTPA administration. When Gd-DTPA is utilized in conjunction with RASE, the T1-shortening effects of Gd-DTPA provide a marked increase in SNR and CAR that significantly exceeds that present in noncontrast conventional images. Other limitations of RASE include the inability of every patient to comply with suspension of respiration for 23 s. Our experience has been that in excess of 90 percent of patients can cooperate if proper instruction before and during the examination is given. However, patients who are critically ill or those with severe pulmonary disease, large abdominal masses, or ascites may have difficulty. A reduction in TE from 10 to 8 ms will allow more imaging slices to be acquired per unit time, and consequently, the TR can be decreased from 275 to 210 ms. This will allow the same 11 imaging slices to be acquired in 18 rather than 23 s. Alternatively, in compliant patients with hepatomegaly, this reduced TE can be used in conjunction with a TR of 275 ms to obtain additional imaging slices with which to cover the enlarged liver while simultaneously improving SNR. Acquisition of a large number of imaging slices during a short imaging time using spin-echo technique can be expected to result in increased power deposition to the patient. However, the specific absorption rate (SAR) required to perform this sequence is well within recommended guidelines for the vast majority of patients using a TE of 10 ms. With use of shorter TE times and acquisition of even more imaging slices, SAR considerations may limit applicability in some patients. Finally, use of a reduced number of phase-encoding steps with RASE results in increased conspicuity of truncation artifacts, which are manifested as one to three linear signal bands immediately adjacent to high tissue contrast interfaces, such as at the interface between air outside the patient and the anterior abdominal wall. Such artifacts are not detrimental to image interpretation and generally do not propagate throughout the image.

The net impact of these various factors on the MRI image cannot be determined solely by quantitative data. Therefore, we undertook a study in which three experienced MRI readers who were blinded to all information regarding imaging parameters were asked to rate both conventional multiacquisition spin-echo and RASE examinations performed in 20 patients (3). The severity of phase encoding errors, edge sharpness, and overall image quality were evaluated on a four-point scale. Excellent to good performances were recorded for 89, 88, and 86 percent of RASE examinations, respectively, versus 41, 59, and 47 percent of conventional examinations. All results were statistically significant with $p < 0.001$.

RASE TECHNIQUE: CLINICAL APPLICATION

As previously discussed, the utility of RASE for evaluation of focal hepatic lesions is improved by its ability to allow for dynamic contrast-enhanced studies. Our method for performing dynamic RASE examinations is as follows: Breathing instructions are carefully reinforced, and a 20-gauge catheter is placed in an antecubital vein before the patient enters the MRI imager. An extra set of extension tubing is connected to the intravenous line and perfused with normal saline. Following performance of a single-slice coronal localizing image using gradient-echo technique, we perform a long TR dual-echo sequence (TR of 2500 ms, TE of 22 ms/90 ms) with a single data acquisition. The purpose of this sequence is to assist in characterization of any lesions that may be detected. This is followed by another single-slice gradient-echo coronal localizer image performed during suspended respiration. The initial RASE sequence is then performed in the transaxial plane. A standard dosage of 0.1 mmol/kg of body weight Gd-DTPA is then injected by means of a three-way stopcock into the intravenous line. Contrast material is injected rapidly, over approximately 20 to 30 s. The Gd-DTPA that remains within the intravenous tubing is rapidly flushed with 20 cc normal saline. RASE imaging is begun immediately following delivery of the contrast material bolus. Results are optimized when there is close communication between the patient, the radiologist administering contrast material, and the technologist responsible for commencing the sequence. As soon as the images from the initial postcontrast RASE sequence are calculated, a second RASE sequence is started without changing any parameters. We usually acquire between three and five separate postcontrast RASE sequences, performed for up to 5 min following contrast material infusion. This is done in order to observe the dynamic contrast enhancement patterns of various lesions, which can assist in their characterization. For lesion detection alone, one or two sets of postcontrast RASE images are sufficient. Total examination time using this protocol is approximately 15 min.

RESULTS

We have evaluated the performance of this dynamic Gd-DTPA–enhanced RASE protocol in a series of 20 patients with a total of 62 focal hepatic lesions (11). The types of lesions represented included hypovascular and hypervascular metastases, hepatocellular carcinomas, cavernous hemangiomas, and hepatic cysts. Measurements of contrast-to-artifact ratios (CAR) were made as follows: (mean signal intensity of lesion − mean signal intensity of uninvolved liver parenchyma)/mean signal intensity of noise in the phase-encoding direction. This measurement provides a quantitative comparison of the performance of various pulse sequences in terms of lesion conspicuity. Our initial data indicate that the dynamic RASE sequence provides significantly greater lesion conspicuity than that of standard sequences. Furthermore, the dynamic RASE sequence allowed lesion characterization based on contrast enhancement patterns similar to those used in dynamic contrast-enhanced CT.

CONCLUSIONS

We have described a method for screening the entire liver during a single breath-holding interval using spin-echo technique. This method is successful in eliminating respiratory-related ghost artifacts and edge blurring and can be effectively implemented with bolus injection of Gd-DTPA resulting in dynamic spin-echo MRI liver imaging. Our results thus far indicate that this technique offers considerable improvements in lesion conspicuity, as well as time efficiency, over conventional T1-weighted and T2-weighted sequences. While further study is necessary, we anticipate that this method will prove to be a highly sensitive means of performing rapid MRI screening examinations of the liver.

REFERENCES

1. Heiken JP, Weyman PJ, Lee JKT, et al: Detection of focal hepatic masses: Prospective evaluation with CT, delayed CT, CT during arterial portography, and MR imaging. Radiology 171:47, 1989.
2. Stark DD, Wittenberg J, Butch RJ, Ferruci JT Jr: Hepatic metastases: Randomized, controlled comparison of detection with MR imaging and CT. Radiology 165:399, 1987.
3. Mirowitz SA, Lee JKT, Brown JJ, et al: Rapid acquisition spin-echo (RASE) MR imaging: A new technique for reduction of artifacts and acquisition time. Radiology 175:131, 1990.
4. Haacke EM, Patrick JL: Reducing motion artifacts in two-dimensional Fourier transform imaging. Magn Reson Imaging 4:359, 1986.

5. Wood ML, Henkelman RM: Suppression of respiratory motion artifacts in magnetic resonance imaging. Med Phys 13:794, 1986.
6. Axel L, Summers RM, Kressel HY, Charles C: Respiratory effects in two-dimensional Fourier transform MR imaging. Radiology 160:795, 1986.
7. Carr DH, Graif M, Niendorf HP, et al: Gadolinium-DTPA in the assessment of liver tumours by magnetic resonance imaging. Clin Radiol 37:347, 1986.
8. Foley WD, Berland LL, Lawson TL, et al: Contrast enhancement technique for dynamic hepatic computed tomographic scanning. Radiology 147:797, 1983.
9. Alpern MB, Lawson TL, Foley WD, et al: Focal hepatic masses and fatty infiltration detected by dynamic CT. Radiology 158:45, 1986.
10. Tweedle MF, Eaton SM, Eckelman, et al: Comparative chemical structure and pharmacokinetics of MRI contrast agents. Invest Radiol 23:S236, 1988.
11. Mirowitz SA, Lee JKT, Gutierrez E, et al: Dynamic gadolinium-DTPA enhanced rapid acquisition spin echo (RASE) MR imaging of the liver. Radiology (in press).

XIV. BILIARY AGENTS

42

Hepatobiliary Agents for MRI: Rationale and Preliminary Evaluation

RANDALL B. LAUFFER

The proper role of magnetic resonance imaging (MRI) in assessing liver disease is not well defined. MRI faces stiff competition from other well-established liver imaging modalities such as ultrasound, liver-spleen scintigraphy, and computed tomography (CT). With further improvements in MRI likely, however, it is far too premature to attempt to select the "gold standard" today.

One of the most important developments that will determine the proper position of MRI is the imminent availability of new liver-selective contrast agents. Since a number of interesting pharmaceutical strategies exist for contrast enhancement in liver MRI, the development and regulatory approval of several agents are possible. The exquisite sensitivity and resolution of MRI coupled with appropriate pharmaceutical probes of liver function could be an unbeatable combination. Although MRI is more expensive than other liver imaging modalities, such as ultrasound or scintigraphy, the determination of cost-effectiveness in the future will have to address the need for multiple "complementary" scans when one good examination may suffice. We also can anticipate a healthy debate concerning the relative value of CT, for which no liver-selective contrast media are available, versus MRI.

POTENTIAL LIVER MRI CONTRAST AGENTS

The large blood supply and avid detoxification activity of the liver make it one of the easiest organs to target with diagnostic imaging agents. (In the development of imaging agents for other tissues, it is often difficult to *prevent* liver uptake.) Three distinct strategies exist:

1. *Nonspecific, extracellular agents.* This class of agents, typified by gadolinium (III)-diethylenetriaminepentaacetic acid (gadolinium-DTPA), quickly distributes in the intravascular and interstitial fluid compartments of all tissues (except the brain) and is rapidly excreted by glomerular filtration (Fig. 42-1). Although these agents possess no liver specificity, they can be used in conjunction with rapid imaging sequences to achieve significant, albeit modest, contrast enhancement of liver lesions.

2. *Particulates, or reticuloendothelial (RE) agents.* These agents, which include various preparations of iron oxide, paramagnetically loaded liposomes, and perfluorocarbon emulsions, have good liver specificity, distributing to the resident macrophage system of that organ (the Kupffer cells) as well as to the RE cells in the spleen, bone marrow, and lungs.

3. *Hepatobiliary agents.* These agents, like gadolinium-DTPA, are small-molecular-weight metal complexes that are selectively extracted by

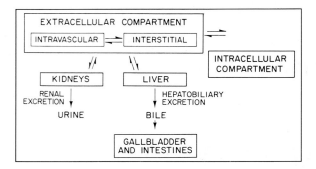

FIGURE 42-1
Principal distribution sites and excretion pathways for intravenously administered soluble metal complexes.

hepatocytes and excreted into the bile. The active derivatives currently being examined, including the prototype agent iron (III)-ethylenebis-(2-hydroxyphenylglycine) (iron-EHPG), also exhibit varying degrees of renal excretion.

The remainder of this chapter focuses on potential hepatobiliary agents for MRI. For a number of reasons discussed in the final section, I believe that these agents hold the most promise for liver (and perhaps biliary) MRI.

HEPATOBILIARY AGENTS IN DIAGNOSTIC MEDICINE

Hepatobiliary pharmaceuticals have been developed and often are used clinically in a number of diagnostic modalities ranging from simple blood tests of liver function to imaging of the gallbladder and biliary tree. While a few of these agents are still used today, most have been replaced by more specific blood tests and improved imaging modalities.

The history of hepatobiliary agents reaches back to 1866, ten years after the first organic dye was synthesized, when Chrzonszczewsky (1) discovered that certain injected dyes localized in both the liver and kidney while others distributed only to the latter organ. Between 1909 and 1913, Rowntree and coworkers (2,3) developed the first liver function test, which involved the measurement of the amount of phenol tetrachlorophthalein excreted in the feces. In 1924–1925, Rosenthal and White (4,5) substituted this dye with a more suitable compound, bromosulfophthalein (BSP). For some 50 years, the BSP liver function test (6), wherein the rate of disappearance from plasma is measured, was an important part of the diagnosis of hepatobiliary disease. Its use declined in the 1970s with the advent of specific enzyme assays.

While phenolphthalein derivatives were being used clinically in liver function tests and as cathartics, Graham and Cole (7) in 1924 utilized the biliary excretion of various halogenated analogues and performed the first intravenous cholecystogram: the radiographic opacification of the gallbladder. These studies paved the way for the development of iodine-containing oral cholecystographic contrast media as well as similar agents for intravenous cholangiography (used primarily for the visualization of the cystic and common bile ducts). Although used successfully for many years, the toxicity of these materials and the advent of ultrasound, CT, scintigraphy, and more direct cholangiographic procedures (such as endoscopic retrograde cholangiopancreatography and percutaneous transhepatic cholangiography) have diminished their importance in the workup of patients with suspected liver or biliary disorders.

The use of hepatobiliary radiopharmaceuticals began with Taplin et al. (8), who in 1955 used [^{131}I]rose bengal in conjunction with external monitoring to evaluate hepatocellular uptake and excretion. Over the years, scores of radiolabeled hepatobiliary agents were tested. In 1975, Loberg and coworkers (9) introduced the [^{99m}Tc]iminodiacetic acid (^{99m}Tc-IDA) complexes that are currently used for cholescintigraphy (10,11).

MRI HEPATOBILIARY AGENTS COMPARED WITH ESTABLISHED MEDIA

In evaluating the potential of paramagnetic MRI hepatobiliary agents, it is helpful to compare various prototypes with the more established hepatobiliary agents just discussed, particularly with regard to dosage and safety considerations (Table 42-1). Although the range of active doses of iron-EHPG and other MRI agents (shown here as 10 to 200 µmol/kg) greatly exceeds the tracer levels needed for cholescintigraphy, the lower end of the range is only slightly higher than the dose in

TABLE 42-1. Hepatobiliary Agents in Medicine: Dose, Safety, and Use

Agent Category	Use	Active IV Dose (μmol/kg)	LD_{50} (μmol/kg)	Apparent Margin of Safety (LD_{50}/dose)	Current Status
Diagnostic tests: Bromosulfophthalein (BSP)	Liver function test	5	100* (IV, dog)	20	Largely replaced by modern tests
Imaging agents: Radionuclide ^{99m}Tc-IDA	Biliary imaging	(Trace)	—	High	Moderate use
X-ray agents: Oral cholecystography (e.g., iopanoic acid)	Enhancement of gallbladder	75 (oral)	11,300† (oral, rat)	150	Declining use
Cholangiography (e.g., iodipamide)	Enhancement of bile ducts	100	2600‡ (IV, mice)	26	Rarely used
Liver enhancement (CT) (e.g., iosefamate)	Enhancement of liver parenchyma	200	7500§ (IV, mice)	38	Too toxic for clinical use
Paramagnetic (MRI)	Liver and biliary enhancement	10–200	2000–5000¶ (IV est.)	10–500 (est.)	Still in preclinical and clinical trials

*Ref. 5
†Ref. 12
‡Ref. 13
§Ref. 14
¶Ref. 15

the safe and successful BSP test. The estimated margin of safety for the proposed MRI agents is equal to or higher than that for BSP. This alone is a favorable sign that safe MRI agents can be developed.

The dosage and margin of safety of the MRI agents are also comparable with those of the iodinated x-ray agents. However, it is important to point out that the cholecystographic and cholangiographic media are used only for biliary enhancement. Since the more likely role of MRI agents is in the enhancement of liver parenchyma, it is more useful to compare MRI agents with the iodinated compounds developed for liver enhancement in CT. The leading compound for this purpose was iosefamate (14,16,17). This agent never reached clinical trials because of excessive toxicity, despite a relatively high apparent margin of safety in acute administration. Since this chemotoxicity most likely stems from the highly iodinated status of the molecule, the failure of this agent has little bearing on the structurally distinct MRI agents. In addition, the required dose of iosefamate (200 μmol/kg) is near the upper limit of the active doses of MRI agents. As I discuss further below, a suitable high-relaxivity gadolinium complex would be used at relatively low doses (perhaps 10 to 50 μmol/kg).

IRON-EHPG, THE PROTOTYPE HEPATOBILIARY AGENT FOR MRI

Iron-EHPG was selected for initial feasibility studies (18). The complex, shown in Figure 42-2, contains coordinated carboxylates, two phenolate rings, net anionic charge, and octahedral coordination to the metal center. The net charge and overall structural properties are similar to those of the ^{99m}Tc-IDA agents, which are thought to be octahedral bis-IDA complexes with two phenyl rings and a -1 charge (10,11). Similar features are also present in BSP and most of the hepatobiliary x-ray compounds.

The water-relaxation ability (relaxivity) of iron-EHPG is moderate, roughly one-fourth that of gadolinium-DTPA. This is due to two factors: (1) the gadolinium (III) ion possesses seven unpaired electrons and a stronger magnetic moment than iron(III), which has only five unpaired electrons,

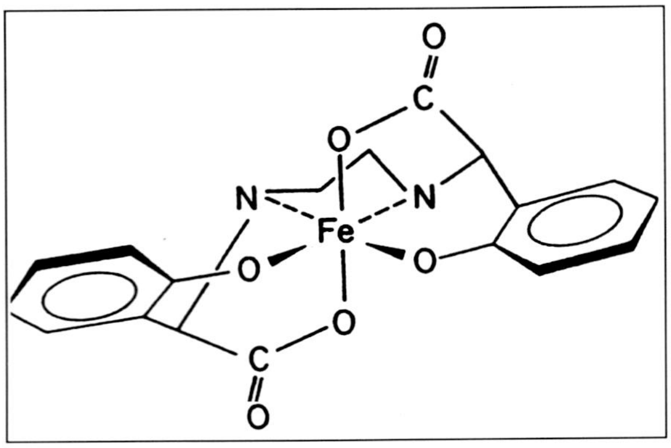

FIGURE 42-2
Structure of one isomer of iron-EHPG.

and (2) while gadolinium-DTPA has one open coordination site for water that communicates the paramagnetic effect to the bulk water protons, iron-EHPG has none. Nonetheless, it was thought that the moderate relaxivity of iron-EHPG would be sufficient if the complex localizes in the liver and bile. (See references 19 and 20 for more on relaxivity and the design of MRI contrast agents.)

A more important reason for the selection of iron-EHPG is its superb stability. The metal-ligand association constant, $\log K = 34$, is one of the highest known. The dissociation of the complex in vivo to form relatively toxic free iron is therefore extremely unlikely.

The initial MRI and biodistribution studies of Fe(EHPG)$^-$ were encouraging (18). At a dose of 200 μmol/kg, the complex increases the $1/T_1$ of rat liver from approximately 3.2 to 4.3 s^{-1} (20 MHz, 37°C) at 10 min postinjection, corresponding to a concentration of approximately 1 mM in the water space of the tissue. This localization yields a 200 percent increase in MRI signal intensity on a 60-MHz imaging system. [It was demonstrated later that the degree of enhancement is dependent on the choice of pulse-sequence parameters in accordance with theoretical expectations (21).] In other studies, the biliary clearance of the intact agent from the liver was observed in several animal species.

Further work focused on various phenyl ring–substituted derivatives of iron-EHPG (22). It was observed that, like the ^{99m}Tc-IDA complexes (10,11), the liver uptake and excretion rates of the paramagnetic complexes are effectively modulated by simple chemical alterations (Fig. 42-3). This strategy will most likely play an important role in the optimization of candidates for clinical trials. This work also showed that considerable enhancement of liver MRI signal intensity could be achieved with doses as low as 50 μmol/kg.

Additional studies addressed the structural basis for the hepatocellular excretion of complexes such as iron-EHPG. As has been discussed previously (19,20), it is thought that hepatobiliary agents may be taken up by the same hepatocellular membrane receptor that is responsible for bilirubin uptake. Since this receptor has not been reconstituted into a soluble form for binding studies, the binding of iron-EHPG derivatives to the bilirubin binding site on human serum albumin (HSA) was explored (23–25). These studies showed that the iron complex indeed does bind to this site; thus iron-EHPG and bilirubin are biochemically similar. Indeed, a molecular graphics analysis revealed considerable correspondence between the structure of iron-EHPG and certain molecular conformations of bilirubin.

IRON-EHPG–ENHANCED MRI OF LIVER METASTASES IN ANIMAL MODELS

To properly evaluate the potential of iron-EHPG to enhance the detection of liver tumors, Shtern et al. (26) modified existing animal models of liver metastases. M5076 sarcoma or C-26 colon tumor cells are injected into the spleen of a mouse and allowed to spread through the blood supply to the liver. This creates multiple, well-defined metastatic lesions in the liver, much like that seen clinically.

The intravenous administration of iron-EHPG (100 μmol/kg) results in considerable contrast enhancement of the metastatic tumors on T1-weighted MRI scans (Fig. 42-4). Little or no signal enhancement is seen in the tumors. The preferential distribution of the agent to the liver also was demonstrated in separate biodistribution studies in animals with direct intrahepatic tumor implants; a liver-to-tumor concentration ratio of 5.2 is obtained at 20 min postinjection.

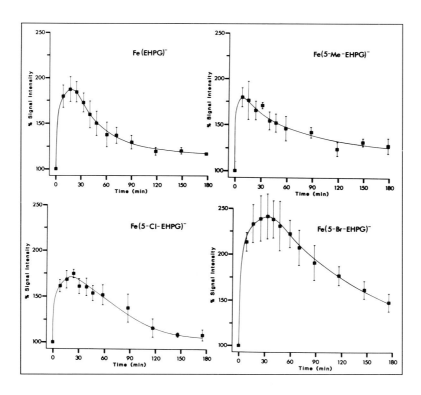

FIGURE 42-3
Time dependence of the average rat liver MRI (1.4 Tesla, IR 1460/400/15) intensities (in terms of percentage of initial preinjection intensity) observed after injection of 50 μmol/kg of the ring-substituted iron-EHPG derivatives shown. Data points displayed represent averages of three animals in each group (± SD). The most lipophilic derivative, iron-5-Br-EHPG, has the greatest liver uptake and longest clearance time. (From Lauffer RB, Vincent AC, Padmanabhan S, et al: New hepatobiliary MR contrast agents: 5-Substituted iron-EHPG derivatives. Magn Reson Med 4:582, 1987. Reprinted by permission.)

An analysis of liver/tumor contrast-to-noise ratios seen in the 2.0-Tesla MRI scans shows that, for relatively small lesions (<5 mm), the T1-weighted iron-EHPG–enhanced scans are significantly better than either unenhanced T1-weighted scans or T2-weighted scans (Fig. 42-5). When the data from both metastases models are combined, it is apparent that while large lesions (>5 mm) are detected by all three imaging strategies, smaller lesions are best detected by the contrast-enhanced scan (Fig. 42-6).

These preliminary results indicate that the enhancement of T1 contrast in MRI of the liver holds great promise for early detection of metastases in cancer patients.

OTHER CANDIDATES FOR HEPATOBILIARY MRI

In addition to the iron-EHPG derivatives, several other iron (III), gadolinium (III), and manganese (II) complexes are currently being examined as hepatobiliary agents (15,27). The manganese complexes currently being examined, while exhibiting good liver enhancement capability, do appear to suffer some degree of dissociation in vivo. In the case of divalent (+2) metal ions, the lower positive charge [compared with iron (III) and gadolinium (III)] and thus reduced affinity for negatively charged ligands presents a challenge in the area of ligand design. Animal studies have shown that manganese (II) ions released

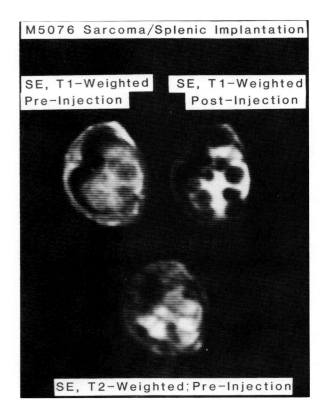

FIGURE 42-4
MR images (2.0 Tesla) of a mouse exhibiting multiple liver metastases. M5076 sarcoma cells were implanted in the spleen of mice and allowed to metastasize to the liver. Figure shows enhancement of normal liver parenchyma on T1-weighted images (SE 200/15) with 100 μmol/kg iron-EHPG, facilitating the detection of the lesions (image at top right was obtained 15 min postinjection). For comparison, a T2-weighted image (SE 2000/60) is shown. (From Shtern F, Garrido L, Compton C, et al: MR imaging of blood-borne liver metastases in mice: Contrast enhancement with iron-EHPG. Radiology [in press]. Reprinted by permission.)

from such agents can have a wide range of subacute physiologic effects (28,29). It is also important to question whether the image-enhancement effects of manganese complexes are due to the intact complex or the free manganese (II) ion itself. The latter has been shown to be an effective hepatobiliary and myocardial perfusion agent (30–32). Whether these considerations will limit the clinical utility of such agents or, alternatively, present new opportunities (i.e., the safe delivery of "free" manganese to tissues) remains to be seen.

While the iron complexes have been useful in initial feasibility studies, a gadolinium derivative would be most useful clinically. Since gadolinium complexes usually exhibit two- to fourfold greater relaxivity than iron complexes, the correspondingly lower doses of the former would be expected to yield a higher margin of safety. A number of attractive gadolinium chelates for hepatobiliary use have been proposed (33,34).

COMPARISON OF HEPATOBILIARY AGENTS WITH OTHER MRI AGENTS FOR LIVER IMAGING

In the search for optimal liver MRI contrast agents, one must consider nonspecific/extracellular and RE-avid compounds in addition to hepatobiliary candidates. From a number of practical viewpoints, the latter category appears to be most attractive for clinical use (Table 42-2).

The nonspecific agents, such as gadolinium-DTPA, enhance both normal liver tissue and lesions, at times obscuring the inherent (preinjection) contrast available with MRI. The pharmacokinetic profile of these agents often differs in the two tissues of interest, enough so that contrast enhancement is available during the first few minutes

TABLE 42-2. *Advantages of Hepatobiliary Agents Over Other Possible Liver MRI Contrast Agents*

			Particulates	
	Hepatobiliary	Extracellular	Iron Oxide	Liposomes
Liver specificity	X		X	X
Enhancement of biliary tree and gallbladder	X			
Use with optimal T1-weighted sequences	X	X		X
Efficient clearance	X	X		
Straightforward formulation	X	X		

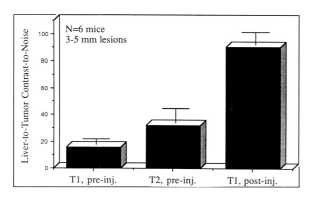

FIGURE 42-5
Liver/tumor contrast in MRI scans of the M5076 metastases model. The T1-weighted iron-EHPG–enhanced images exhibit significantly greater contrast than the unenhanced T1- or T2-weighted scans. (See Fig. 42-4 for experimental details.)

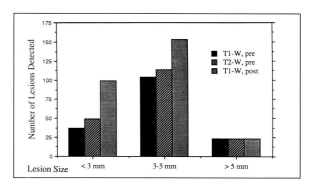

FIGURE 42-6
Combined tumor-detection data from the MRI studies of C-26 and M5076 metastases models. The three bars for each lesion size represent, from left to right, unenhanced T1-weighted scans, unenhanced T2-weighted scans, and iron-EHPG–enhanced T1-weighted scans. The contrast enhancement provided by iron-EHPG was important in the detection of small metastatic lesions (<5 mm). (See Fig. 42-4 for experimental details.)

after injection. However, the added challenge of this procedure may inhibit wide acceptance, especially if more specific agents become available.

With regard to the liver-specific (or liver-selective) candidates, the hepatobiliary approach offers several distinct advantages over RE agents such as iron oxide formulations or paramagnetically loaded liposomes. The ability to enhance the biliary tree and gallbladder is a unique feature of the hepatobiliary agents that is not available with the particulates. However, further investigation will be required to determine the value of biliary imaging with MRI in light of several competing technologies.

A more important advantage of the hepatobiliary agents over the iron oxide particles is that the former, which act on MRI signal intensity by reducing T1, can be used in conjunction with the best MRI pulse sequences for imaging the liver: the highly T1-weighted short TR/short TE sequence. Iron oxide particles, on the other hand, are T2 agents and must be used with long TR/long TE sequences. While the role of field strength and novel pulse sequences still dominates discussions of liver MRI, the fact is that when significant T1 differences between liver and lesion can be induced by a contrast agent, the short TR/short TE sequence will provide superior contrast and image quality. This is so because the short TR allows extensive signal averaging and, more important, the short TE provides high signal intensity, fewer motion artifacts, and strong T1 weighting (21,26).

RE agents in general possess certain disadvantages when compared with the types of molecules suitable for hepatobiliary imaging. First, the particulate media must involve some supermolecular structure, which leads to potential complications in manufacturing and formulation processes as well as important questions with regard to shelf stability. Second, the clearance of these agents from the body can be quite slow, often requiring metabolic breakdown, which increases the number of chemical species that one must prove are safe to the patient. The iron oxide particles, for example, release free iron ions, which are known to be excellent catalysts for oxygen free-radical tissue damage. These concerns may limit the number of repeat examinations that could be performed with such contrast media. It should be noted that despite intense investigation, no particulate-based liver contrast agents for CT have achieved regulatory approval.

Hepatobiliary agents, on the other hand, will bear a strong resemblance to gadolinium-DTPA and the other nonspecific agents currently in clinical trials: They will be simple, small-molecular-weight metal complexes with fairly straightforward preparation and efficient clearance (as the intact complex) from the body. Practical pharmacologic considerations such as these, although mundane to many investigators, may play an important role in the final selection of optimal liver MRI contrast agents.

CONCLUSIONS

Hepatobiliary agents are an important new class of potential MRI contrast agents. By virtue of their efficient excretion from the body, the development of safe derivatives of this class seems likely. Additionally, in contrast with the nonspecific renal agents, hepatobiliary agents may give an indication of the status of specific cellular function: that of the hepatocytes of the liver.

The potential diagnostic utility of this class of MRI agents includes

1. Selective enhancement of normal, functioning liver tissue to aid in the detection of small lesions, such as metastatic tumors (focal liver disease)
2. Indication of the status of liver function in order to detect diffuse liver disease such as cirrhosis
3. High-resolution visualization of bile ducts and the gallbladder.

REFERENCES

1. Chrzonszczewsky N: Zur anatomie und physiologie der leber. Arch Pathol Anat Physiol 35:153, 1866.
2. Abel JJ, Rowntree LG: On the pharmacological action of some phthaleins and their derivatives, with especial reference to their behavior as pergatives. J Pharmacol Exp Ther 1:231, 1909.
3. Rowntree LG, Hurvitz SH, Bloomfield AL: An experimental and clinical study of the value of phenol tetrachloro-phthalein as a test for hepatic function. Bull Johns Hopkins Hosp 24:327, 1913.
4. Rosenthal SM, White EC: Studies in hepatic function: VI. A. The pharmacological behavior of certain phthalein dyes. B. The value of selected phthalein compounds in estimation of hepatic function. J Pharmacol Exp Ther 24:265, 1924.
5. Rosenthal SM, White EC: Clinical application of the bromsulfophthalein test for hepatic function. JAMA 84:1112, 1925.
6. Jablonski P, Owen JA: The clinical chemistry of bromsulfophthalein and other cholephilic dyes. Adv Clin Chem 12:309, 1969.
7. Graham EA, Cole WH: Roentgenologic examination of the gallbladder. JAMA 82:613, 1924.
8. Taplin GV, Meredith OM, Kade H: The radioactive I-131 tagged rose bengal uptake excretion test for liver function using external gamma ray scintillation counting techniques. J Lab Clin Med 45:665, 1955.
9. Harvey E, Loberg MD, Cooper M: Tc-99m-HIDA: A new radiopharmaceutical for hepatobiliary imaging. J Nucl Med 16:533, 1975.
10. Loberg MD, Nunn AD, Porter DW: Development of hepatobiliary imaging agents, in Nuclear Medicine Annual. New York, Raven, 1981, pp 1–33.
11. Chervu LR, Nunn AD, Loberg MD: Radiopharmaceuticals for hepatobiliary imaging. Semin Nucl Med 12:5, 1982.
12. Harnish P: Sterling Drug, personal communication, 1990.
13. Marshall TR, Ling JT: Clinical evaluation of a new intravenous cholangiographic medium: 5,5'-sebacoyl-diimino-bis (2,4,6-triiodo-N-methylisophthalamic acid). AJR 90:854, 1963.
14. Seltzer SE, Hamilton C, VanDeripe D: Experimental evaluation of iosefamate meglumine and its derivatives as hepatobiliary CT contrast agents. AJR 145:67, 1985.
15. Elizondo G, Fretz CJ, Stark DD, et al: Preclinical Efficacy Studies of Gadolinium-BOPTA as an Hepatobiliary Contrast Agent for MRI. Presented at the Eighth Annual Meeting of the Society of Magnetic Resonance in Medicine, Amsterdam, 1989.
16. Koehler RE, Stanley RJ, Evans RG: Iosefamate meglumine: An iodinated contrast agent for hepatic computed tomography scanning. Radiology 132:115, 1979.
17. Moss AA: Computed tomography of the hepatobiliary system, in Moss AA, Gamsu G, Genant HK (eds): Computed Tomography of the Body. Philadelphia, Saunders, 1983, p 615.
18. Lauffer, RB, Greif WL, Stark DD, et al: Iron-EHPG as an hepatobiliary MR contrast agent: Initial imaging and biodistribution studies. J Comput Assist Tomogr 9:431, 1985.
19. Lauffer RB: Paramagnetic metal complexes as water proton relaxation agents for NMR imaging: Theory and design. Chem Rev 87:901, 1987.

20. Lauffer RB: Magnetic resonance contrast media: Principles and progress. Magn Reson Q 6:65, 1990.
21. Greif WL, Buxton RB, Lauffer RB, et al: Pulse sequence optimization for MR imaging using a paramagnetic hepatobiliary contrast agent. Radiology 157:461, 1985.
22. Lauffer RB, Vincent AC, Padmanabhan S, et al: New hepatobiliary MR contrast agents: 5-Substituted iron-EHPG derivatives. Magn Reson Med 4:582, 1987.
23. Lauffer RB, Vincent AC, Padmanabhan S, Meade TJ: Stereospecific binding of rac-iron(III)-N,N'-ethylene-bis[(5-bromo-2-hydroxyphenyl)glycinate] to the bilirubin site on human serum albumin. J Am Chem Soc 109:2216, 1987.
24. Larsen SK, Jenkins BG, Memon NG, Lauffer RB: Structure-affinity relationships in the binding of unsubstituted iron phenolate complexes to human serum albumin: Molecular structure of iron(III)-N,N'-bis(2-hydroxybenzyl)ethylenediamine-N,N'-diacetate. Inorg Chem 29:1147, 1990.
25. Jenkins BG, Armstrong E, Lauffer RB: Site-specific water proton relaxation enhancement of iron(III) chelates bound noncovalently to human serum albumin. Magn Reson Med (in press).
26. Shtern F, Garrido L, Compton C, et al: MR imaging of blood-borne liver metastases in mice: Contrast enhancement with iron-EHPG. Radiology (in press).
27. Elizondo G, Tsang YM, Rocklage SM, et al: Hepatobiliary Contrast Agents: Preclinical Efficacy Studies. Presented at the Seventh Annual Meeting of the Society of Magnetic Resonance in Medicine, San Francisco, 1988.
28. Luckey TD, Venugopal B: Metal Toxicity in Mammals, vol 1. New York, Plenum, 1977.
29. Wolf GL, Baum L: Cardiovascular toxicity and tissue proton T1 response to manganese injection in the dog and the rabbit. AJR 141:193, 1983.
30. Wolf GL, Burnett KR, Goldstein EJ, Joseph PM: Contrast agents for magnetic resonance imaging, in Magnetic Resonance Annual. New York, Raven, 1985, pp 231–266.
31. Lauterbur PC, Mendoca-Dias MH, Rudin AM: Augmentation of tissue water proton spin-lattic relaxation rates by in vivo addition of paramagnetic ions, in Dutton PL, Leigh LS, Scarpa A (eds): Frontiers of Biological Energetics. New York, Academic, 1978, p 752.
32. Brady TJ, Goldman MR, Pykett IL, et al: Proton nuclear magnetic resonance imaging of regionally ischemic canine hearts: Effect of paramagnetic proton signal enhancement. Radiology 144:343, 1982.
33. Lauffer RB, Brady TJ: Hepatobiliary NMR Contrast Agents. U.S. Patent No. 4,899,755.
34. Lauffer RB: In Vivo Enhancement of NMR Relaxivity. U.S. Patent No. 4,880,008.

43

Hepatobiliary Contrast Agents: An Overview of the Development of Manganese Dipyridoxyl Diphosphate (Mn-DPDP)

SCOTT M. ROCKLAGE and
MICHELLE VANWAGONER

One of the most important clinical areas in which magnetic resonance imaging (MRI) has yet to have a major impact is within the upper abdomen. Contrast-enhanced CT remains the accepted "gold standard" for liver imaging, primarily because of its ability to demonstrate liver metastases with greater sensitivity and specificity than either ultrasound or radiopharmaceutical-based nuclear medicine (1), although major limitations remain (2). Freeny et al. (3) demonstrated that despite use of state-of-the-art dynamic bolus-enhanced CT of the liver in staging colorectal carcinoma, 27 percent of liver metastases confirmed at surgery went undiscovered by CT. An additional study by Heiken et al. (4) indicated that only 14 of 37 lesions (38 percent) confirmed by pathologic correlation were detected by contrast-enhanced CT.

To date, MRI has had limited application within the upper abdomen owing to image artifacts resulting from various biologic motions and the lack of a suitable liver contrast agent. An additional complication is the lack of an accepted MRI liver imaging protocol that will yield consistent results within a window of instrument parameters. If one simply considers spin-echo imag-

The authors would like to acknowledge the technical contributions of David Stark, Kelvin Lim, Philip Leese, and Dilip Worah.

ing, which is the most frequently used pulse sequence in hepatic MRI, the capacities of individual systems vary to such a degree that MRI images obtained with similar echo times from two different systems may yield differing results. The use of hepatic contrast media in MRI is expected to make the technique substantially more robust so that small differences in instruments or their data-acquisition/processing capabilities may be rendered insignificant.

MRI contrast agents for liver imaging will likely lead to increased sensitivity and specificity in clinical diagnosis. These agents may be necessary to enhance the contrast difference between pathologic and normal tissues that do not inherently possess the proton density or T1 and/or T2 differences to allow for effective visualization regardless of the pulse sequence used. The hepatic contrast agents investigated to date fall into the categories of hepatocyte-specific, reticuloendothelial-specific, and vascular agents (5). Although overlap exists between these categories, the hepatic agents contain either manganese, iron, or gadolinium as the source of paramagnetic or superparamagnetic/ferromagnetic potency. Table 43-1 is a partial list of some of the hepatic contrast agents that have been evaluated in animal and, in some cases, human studies.

TABLE 43-1. Hepatic Contrast Agents

Hepatobiliary	Reticuloendothelial	Vascular
$MnCl_2$	Gd_2O_3	Gd-DTPA
Mn-DPDP	Iron particles	Gd-DTPA-BMA
Gd-BOPTA	Liposomes	Gd-DOTA
Fe-EHPG		Gd-HP-DO3A
Fe-HBED		

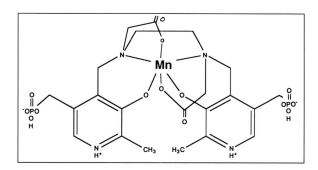

FIGURE 43-1
Structure of Mn-DPDP.

Mn-DPDP

Manganese(II) N,N'-dipyridoxylethylenediamine-N,N'-diacetate-5,5'-bis(phosphate), Mn-DPDP, has been developed as a paramagnetic contrast agent for MRI of the hepatobiliary system. Mn-DPDP, commonly referred to as *manganese dipyridoxyl diphosphate*, is a manganese chelate derived from pyridoxal-5'-phosphate, a catalytically active form of vitamin B_6 and a coenzyme in the breakdown of amino acids and the metabolism of fats and carbohydrates (6). Mn-DPDP has a molecular weight of 691.4 (as the free acid), a molecular formula of $MnC_{22}H_{30}N_4O_{14}P_2$, and the structural formula illustrated in Figure 43-1.

The manganese coordination site is a distorted octahedron made up of two phenolate oxygen atoms, two carboxylate oxygen atoms and two tertiary nitrogen atoms. The manganese atom is in the +2 oxidation state based on the charge inventory, magnetic susceptibility measurements (5.93 μ_B, theoretical for high-spin Mn^{2+} is 5.92 μ_B), and structural parameters (7). The thermodynamic stability constant has been determined to be log K = 15.1. Reference 7 describes the complete synthesis, as well as providing a structural and thermodynamic characterization of Mn-DPDP.

Longitudinal and transverse relaxivities of Mn-DPDP in aqueous solution are similar to those of other paramagnetic agents (R_1 = 2.4 mM^{-1}s^{-1}, R_2 = 3.0 mM^{-1}s^{-1} at 10 MHz, 37°C).

PRECLINICAL EVALUATION

Imaging, pharmacology, toxicology, and drug metabolism studies have been conducted to evaluate Mn-DPDP. The ability of Mn-DPDP to produce image enhancement has been demonstrated in rodents and rabbits. Mn-DPDP administered intravenously at dosages of 10 to 50 μmol/kg enhanced the visualization of pathologic conditions such as liver tumors and increased the signal-to-noise ratio (SNR) from the liver by up to 200 percent. Enhancement studies using a spin-echo (SE 250/18) pulse sequence were conducted using rats with mammary adenocarcinoma implanted directly in the liver (8). Baseline unenhanced images showed tumor/liver contrast-to-noise ratios (CNRs) of −7.6 ± 3.2. Following injection of Mn-DPDP (50 μmol/kg), both hepatic and tumor signal intensities increased immediately. Thirty minutes after injection, the liver signal-to-noise ratio (SNR) was 100 percent greater than baseline and the tumor/liver CNR magnitude had increased to −35.3 ± 7.5. These values remained essentially unchanged for 1 hour and then slowly returned toward baseline (9).

Hemodynamic studies were conducted using 10 normal, fasted dogs anesthetized with sodium pentothal and maintained on a mixture of halothane-O_2-N_2O anesthesia after tracheal intubation. Intravenous doses of 58, 116, 232, and 464 μmol/kg Mn-DPDP were administered intravenously to eight of the dogs over a 60-s period. These dosages represent a 6- to 46-fold range over the anticipated clinical dosage (10 μmol/kg) and cumulatively up to 87 times the anticipated clinical dosage. A saline solution iso-osmolar (1000 mOsmol/kg) to the Mn-DPDP solution was administered to two control dogs at the same volume (ml/kg), rate, and intervals as the Mn-DPDP solution.

There were no physiologically significant hemodynamic changes (aortic, left ventricular, pulmonary artery, and right atrial blood pressure, $dLVP/dt$, mean aortic blood flow, heart rate) observed at dosages up to 23 times the anticipated clinical dosage. At the 58 and 116 μmol/kg dosages, mean aortic pressure values were indistinguishable from those of saline controls. At 464 μmol/kg (46 times the anticipated human dosage), transient decreases in aortic and left ventricular pressures were detected. The systemic and pulmonary vascular resistances showed transient decreases in the presence of minimal changes in the heart rate and filling pressure. Control dogs demonstrated a 10 percent mean aortic pressure decrease when saline was injected at the same volume. All observed changes were transient, with values usually returning to pretreatment levels within 12 minutes after dosing. Similar studies with $MnCl_2$ have shown significant hemodynamic toxicity resulting in death at dosages of 0.02 and 0.1 mmol/kg (10).

Acute lethality is an important and traditional index of toxicity used to evaluate new drug candidates. No deaths occurred at 2893 μmol/kg (290 times the anticipated clinical dosage) in studies in mice and rats when Mn-DPDP was administered as an infusion for periods ranging from 5 to 8 minutes and 41 seconds. When administered as an intravenous bolus injection in mice, the LD_{50} of Mn-DPDP was 1901 μmol/kg (approximately 190 times the anticipated clinical dosage). The LD_{50} of $MnCl_2$ in mice was 0.3 mmol/kg compared with 5.5 to 10 mmol/kg for Gd-DTPA (11,12) and 10.6 mmol/kg for Gd-DOTA (11). The range of safety factors, expressed as the ratio of LD_{50} to the dose used for imaging, was 200 for Mn-DPDP, 15 for $MnCl_2$, 60 to 100 for Gd-DTPA (11,12), and 100 for Gd-DOTA (11).

Subchronic toxicity of Mn-DPDP was studied in Sprague-Dawley rats and cynomolgus monkeys. Mn-DPDP was injected intravenously 3 times a week for 3 consecutive weeks at dosages of 29, 116, or 290 μmol/kg in the rat study and 29 and 290 μmol/kg in the monkey study. Both studies included a control group receiving normal saline.

In the rat study, there were no positive findings with respect to clinical observations, food consumption, clinical chemistry (including alanine aminotransferase, alkaline phosphatase, lactate dehydrogenase, gamma glutamyltransferase, bilirubin, albumin, creatinine, and blood urea nitrogen), urinalysis, body and organ weights, and gross and microscopic pathology. Treatment-related effects were limited to the high-dosage group (29 times the anticipated clinical dosage). Noteworthy findings included a significantly higher mean eosinophil count in the high-dosage females, lower absolute testes weight in the high-dosage males with no remarkable microscopic findings, and an increased incidence of hepatic microgranulomas in the high-dosage females. No animals died in the study.

In the monkey study, transient flushing of the face, vomiting, and increases in clinical chemistry values (including alanine aminotransferase, aspartate aminotransferase, gamma glutamyltransferase, bilirubin, creatinine, and blood urea nitrogen) were noted in the high-dosage animals. It was demonstrated that the liver was a target organ, with some involvement of the kidney. When examined after a 2-week treatment-free period, treatment-related changes appeared to be reversing. All but one of the 22 monkeys survived at dosages up to 29 times the anticipated clinical dosage.

The pharmacokinetic data for Mn-DPDP was best described by a two-compartment model when administered intravenously at 29 μmol/kg to cynomolgus monkeys. The distribution half-life of Mn-DPDP, measured as total manganese, was rapid (7.89 min), with an elimination half-life of approximately 43 h. The pharmacokinetics of a single intravenous dose (29 μmol/kg) of Mn-DPDP administered to Sprague-Dawley rats followed an open one-compartment model with an elimination half-life of 13.2 min and a plasma clearance rate of 76.4 ml/h.

Biodistribution studies in Sprague-Dawley rats demonstrated that 30 minutes after injection 13 ± 3 percent of the ^{54}Mn administered as [^{54}Mn]-DPDP was present in the liver; 9 ± 5 percent in the small intestine, 3 ± 1 percent in the blood, 1.3 ± 0.3 percent in the kidneys, and less than 1 percent in the cecum, heart, lungs, spleen, brain, large intestine, and stomach. [^{54}Mn]Cl_2 demonstrated higher liver extraction efficiency with 38 ± 6 percent of the administered dose in the liver, 14 ± 7 percent in the small intestine, 3 ± 1 percent in the blood, 1.1 ± 0.1 percent in the kidneys, 1.4 ± 0.4 percent in the cecum, 1.2 ± 0.2

percent in the heart, and less than 1 percent in the lungs, spleen, brain, large intestine, and stomach. The biliary system, measured as the sum of the liver and small intestine percentage dose per organ values, contained a higher concentration of ^{54}Mn administered as [^{54}Mn]Cl$_2$ (52 percent) than as [^{54}Mn]-DPDP (22 percent) 30 minutes postinjection. The total is less than 100 percent of the dose owing to distribution of ^{54}Mn in tissues that were not measured (e.g., muscle) as well as urinary and fecal losses during the first 30 minutes.

In a whole-body clearance study in rats, [^{54}Mn]-DPDP demonstrated 43 percent renal excretion after 6 hours, with 47 percent fecal excretion and 6 percent body retention 7 days after administration. [^{54}Mn]Cl$_2$ showed no measurable renal excretion, with 50 percent fecal excretion and 50 percent whole-body retention 7 days after administration (Fig. 43-2).

Manganese is a trace metal considered to be nutritionally essential with a normal whole-body content of 12 to 20 mg (218 to 364 μmol) (13–16). Although a formal recommended dietary allowance (RDA) has not been established, the estimated adequate daily allowance of manganese for adults is 2.5 to 5.0 mg (45.5 to 91.0 μmol) (17). Dietary absorption of manganese occurs through the small intestine. Mn^{2+} in the blood, whether free or bound to proteins, is efficiently cleared by the liver, and excess Mn^{2+} is normally excreted in the bile (14). Excretion of manganese also occurs through the gastrointestinal mucosa and pancreatic secretions (18–22), with virtually none excreted through the kidney (23), consistent with the whole-body excretion study mentioned earlier. Within the cell, Mn^{2+} is incorporated into mitochondria (24), where it functions as a coenzyme in the synthesis of proteins (25). Tissues rich in mitochondria, such as liver, kidney, heart, and pancreas, are those which contain the highest levels of Mn^{2+} (26,27).

Results from the preclinical evaluation supported the evaluation of Mn-DPDP in humans as a hepatobiliary contrast-enhancing agent with MRI.

CLINICAL EVALUATION

A phase I clinical trial to evaluate Mn-DPDP was conducted at Quincy Research Center in Kansas City, Missouri. The objectives of this study were

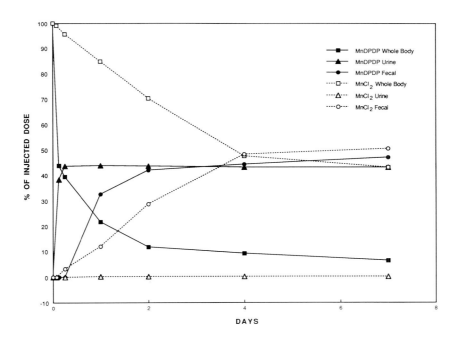

FIGURE 43-2
Seven-day whole-body clearance study in rats, [^{54}Mn]-DPDP and [^{54}Mn]Cl$_2$.

to determine the safety, tolerance, pharmacokinetics, and MRI contrast-enhancement ability of Mn-DPDP when administered intravenously to healthy male subjects.

Materials and Methods
Fifty-four subjects were entered into this randomized, double-blind, ascending-dosage study. Mn-DPDP at a concentration of 145 mM (100 mg/ml) was administered at dosages of 3, 10, 15, 20, and 25 µmol/kg. Forty-two subjects were studied in a randomized double-blind manner; 28 were administered Mn-DPDP and 14 were administered placebo. The remaining 12 subjects received Mn-DPDP in a nonblinded manner and were imaged. The dosages administered to subjects imaged were 3, 10, and 15 µmol/kg, and the injection rates were 0.016, 0.08, 0.12, and 0.25 ml/s. Subjects were consenting, healthy, adult males between 18 and 45 years of age and were confined to the research facility from 36 hours before to 72 hours after the administration of Mn-DPDP.

Safety parameters focusing on potential cardiovascular, hematologic, renal, and hepatobiliary effects were measured and recorded throughout the study period. Laboratory tests consisted of serum chemistry, hematology, differential count, urine chemistry, and urinalysis. Serum, urine, and feces were collected for pharmacokinetic evaluation. Clinical measures included vital signs, ECG, and recording of discomforts and adverse events.

MRI was performed at 1.5 Tesla (GE Signa). Transaxial abdominal sections through the liver were obtained in a single-breath-hold interval of 21 s using spin-echo saturation pulse sequences. Imaging parameters were as follows: TR = 150 ms, TE = 20 ms, section thickness = 20 mm, field of view = 48 cm, 128 phase-encoding steps, and 1 excitation per step. RF transmit and receive attenuations were set for the preinjection scans and were not changed for the postinjection scans. The use of a single-breath-hold acquisition and application of presaturation pulses superior and inferior to the acquired transaxial slice greatly reduced breathing and flow artifacts. Preadministration scans were obtained 7 min prior to injection. After administration of Mn-DPDP, scans were obtained every 1 to 5 min for a mean period of 28 min.

Signal-intensity values for liver and spleen were obtained by using an operator-defined rectangular region of interest (ROI). Owing to slight movement of the subjects between scans, measurement ROIs were manually defined on each image in roughly the same region of homogeneous organ parenchyma. Approximately 500 pixels (range 200 to 700) were used for the liver ROI, and approximately 110 pixels (range 48 to 216) were used for the spleen. The signal-intensity values for each organ were normalized to the average of the three precontrast values.

Safety Results
Mn-DPDP induced transient increases in blood pressure and pulse rate immediately after injection that were dose-dependent and in some instances administration-rate-dependent. These increases, which were observed at all dosage levels, peaked at 1 to 3 min after injection and generally returned toward baseline 5 to 10 min after injection. None of the individual subject increases in blood pressure or pulse rate persisted or were considered serious by the investigator. No clinically significant changes were reported in ECG parameters.

No clinically significant drug- or dose-related trends in any blood or urine laboratory parameters were noted. Several serum chemistry parameters, however, did show a greater frequency of values that increased above the normal range: alanine aminotransferase (ALT), serum iron, and serum triglycerides. Four subjects experienced increases in ALT that went from within the normal range at baseline to above the normal range at two or more time periods following administration of Mn-DPDP. The maximum ALT value observed in any subject was 70 IU/liter (the upper limit of the normal range is 45 IU/liter). Increases in serum iron and triglycerides were seen in subjects receiving placebo and Mn-DPDP with a similar frequency.

Drug-related adverse events were observed at all dosages and were generally limited to transient warmth and flushing in the face, ears, and/or head. This event occurred shortly after administration of Mn-DPDP, usually lasting less than 1 min. There was a tendency for severity and occurrence of flushing and warmth to increase with increasing dose and administration rate. Nausea was experienced by one subject in the 10 μmol/kg dosage group; this event increased in frequency with increasing dose. Vomiting was experienced by one subject receiving a dosage of 25 μmol/kg.

Efficacy Results

Liver parenchyma enhancement was observed as early as 1 min following injection, reaching a plateau at 10 min (Fig. 43-3); signal intensity remained high 30 min following injection. Variable enhancement (−24 to +52 percent) was demonstrated in the spleen during the first few minutes following injection and then returned toward preinjection levels (Fig. 43-4). The greater variability in the spleen data is probably due to the nonspecific mechanism of drug delivery and normal variations in splenic blood volume and perfusion. In all cases in which the gallbladder was visualized on preinjection images, gallbladder enhancement was observed within 15 min of administration of Mn-DPDP, demonstrating clearance of the agent into the gallbladder (Fig. 43-5).

Figures 43-6 and 43-7 summarize the data for relative signal intensity in liver for the three dosage groups. A machine malfunction occurred while imaging one subject in the 15 μmol/kg dosage group, reducing the number of subjects in the group to two. The mean value for relative signal intensity across subjects at 10 min postinjection, at each dosage, was determined. While there was an increase in the relative signal intensity between 3 μmol/kg (+36 percent, range 21 to 50 percent, n = 2) and 10 μmol/kg (+97 percent, range 65 to 120 percent, n = 7), there was no further relative signal-intensity increase at a dosage of 15 μmol/kg (+92 percent, range 85 to 99 percent, n = 2), although the data set is limited.

Administration rate was varied only in the 10 μmol/kg dosage groups. The mean value for relative signal intensity across subjects at 10 min postinjection, at each administration rate, was determined. At a rate of 0.25 ml/s, the mean increase in relative signal intensity was 76 percent (65 to 86 percent, n = 2), at 0.08 ml/s it was 91 percent (n = 1), and at 0.016 ml/s it was 109 percent (94 to 120 percent, n = 4).

CONCLUSION

Mn-DPDP is a paramagnetic contrast agent that employs a chelate based on vitamin B_6, pyridoxal-5′-phosphate (PLP). While preclinical studies have shown $MnCl_2$ to be an effective hepatobiliary contrast agent owing to selective uptake of Mn^{2+} by the liver, the use of manganese salts as contrast agents has been limited by their cardiotoxicity (10,28–30). Manganese can act as a

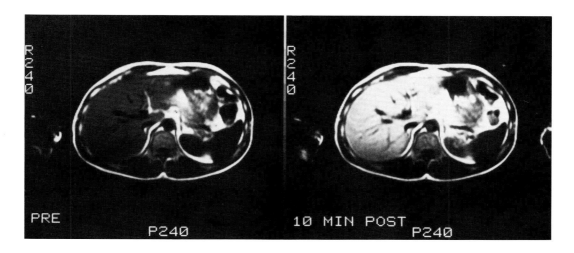

FIGURE 43-3

Transaxial images (TR 150/TE 20) demonstrate preinjection and 10 min postinjection; subject administered Mn-DPDP at 10 μmol/kg, 0.016 ml/s.

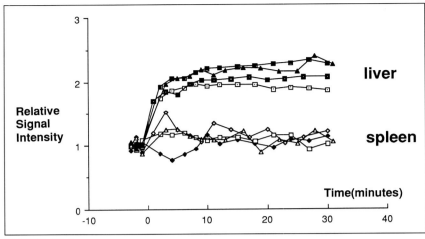

FIGURE 43-4

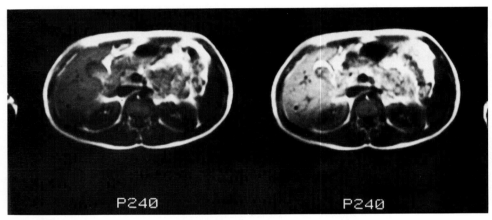

FIGURE 43-5

FIGURE 43-4
Relative signal intensity of liver and spleen for subjects receiving Mn-DPDP at 10 μmol/kg, 0.016 ml/s. Scans obtained preinjection to 30 min postinjection.

FIGURE 43-5
Transaxial images (TR 150/TE 20) demonstrate pre- and postinjection; subject administered Mn-DPDP at 3 μmol/kg. The relative increase in signal intensity in the gallbladder indicates clearance of the agent into the gallbladder.

calcium-channel blocking agent and thus have effects on cardiac contractility and muscle electrophysiology (10). The chelation of manganese by DPDP decreases the acute toxicity of Mn-DPDP (measured by LD_{50} determination, IV administration in mice) compared with $MnCl_2$ by a factor of 10. In animal studies, the safety factor (defined as the ratio of the acute toxicity to the dosage used for imaging) of Mn-DPDP, 200, was superior to that of Gd-DTPA, 60 to 100 (12).

Gd-DTPA behaves as an extracellular paramagnetic contrast agent with rapid renal clearance. Rapid equilibration of Gd-DTPA into the interstitium of both normal and pathologic tissues can

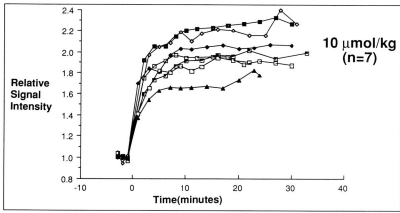

FIGURE 43-6

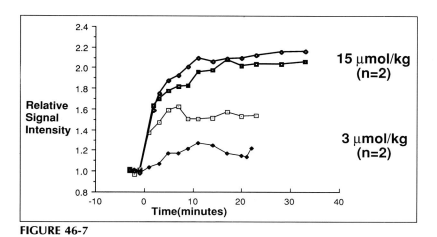

FIGURE 46-7

FIGURE 43-6
Relative signal intensity in liver for seven subjects administered Mn-DPDP at 10 μmol/kg.

FIGURE 43-7
Relative signal intensity in liver for two subjects administered Mn-DPDP at 3 μmol/kg and two subjects administered Mn-DPDP at 15 μmol/kg.

result in the loss of contrast between the two tissues, demonstrated by Saini et al. (31) using a dynamic MRI scanning technique. They observed maximum tumor/liver contrast 1 to 2 min after administration of the contrast agent, with complete loss of contrast in as little as 8 min. Hence, with extracellular contrast agents, timing of the imaging protocol is critical to take advantage of the signal-enhancing effect of the agent. This short "imaging window" limits the clinical use of nonspecific, extracellular contrast agents in the liver. In the current study, full signal enhancement with Mn-DPDP was present at the end of the 30-min imaging period. Preclinical animal studies showed this effect to be present even after 4 h (9). This extended imaging window should provide adequate time for all necessary clinical imaging sequences to be acquired.

Preclinical imaging studies of Mn-DPDP in rats at a dosage of 50 μmol/kg achieved signal enhancements of 200 percent (9). In the phase I study, there appeared to be no difference between the 10 and 15 μmol/kg dosages, although the number of subjects was small. If the signal enhancement observed in rat liver can be extrapolated to human liver, the failure to demonstrate increased signal intensity from 10 to 15 μmol/kg might be explained by a nonlinear response at higher dosages, such as would occur if cellular uptake mechanisms became saturated. Another explanation might be the dose-dependent, competing effect of T1 and T2 shortening, resulting in reduced contrast enhancement.

The results of this phase I clinical trial suggest that an intravenous dosage of up to 10 μmol/kg of Mn-DPDP was generally well tolerated and produced substantial signal enhancement, effectively increasing liver parenchyma signal-to-noise ratios. The utility of Mn-DPDP for cancer detection will depend on the relative uptake kinetics of normal liver parenchyma versus tumor (9); efficacy for cancer detection will be evaluated in the phase II clinical trials. The combination of hepatobiliary specificity, preclinical safety, significant liver enhancement (97 percent) at 10 μmol/kg in the phase I clinical study, and a long imaging window make Mn-DPDP a potentially superior MRI hepatobiliary contrast agent when compared with currently available nonspecific, extracellular contrast agents. The overall results of this study suggest that Mn-DPDP may be a safe and useful MRI contrast agent for the liver (32), and phase II clinical studies are in progress to evaluate safety and efficacy in patients with focal liver disease.

REFERENCES

1. Taveras JM, Ferrucci JT: The liver: Anatomy and examination techniques, in Bernardino ME (ed): Radiology: Diagnosis/Imaging Intervention, vol 4. Philadelphia, Lippincott, 1986, p 3.
2. Clinical MR Group, University of Aberdeen and Grampian Health Board: Magnetic resonance imaging of parenchymal liver disease: A comparison with ultrasound, radionuclide scintigraphy and x-ray computed tomography. Clin Radiol 38:495, 1987.
3. Freeny PC, Marks WM, Ryan JA, et al: Colorectal carcinoma evaluation with CT: Preoperative staging and detection of postoperative recurrence. Radiology 158:347, 1986.
4. Heiken JP, Weyman PJ, Lee JKT, et al: Detection of focal hepatic masses: Prospective evaluation with CT, delayed CT, CT during arterial portography, and MR imaging. Radiology 171:47, 1989.
5. Wolf GL, Burnett KR, Goldstein EJ, et al: Contrast agents for magnetic resonance imaging, in Kressel HY (ed): Magnetic Resonance Annual 1985. New York, Raven Press, 1985, p 231.
6. Dolphin D, Poulson R, Avramovic O: Vitamin B_6 pyridoxal phosphate: Chemical, biochemical, and medical aspects, in Coenzymes and Cofactors. vol 1, part B. New York, Wiley-Interscience, 1986.
7. Rocklage SM, Cacheris WP, Quay SC, et al: Manganese(II)-N,N'-dipyridoxylethylenediamine-N,N'-diacetate-5,5'-bis(phosphate): Synthesis and characterization of a paramagnetic chelate for magnetic resonance imaging enhancement. Inorg Chem 28:477, 1989.
8. Saini S, Stark DD, Wittenberg J, et al: A rat model of liver cancer for imaging research. Invest Radiol 22:149, 1987.
9. Elizondo G, Fretz CJ, Stark DD, et al: Preclinical evaluation of Mn-DPDP: A new paramagnetic hepatobiliary contrast agent for MRI. Radiology (in press).
10. Wolf G, Baum L: Cardiovascular toxicity and tissue proton T1 response to manganese injection in the dog and rabbit. AJR 141:193, 1983.
11. Bousquet JC, Saini S, Stark DD, et al: Gd-DOTA: Characterization of a new paramagnetic complex. Radiology 166:693, 1988.
12. Weinmann HJ, Brasch RC, Press WR, et al: Characteristics of Gd-DTPA complex: A potential NMR contrast agent. AJR 142:619, 1984.
13. Cotzias GC: Manganese in health and disease. Physiol Rev 38:503, 1958.
14. Leach RM, Liburn MS: Manganese metabolism and its function. World Rev Nutr Diet 32:123, 1978.
15. Schroeder HA, Balassa JJ, Tipton IH: Essential trace metals in man: Manganese. J Chronic Dis 19:545, 1966.
16. Borg D, Cotzias GC: Manganese metabolism in man: Rapid exchange of Mn-56 with tissue as demonstrated by blood clearance and liver uptake. J Clin Invest 37:1269, 1958.
17. National Academy of Sciences: Recommended Dietary Allowances, 9th ed. Washington, National Academy of Sciences, 1980.

18. Kato M: Distribution and excretion of radiomanganese administered to the mouse. Q J Exp Physiol 48:355, 1963.
19. Papavasiliou PS, Miller ST, Cotzias GC: Role of liver in regulating distribution and excretion of manganese. Am J Physiol 211:211, 1966.
20. Bertinchamps AJ, Miller ST, Cotzias GC. Interdependence of routes excreting manganese. Am J Physiol 211:217, 1966.
21. Cotzias GC, Greenough JJ: The high specificity of the manganese pathway through the body. J Clin Invest 37:1298, 1958.
22. Mahoney JP, Small WJ: Studies on manganese: III. The biological half-life of radiomanganese in man and factors which affect this half-life. J Clin Invest 47:643, 1968.
23. Burnett WT, Bigelow RR, Kimbal AW, et al: Radiomanganese studies on the mouse, rat and pancreatic fistula dog. Am J Physiol 168:620, 1952.
24. Maynard LS, Cotzias GC: The partition of manganese among organs and intracellular organelles of the rat. J Biol Chem 214:489, 1955.
25. Martin DW, Mayes PA, Rodwell VW, et al (eds): Harper's Review of Biochemistry, 28th ed. California, Lange, 1985, pp 659–678.
26. Tipton IH, Cook, MJ: Trace elements in human tissue: II. Adult subjects from the United States. Health Phys 9:103, 1963.
27. Fore H, Morton RA: Manganese in rabbit tissue. Biochem J 51:600, 1952.
28. Mena J, Meurin O, Feunzoba S, et al: Chronic manganese poisoning: Clinical picture and manganese turnover. Neurology 17:128, 1967.
29. Kang YS, Gore JC: Studies of tissue NMR relaxation enhancement by manganese: Dose and time dependences. Invest Radiol 19:399, 1984.
30. Pflugfelder PW, Wendland MF, Holt WW, et al: Acute myocardial ischemia: MR imaging with Mn-TP. Radiology 167:129, 1988.
31. Saini S, Stark DD, Brady TJ, et al: Dynamic spin-echo MRI of liver cancer using gadolinium-DTPA: Animal investigation. AJR 147:357, 1986.
32. Lim KO, Stark DD, Leese PT, et al: MR hepatobiliary imaging: First human experience with Mn-DPDP. Radiology (in press).

44

Hepatobiliary Contrast Agents for MRI

FRIEDRICH CAVAGNA, PIERO TIRONE,
ERNST FELDER, and CHRISTOPH DE HAËN

The liver is the organ to which primary cancers in other parts of the body most frequently metastasize. On autopsy, hepatic metastases are found in 36 percent of all cancer patients and in 48 percent of those with primary tumors drained by the portal venous system (1). A number of imaging tests are available for detection of focal masses in the liver. Their first goal is survey scanning, i.e., the separation of normal patients from those with one or more liver lesions. Their second goal is the detection of individual hepatic lesions, i.e., the exact determination of their number and anatomic location in view of a hepatic resection or of local chemotherapy. In both cases, the sensitivities of the modern imaging modalities are unsatisfactory. For survey scanning, sensitivities of 80 percent for contrast-enhanced CT and of 82 percent for MRI have been reported (2). On a lesion-by-lesion basis, a recent study (3) comparing CT during arterial portography (CTAP), MRI, delayed CT, and contrast-enhanced CT has shown their sensitivities to be 81, 57, 51, and 38 percent, respectively. In the case of metastases of less than 1 cm in size, the sensitivities are dramatically lower and amount to 61 percent for CTAP, 17 percent for MRI, and 0 percent for delayed and contrast-enhanced CT.

In view of the impact that the detection of a single metastasis has on both prognosis and therapy, and in view of the invasiveness of the CTAP technique, this can hardly be called a satisfactory situation. Lesion conspicuity can be quantitatively related to the contrast-to-noise ratio (CNR), and the threshold size for lesion detection decreases when the CNR is enhanced. The accuracy of lesion-size measurements also correlates directly with CNR magnitude (4). The CNR may be enhanced by the development of instruments with higher sensitivity and/or with artifact-suppression techniques. For any given instrumentation, the CNR may be further increased by the administration of appropriate contrast agents. Early approaches to the problem of contrast-enhanced tumor imaging in the liver have relied on a differential kinetics of distribution of Gd-DTPA^{2-} in tumor and healthy tissue. Success has been hampered by the rapidity with which extracellular spaces of liver and tumor equilibrate, resulting in isointense images within 8 min (5). More promising approaches are based on tissue-specific contrast agents. While interesting possibilities exist for particulate contrast agents that target the reticuloendothelial system, we restrict our attention here to the design of hepatobiliary contrast agents and present a compound that provides for prolonged enhancement of liver/lesion CNR.

DESIGN CRITERIA FOR HEPATOBILIARY AGENTS

Hepatobiliary agents must first cross the sinusoidal and then the canalicular plasma membrane of hepatocytes. Transport of small bilitropic molecules across the sinusoidal plasma membrane is of the facilitated type and thus reversible. There exists also some small nonspecific leakage. Transport may be driven by the concentration gradient of the compound itself or by the concentration gradient of a cotransported sodium ion, both further modulated by the membrane potential. In the second case, a pronounced transport against a concentration gradient of the bilitropic substance is possible (secondary active transport).

Transporters are sinusoidal membrane proteins that recognize certain molecular features of hepatobiliary agents, the recognition showing a poor specificity. To date, four transport systems have been identified: the transporter of conjugated bile acids, the fatty acid transporter, the organic cation transporter, and the transporter for non-biliary acid, nonfatty acid, and albumin-binding organic anions. The first two involve secondary active transport, whereas the latter two are driven by the concentration gradient of the substance itself.

Much less is known about the export of molecules into bile (6), even though this step is usually rate-limiting. Many bilitropic substances are enzymatically modified before biliary excretion. Inevitably, this process requires indirectly ATP and directly other cellular resources that may be limited, e.g., glutathione. A contrast agent that does not require enzymatic modification for biliary excretion thus may be less noxious to the liver than one that requires modification.

Export of molecules from hepatocytes into bile is an ATP-requiring process involving pumps in the canalicular plasma membrane or in cytoplasmic vesicles that are later exocytosed into the canalicular space (7). In general, these pumps do not recognize the same molecular features as the sinusoidal transporters, although in special cases they may do so. More frequently, they seem to recognize features deriving from enzymatic processing of the molecules. One way of facilitating transfer from the cytoplasm to the bile without enzymatic modification is to incorporate into the bilitropic molecule features of the type created by the typical hepatic drug transformation reactions or features that mimic them.

Many bilitropic substances bind reversibly to some liver proteins, among others (8) also to glutathione transferase B (9) (formerly called protein Y), the best-known binding protein. The latter is part of the cellular biotransformation machinery, but it also binds bilitropic compounds that do not serve as substrate, e.g., iodipamide (10).

For bilitropic compounds that do not suffer biotransformations, these proteins may not play a significant role in transhepatic traffic. For example, ioglycamic acid, although bilitropic, does not bind measurably to these proteins. However, binding to intracellular proteins of the hepatocyte reduces the rotational correlation times of paramagnetic contrast agents, resulting in increased longitudinal relaxation rates. Thus affinity for these proteins is a desirable property of a hepatobiliary MRI imaging agent not only because it affects the relative concentrations of contrast agent in liver and lesion, but also because it produces a hepatocyte-specific enhancement of the contrasting efficacy of the agent. It therefore should be borne in mind that biodistribution parameters such as liver-blood and intestine-liver ratios, fractional biliary excretion rate, octanol/water partition coefficient, indices of hydrophobicity, and so on (11,12) or the parameters used for the general characterization of MRI contrast agents, such as the relaxivity in water, are of little value in predicting the efficacy of liver specific contrast agents.

Many bilitropic compounds bind reversibly to serum albumin. This binding slows down biliary excretion (13,14) and is not a prerequisite for it, as shown by the case of p-aminohippuric acid (15). Except for the fact that hepatocytes contain serum albumin in various stages of preparation for secretion, which may contribute to longitudinal relaxation through binding of contrast agents, affinity for albumin is not a prerequisite for a hepatobiliary agent.

PROTOTYPE HEPATOBILIARY CONTRAST AGENTS AND AGENTS IN DEVELOPMENT

Various complexes have been studied as potential paramagnetic hepatobiliary agents, including iron(III)-based analogues of hepatobiliary agents for scintigraphy. Among these are the iron(III) complex of N,N'-ethylene-bis [2-(2-hydroxyphenyl) glycine] (Fe-EHPG$^-$), the iron(III) complex of N,N'-bis(2-hydroxybenzyl)-ethylenediamine-N,N'-diacetic acid (Fe-HBED$^-$), a manganese(II) complex of the vitamin B_6 analogue dipyridoxal diphosphate (Mn-DPDP^{2-}), and gadolinium(III)-based Gd-BOPTA^{2-}, the ligand of which shares a common backbone with Gd-DTPA^{2-} (Fig. 44-1). Some basic physicochemical and pharmacologic properties of these agents are summarized in Table 44-1. Fe-EHPG$^-$ and Fe-HBED$^-$ are prototype agents (16–19). They are coordinatively saturated hexacoordinate compounds without any water molecule in the first coordination sphere, and therefore, they feature low magnetic water proton relaxivities (Table 44-1). Mn-DPDP^{2-} is a hexacoordinate complex, Gd-BOPTA^{2-} is an octacoordinate complex, and both have one water molecule in the first coordination sphere. Mn-DPDP^{2-} appropriately salified (20–23) and Gd-BOPTA/Dimeg (19,24–28) are currently both undergoing clinical trials. In the following we will focus mainly on Gd-BOPTA/Dimeg, the most recent of these agents.

Gd-BOPTA/Dimeg

Physicochemical Properties

Gd-BOPTA/Dimeg differs from the already widely used Gd-DTPA/Dimeg in that one of the eight methylene protons of the four equivalent acetate moieties of DTPA is replaced by the benzyloxymethyl group. The two structures are shown in Figure 44-1. Since Gd-BOPTA^{2-} enters the bile efficiently while Gd-DPTA^{2-} does so barely, and since Gd-BOPTA remains unchanged in the process, the benzyloxymethyl group must constitute the molecular handle that enables Gd-BOPTA^{2-} to be recognized by a hepatic transporter in the sinusoidal membrane. It is less clear whether the same group is also responsible for recognition by the pump responsible for export from the cytoplasm into the bile. As the value of

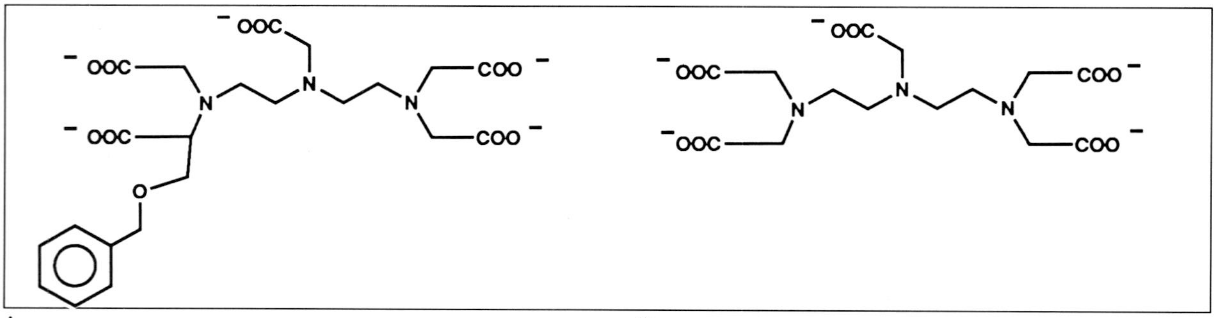

FIGURE 44-1
The structure of Gd^{3+} ligands. Kinks in the lines indicate $-CH_2-$ units. (A) BOPTA^{5-}. (B) DTPA^{5-}.

TABLE 44-1. *Some Physicochemical and Pharmacological Properties of Hepatobiliary Contrast Agents and Gd-DTPA*

	Fe-HBED	Fe-EHPG	Mn-DPDP	Gd-BOPTA	Gd-DTPA
Relaxivity R1 mM^{-1}s^{-1}	1.1	1.0	2.5	4.4	3.8
Relaxivity R2 mM^{-1}s^{-1}	1.0	1.1	3.9	5.6	4.7
Stability constant (M^{-1})	10^{29}	10^{33}	10^{15}	10^{22}	10^{23}
Partition coefficient (octanol/buffer)	0.002	0.019	—	0.0016	0.0001*
Biliary excretion (rat, %)	52	17	22	50	5.0

*Butanol/buffer

the partition coefficient in Table 44-1 shows, bilitropism in Gd-BOPTA/Dimeg is obtained without unduly augmenting the lipophilicity of the compound, which might have led to an increased retention in fat deposits and in the membrane lipid bilayers with a consequent increase in toxicity. The crystal structure of Gd-BOPTA^{2-} (Fig. 44-2A) shows the Gd^{3+} ion in the center of a distorted capped square antiprism, eight of the corners being formed by three nitrogens and five oxygens of the ligand and the cap in the axial position being a H$_2$O molecule in the first coordination sphere (Fig. 44-2B). This geometry of ligand atoms is shared by both linear and cyclic polyaminocarboxylate Gd^{3+} chelates such as Gd-DTPA^{2-} and Gd-DOTA^{2-}.

Pharmacokinetics

The pharmacokinetics of Gd-BOPTA^{2-} were studied in experimental animals with respect to plasma kinetics, tissue distribution, and excretion. The quantitative assay was performed by HPLC, x-ray fluorescence analysis, and radioisotopic assay ([^{153}Gd]-BOPTA^{2-}). The compound is quickly removed from blood. The plasma kinetics in both rat and rabbit show a biphasic pattern with distribution and elimination half-lifes of 5.5 and 22 min (rat, 250 μmol/kg) and of 6 and 40 min (rabbit, 200 μmol/kg). The compound is distributed in the plasma and in the extracellular space.

In the rat at a dosage of 0.25 mmol/kg, elimination takes place almost to the same extent (50 percent in the first 8 h) through biliary and urinary excretion, while in the rabbit at a dosage of 0.2 mmol/kg, at 8 h the cumulative urinary excretion (70 percent) is higher than the cumulative biliary excretion (25 percent). In both species, the compound is excreted entirely unchanged. The biliary excretion of Gd-BOPTA^{2-} was proved to be a saturable process by studying its dependence on the intravenous infusion rate in the rabbit. As shown in Figure 44-3, the biliary excretion rate approaches a maximum (transport maximum) of $T_m = 0.92$ μmol·kg^{-1}·min^{-1} at an infusion rate of 15 μmol·min^{-1}, above which a steep increase in the urinary excretion rate and in the plasma level compensate for the lack of biliary excretion capacity. In the rat, the hepatic clearance of the compound was inhibited by the coinjection of bromosulfophthalein, while it was not affected by coinjection of either oxyphenonium or taurocholate. These compounds are known to be subject to distinct carrier-mediated transport systems. The preceding experiments are therefore consistent with the hypothesis that Gd-BOPTA^{2-} enters hepatocytes by the facilitated transport system for nonbiliary acid, nonfatty acid, albumin-binding organic anions, but the observation does not preclude the possibility that the inhibition occurred at a different step.

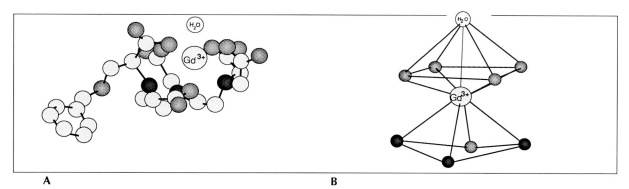

FIGURE 44-2

Structure of Gd-BOPTA^{2-} as obtained by single crystal x-ray diffraction analysis of Gd-BOPTA/2Na. The two sodium counterions are not shown. Light gray balls are carbon atoms, intermediate gray balls are oxygen atoms, and dark gray balls are nitrogen atoms. (A) Ball model of anion. (B) First sphere of coordination around Gd^{3+} only. (Data obtained in collaboration with Dr. Paula Paoli and Dr. Mauro Micheloni, University of Florence, Italy.)

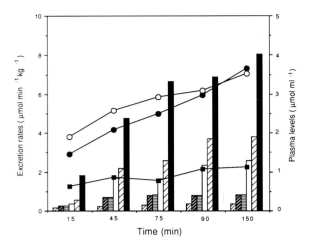

FIGURE 44-3

Plasma levels, biliary excretion rates, and urinary excretion rates of Gd-BOPTA^{2-} during IV infusion of Gd-BOPTA/Dimeg at different rates into the rabbit. Plasma levels are indicated with closed squares, closed circles, and open circles for infusion rates of 7.5, 15.0, and 22.5 μmol/min, respectively. The bars represent measurements of excretion rates at the points of time of the measurements of the plasma levels. At each point of time the six bars are, from left to right, biliary excretion rates at infusion rates of 7.5, 15.0, and 22.5 μmol/min and urinary excretion rates at infusion rates of 7.5, 15.0, and 22.5 μmol/min.

MRI Signal-Intensity Enhancement Kinetics

In normal rats, the liver parenchymal signal-intensity enhancement after IV administration of Gd-BOPTA/Dimeg was found to be quick, strong, and persistent. We observed that peak enhancement of 70 percent was reached 4 min after injection of Gd-BOPTA/Dimeg at the dosage of 250 μmol/kg into the tail vein of the rat. After staying for 15 min at this plateau level, the enhancement decayed only very slowly to retain a value of 53 percent after 120 min (Fig. 44-4). We used the ultrafast inversion-recovery snapshot flash technique (29) to acquire images with a scan time of 200 ms at 2-s intervals in order to characterize the early phases of the hepatic uptake of Gd-BOPTA^{2-}. The liver signal enhancement reached its maximum 8 s after injection into the jugular vein (Fig. 44-5A) and remained unchanged afterwards. In a similar experiment, Gd-DTPA^{2-} reached even faster (5 s) its maximum enhancement (Fig. 44-5B), which, however, was lower and was immediately followed by a decay due to the washout of the contrast agent that resulted in isointensity of liver and tumor after some minutes. These experiments provide evidence for very fast hepatocellular uptake of Gd-BOPTA^{2-}.

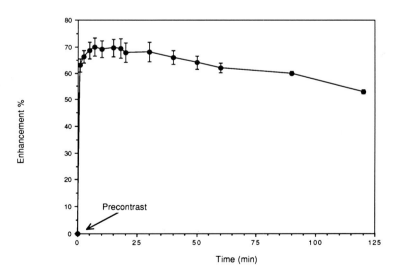

FIGURE 44-4

Time course of liver parenchyma signal-intensity enhancement by Gd-BOPTA/Dimeg. After administration of 250 μmol/kg Gd-BOPTA/Dimeg into the tail vein of the rat, SE 200/16 images were taken at 0.5 Tesla on an Esatom MR 5000 instrument.

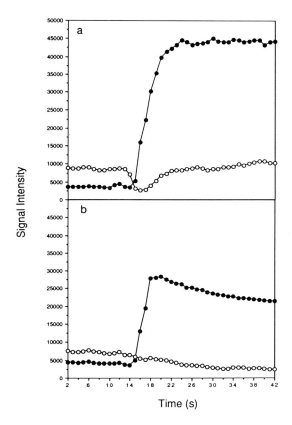

FIGURE 44-5
Time course of liver and tumor signal-intensity enhancement by Gd-BOPTA/Dimeg and Gd-DTPA/Dimeg. Gd-BOPTA/Dimeg was injected at the dose of 250 µmol/kg into the jugular vein of the rat. Inversion-recovery snapshot flash images were taken on a Bruker Biospec 47/40 4.7-Tesla instrument. Liver is indicated by open circles and tumor by closed circles. (A) Gd-BOPTA/Dimeg. (B) Gd-DTPA/Dimeg. Data obtained from the study described in reference 29.

Liver/Tumor CNR and Relaxation-Rate Enhancement
The performance of the four contrast agents Fe-HBED$^-$, Fe-EHPG$^-$, Mn-DPDP^{2-}, and Gd-BOPTA^{2-} in focal liver lesion detection has been the subject of preclinical investigations (18–20,22,23,28). Most of these studies used the rat mammary adenocarcinoma (R3230 AC) tumor model, which duplicates the histology and physiology of metastatic human breast cancer. Recently, experiments also have been carried out in our laboratories using a Walker carcinoma 256 line B rat liver tumor model. In all these investigations, the efficacy of an agent was assessed by measuring the percentage enhancement of CNR in heavily T1-weighted images per unit time and per amount of the compound administered. Furthermore, T1 and T2 were measured on excised liver and tumor tissues. In our study, in vivo T1 and T2 measurements were carried out to determine the extent and tissue selectivity of the relaxation-rate enhancement. Table 44-2 shows the results.

It is noteworthy that Gd-BOPTA^{2-} produced both the highest relaxation-rate enhancements in the liver and by far the highest tissue specificities in both the adenocarcinoma and Walker carcinoma tumor models. The CNR results summarized in Table 44-2 again show that Gd-BOPTA/Dimeg produced the highest increment for both tumor types, rendering this agent very promising for focal liver lesion detection. Three images taken prior to and 30 and 120 min after IV injection of 250 µmol/kg Gd-BOPTA/Dimeg are shown in Figure 44-6A. They demonstrate the persistence of the CNR enhancement, which reaches a peak of 370 percent after 30 min and still amounts to 240 percent after 2 h. For comparison, Figure 44-6B shows the rapid loss of contrast that occurs after injection of the same dosage of the extracellular contrast agent Gd-DTPA/Dimeg. The CNR time course for both agents is shown in Figure 44-7. In the case of Gd-DTPA^{2-}, liver/lesion isointensity is reached after only 2 min. This is much faster than reported by Saini et al. (5) and is probably due to the smaller size and the higher vascularity of the lesions studied by us.

In Vivo Relaxation Times and Relaxivities
Usually, in vivo as well as in vitro relaxation times are determined by applying specific pulse sequences such as the Carr-Purcell-Meiboom-Gill sequence for T2 and the inversion recovery sequence for T1 measurements. We took advantage of the new software program MacMRI (30) to perform the coupled measurements of T1 and T2 from a number (usually five) of spin-echo images with appropriately varied TR and TE parameters. By carefully choosing these parameters high precision of the data could be obtained, as shown in Table 44-3.

TABLE 44-2. *Contrast-Induced Increases in Longitudinal Relaxation Rates and Contrast-to-Noise Ratio (CNR)*

	Fe-HBED	Fe-EHPG	Mn-DPDP	Gd-BOPTA	Gd-BOPTA	Gd-DTPA
Dose (μmol/kg)	100	300	50	250	250	200
Tumor model*	AC	AC	AC	AC	W256	AC
Relaxation-rate increment percentage at 0.5 Tesla:						
$\Delta\%$ R1 of liver †	26	77	454	667	524‡	155
$\Delta\%$ R1 of tumor	16	8	200	6	21‡	95
CNR increment percentage	52§	55§	110§	346§	370¶	12§
MR sequence	SE250/18	SE250/18	SE250/21	SE250/18	SE200/16	SE250/18

*AC = rat mammary adenocarcinoma liver tumor model; W256 = Walker 256B rat liver tumor model.
†$\Delta\%R1 = 100[(1/T1)_+ - (1/T1)_-]/(1/T1)_-$, where + and − indices indicate with and without contrast agent, respectively.
‡In vivo studies.
§Data are taken from Ref. 19 and Ref. 20 and are measured at 0.6 Tesla.
¶Measured at 0.5 Tesla with NEX = 8.

TABLE 44-3. *In Vivo Tumor and Liver Pre- and Postcontrast T1 and T2 Relaxation Times*

	T1 (ms)	± SD	T2 (ms)	± SD	No. of Animals
Tumor precontrast	901	±70	72	±2	9
Tumor postcontrast	748	±73	55	±3	5
Liver precontrast	362	±22	49	±3	10
Liver postcontrast	58	±8	42	±3	11

Combining the data on the biodistribution of [^{153}Gd]-BOPTA^{2-} in the liver at 15 min with the relaxation times given earlier, one can estimate crudely the in vivo relaxivity of Gd-BOPTA^{2-} in the liver, although the two sets of data have been obtained from different groups of animals. The value of about 30 mM^{-1}s^{-1} at that point of time represents a roughly sixfold increase with regard to the value in water.

The Influence of the Pulse Sequence on Contrast Agent Performance

When evaluating the CNR performance of a contrast agent, one has to be aware of the strong bearing that the choice of the pulse sequence has on the results. This prompted us to investigate the tumor/liver CNR performance at 0.5 Tesla of spin-echo (SE) and inversion-recovery (IR) pulse sequences prior to and after IV administration of 250 μmol/kg Gd-BOPTA/Dimeg in the rat.

Starting from the four pairs of in vivo T1 and T2 values of tumor and liver, pre- and postcontrast, shown in Table 44-3, we generated theoretical three-dimensional contrast plots with the program MacMRI (30), where the CNR value is plotted on the vertical axis against TR and TE for SE sequences and against two of the three parameters TR, TI, and TE for IR sequences. The program takes care of normalizing the CNR with respect to total acquisition and signal sampling times. One therefore can quickly inspect the CNR behavior of various classes of pulse sequences for a given pair of tissues, which might otherwise be difficult to predict for unusual sequences or combinations of relaxation times.

Two such plots for SE sequences are displayed in Figure 44-8. They are drawn to scale so that the CNR enhancement for any sequence can be assessed by direct comparison of the two plots. The precontrast plot shows two maxima with about the same CNR value, one for T1-weighted (SE 200/16) and one for T2-weighted (SE 2250/80) sequences. The CNR of the former is greatly increased (360 percent) in the postcontrast plot, while that of the latter is increased only marginally. In the postcontrast plot, the steepness around the maximum in all directions emphasizes the importance of both short TR and TE. The experimental data (370 percent) are in good agreement with the theoretically expected value

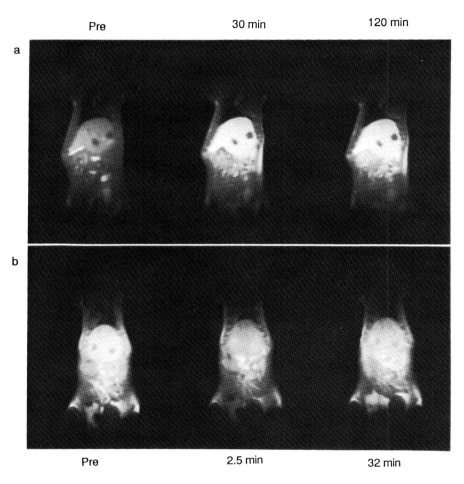

FIGURE 44-6

MRI of rats bearing implanted Walker carcinoma 256 line B tumors in the liver. Images (SE 200/16) are taken on an Esatom MR 5000 0.5 Tesla instrument prior (Pre) to contrast agent injection and at two times of interest after injection of 250 μmol/kg contrast agent. NEX = 8, FOV = 15.5 cm, matrix size 128 × 256, 8-cm receiver coil. (A) Gd-BOPTA/Dimeg: Precontrast enhancement (Pre), at the maximum of contrast enhancement (30 min), and at a late time (120 min). (B)Gd-DTPA/Dimeg: Precontrast enhancement (Pre), at the time of isointensity following the initial but short-lasting tumor/liver contrast enhancement (2.5 min), and at the time of return to initial conditions (32 min).

(360 percent). We have also investigated the postcontrast behavior of STIR (short TI inversion-recovery) pulse sequences, in which T1- and T2-dependent contrasts add constructively to each other (31). At a TI value of 50 ms (close to the "null point" of the liver and the shortest TI implementable on our imager), the highest CNR was computed for 1350/50/30 (TR/TI/TE) sequences, with only a modest (66) percent contrast increase above that obtained with the standard precontrast SE 200/16 sequence. This was again in good agreement with the experimental contrast. The highest postcontrast CNR of all, even higher than that for the SE 200/16 sequence, was computed for strongly T1-weighted IR sequences with a TI of 100 ms. However, this contrast cannot be achieved in practice because, owing to the very short T1 of the liver, the longitudinal magnetization of tumor

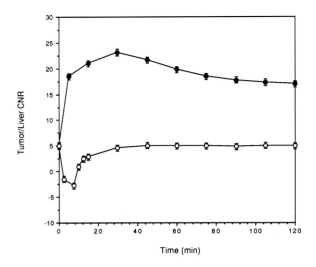

FIGURE 44-7
Time course of tumor/liver CNR after IV injection of Gd-BOPTA/Dimeg and Gd-DTPA/Dimeg. Both contrast agents were given by IV injection of 250 μmol/kg into the tail vein of rats. The CNR was measured for an imaging time of 3.4 min at 0.5 Tesla.

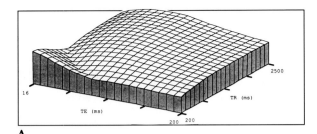

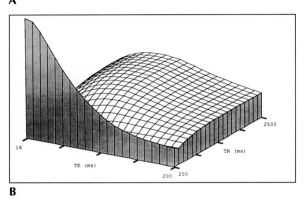

FIGURE 44-8
Tumor/liver contrast for spin-echo pulse sequences at 0.5 Tesla calculated from measured T1 and T2 values. (A) Without contrast agent. (B) With Gd-BOPTA^{2-} present at the concentrations reached 15 min after IV injection into the tail vein of rats of 250 μmol/kg Gd-BOPTA/Dimeg.

and liver are of opposite sign at this point of time. Therefore, imagers operating in the phase-sensitive image-reconstruction mode are required to take advantage of this contrast, while it is lost by the magnitude reconstruction implemented in most commercial instruments.

Hence, at least as far as SE and IR pulse sequences are concerned, there is no real alternative to short TR/short TE sequences in the evaluation and exploitation of the efficacy of tissue specific T1-relaxing paramagnetic contrast agents in the detection of metastatic focal liver disease.

REFERENCES

1. Willis RA: The Spread of Tumors in the Human Body. London, Butterworth, 1973, pp 175–192.
2. Stark DD: MR imaging of focal liver masses. Radiology 168:323, 1988.
3. Heiken JP, Weyman PJ, Lee JKT, et al: Detection of focal hepatic masses: Prospective evaluation with CT, delayed CT, CT during arterial portography, and MR imaging. Radiology 171:47, 1989.
4. Tsang YM, Stark DD, Chen MC, et al: Hepatic micrometastases in the rat: Ferrite-enhanced MR imaging. Radiology 167:21, 1988.
5. Saini S, Stark DD, Brady TJ, et al: Dynamic spin-echo MRI of liver cancer using gadolinium-DTPA: Animal investigation. AJR 147:357, 1986.
6. Moseley RH: Mechanisms of bile formation and cholestasis: Clinical significance of recent experimental work. Am J Gastroenterol 81:731, 1986.
7. Jones AL, Schmucker DL, Mooney JS, et al: Alteration in hepatic pericanalicular cytoplasm during enhanced bile secretory activity. Lab Invest 40:512, 1979.
8. Sugiyama Y, Yamad T, Kaplowitz N: Newly identified bile acid binders in rat liver cytosol: Purification and comparison with glutathione S-transferases. J Biol Chem 258:3602, 1983.
9. Arias IM, Fleischner G: On the structure, regulation, and function of ligandin, in Arias IM, Jakoby WB (eds): Glutathione: Metabolism and Function. New York, Raven Press, 1976.
10. Kaplowitz N: Physiological significance of glutathione S-transferases. Am J Physiol 239:G439, 1980.
11. Smith RL: The Excretory Function of Bile. London, Chapman and Hall, 1973, p 33.

12. Loberg MD, Nunn AD, Porter DN: Development of hepatobiliary imaging agents, in Nuclear Medicine Annual 1981. New York, Raven Press, 1981, pp 1–33.
13. Rosati G, Schiantarelli P: Biliary excretion of contrast media. Invest Radiol 5:232, 1970.
14. Song CS, Beranbaum ER, Rothschild MA: The role of serum albumin in the hepatic excretion of iopamide. Invest Radiol 11:39, 1976.
15. Taggart JV: Protein binding of p-aminohippurate in human and dog plasma. Am J Physiol 167:248, 1951.
16. Lauffer RB, Vincent AC, Padmanabhan S, et al: Hepatobiliary MR contrast agents: 5-Substituted iron-EHPG derivatives. Magnet Reson Med 4:582, 1987.
17. Shtern F, Garrido L, Compton C, et al: Comparison of Fe-EHPG, a prototype hepatobiliary agent, with Gd-DTPA in MR imaging of blood-borne metastases in mice. Radiology 165(suppl P):316, 1987.
18. Lauffer RB, Betteridge DR, Padmanabhan S, Brady TJ: Albumin binding of paramagnetic hepatobiliary contrast agents: Enhancement of outer sphere relaxivity. Nucl Med Biol 15:45, 1988.
19. Elizondo G, Fretz CJ, Stark DD, et al: Preclinical efficacy studies of gadolinium BOPTA as an hepatobiliary contrast agent for MRI, in Eighth Annual SMRM Meeting, Book of Abstracts, Amsterdam, 1989, p 350.
20. Tsang YM, Chen M, Elizondo G, et al: Hepatobiliary contrast agent for hepatic MR: Tissue-specific biodistribution of Mn-S095, in Sixth Annual SMRI Meeting, Book of Abstracts, Boston, 1988, p 124.
21. Worah D, Rocklage SM, Quay SC, et al: MR hepatobiliary imaging with a paramagnetic manganese chelate derived from pyridoxal-5-phosphate, in Sixth Annual SMRM Meeting, Book of Abstracts, New York, 1987, p 16.
22. Elizondo G, Tsang YM, Rocklage SM, et al: Hepatobiliary contrast agents: Preclinical efficacy studies, in Seventh Annual SMRM Meeting, Book of Abstracts, San Francisco, 1988, p 798.
23. Stark DD, Elizondo G, Fretz C, Weissleder R: Tissue-specific contrast agents for MRI of the liver, in CMR 1989, Book of Abstracts, Sidney, 1989, MR17.
24. Felder E, Uggeri F, Fumagalli L, Vittadini G: Paramagnetic chelates useful for NMR imaging. U.S. Patent No. 4,916,246 (C07F13/00; 556/1), April 10, 1990, IT 19236A/86, January 30, 1986.
25. Pavone P, Passariello R, Musu C, et al: A potential liver contrast agent for MRI: Preliminary in vivo evaluation, in Sixth Annual SMRM Meeting, Works in Progress, Boston, 1988, p 511.
26. Musu C, Felder E, Tirone P, et al: New MRI contrast agents. Diagn Imaging Int 4(suppl):72.
27. Vittadini G, Felder E, Musu C, Tirone P: Preclinical profile of Gd-BOPTA, a liver-specific contrast agent, in CMR 1989, Book of Abstracts, Sidney, 1989, MR 19.
28. Elizondo G, Fretz CJ, Stark DD, et al: Gd-BOPTA: Preclinical efficacy evaluation as a hepatobiliary contrast agent for MR imaging, in 75th RSNA Meeting, Book of Abstracts, Chicago, 1989, p 253.
29. Syha J, Bartkowsky R, Cavagna F, et al: High-Speed Dynamic Observation of the Early Phases of Vascular Distribution and Hepatocyte Uptake of Gd-BOPTA by Inversion Recovery Snapshot-Flash MRI. Presented at the Ninth Annual SMRM Meeting, New York, 1990.
30. Weissleder R: MacMRI: An interactive software program for MR image analysis, personal communication, 1989.
31. Dwyer AJ, Frank JA, Sank VJ, et al: Short-TI inversion-recovery pulse sequence: Analysis and initial experience in cancer imaging. Radiology 168:827, 1988.

XV. PARTICULATES

45

Particulate Biodegradable Contrast Medium for CT of the Liver

T. GJØEN, E. HOLTZ, P. STRANDE,
J. KLAVENESS, P. LEANDER, and A. BERG

In nuclear medicine, technetium-labeled particles are in wide clinical use for scintigraphic imaging of the liver and spleen (1). Particulate MRI contrast agents have recently been clinically evaluated (2). However, in x-ray imaging, the oldest imaging technology, there is no particulate liver contrast medium on the market. Almost all available parenteral iodinated x-ray contrast agents are hydrophilic water-soluble substances with the same pharmacokinetic properties: extracellular distribution and renal elimination (3). There is, however, a need for a good x-ray contrast agent for the diagnosis of focal liver disease. Various approaches for water-insoluble liver x-ray contrast agents like iodinated fat emulsions (4), liposome encapsulated x-ray contrast agents (5), and various iodinated solid particles (6) have been evaluated, but most of these products have not yet been developed further.

From a theoretical point of view, the ideal particulate x-ray contrast agent should be stable in an aqueous suspension with long shelf life, be selectively taken up by the liver and spleen, stay in the target organs long enough for visualization of the organ (approximately 1 h), and then effectively degraded to nontoxic metabolites and excreted. One interesting approach involves particles made from water-insoluble derivatives of ionic x-ray contrast agents. Violante and coworkers have evaluated particulate contrast agents made of iothalamate ethyl ester (IEE) and iodipamide ethyl ester (IDE) (6–12). Following intravenous infusion of IDE particles, approximately 60 percent of the injected dose accumulated in the rat liver and cleared from this organ with a half-life of approximately 11 h (9).

In the field of antibiotics, the prodrug concept in drug design has improved the poor absorbtion of ampicillin from the gastrointestinal tract. Using special double esters or carbonate esters of ampicillin, the absorbed prodrug is rapidly hydrolyzed to the active compound by nonspecific esterases. Thus these enzyme-catalyzed, degradable esters are attractive in prodrug approaches because of the significant difference between in vitro and in vivo stability. Although double esters and carbonate esters are hydrolyzed very rapidly in vivo by nonspecific esterases, the stability in storage is high. We have introduced the prodrug concept in design of particulate x-ray contrast agents that are rapidly hydrolyzed in vivo. Different water-insoluble double esters and carbonate esters of metrizoic acid have been synthesized, formulated as homogeneous particle suspensions, and evaluated as potential particulate x-ray liver contrast agents. The most promising of them is IEEC (Fig. 45-1), which is the compound reported in this chapter. This prodrug is a carbonate ester of metrizoic acid—the same carbonate ester applied in the antibioticum bacampicillin (13).

MATERIALS AND METHODS

Chemical Synthesis

IEEC [1'-(ethyloxycarbonyloxy)-ethyl-5-acetylamino-3-(N-methyl-acetylamino)-2,4,6-triiodobenzenecarboxylate] was synthetized as follows: 5-Acetylamino-3-(N-methyl-acetylamino)-2,4,6-triiodobenzenecarboxylic acid (metrizoic acid; 0.6 mol, 377 g) was suspended in water (1.5 liters). A solution of approximately 20 percent potassium hydroxide was added cautiously to pH 7.1. The clear solution was evaporated to dryness and dried in vacuo for 4 days at 50°C to give potassium 5-acetylamino-3-(N-methyl-acetylamino-2,4,6-triiodobenzenecarboxylate.

This compound (0.6 mol, 400 g) and sodium iodide (0.06 mol, 8.99 g) was dissolved in DMF (2 liters) at room temperature. 1-Chloroethyl ethyl carbonate (0.66 mol, 101 g) was added dropwise over 1.5 h at room temperature. The temperature was raised to 50°C, and the suspension was stirred for 26 h. The solvent was removed at reduced pressure and the product was dried in vacuo at room temperature for 3 days to give the product 1'-(ethyloxycarbonyloxy)-ethyl 5-acetylamino-3 (N-methyl-acetylamino)-2,4,6-triiodobenzenecarboxylate, yield 551.6 g. The residue was dissolved in chloroform (1.2 liters) and washed four times with 0.3 liter of a saturated sodium hydrogen carbonate solution and twice with 0.3 liter water. The organic phase was stirred with magnesium sulfate and activated charcoal (10 g) at room temperature for 1.5 h. After filtration the product was crystallized by concentrating the solution at reduced pressure to 250 milliliters. After 1 day at room temperature, the precipitate was filtrated off, washed with chloroform, and dried in vacuo at 50°C for 1 day. The product was suspended in acetone (0.5 liter) and refluxed for 2 h. After 1 day at room temperature, the precipitate was filtrated off and washed with acetone. The product was dried in vacuo at 50°C for 4 days. The yield was 77 percent and the HLPC purity 99.5 percent.

Preparation of Particles

A 3 percent solution of human albumin (HSA) in distilled water was prepared (150 ml) and filtered through a membrane filter (0.45 μm). A filtered solution (0.22 μm) of IEEC (1.2 g) in 96 percent ethanol (30.0 ml) was slowly added to the HSA solution under vigorous stirring. The microparticles formed were centrifuged and washed repeatedly before resuspending in sterile phosphate-buffered saline (10.7 ml) (Fig. 45-1). The size and distribution of the particles were analyzed by Coulter counter multisizer. The mean diameter was 2.13 μm (number based), with 95 percent in the range between 1.28 μm and 3.57 μm (number based). The iodine content of the particles is 51.2 percent w/w.

Experimental Animals

Male Wistar rats weighing 150 to 300 g and male NMRI mice weighing 18 to 22 g were obtained from Møllegård and Bomholtgaard Breeding Centers (Denmark), respectively. Male ChbbHM rabbits (1.7 to 2.2 kg) were obtained from Dr. K. Thomae Breeding Center (West Germany) and housed individually at 18 ± 2°C. The animals were given tap water and pellets ad libitum. The rodents were housed in plastic cages at 21 ± 2°C and at a relative humidity of 55 ± 10 percent. A 12-h light-dark cycle was maintained. The acclimatization period was at least 5 days.

Administration of Test Substance

The particle suspension was routinely agitated on a whirl mixer for at least 2 min. The absence of aggregates in the final suspension was controlled by light microscopic inspection. The concentration of the particles was 100 mg IEEC per milliliter, corresponding to 50 mg iodine per milliliter. The particles were injected at a rate of about 150 mg iodine per minute per kilogram of body weight in the experiments.

Pharmacokinetics

The biodistribution and excretion of the IEEC particles were investigated in rats after intravenous injection of 100 mg I/kg. After different intervals, the animals were sacrificed by cervical dislocation, and the liver and lungs were excised, weighed, and stored at −20°C for iodine analysis. Groups of three rats were anaesthetized, and the bile duct and the urinary bladder were cannulated for sampling of excreta the first 3 hours after injection. Finally, three rats were placed in metabolic

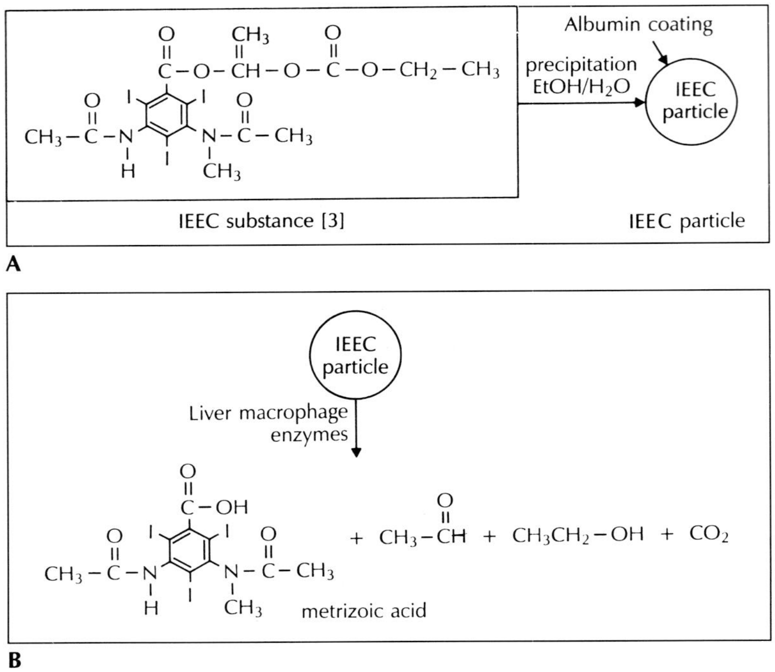

FIGURE 45-1
(A) *IEEC particle production principle.* (B) *Degradation of the IEEC particle.*

cages for daily sampling of urine and feces for 7 days after injection. Urine, bile, and feces were analyzed for iodine and/or IEEC content by x-ray fluorescence or HPLC. The plasma half-life of the particles was investigated in five rabbits after an injection of 100 mg I/kg. Blood samples were drawn at different time intervals from a lateral ear vein and stored in heparinized vials at $-20°C$. The rabbits were placed in metabolic cages for urine and feces sampling. Urine, feces, and whole blood was analyzed for iodine by x-ray fluorescence. For the pharmacokinetic calculations, the Siphar kinetics software (Mimed, France) was used.

Acute Intravenous Toxicity

Mice. A group of 39 mice was injected IV in a lateral tail vein with increasing doses of IEEC particles. The observation period for clinical signs and mortality was 7 days. For the higher dose levels, a particle suspension containing 100 mg I/ml was used.

Rats. The single dose intravenous toxicity was investigated in rats after administration of 100, 500, or 1000 mg I/kg. After 6 h and 1, 2, and 7 days,

a 0.5-ml blood sample was collected from a tail vein incision. Serum was stored at $-70°C$ before analysis of alanine aminotransferase (ALAT), aspartate aminotransferase (ASAT), alkaline phosphatase (ALP), urea, and creatinine on a Cobas Fara autoanalyzer (Roche Diagnostica, N.J.) using standard commercial kits. After the last blood sample, the animals were fasted overnight before sacrifice. The liver, spleen, lungs, and kidneys were excised, weighed, and specimens fixed in buffered Formalin. The specimens were processed by standard methods for light microscopy.

Reticuloendothelial Clearance Capacity

The capacity of the liver to phagocytose particulate matter after IEEC particle pretreatment was studied in rats. As an indicator for phagocytic activity, heat-denatured albumin aggregates (Albures) were used. This colloid suspension was radiolabeled with [^{125}I]tyramine cellobiose (14).

Five rats each were injected IV with 200 mg I/kg IEEC particles or 0.9 percent saline. One hour after the injection, the animals were anesthetized with 50 mg/kg pentobarbital IP and injected with

Albures. Blood samples (50 µl) were drawn at different time intervals and analyzed for radioactivity. Sixty minutes after the Albures injection, the animals were sacrificed and the liver and spleen were excised and analyzed for radioactivity.

CT Study in Rabbit Tumor Model
Two groups of four and five New Zealand rabbits, respectively, were inoculated with VX2 adenocarcinoma (kindly provided by Prof. Kethura, National University of Tokyo, Japan) directly into the liver by laparotomy. Each rabbit received two inoculations of 0.5 ml VX2-saline cell suspension. After 11 to 19 days, imaging studies were carried out. During laparotomy and imaging, the animals were anaesthetized with pentobarbital (Mebumal Vet, 60 mg/ml) at a dose of 60 mg/kg IV. In addition, two animals were inoculated as described above but imaged after 7 days to visualize small tumors. After sacrifice, the liver was excised, and CT findings were correlated with macroscopic findings. Four rabbits were given a particle dose of 50 mg I/kg, and five rabbits were given 100 mg I/kg.

The additional two rabbits imaged after 7 days received the higher dose. All images were obtained on a clinical CT, Siemens Somatom DRG. Imaging parameters were as follows: 125 kV, 350 mA, 480 projections, 4-s scan time, 4-mm slice thickness without interslice gaps, and 256 matrix. Six to eight slices covered the entire liver of each animal. Imaging procedures were performed before and 10 min after intravenous contrast medium administration. Image attenuation expressed in Hounsfield Units (HU) was measured by the region of interests (ROIs) facility for nine rabbits. Contrast was calculated as the difference in Hounsfield Units between liver and tumor tissue.

RESULTS

Biodistribution and Excretion

Rats. Fifteen minutes after intravenous injection of 100 mg I/kg IEEC particles into rats, more than 70 percent of the dose was localized in the liver (Fig. 45-2A). The liver uptake corresponded to a concentration of 1.4 mg I/g liver (Fig. 45-2B). The liver iodine content remained constant for at least 3 h and then decreased steadily. At 24 h, only 4.5 percent of the iodine dose was found in the liver, while no iodine could be detected later than 3 days after injection. In the lungs, a maximum of 1.3 percent of the dose was found after 15 min. No iodine could be detected in the lungs later than 6 h after injection. Figure 45-2C shows the excretion pattern in rats during the first week after injection. Within 24 h after injection, 85 percent of the dose was already eliminated from the body. Urinary excretion accounted for 47 ± 2 percent, whereas 48 ± 4 percent of the iodine dose was fecally excreted. In the anaesthetized rats with cannulated bile duct and urinary bladder, 8.1 ± 6.2 percent and 3.6 ± 2.1 percent of iodine was excreted in bile and urine, respectively, during the first 3 h after injection. This may be due to reduced urine flow in the laparotomized animals, with a urine output in the cannulated animals of 0.19 ± 0.07 ml/h, while the rats in metabolic cages excreted 0.55 ± 0.10 ml/h on average. HPLC analyses of urine and bile samples showed that the iodine is excreted as metrizoic acid salt.

Rabbits. A typical plasma clearance curve after IV injection of 100 mg I/kg to a rabbit is shown in Figure 45-3A. The majority of particulate matter is cleared from the blood within the first 10 min. Using a biexponential (two-compartment) model, the plasma half-life in the α phase was calculated to be 1.8 ± 0.2 min ($n = 5$) and in the β phase 194 ± 55 min ($n = 5$).

The excretion of iodine in rabbits after injection of particles at a dose of 100 mg I/kg is given in Figure 45-3B. Within the first 48 h after injection, 85 ± 3 percent of the dose was excreted in urine and less than 2 percent in the feces. The total recovery of iodine after 7 days was 87 percent ($n = 5$). No iodine was found in the liver, spleen, heart, kidneys, and lungs 7 days after injection, with a detection limit for iodine of 12 ppm.

Acute Toxicity

Mice. The approximate LD_{50} in mice was found to be 2000 mg I/kg, corresponding to 4 g particles per kilogram. At the highest dose levels (4.5 and 6.3 g particles per kilogram), the animals died shortly after injection. The suggested cause of death was pulmonary embolization.

Rats. The acute IV toxicity was studied in rats after a single injection of 100, 500, and 1000 mg I/kg. No difference in body weight gain between the control and low-dose group was observed, with a weight increase of 36 and 38 g, respectively, over 7 days. At the medium- and high-dose levels, a statistically significant ($p < 0.05$) dose-dependent

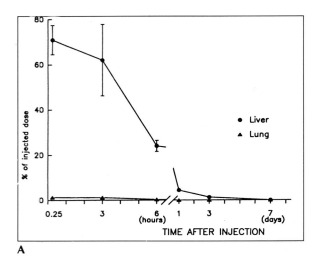

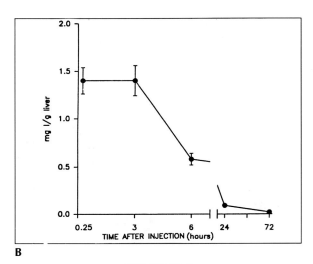

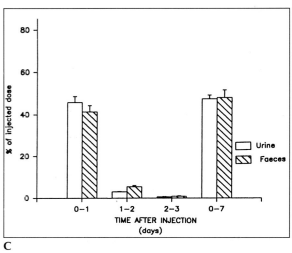

FIGURE 45-2
Organ uptake and excretion of IEEC particles after intravenous injection of 100 mg I/kg in rats. (A) Iodine content of liver and lung in percent of injected dose. (B) Iodine concentration of the liver in milligrams per gram wet tissue. (C) Daily and total excretion of contrast material in urine and feces.

reduction in body weight gain (22 and 12 g, respectively) was found. The relative spleen weight (organ weight in percent of body weight) was increased ($p < 0.05$) at the medium- and high-dose levels. The clinical chemistry analyses revealed alterations related mainly to the function of the target organ liver. The transaminase levels were elevated in a dose-dependent manner in the first blood samples after injection (Fig. 45-4A, B). The level of ASAT was significantly increased in the medium- and high-dose groups and reached about 9 times control in the highest dose group 6 h after injection. A fivefold increase of ALAT was seen in the 1000 mg I/kg group, while this parameter was unchanged in the 100 mg I/kg group.

Phagocytic Capacity

Rats pretreated with 200 mg I/kg IEEC particles 1 h before the clearance of Albures colloids was investigated displayed a significantly different value from control only in the first blood sample (2 min). By then, 8.0 ± 1.8 percent and 17.7 ± 6.1 percent of the injected Albures remained in the blood of the control and IEEC pretreated rats, respectively. In both groups, more than 98 percent of the colloids were cleared within 10 min (Fig. 45-5). One hour after injection the liver had accumulated 71.0 ± 11.5 percent and 62.7 ± 5.9 percent of the injected dose in control and test groups, respectively.

Contrast Efficacy in Rabbit Tumor Model

All rabbits were found to have tumors ranging from 5 to 20 mm in diameter. The size and location of the tumors corresponded well with the CT images. No central necrosis was detected by macroscopic inspection. The attenuation precontrast for liver and tumors tissue for nine rabbits measured was 63 HU (53–84) and 37 HU (10–55) (mean values and range). The attenuation postcontrast at a dose of 50 mg I/kg for four rabbits was 94 HU (79–

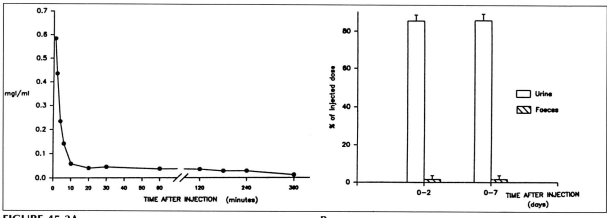

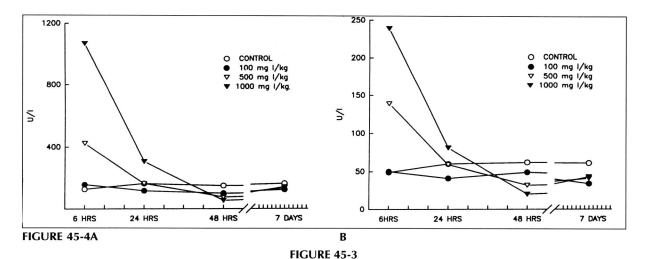

FIGURE 45-3
Blood clearance (A) and excretion (B) of iodine after intravenous injection of 100 mg I/kg IEEC particles in rabbit.

FIGURE 45-4
Serum levels of ASAT (A) and ALAT (B) after different doses of IEEC particles injected intravenously in rats.

129) and 34 HU (23–45) for liver and tumorous tissue, respectively, and at a dose of 100 mg I/kg for five rabbits 106 HU (93–110) and 37 HU (22–46). Calculated contrast was 26, 61, and 68 HU for precontrast and postcontrast at the two doses, respectively (Fig. 45-6).

In the rabbits imaged and dosed 7 days after tumor cell inoculation, small tumors with a diameter of 5 mm were visualized. Owing to the effectiveness of the studied particles in the rabbit tumor model, the anticipated imaging dose was defined as 100 mg I/kg, with good contrast enhancement already at 50 mg I/kg.

DISCUSSION

The current methods for detection and diagnosis of focal disease in liver and spleen (US, MRI, scintigraphy, CT) frequently demonstrate insufficient sensitivity. Small lesions often pass undetected

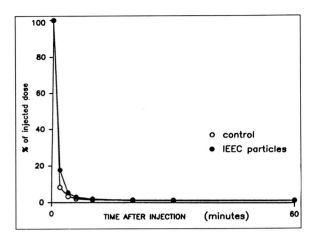

FIGURE 45-5
Plasma clearance of ^{125}I–TC–Albures colloids 1 h after injection of 200 mg I/kg IEEC particles in rats.

after these types of studies. The main purpose of a particulate contrast agent is to increase the sensitivity and comfort of hepatosplenic imaging. Different approaches to solve these questions have been tried during the last two decades. Iodinated oils, liposomes, and solid particles made from derivatized contrast media have all been revealed to be of diagnostic value, but most of these compounds have not yet been developed further.

We have investigated a novel compound, IEEC, for its suitability as a hepatolienographic contrast agent. The biodistribution of the particle and the iodine content of liver and lung were directly comparable with results presented earlier with the iodipamide ethyl ester particle (9). The IEEC particles have short half-life in vivo, owing to hydrolysis by nonspecific esterases. The fast excretion of metrizoic acid indicates that IEEC is cleaved more readily than IDE in vivo (9). In contrast to IDE, IEEC is seen to be metabolized (Fig. 45-1B). From the biodistribution studies, the iodine-containing metabolite was found to be metrizoic acid. The assumed additional metabolites shown in Figure 45-1B are the same as for bacampicillin (13). In an in vitro system, equimolar amounts of metrizoate, acetaldehyde, and ethanol were generated upon incubation of IEEC with liver esterases (CO_2 was not analyzed). Lipophilic substances are generally more toxic than the corresponding hydrophilic counterpart. The rapid degradation of IEEC to water-soluble metabolites, owing to the susceptibility of the carbonate ester to nonspecific esterases, seems advantageous with regard to toxicity compared with other non-degradable or slowly degradable esters, such as IDE.

A species-specific difference in the excretion pattern between rats and rabbits was observed. Similar minor differences can be observed with traditional water-soluble contrast agents, with a tendency toward higher biliary excretion in the rat than in other species (15,16).

The short half-life of the particles in blood reflects adhesion of the particles to membranes of phagocytic cells in the reticuloendothelial system. The clearance rate was comparable with what has been obtained with other types of microspheres, such as latex and albumin aggregates (17). A high ratio between tissue and blood iodine values is therefore quickly established, and maximal specific contrast enhancement is obtained. This particle therefore seems to possess the desired pharmacokinetic properties for a hepatolienographic agent: a high specific targeting combined with rapid excretion of nontoxic metabolites.

The importance of a protein coat on contrast particles has been investigated by Violante and coworkers (6). The albumin coat is necessary to minimize interaction with blood constituents after injection, which may result in aggregation and pulmonary embolism. An approximate LD_{50} in mice of about 20 times the anticipated clinical dose indicates an acceptable low acute toxicity for this agent. This was further corroborated by the findings in the acute toxicity study in rats. The ASAT:ALAT ratio observed in the 6-h blood samples indicates that these elevations are not derived from hepatocellular leakage alone (18). ASAT is more widely distributed in rat tissues than ALAT and may leak to plasma after general systemic perturbations, such as hypoxia or vascular collapse (19). The relatively higher increase of this parameter may therefore reflect hemodynamic changes. Preliminary studies not reported here indicate a dose-related hypotensive effect on systemic blood pressure in rats, but not in rabbits.

No histopathologic changes were observed in liver, spleen, kidneys, or lung 8 days after single injection. However, this does not preclude the

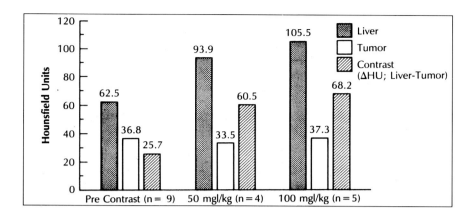

FIGURE 45-6
Rabbit VX2 liver tumor model. Precontrast values from nine rabbits. Postcontrast measurements 10 min after a dose of either 50 of 100 mg I/kg IEEC particles.

existence of transient histologic changes in these organs. Morphologic studies with IDE have demonstrated transient changes occurring a few days after injection, with a recovery to normal morphology within 1 week after injection (8,12).

The results of the Albures colloid clearance study showed that a dose of IEEC particles twice the expected clinical dose did not compromise the phagocytic capacity of the liver. A massive RES blockade was therefore not observed after IEEC exposure.

The imaging studies confirmed the good contrast efficacy of a particulate agent for visualization of focal liver disease. The results were in agreement with earlier studies with the IEE and IDE particles (7,10,11). The agent enhances the contrast difference between normal and malignant liver tissue more than twofold and will therefore improve the detectability of certain liver diseases.

In conclusion, the IEEC particle seems to fulfill the basic criteria for a hepatosplenic contrast agent. Favorable pharmacokinetics, suitable imaging contrast enhancement, and properties indicative of low toxicity make this compound promising for further development as a contrast medium for liver imaging.

REFERENCES

1. Billinghurst MW: Radiopharmaceuticals for imaging the reticuloendothelial system, in Fritzberg AR (ed): Radiopharmaceuticals: Progress and Clinical Perspectives. Boca Raton, Fla., CRC Press, 1986.
2. Hahn PF, Stark DD, Weissleder R, et al: Clinical applications of superparamagnetic iron oxide to MR imaging of tissue perfusion in vascular liver tumors. Radiology 174:361, 1990.
3. Felix R, Fischer HW, Kormano M, et al (eds): Contrast Media from the Past to the Future. Stuttgart, Thieme-Verlag, 1987.
4. Ivancev K, Lunderquist A, Isaksson A, Hochbergs P, Wretlind A: Clinical trials with a new iodinated lipid emulsion for computed tomography of the liver. Acta Radiol 30:449, 1989.
5. Seltzer SE: The role of liposomes in diagnostic imaging. Radiology 171:19, 1989.
6. Violante MR, Fischer HW, Mahoney JA: Particulate contrast media. Invest Radiol 15:329, 1980.
7. Sands MS, Violante MR, Gadeholt G: Computed tomographic enhancement of liver and spleen in the dog with iodipamide ethyl ester particulate suspension. Invest Radiol 22:408, 1987.
8. Lauteala L, Kormano M, Violante MR: Effect of intravenously administered iodipamide ethyl ester particles on rat liver morphology. Invest Radiol 19:133, 1984.
9. Violante MR, Måre K, Fischer HW: Biodistribution of a particulate hepatolienographic CT contrast agent: A study of iodipamide ethyl ester in rat. Invest Radiol 16:40, 1981.
10. Violante MR, Dehn PB, Fischer HW, Mahoney JA: Particulate contrast media for computed tomographic scanning of the liver. Invest Radiol 15:171, 1980.

11. Violante MR, Dean PB: Improved detectability of VX2 carcinoma in the rabbit liver with contrast enhancement in computed tomography. Radiology 134:237, 1980.
12. Lauteala L, Kormano M, Violante MR: Uptake and dissolution of particulate iodipamide ethyl ester in the spleen: A morphologic study. Invest Radiol 22:829, 1987.
13. Bodin NO, Ekstrøm B, Forsgren U, et al: Bacampicillin: A new orally, well-absorbed derivative of ampicillin. Antimicrob Agents Chemother 8:518, 1975.
14. Pittman RC, Carew TE, Glass CK, et al: A radioiodinated, intracellularly trapped ligand for determining the sites of plasma protein degradation in vivo. Biochem J 212:791, 1983.
15. Michelet ÅA, Skinnemoen K: Pharmacokinetics of iopentol in the rat. Acta Radiol [Suppl] 370:101, 1987.
16. Waaler A, Jørgensen NP, Koksvik B, et al: Pharmacokinetics of iopentol in healthy volunteers. Acta Radiol [Suppl] 370:113, 1987.
17. Arthurson P, Laakso T, Edman P: Acrylic microspheres in vivo: IX. Blood elimination kinetics and organ distribution of microparticles with different surface characteristics. J Pharm Sci 72:1415, 1983.
18. Rosalki SB: Enzyme tests in diseases of the liver and hepatobiliary tract, in Wilkinson JH (ed): The Principles and Practice of Diagnostic Enzymology. London, E. Arnold, 1976.
19. Zimmerman HJ, Seef LB: Enzymes in hepatic disease, in Coodley EL (ed): Diagnostic Enzymology. Philadelphia, Lea and Febiger, 1970.

46

Ferrite Particles: Rationale and Clinical Results (Midfield)

JOSEPH T. FERRUCCI

Iron oxide, in the form of superparamagnetic particles, is a powerful tissue-specific MRI contrast agent for enhanced detection of tumors in the liver and spleen. Extensive preclinical studies at the Massachusetts General Hospital (MGH) during 1985–1988 elucidated the biological and pharmaceutical principles for MRI (1–7) and led to the first clinical trial in 1988, in which greatly enhanced liver lesion detection was confirmed (8). Additional clinical trials are now in progress in the United States as well as in France, Belgium, and Japan, and early results from one European center have recently been reported (9).

This chapter reviews the development of iron oxide-enhanced MRI of the liver and spleen over the past 5 years. The emphasis will be on work carried out by the Division of Gastrointestinal Radiology at the MGH. In our studies, clinical imaging has been carried out at midfield (0.3 to 0.6 Tesla). Results at high field (1.5 Tesla) will be presented in the next chapter.

SUPERPARAMAGNETIC IRON OXIDE: PHYSICAL PROPERTIES

Superparamagnetic iron oxides (SPIOs) are crystalline structures with the general formula $Fe_2^{3+}O_3 M^{2+}O$, where M^{2+} is a divalent metal ion such as iron, manganese, nickel, cobalt, or magnesium. SPIO is similar to magnetite, a naturally occurring ferrite, in which the metal ion (M^{2+}) is ferrous iron (Fe^{2+}) with the formula Fe_3O_4 (Fig. 46-1.)

Because of its ubiquitous presence in living tissue, iron is a natural candidate for manipulation of the MRI signal. Indeed, the ferrite magnetite is particularly suitable because this iron oxide has been isolated from certain birds, fish, and bacteria, where its interaction with the magnetic field of the earth has been found to play a critical role in navigation (10).

Pharmaceutical grade preparations suitable for clinical use have evolved rapidly since the earliest characterization studies of magnetic particles for possible medical applications were performed in our laboratory (1–3). Superparamagnetic iron oxide crystals by themselves are 5–50 nm in size. However, these crystals are usually formed by precipitation of iron salts with a coating material to form larger composite particles. Median diameter of composite particle size has been varied from the 1-µm range used in early studies to less than 10 nm (Fig. 46-2). The smaller size of newer particles accelerates degradation of SPIO into paramagnetic forms of iron. Biocompatible coatings such as starch (dextran), protein, glycoprotein, or lipid permit safe intravenous administration and ready biodegradability. The compound used in our initial clinical trials is a stable colloidal

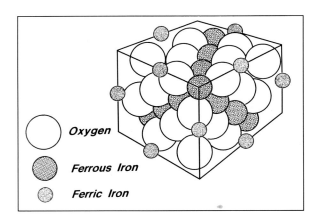

FIGURE 46-1
Spinel crystal structure characteristic of superparamagnetic iron oxides.

aqueous suspension of iron oxide and dextran, reddish brown to black in color, formulated at 0.2 M Fe and designated AMI-25, or Feridex (Advanced Magnetics, Inc., Cambridge, Mass. 02138).

The magnetic properties of these materials were first termed *superparamagnetic* in 1955 (11). The term refers to the extremely large magnetic moments they acquire when placed in external magnetic fields. This sensitivity to magnetic fields is the result of the crystalline matrix, which facilitates alignment of adjoining spins to an applied field. This is so efficient that even at low field strengths, all available spins can be recruited and no further gain in magnetization is achieved by increasing the applied field strength. Superparamagnetic materials differ from ferromagnetic substances because, like diamagnetic and paramagnetic materials, they do not retain any magnetization once the external field is removed. In contrast, once magnetized, ferromagnetic materials show remanence (i.e., they remain partially magnetized even in the absence of an applied field) and are therefore used as recording materials and to make permanent magnets.

In tissue, the large magnetic moments associated with superparamagnetic iron particles result in local magnetic field inhomogeneities. Diffusion of water through these local field disturbances produces rapid proton dephasing, which results in preferential shortening of transverse relaxation time, T2, with little effect on longitudinal relaxation times, T1. The T2 relaxivity (R2) of $1 \times 10^5 \, s^{-1} M^{-1}$

FIGURE 46-2
Electron micrograph of superparamagnetic iron oxide particle (M4125, Advanced Magnetics, Inc., Cambridge, Mass.) magnified ×82,000 showing an irregularly shaped structure approximately 1 μm in size. Particle shape and size are stabilized by coating a cluster of iron oxide crystals with a hydrophilic polymer. Individual superparamagnetic ferrite crystals can be seen. (From Saini S, Stark DD, Hahn PF, et al: Ferrite particles: A superparamagnetic MR contrast agent for the reticuloendothelial system. Radiology 162:211, 1987. Reprinted by permission.)

and T1 relaxivity (R1) of $3 \times 10^4 \, s^{-1} M^{-1}$ of iron oxide are substantially larger than the relaxation of paramagnetic molecules such as Gd-DTPA [R2 6×10^3 and R1 $4 \times 10^3 \, s^{-1} M^{-1}$ (1-7)](Fig. 46-3).

SUPERPARAMAGNETIC IRON OXIDE: PHYSIOLOGIC CONSIDERATIONS

Pharmacokinetic behavior of SPIO is generally comparable in animals and humans (1-7). Since the injected particles are smaller than erythrocytes (which are approximately 7 μm in diameter), they successfully traverse capillary beds in the lung, brain, heart, and kidney. Particles are promptly sequestered by the reticuloendothelial

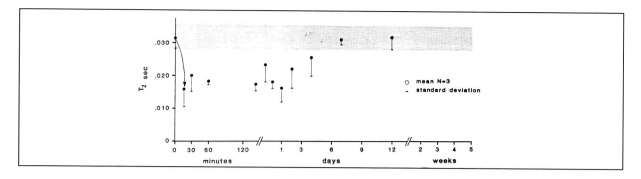

FIGURE 46-3
Magnetic degradation of superparamagnetic iron oxide. T2 relaxivity values of excised rat liver measured 15 minutes to 12 days after injection. Normal T2 relaxivity ± 1 SD shown as the gray zone. An initial prompt decrease reflects uptake by hepatic RES Kupffer cells. The effect persists for approximately 3 days, with gradual return of relaxation values to normal by 1 week. The relaxation data alone cannot distinguish between clearance of intact particles from liver and magnetic degradation of superparamagnetic crystals into paramagnetic forms of iron.

system (RES). The RES cells have a scavenging function and, by phagocytosis, readily remove particulate materials from the circulation. AMI-25 shows a blood clearance half-life of about 10 min, with uptake by hepatic RES Kupffer cells accounting for 80 percent of the injected dose (1-7) (Fig. 46-3). Thus T2 relaxation times of blood, liver, and spleen decrease promptly after IV injection, but only blood quickly returns to normal. The extremely powerful effect that SPIO particles have on proton relaxation is attested to by the observation that even in minute doses (8 μmol/kg) that are located in a very small (approximately 2 percent) portion of the hepatic cellular volume (i.e., Kupffer cells) there is essentially complete signal loss from the entire liver.

Because neoplastic tumor nodules are devoid of the phagocytic Kupffer cells, they do not sequester SPIO (Fig. 46-4). As a consequence, the signal difference between normal RES tissue and tumor is greatly enhanced. Following SPIO administration, there is no change in relaxation times of tumor, whereas normal liver shows a marked decrease in T2 (Table 46-1). This difference in T2 relaxation between tumor and liver, expressed as a percentage of T2 of normal liver, increased from 49 percent to 280 percent in ex vivo studies of a rat liver tumor model (2).

Newer formulations of SPIO have to date been evaluated only in animals. Ferrosomes are a class of SPIO encapsulated in lipid vesicles (liposomes) developed by Vestar, Inc. (San Dimas, Calif.), that exhibit prolonged blood circulation (clearance half-life 4 hours). Prolonged circulation permits increased delivery of SPIO to tissues other than the liver and spleen. For example, ferrosomes show distribution to macrophages located at the periphery of tumors (12).

Metabolically, AMI-25 iron is biodegradable and bioavailable, being rapidly turned over into the body iron stores and incorporated into erythrocytes as hemoglobin (6). Using light microscopy, stainable iron disappears from rat liver within 2 weeks, while radiolabeled ^{59}Fe iron oxide shows a liver/spleen half-life of 3 to 4 days (7). At in vivo MRI in animals as well as humans, liver signal blackening shows a reversal toward normal baseline tissue characteristics over 3 to 7 days (1,8).

Bioavailability is demonstrated by the incorporation of molecular iron into hemoglobin after administration of ^{59}Fe AMI-25. Twenty percent of radiolabeled iron is found in hemoglobin 14 days after IV administration. Similar rates of erythrocyte incorporation (21 percent) occur with administration of radiolabeled ferritin. Bioavailability is also shown by the ability of SPIO to reverse iron-deficiency anemia in rats to an extent similar to that of hematinic iron-dextran (6).

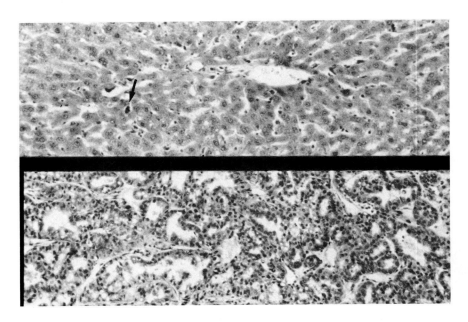

FIGURE 46-4
Reticuloendothelial sequestration of intravenously administered SPIO particles in normal liver but not in tumor tissue. Light microscopic sections stained with iron (Prussian blue) of normal rat liver (top, ×320) and tumor tissue (bottom, ×200). SPIO particles are stained blue and can be readily identified (arrow) in hepatic reticuloendothelial cells. No such particles are present in hepatocytes or in tumor tissue. (From Saini S, Stark DD, Hahn PF, et al: Ferrite particles: A superparamagnetic MR contrast agent for enhanced detection of liver carcinoma. Radiology 162:217, 1987. Reprinted by permission.)

TABLE 46-1. *Tissue Relaxation Times Before and After Administration of SPIO*

	Liver (ms)	Tumor (ms)
Control:		
T1	317 ± 23	540 ± 82
T2	33.3 ± 2.9	50 ± 8.8
Ferrite:		
T1	291 ± 28	580 ± 56
T2	12.7 ± 2.8	48.2 ± 7.1

Source: From Saini S, Stark DD, Hahn PF, et al: Ferrite particles: A superparamagnetic MR contrast agent for enhanced detection of liver carcinoma. Radiology 162:217, 1987. Reprinted by permission.

Extensive toxicity studies in animals have disclosed no acute toxicity (LD_{50} in rats) or chronic injury at doses greater than 100 times the clinically effective dose of 20 μm Fe per kilogram of body weight (3,6). Even at the subcellular level, when a massive dose of 250 mg Fe per kilogram was given to rats, Bacon et al. (3) were unable to detect hepatic mitochondria dysfunction or microsomal lipid peroxidation, both sensitive biochemical indicators of iron induced hepatotoxicity. Despite the large increase in hepatic iron concentration, at 10 weeks after SPIO administration, biochemical and morphologic studies give no evidence of chronic injury.

HUMAN TOXICITY

Despite these wide margins of safety in animals, dose escalation in human clinical trials with AMI-25 have shown dose-dependent acute hypotensive reactions when more than 40 μmol kg is administered at rates greater than 1000 μmol per minute (8). In the U.S. trials to the present, 40 patients have received 20 μmol Fe per kilogram administered at the recommended rate of 200 μmol per minute, and only one patient was found to have a 20-mmHg drop in systolic blood pressure; no treatment was required. The mechanism of these adverse reactions in unknown. They have been reversed by infusions of saline. Further clinical trials are being conducted to explore safety and efficacy. Newer formulations with enhanced safety profiles also can be anticipated.

EFFECTS AT MRI

Numerous beneficial effects of SPIO MRI contrast agents have been documented at in vivo imaging. Liver and spleen signal intensity decreases, whereas tumor nodules are displayed as high-signal-intensity areas with a variety of pulse sequences (2) (Fig. 46-5). Quantitative measurements of signal-to-noise ratio (SNR) and contrast-to-noise ratio (CNR) demonstrate marked enhancement after SPIO administration (Table 46-2). Maximal decrease in signal from liver occurs on more heavily T2-weighted pulse sequences (spin-echo TR > 1000, TE > 50 ms), although relaxation effects can be demonstrated using a wide variety of sequences. Pulse sequences where tumor and liver appear essentially isointense before SPIO administration, such as SE 500/30, show great increase in tumor conspicuity after SPIO administration.

A further beneficial effect of increased lesion conspicuity is reduction in threshold size for lesion detection. Tsang et al. (5) conducted a detailed MRI pathologic correlation of implanted mammary tumors under 1 cm in size in rat livers. They studied 39 separate tumor nodules measuring 1 to 10 mm imaged before and after SPIO administration and correlated MRI appearances with thin-slice necropsy measurements. With

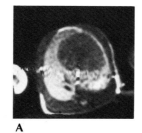 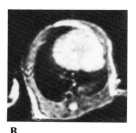

A B

FIGURE 46-5

Effects of SPIO (30 μmol Fe per kilogram) on liver/tumor visibility. Implanted mammary carcinoma in a rat. (A) SE 500/15 T1-weighted image. Bright signal from liver outlines tumor nodule, which has slightly longer T1 relaxation time. (B) SE 500/30 sequence after SPIO administration shows complete loss of signal intensity from normal hepatic parenchyma. The tumor nodule has slightly brighter signal compared with the precontrast image because of the longer TE and greater T2 weighting. The overall liver tumor contrast is markedly increased after SPIO administration.

contrast enhancement, the threshold size for lesion detectability decreased from 1 cm to less than 3 mm in diameter. This increase in sensitivity was obtained with a 0.6-Tesla clinical MRI system using a widely available SE 500/32 pulse sequence. These investigators further noted that even these tiny millimeter-sized nodules were not obscured on imaging nor underestimated in size. Comparison of actual pathologic measurements with MRI images confirmed that extremely high accuracy can be expected for clinical MRI lesion assessment. Furthermore, this study showed that enhanced contrast-to-noise ratios (CNR) correlate with improved lesion detection.

TABLE 46-2. *Quantitative MRI Image Analysis: CNR and SNR*

Pulse Sequence	Cancer SNR	Liver SNR	Spleen SNR	Cancer/Liver CNR
Unenhanced (prior to drug administration):				
SE 260/14	28.7 ± 17.5	39.5 ± 12.5	27.4 ± 11.4	−10.8 ± 9.6
SE 500/28	28.1 ± 10.7	31.4 ± 9.4	26.2 ± 9.4	− 3.3 ± 4.4
SE 1500/40	24.6 ± 10.9	23.9 ± 9.3	25.6 ± 13.3	+ 0.6 ± 4.9
SE 1500/80	19.4 ± 6.3	14.9 ± 3.9	21.3 ± 6.4	+ 3.4 ± 3.8
Ferrite-enhanced (1 to 2 hours after administration):				
SE 500/28	37.3 ± 14	21.8 ± 10.6*	28.5 ± 11.3	+15.9 ± 7.6*
SE 1500/40	24.4 ± 11.6	8.1 ± 3.7*	11.6 ± 4.9*	+16.3 ± 9.6*
SE 1500/80	18.9 ± 10.8	4.3 ± 3.1*	4.8 ± 2.3*	+14.5 ± 9.8*

*$p < 0.01$; ferrite-enhanced values are significantly different from unenhanced values.

Kawamura et al. (13) confirmed these results in similar studies using a slightly larger 100-nm particle obtained from a Japanese supplier. The detection rate for 89 implanted rat tumors, including some less than 2 mm in diameter, increased from 10 percent (9 of 89) before ferrite administration to 65 percent (58 of 89) after injection.

The breadth of clinically advantageous SPIO effects with a variety of pulse-sequence parameters was stressed in another study from our laboratory by Fretz et al. (14). A range of conventional mildly T2-weighted spin-echo sequences (TRs of 500 to 1500 ms and TEs of 30 to 80 ms) showed excellent enhancement of liver/tumor CNR at 0.6 Tesla. Gradient echo techniques, irrespective of echo time and flip angle, showed the greatest benefit after iron oxide administration. Gradient echo techniques are well known to be exceptionally sensitive to the presence of local field inhomogeneities such as those produced by the presence of iron particles. Local magnetic field disturbances caused by the particles create both irreversible (T2) and reversible dephasing of transverse coherence. Together, this transverse relaxation enhancement (T2* effect) causes extra signal loss detectable by gradient echo techniques. The added sensitivity of gradient echo methods may be superior to the exploitation of T2 effects with SE imaging. In our initial clinical study (8), we confirmed this effect in humans.

CLINICAL RESULTS

Our group has imaged more than 40 patients with liver tumors at two sites using midfield systems (0.3 and 0.6 Tesla), and detailed analysis of the results of 15 patients has been reported previously (8). Initially, doses of SPIO ranging from 10 to 50 μmol/kg were administered intravenously at a rate of 1 ml (11.2 mg Fe) per minute in a dose-escalation study. Based on analysis of toxicity data, the recommended clinical dose for AMI-25 has been set at 10 to 20 μmol Fe per kilogram of body weight. The ultimate dose of SPIO that will be allowed by the FDA (if approved) has yet to be established. Imaging usually has been performed within 1 hour of injection, although satisfactory clinical imaging results could be achieved easily as late as 48 hours.

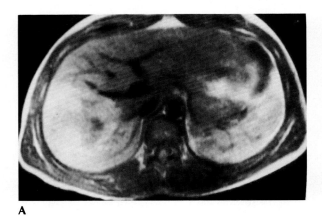
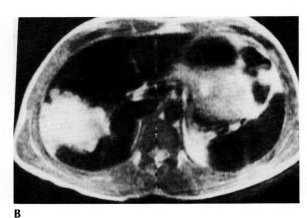

FIGURE 46-6
Metastatic colon cancer. (A) Unenhanced SE 1500/40 image shows a mass displacing vessels in the posterior segment of the right hepatic lobe. Contrast between tumor and liver is low, and the exact margins of the tumor are difficult to delineate. (B) One hour following intravenous administration of superparamagnetic iron oxide (AMI-25, 40 μmol Fe per kilogram). Tumor is now easily detected, sharply delineated, and distinguished from adjacent blackened liver tissue. Note corresponding signal decrement in the spleen. (From Weissleder R, Elizondo G, Stark DD, et al: The diagnosis of splenic lymphoma by MR imaging: Value of superparamagnetic iron oxide. AJR 152:175, 1989. Copyright © by American Roentgen Ray Society. Reprinted by permission.)

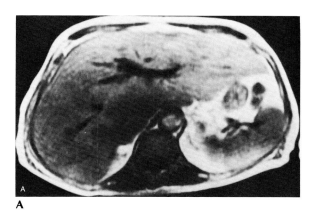
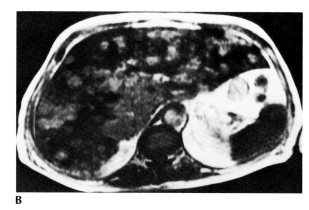

FIGURE 46-7
Improvement in sensitivity for lesion detection. Patient with metastatic renal cell carcinoma. (A) SE 500/28/T1-weighted image before ferrite administration shows normal upper abdominal anatomy. An ill-defined low-intensity region is seen near the caudate lobe of the liver. (B) Image at the same anatomic level with same sequence 15 minutes after administration of AMI-25 (20 μmol/kg). Diffuse hepatic metastases, many smaller than 0.5 cm in diameter, can be identified. The large lesion in the region of the caudate lobe corresponds to the area of abnormal signal on the unenhanced image. Note the reduction in signal of the spleen. (From Stark DD, Weissleder R, Elizondo G, et al: Superparamagnetic iron oxide: Clinical application as a contrast agent for MR imaging of the liver. Radiology 168:297, 1988. Reprinted by permission.)

Profound reduction in both liver and spleen signal intensity was seen in all patients, even as early as 5 minutes after SPIO administration (Fig. 46-6). As expected, cancer tissue was unaffected, and striking improvements in the sensitivity of lesion detection occurred when compared with precontrast images (Fig. 46-7). The beneficial effect on lesion detection occurred with a range of conventional pulse sequences. Overall, there was an increase in the number of lesions detected after contrast material administration from 89 to 349 on SE 500/28 images, from 21 to 325 on SE 1500/40 images, and from 20 to 271 on SE 1500/80 images (out of a total of 370 lesions identified). Quantitative analyses of cancer/liver CNR values confirm the subjective visual appearances, as shown in Table 46-2.

In patients with known hepatic metastases, lesions smaller than 1 cm in diameter were not visible on unenhanced SE TR 500 and 1500 images, while threshold size for lesion detection on unenhanced SE 260/14 images was 0.5 cm using a 0.6-Tesla MRI system. Following contrast material administration, many 0.3 to 1.0-cm lesions could be identified (Fig. 46-8). The size threshold for lesion detectability decreased from 1.5 to 0.3 cm on SE 500/28 images, from 2.1 to 0.3 cm on SE 1500/40 images, and from 1.9 to 0.4 cm on SE 1500/80 images. These results were statistically significant at $p < 0.005$.

In order to provide more objective documentation of the benefits of SPIO for liver cancer detection, quantitative comparisons of diagnostic accuracy were made using receiver operating characteristic (ROC) analysis. Fretz et al. (15) performed a controlled observer performance test of contrast-enhanced CT, unenhanced MRI, and MRI after AMI-25 administration on 731 individual images from our clinical trial material. Contrast-enhanced MRI showed significantly better observer performance scores than bolus contrast-enhanced CT, while enhanced SE 1500/40 and 1500/80 sequences yielded significantly greater areas under the ROC curve than standard MRI sequences. The superiority of SPIO-enhanced MRI over iodine-enhanced CT and unenhanced MRI was statistically significant for both ($p < 0.01$).

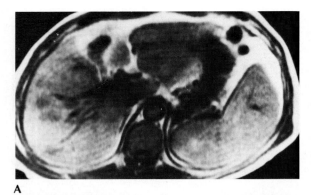

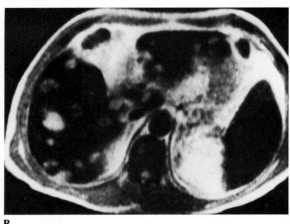

FIGURE 46-8
Demonstration of hepatic and splenic metastases following AMI-25 administration. (A) Precontrast SE 500/28 T1-weighted image. Several 1- to 3-cm metastases are visible in the right hepatic lobe. Questionable area of reduced signal intensity in the medial portion of the spleen was thought to be an artifact. (B) One hour after injection of contrast material with SE 1500/42 sequence containing mild T2 weighting. Multiple additional small hepatic lesions measuring 5 to 10 mm are evident in both the right and left hepatic lobes. In addition, the entire medial portion of the spleen is replaced by a large solitary metastatic deposit. The splenic tumor was confirmed at splenectomy. (From Weissleder R, Hahn PF, Stark DD, et al: Superparamagnetic iron oxide: Enhanced detection of focal splenic tumors with MR imaging. Radiology 169:399, 1988. Reprinted by permission.)

SPLEEN IMAGING ENHANCED BY SPIO

None of the currently available modalities, including CT scanning, is very sensitive to either metastatic disease or lymphomatous involvement of the spleen. Detection of splenic deposits by MRI also has been unreliable because of the similarity of spleen relaxation times (T1 and T2) and proton density to the MRI characteristics of tumor tissue. As a result, there is little net tumor/spleen signal-intensity difference on most pulse sequences. However, as in the case of hepatic metastases, SPIO selectively alters the tissue characteristics (T2) of spleen without affecting tumor, producing a marked increase in image contrast and detectability of splenic tumor deposits.

Early studies by Weissleder et al. (4) from our group showed in animal models that implanted splenic tumors 4 to 6 mm in size become readily visible after SPIO administration (Fig. 46-9). Tumors appear hyperintense against the black background of spleen tissue because, again, the SPIO is not sequestered by tumor tissue. Quantitative measurements of lesion conspicuity assessed by tumor/spleen CNR ratios also showed 40- to 50-fold increases. In a subsequent series of 18 patients, SPIO-enhanced MRI disclosed 45 individual splenic nodules (4 patients were positive) as opposed to 4 lesions (2 patients were positive) on unenhanced images (16) (Table 46-3 and Fig. 46-10). Because the effect of SPIO is less in splenic pulp than in liver, the dose of iron necessary to achieve comparable degrees of spleen blackening may be slightly larger, that is, 20 to 30 μmol Fe per kilogram of body weight.

Of perhaps even greater clinical significance is the ability of SPIO to disclose diffuse lymphomatous involvement of the spleen. In lymphoma patients, splenomegaly per se is an unreliable indicator of active neoplastic infiltrate. Our group developed techniques for SPIO-enhanced MRI to detect both micronodular lymphoma and diffuse lymphoma in animal models (7). Moreover, benign splenomegaly was differentiated by its

TABLE 46-3. *SPIO-Enhanced Detection of Splenic Metastases (N = 18 Patients)*

	US	CT	MRI	SPIO MRI
Patients	2	2	2	4
Tumors	8	21	4	45

Source: From Weissleder R, Hahn PF, Stark DD, et al: Superparamagnetic iron oxide: Enhanced detection of focal splenic tumors with MR imaging. Radiology 169:399, 1988. Reprinted by permission.

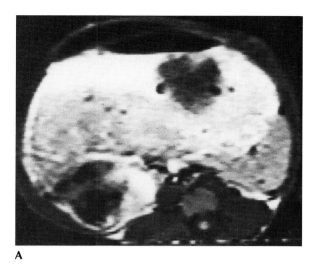
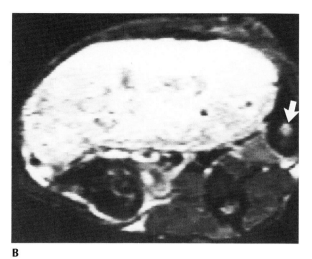

FIGURE 46-9
Demonstration of splenic tumor in animal model following ferrite administration. (A) Pre-SPIO SE 500/32 image showing no abnormality within the spleen. (B) After administration of SPIO, blackening of the spleen parenchyma discloses a tumor nodule due to markedly enhanced tumor/spleen contrast (arrow).

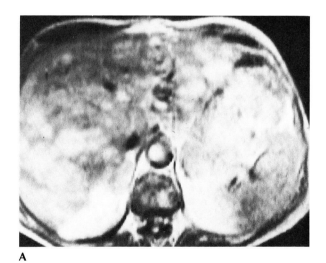
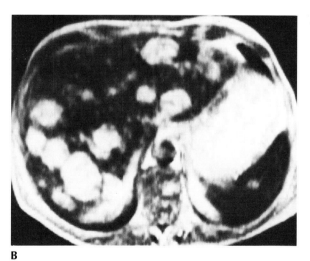

FIGURE 46-10
Enhanced detection of splenic tumor nodules in a patient with widespread hepatic metastases. (A) 1500/40 spin-echo image faintly shows several high-signal-intensity liver metastases. No definite abnormality evident in the spleen. (B) After AMI-25 administration, a single discrete tumor nodule is visible in the spleen. The liver metastases are greatly increased in visibility and in number with numerous small subcentimeter nodules now evident.

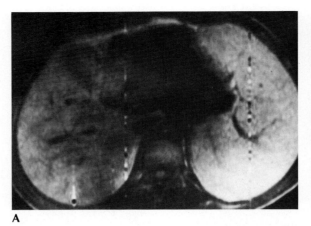 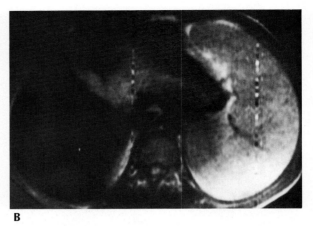

FIGURE 46-11
Malignant splenomegaly due to lymphoma. (A) Prior to AMI-25 administration, there is normal signal intensity in liver and spleen. (B) After contrast, liver blackening proceeds normally, but there is no uptake of administered agent by the spleen and signal intensity does not diminish. The effect is presumed to reflect diffuse neoplastic blockade of splenic RES elements.

preservation of complete blackening after SPIO, whereas spleens with diffuse malignant lymphoma showed no iron uptake. Lymphomatous spleens retained their diffuse bright signal after SPIO presumably owing to blockade of RES phagocytic activity by malignant infiltrate (Fig. 46-11). In patients with normal spleens and those with benign splenomegaly, spleen signal intensity showed the typical marked blackening after ferrite. These findings were confirmed in four patient subjects in a preliminary clinical investigation (17).

The results suggest that both metastatic and lymphomatous neoplasms of the spleen, whether focal or diffuse, may be diagnosed with improved accuracy with SPIO-enhanced MRI.

CIRRHOSIS AND HEPATITIS

Striking morphologic and functional effects were seen after SPIO administration in a small pilot series of seven patients with cirrhosis and active alcoholic hepatitis (18). Cirrhotic liver tissue showed an inhomogeneous decrease in liver signal intensity with a superimposed reticular nodular pattern of thin septa of high signal intensity believed to represent collagenous bands. Splenomegaly with marked signal loss confirmed the well-known redistribution of particulate matter occurring in cirrhotic portal hypertension. Patients with active hepatitis showed a markedly reduced hepatic response to iron oxide with effective preservation of normal signal intensity. This effect was believed to reflect diminished Kupffer cell activity. The results were believed highly promising as a means to further characterize diffuse liver disease.

SPIO MRI INTERPRETATION

As with any fundamentally new imaging modality, SPIO-enhanced MRI raises complex interpretative issues for the radiologist. Since the liver turns dark on all pulse sequences, tumor nodules are always higher in signal intensity than surrounding liver. However, signal in blood vessels viewed in cross section may resemble millimeter size tumors. To overcome this pitfall, Hahn et al. (19) performed imaging during the first 12 minutes after ferrite injection, while the contrast agent remains in circulation (distribution phase). Hahn et al. showed reduction of signal from small intrahepatic blood vessels as the entire liver became uniformly blackened, allowing greater confidence in distinguishing tumor from vessels in cross section. Distribution-phase images showed little or no signal loss from cancer tissue. Vascular

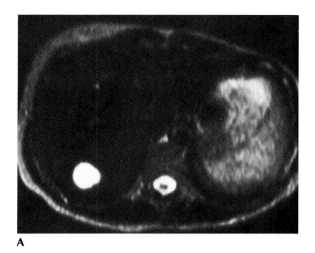 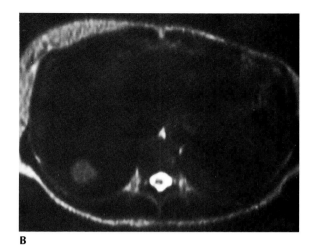

FIGURE 46-12
Cavernous hemangioma showing negative contrast enhancement after AMI-25 administration. The lesion was considered atypical because of poor contrast enhancement on CT. Heavily T2-weighted SE 2350/180 MRI images before (A) and 2 hours after (B) injection of AMI-25 (20 μmol Fe per kilogram). The hemangioma loses signal because of retention of agent in the vascular pool of the lesion. (From Hahn PF, Stark DD, Weissleder R, et al: Clinical application of superparamagnetic iron oxide to MR imaging of tissue perfusion vascular liver tumors. Radiology 174:361, 1990. Reprinted by permission.)

signal was restored on images at 1 to 2 hours (retention phase).

A further major problem in clinical cancer imaging is differentiation of malignant nodules from incidental coexisting benign tumors, especially the common cavernous hemangioma. In the same study described above, Hahn et al. found that hemangiomas showed greater signal loss in retention-phase images (1 to 2 hours after injection) than metastatic lesions (Fig. 46-12). Intralesional signal-intensity loss of 60 percent or more of the precontrast intensity was characteristic of cavernous hemangioma. These findings confirm the slower and prolonged perfusion of cavernous hemangiomas observed by other imaging modalities. Although SPIO perfusion effects promise significant potential to provide tissue characterization, more studies are required for confirmation. Similar strategies are utilized to diagnose hemangiomas by blood pool imaging of iodine (CT), [99mTc]-labeled erythrocytes (nuclear medicine), or Gd-DTPA–enhanced MRI.

In the context of tissue characterization by MRI there are two further caveats. First, it should be pointed out that the use of signal-intensity measurements or calculated T2 relaxation times may give spurious results when lesion/liver ratios are applied to patients with liver T2 shortened by iron (20). Specifically, the presence of exogenously administered iron oxide variably alters both hemangioma and liver signal intensities, eliminating the very long T2 of hemangiomas while varying (unpredictably) their signal-intensity ratio relative to liver.

Second, certain primary liver tumors or tumor-like conditions such as hepatic adenoma and focal nodular hyperplasia may contain Kupffer cells. SPIO may cause such lesions to lose signal, even in the retention phase. This would tend to obscure the lesion, but it might have diagnostic value in suggesting a tissue-specific diagnosis.

CONCLUSIONS

The value of SPIO-enhanced MRI imaging of the liver and spleen has been rapidly accepted by the medical research community. Further clinical experience must be accumulated to validate its clinical role. As a first priority, it will be necessary to establish a clear safety profile for the various formulations under development. New commercial formulations may extend the safety margins. Biodistribution, clearance, and protocols for clinical administration may or may not be altered for various SPIOs.

Future research directions will involve the use of SPIO for splenic neoplasia, especially lymphomas, and diffuse liver diseases, as well as bone marrow and lymph node imaging and perfusion studies. Cardiac studies offer an especially interesting possibility when combined with high-speed gradient echo or echo-planar imaging techniques. The ability of these methods to permit further reduction of the SPIO dose will certainly be studied extensively in near-term clinical trials. Finally, in the liver, where the first clinical applications are likely, more detailed definition of cellular function and temporal profiles of SPIO retention within benign and malignant liver tumors will be necessary to refine diagnostic criteria for clinical use. The agent appears to have a promising future in clinical MRI.

REFERENCES

1. Saini S, Stark DD, Hahn PF, et al: Ferrite particles: A superparamagnetic MR contrast agent for the reticuloendothelial system. Radiology 162:211, 1987
2. Saini S, Stark DD, Hahn PF, et al: Ferrite particles: A superparamagnetic MR contrast agent for enhanced detection of liver carcinoma. Radiology 162:217, 1987.
3. Bacon BR, Stark DD, Park CH, et al: Ferrite particles: A new magnetic resonance imaging contrast agent. Lack of acute or chronic hepatotoxicity after intravenous administration. J Lab Clin Med 110(2):164, 1987.
4. Weissleder R, Hahn PF, Stark DD, et al: MR imaging of splenic metastases: Ferrite-enhanced detection in rats. AJR 149:723, 1987.
5. Tsang YM, Stark DD, Chen MCM, et al: Hepatic micrometastases in the rat: Ferrite-enhanced MR imaging. Radiology 167:21, 1988.
6. Weissleder R, Stark DD, Engelstad BL, et al: Superparamagnetic iron oxide: Pharmacokinetics and toxicity. AJR 152:167, 1989.
7. Weissleder R, Stark DD, Rummeny EJ, et al: Splenic lymphoma: Ferrite-enhanced MR imaging in rats. Radiology 166:423, 1988.
8. Stark DD, Weissleder R, Elizondo G, et al: Superparamagnetic iron oxide: Clinical application as a contrast agent for MR imaging of the liver. Radiology 168:297, 1988.
9. Marchal G, Van Hecke P, Demaerel P, et al: Detection of liver metastases with superparamagnetic iron oxide in 15 patients: Results of MR imaging at 1.5 T. AJR 152:771, 1989.
10. Blakemore RP, Frankel R: Magnetic navigation in bacteria. Sci Am 246:58, 1981.
11. Bean CP: Hysteresis loops of mixtures of ferromagnetic micropowders. J Appl Physiol 26:1381, 1955.
12. Patrizio G, Elizondo G, Fretz C, et al: Cancer targeted liposomes containing superparamagnetic iron oxide: Ferrosomes, in Abstracts of the Society Magnetic Resonance in Medicine Eighth Annual Meeting, 1989, p. 327.
13. Kawamura Y, Endo Y, Watanabe Y, et al: Use of magnetite particles as a contrast agent for MR imaging of the liver. Radiology 174:357, 1990.
14. Fretz CJ, Elizondo G, Weissleder R, et al: Superparamagnetic iron oxide–enhanced MR imaging: Pulse sequence optimization for detection of liver cancer. Radiology 172:393, 1989.
15. Fretz CJ, Stark DD, Ferrucci JT, et al: ROC analysis of scan oxide enhanced MRI, scan contrast MRI and contrast enhanced CT for the detection of focal hepatic lesions. (in press).
16. Weissleder R, Hahn PF, Stark DD, et al: Superparamagnetic iron oxide: Enhanced detection of focal splenic tumors with MR imaging. Radiology 169:399, 1988.
17. Weissleder R, Elizondo G, Stark DD, et al: The diagnosis of splenic lymphoma by MR imaging: Value of superparamagnetic iron oxide. AJR 152:175, 1989.
18. Elizondo G, Weissleder R, Stark DD, et al: Hepatic cirrhosis and hepatitis: MR imaging enhanced with superparamagnetic iron oxide. Radiology 174:797, 1990.
19. Hahn PF, Stark DD, Weissleder R, et al: Clinical application of superparamagnetic iron oxide to MR imaging of tissue perfusion vascular liver tumors. Radiology 174:361, 1990.
20. Mirowitz S, Heiken JP, Lee JKT: Potential MR pitfall in relying on lesion/liver ratio in presence of hepatic hemochromatosis. J Comput Assist Tomogr 12:323, 1988.

47

Iron Oxide: High-Field MRI Clinical Results

G. MARCHAL, P. VAN HECKE, P. DEMAEREL,
E. DECROP, and A. L. BAERT

The ideal modality for the diagnostic workup of focal liver lesions should combine the following characteristics: optimal lesion detection and reliable characterization. In MRI, the strategy to reach both goals depends on the field strength. In low- and middle-field-strength systems, T1-weighted images provide the best detection rate, whereas T2 images are needed for tissue characterization. However, in high-field-strength systems, both optimal detection and tissue characterization are obtained with the same T2-weighted sequence. (1)

The purpose of the additional use of contrast medium is to improve either the detection or the tissue characterization or both. Different classes of contrast agents have been explored. The nonspecific agents (e.g., the water-soluble gadolinium derivatives) exploit the temporal differences in contrast material uptake by lesion and liver, an approach similar to dynamic CT (2–5). Organ-specific contrast agents (ferrites, labeled liposomes) are particulate substances that are actively cleared from the blood by the Kupffer cells of the liver. Therefore, they label the nondiseased liver parenchyma (6–9). Pathology-specific contrast agents are exemplified by labeled monoclonal antibodies. These should selectively attach to the pathologic cells.

When the efficacy of a new contrast agent is to be evaluated, its effect on both detection and tissue characterization has to be assessed. Any drug used as contrast agent should definitely improve at least one of these aspects. Possible advantages, but also drawbacks have to be established.

This chapter is a preliminary evaluation of the effects of crystalline iron oxide as contrast agent for MRI of the liver at 1.5 Tesla.

PHARMACOLOGY OF FERRITES

Crystalline superparamagnetic iron oxide (AMI-25, Guerbet) is an organ-specific contrast agent. Particles of an appropriate size (0.035 to 1 μm) can be injected intravenously as a suspension. These particles are rapidly cleared from the blood, about 80 percent by the Kupffer cells of the liver, and the rest by the spleen and the bone marrow (10,11). When the function of the reticuloendothelial system (RES) is normal, the blood half-life is about 30 min (12). Liver tumors, which do not possess RES cells, do not take up the contrast agent and, therefore, can be differentiated from normal liver parenchyma on postcontrast scans. Because of the high sensitivity of MRI to the effect of ferrites, they can be used at a dose as low as 1 mg iron per kilogram of body weight (10,12). To avoid side effects, it is recommended that the drug be injected slowly at a rate of 1 ml/min. Once in the

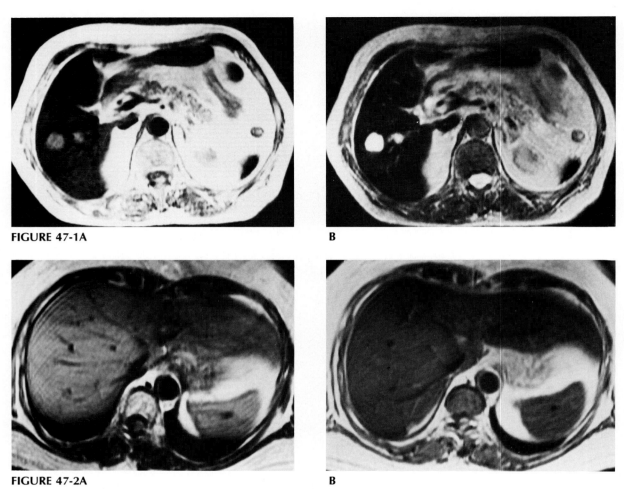

FIGURE 47-1
Metastases of unknown origin in a patient with hemochromatosis. (A) Intermediate SE sequence (TR/TE: 820/30 ms). (B) Strongly T2-weighted SE sequence (TR/TE = 2200/70 ms). Typical appearance of hemochromatosis with decrease of signal intensity of liver and spleen on both sequences. The obtained liver/lesion contrast is similar to that of iron oxide–enhanced images.

FIGURE 47-2
Low iron oxide uptake 3 weeks after chemotherapy. (A, B) Plain and iron oxide–enhanced proton density images (TR/TE = 2200/22 ms). In comparison with Fig. 47-7, there is only a minimal contrast enhancement.

Kupffer cells, the ferrites remain clinically active for several hours and are then progressively metabolized and incorporated in the normal body iron store (10–12).

Superparamagnetic particles cause local field inhomogeneities in their immediate vicinity. Diffusion of tissue water through these magnetic gradients produces spin dephasing of the transverse magnetization. The resultant shortening of T2 causes a blackening of the normal parenchyma, similar to the effect of liver iron in patients with hemochromatosis (13) (Fig. 47-1).

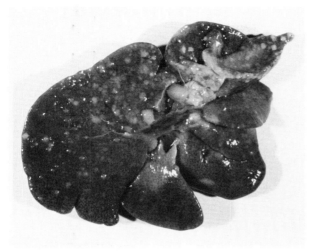
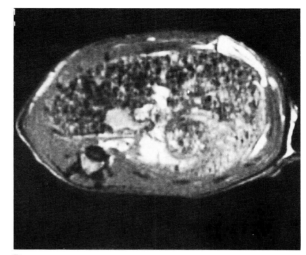

FIGURE 47-3A B

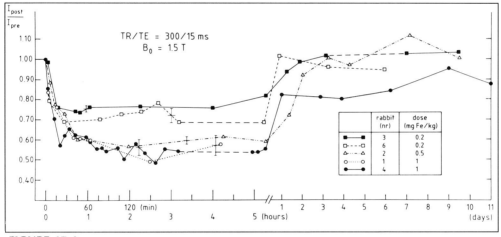

FIGURE 47-4

FIGURE 47-3
Nitrosodimethylamine-induced tumor in rat liver. (A) Macroscopic appearance of the liver containing multiple small focal lesions. (B) Iron oxide–enhanced image (TR/TE = 600/22 ms). The diffuse involvement by millimeter-sized lesions is obvious.

FIGURE 47-4
Rabbit liver signal intensity (normalized to the intensity before injection) as a function of time after intravenous injection of ferrite.

IMAGING PARAMETERS AND TIMING AT 1.5 TESLA

Before being effective as a specific contrast agent, iron oxide has to accumulate in the liver RES (14) (Figs. 47-2 and 47-3). When RES activity is normal, the effect is maximum ½ h after an intravenous injection (10,12) (Fig. 47-4). According to the transfer modulation curve, lesion detection not only depends on size, but also on lesion-to-liver contrast.

To optimize lesion detection after contrast enhancement with iron oxide, therefore, the image-acquisition parameters should be chosen to:

1. Further improve lesion-to-liver contrast by enhancing the T2 effect by the use of T2-weighted or gradient-echo sequences and by reducing, if possible, volume-averaging effects by breath-hold imaging.
2. Preserve the maximal image resolution achievable within the chosen acquisition time.

For fast breath-hold imaging, different types of sequences are available. Rapid-acquisition spin-echo (RASE) imaging produces breath-hold strongly T1-weighted images, with focal lesions appearing dark on unenhanced images (15). Unenhanced FLASH or FISP gradient-echo sequences suffer from poor inherent contrast (3) (focal lesions appearing isointense on unenhanced images) but are very sensitive to the T2 effect induced by the ferrite. The combination of both effects results in an excellent lesion-to-liver contrast (Fig. 47-5). The liver intensity is reduced to the noise level, whereas the relatively high signal of the lesions remains unaffected. In addition, breath-hold images with full resolution can be acquired within less than 10 s. Gradient-echo imaging should necessarily be combined with spatial presaturation pulses to avoid misinterpretation of high signal from intrahepatic vessels as focal lesions. Despite saturation pulses, remaining signal from vessels, periportal fatty tissue, or dilated bile ducts can still interfere with interpretation.

DETECTION OF LIVER METASTASES WITH SUPERPARAMAGNETIC IRON OXIDE IN 15 PATIENTS: RESULTS OF MRI AT 1.5 TESLA WITH SE SEQUENCES

The first clinical results on the use of superparamagnetic ferrite particles as a tissue-specific contrast agent for MRI of the liver at high fields (1.5 Tesla) were reported by our group in 1989 (9). Fifteen patients with proven secondary liver malignancies were studied with plain and contrast-enhanced MRI. Superparamagnetic iron oxide was administrated IV in a dose of 20 µmol/kg. Intermediate TR (TR/TE = 820/30, 60 ms) and long TR (TR/TE = 2200/22, 70 ms) spin-echo sequences were used before and 1 h after injection of contrast material. Before injection, the largest number of lesions (437) was detected with the T2-weighted sequence. Lesion-to-liver contrast, expressed as the difference between the tumor and the liver signal-to-noise, improved after ferrite administration in both sequences from −1 to 20 and from 7 to 15 for the 820/30, 60 sequence and from 9 to 34 and 15 to 21 for the 2200/22, 70 sequence (Table 47-1). Despite this significant improvement in terms of lesion-to-line contrast, ferrite-enhanced images did not show significantly more metastases than the unenhanced T2-weighted images (383, 421, 407, and 407 versus as many as 437, respectively) (Table 47-2).

TABLE 47-1. *Effect of Ferrite Enhancement on Signal-to-Noise (SNR) and Contrast-to-Noise (CNR) Ratios in 13 Patients*

Spin-Echo Pulse Sequence (TR/TE)	Mean Ratio ± SD		
	Tumor SNR	Liver SNR	Tumor/Liver CNR
820/30:			
Precontrast	28 ± 7	28 ± 8	−1 ± 5
Postcontrast	29 ± 12	8 ± 4	20 ± 10
820/60:			
Precontrast	20 ± 6	13 ± 6	7 ± 6
Postcontrast	19 ± 2	3 ± 2	15 ± 6
2200/22:			
Precontrast	49 ± 20	40 ± 12	9 ± 9
Postcontrast	46 ± 21	12 ± 6	34 ± 17
2200/70:			
Precontrast	30 ± 11	14 ± 6	15 ± 7
Postcontrast	27 ± 12	6 ± 9	22 ± 11

Note: Postcontrast images were obtained 1 h after administration of ferrite.

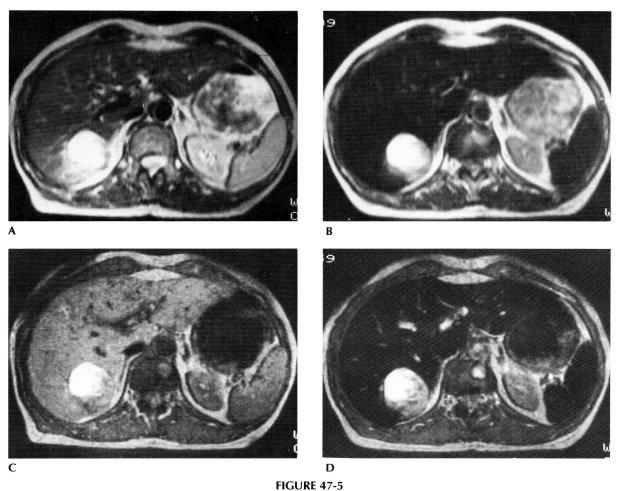

FIGURE 47-5

Focal mass with central bleeding. (A) Intermediate SE sequence (TR/TE = 820/60 ms, 128/256 matrix, 4 acquisitions). Spontaneously hyperintense lesion at the posterior aspect of the right liver lobe. (B) Identical sequence parameters. Examination 1 h after iron oxide administration. Notice the improved liver/lesion contrast-to-noise ratio. Limited spatial resolution due to rectangular matrix used and long imaging time (± 5 min). (C) Breath-hold FLASH image (TR/TE = 50/18 ms, flip angle 35 degrees, 1 acquisition, 256/256 matrix, axial saturation pulses cranial and caudal of the imaged volume). The solid parts of the tumor are hard to distinguish from the adjacent normal parenchyma. The bleeding appears hyperintense. (D) Identical sequence parameters. Examination ± 1 h after iron oxide injection. Dramatic improvement of image detail in comparison with image in Fig. 47-1B. Despite the applied saturation pulses, the portal veins still generate intraheptic signal.

DISCUSSION

The efficiency of liver MRI in detecting liver tumors largely depends on the sequence used. In general, both T1 and T2 are increased in tumor tissue. Therefore, liver tumors are generally shown as hypointense areas on T1-weighted images and as hyperintense areas on T2-weighted images. Although, theoretically, T2-weighted images yield the highest diagnostic sensitivity, such sequences suffer from drawbacks, including long acquisition times, low SNRs, and high susceptibility to motion artifacts. Some of these problems

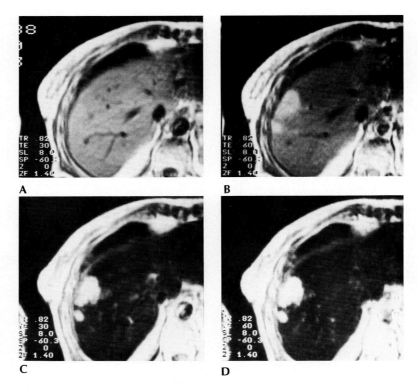

FIGURE 47-6
Metastases from breast carcinoma. (A,B) Intermediate sequence (TR/TE = 2200/22/70). (C,D) Long TR sequence (TR/TE = 2200/30/60). (E to H) Intermediate and long TR sequences after iron oxide enhancement. Despite the improved liver/lesion contrast-to-noise ratio, the enhanced images do not show more lesions than the strongly T2-weighted SE image (part D).

TABLE 47-2. *Effect of Ferrite Enhancement on the Detection of Lesions in 13 Patients*

Spin-Echo Pulse Sequence TR/TE	No. of Lesions	
	Unenhanced Image	Enhanced Image
830/30	114	383
820/60	280	421
2200/22	221	407
2200/70	437	407

Note: Enhanced images were obtained 1 h after administration of ferrite. Scan times: 820/30, 60, 7 min; 2200/22, 70, 19 min.

can be avoided by the combination of a reduced image resolution (128/256), signal averaging (four acquisitions), and gradient nulling sequences for motion-artifact reduction. However, these techniques also affect lesion-to-liver contrast by the decreased image resolution and volume averaging due to respiration.

In this study we analyzed how ferrite either improved the diagnostic content of the MRI scan or reduced the examination time. By using a contrast-enhanced intermediate TR/long TE sequence (820/30, 60), similar lesion-to-liver contrast ratios were achieved in a much shorter acquisition time than with an unenhanced (heavily T2-weighted) long TR/long TE sequence (2200/70) (Table 47-2 and Fig. 47-6).

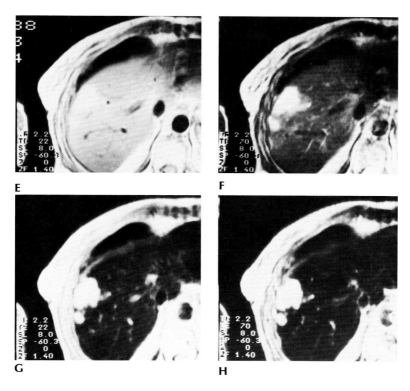

FIGURE 47-6 *(continued)*

Although counting the number of lesions detected provides only a very crude estimation of diagnostic efficacy and is compounded by a number of methodologic difficulties, the trends in these figures allow us to draw some conclusions. The number of lesions detected by the intermediate TR sequences (820/30, 60) after contrast material administration was almost as high as the number detected before contrast administration with the 2200/70 sequence (383 and 421 versus 437). The use of contrast material in the sequence with a longer TR (2200/22, 70) did not further improve the number of tumors detected (407 and 407 versus 437) (see Table 47-2). The latter finding is in agreement with the observation that for only 1 of 13 patients, more lesions were detected with the T2-weighted sequence (2200/70) after ferrite administration.

It also should be noted that the 2200/22 sequence, which showed the highest tumor to liver contrast after ferrite injection, did not provide better tumor detection than the other contrast-enhanced sequences (see Table 47-2). In one patient, the use of ferrite obscured one of the signs of the metastases, making the diagnosis somewhat more difficult (Fig. 47-7).

Our observations on the effects of ferrite for liver tumor detection at high field strength clearly differ from those of Stark et al. (7) for low and intermediate field strengths (0.3 and 0.6 Tesla). The dramatic improvement (four- to sixteen-fold) in tumor detection numbers obtained by Stark et al. with ferrite for both T1 (500/28) and T2 (1500/40, 80) sequences was not observed in our high-field-strength system. Compared with our standard T2 sequence (2200/70) for clinical evaluation of liver lesions, none of the SE sequences used with the ferrite contrast agent susbstantially improved detection. On the other hand, the same sensitivity was obtained with the contrast-enhanced intermediate

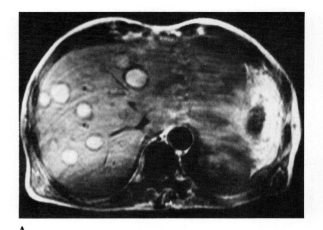

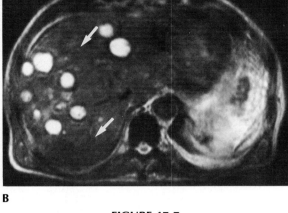

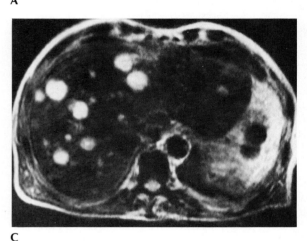

FIGURE 47-7
Metastases of unknown origin. (A) Proton density image (TR/TE = 2200/22 ms). Rather high-intensity lesions limited by a hypointense halo. (B) T2-weighted SE image (TR/TE = 2200/70 ms). Improved liver-to-tumor contrast. Additional small lesions (arrows) also bordered by a hypointense halo are visualized. (C) Iron oxide–enhanced image (TR/TE = 2200/70 ms). Because of the blackening of the adjacent normal liver parenchyma by the iron oxide, the halo sign, well seen on the unenhanced images, is lost.

TR sequence (820/30, 60). The high performance of our standard T2 sequence (2200/70) is due to the improved SNR at high field strengths and the use of gradient nulling motion compensation. This is reflected in the much larger tumor-to-liver CNR at high field strengths (15 ± 7) compared with the value (3.4 ± 3.8) obtained at lower field strengths by Stark et al. As a result, we obtained the highest tumor detection before contrast material administration with T2-weighted sequences, while Stark et al. reported a progressive decrease in detection with progressive T2 weighting.

In the present study only the influence of the ferrite on lesion-to-liver contrast could be evaluated, since for both pre- and postcontrast studies the same SE sequences were used. However, one can easily foresee that with the use of breath-hold images at full matrix resolution, the detection rate for small lesions will improve. Here again, the results will probably differ according to the imaging strategy used, consecutive single slices or multislice volume scanning.

Besides the effect on detection, the effect on tissue characterization is the second aspect to be evaluated. As long as tissue differentiation remains based on their T1 and T2 values, good T2-weighted sequences remain mandatory. This information is not available when postferrite images are acquired with intermediate SE or T1-weighted fast-imaging sequences (Fig. 47-8).

The potential of ferrite as a perfusion agent or as a tissue-specific contrast agent has still to be established. Some promising results in this area have been reported. Hahn et al. (16) report a decreased signal in hemangiomas during the early vascular phase after injection.

Tolerance for ferrite was excellent in this study, since no side effects were detected. However, it has to be emphasized that the drug was given by a slow IV injection and that patients with allergic predispositions were excluded from the study.

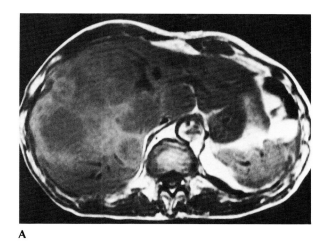 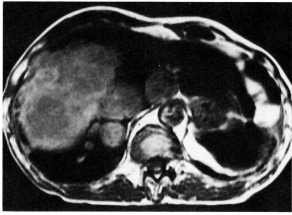 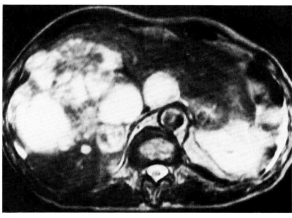

FIGURE 47-8
Metastases of breast carcinoma. (A,B) Intermediate sequence (TR/TE = 820/30 ms) before and after iron oxide enhancement. (C) Heavily T2-weighted SE sequence (TR/TE = 2200/70 ms). Improved detection of focal masses on postcontrast image (B). However, tissue characterization is poor compared with the standard unenhanced T2-weighted sequence (C).

CONCLUSIONS

At 1.5 Tesla, ferrite can effectively be used to improve lesion-to-liver contrast. Optimal lesion detection should be obtained with high-resolution breath-hold images.

REFERENCES

1. Reinig JW, Dwyer AJ, Miller DL, et al: Liver metastases: Detection with MR imaging at 0.5 and 1.5 T. Radiology 170:149, 1989.
2. Yoshida H, Itai Y, Ohtomo K, et al: Small hepatocellular carcinoma and cavernous hemangioma: Differentiation with dynamic FLASH MR imaging with Gd-DTPA. Radiology 171:339, 1989.
3. Marchal G, Demaerel PH, Decrop E, et al: Gadolinium-DOTA enhanced fast imaging of liver tumors at 1.5 T. J Comput Assist Tomogr 14:217, 1990.
4. Van Beers B, Demeure R, Pringot J, et al: Dynamic spin-echo imaging with Gd-DTPA: Value in the differentiation of hepatic tumors. AJR 154:515, 1990.
5. Edelman RR, Siegel JB, Singer A, et al: Dynamic MR imaging of the liver with Gd-DTPA: Initial clinical results. AJR 153:1213, 1989.
6. Unger EC, Winokur T, MacDougall P, et al: Hepatic metastases: Liposomal Gd-DTPA–enhanced MR imaging. Radiology 171:81, 1989.
7. Stark DD, Weissleder R, Elizondo G, et al: Superparamagnetic iron oxide: Clinical application as a contrast agent for MR imaging of the liver. Radiology 168:297, 1988.
8. Kawamura Y, Endo K, Watanabe Y, et al: Use of magnetic particles as a contrast agent for MR imaging of the liver. Radiology 174:357, 1990.
9. Marchal G, Van Hecke P, Demaerel P, et al: Detection of liver metastases with superparamagnetic iron oxide in 15 patients: Results of MR imaging at 1.5 T. AJR 152:771, 1989.
10. Saini S, Stark DD, Hahn PF, et al: Ferrite particles: A superparamagnetic MR contrast agent for the reticuloendothelial system. Radiology 162:211, 1987.

11. Mendonca-Dias MH, Lauterbur PD: Ferromagnetic particles as contrast agents for magnetic resonance imaging of the liver and spleen. Magn Reson Med 3:328, 1986.
12. Van Hecke P, Marchal G, Decrop E, and Baert AL: Experimental study of the pharmacokinetics and dose response of ferrite particles used as a contrast agent in MRI of the normal liver of the rabbit. Invest Radiol 24:397, 1989.
13. Stark DD, Moseley ME, Bacon BR, et al: Magnetic resonance imaging and spectroscopy of hepatic iron overload. Radiology 154:137, 1985.
14. Elizondo G, Weissleder R, Stark DD, et al: Hepatic cirrhosis and hepatitis: MR imaging enhanced with superparamagnetic iron oxide. Radiology 174:797, 1990.
15. Mirowitz SA, Lee JKT, Brown JJ, et al: Rapid acquisition spin-echo (RASE) MR imaging: A new technique for reduction of artifacts and acquisition time. Radiology 175:131, 1990.
16. Hahn PF, Stark DD, Weissleder R, et al: Clinical application of superparamagnetic iron oxide to MR imaging of tissue perfusion in vascular liver tumors. Radiology 174:361, 1990.

48

Superparamagnetic Starch Microspheres: A Reticuloendothelial MRI Contrast Agent

ANNE K. FAHLVIK,
ECKART HOLTZ, and
JO KLAVENESS

There has for many years been a great interest in development of safe and efficient contrast agents for clinical imaging of the liver. Various approaches such as particulate carriers, passive targeting to hepatocytes using lipophilic water-soluble compounds, and finally, receptor-mediated targeting of contrast agents to liver tissue have been evaluated.

In radioisotope imaging, lipophilic technetium chelates such as ^{99m}Tc-HIDA derivatives are widely used in clinical practice for evaluation of the hepatobiliary pathway (1), and various technetium-labeled particles are used in scintigraphic examinations of liver and other organ systems (2). Technetium-labeled radiopharmaceuticals can also be actively targeted to hepatocytes using galactose conjugates (3).

In the x-ray field, both lipophilic water-soluble iodinated compounds (4) and various approaches for particulate carriers such as iodinated fat emulsions, liposome-encapsulated agents, and iodinated solid particles have been suggested and evaluated for liver diagnosis (5). However, to date no efficient liver-specific x-ray contrast agent for parenchymal enhancement is in clinical use.

With MRI's large potential in liver diagnosis, there has been great interest in development of liver-specific MRI contrast agents (6). Both paramagnetic hepatobiliary agents (7) and particulate carriers of paramagnetic and superparamagnetic compounds (8) have been evaluated in liver MRI. Recently, receptor-mediated MRI contrast agents for selective uptake in hepatocytes also have been suggested (9). Superparamagnetic particles seem to have a greater potential than paramagnetic particles for liver imaging based on the high efficacy and low toxicity of this material.

Stark and coworkers (10) have evaluated the potential of a superparamagnetic liver MRI contrast agent (Feridex) in many animal models as well as in humans. Further clinical trials with the dextran-based superparamagnetic particles have to some extent been delayed due to hemodynamic effects (11). However, superparamagnetics probably have a great potential in liver imaging, and different superparamagnetic agents are at the moment under preclinical development. Here we summarize initial preclinical studies with 0.4-μm superparamagnetic microspheres based on a starch matrix.

MATERIALS AND METHODS

Magnetic starch microspheres (MSM) were produced by controlled precipitation of iron oxide in an aqueous solution of starch and then suspended in saline solution (12). The diameter of MSM was in the range of 0.1 to 0.5 μm, mean 0.4 μm. Approximately 40 percent (w/w) of the microsphere weight represented magnetically active iron oxide.

Male Wistar rats and female BALB/c and NMRI mice were used. The MSM suspension was injected into the tail vein.

The in vitro relaxation analysis was performed at 37°C and 0.24 Tesla on a Radx tabletop spectrometer (Radx, Texas), and imaging experiments were performed in a 2.4-Tesla Medspec 24/30 system (Bruker, Germany).

Radioactivity measurements of various tissues were done on a gamma counter (Clini Gamma, Finland). Light and electron microscopic evaluations of liver and spleen after MSM administration and of cultured macrophages exposed to MSM in vitro were performed.

The cellular toxicity of MSM was determined after incubation of the microspheres with cultured murine macrophages (J774 cells) by a modified MTT cytotoxicity assay (13).

RESULTS AND DISCUSSION

Iron oxides are known to be high-potent relaxation enhancers both in vitro and in vivo (14–16). The in vitro relaxivity values of MSM in different media are given in Table 48-1. The relaxivity of MSM seems to be relatively independent of the nature of the suspension media, although, when MSM was added to homogenized liver in vitro, the efficacy was reduced compared with the effect in the other test media.

TABLE 48-1. Relaxivity Values of MSM in Various Media at 0.24 Tesla and 37°C

Medium	r_1*	r_2†	r_2/r_1
Agar gel	51	226	4.4
Distilled water	41	208	5.1
Serum	30	204	6.8
Blood	32	261	8.2
Liver homogenate	13	114	8.8

*r_1 = T1 relaxivity, s^{-1} $mmol^{-1}$ Fe L.
†r_2 = T2 relaxivity, s^{-1} $mmol^{-1}$ Fe L.

This observation is in accordance with what has been observed when the liver was homogenized after intravenous injection of MSM to mice (17). After administration of MSM, the intrinsic liver relaxation effect of MSM was high, but further increased in response to the homogenization process. In the in vivo experiment, the efficacy seemed to be limited by compartmentalization of MSM, while intracellular entrapped water could probably explain the lower effect of MSM added to a liver homogenate in vitro. However, both the T1 and the T2 in vitro relaxivity were high, and the ratios of T2 relaxivity to T1 relaxivity (r_2/r_1) were within the typical range of superparamagnetic materials (15).

The in vivo efficacy of MSM per injected dose was quantitated by in vitro relaxation analysis and MRI (12). The liver ED_{50} doses, i.e., doses causing a T2 reduction to 50 percent of the control T2 and a signal intensity reduction to 50 percent of control signal intensity, were calculated to be approximately 1 mg Fe per kilogram from the relaxation analysis and to about 0.3 mg Fe per kilogram from imaging analysis. Liver T2 was dose-dependently decreased, while T1 remained unchanged as the dose increased (Fig. 48-1).

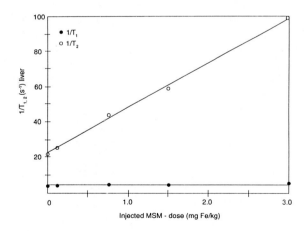

FIGURE 48-1

Relaxation rates of liver tissue with increasing doses of MSM after intravenous injection to mice (0.24 Tesla, 37°C). Mean values of 5 to 8 mice are plotted. (From Fahlvik AK, Holtz E, Leander P, et al: Magnetic starch microspheres: Efficacy and elimination. Invest Radiol 25:113, 1990. Reprinted by permission.)

In the imaging experiment, the signal intensity was decreased until tissue intensity reached the background noise level, and no further effect was obtained in the liver with MSM doses above 1.5 mg Fe per kilogram (Fig. 48-2). In the spleen, both T1 and T2 were shortened in a dose-dependent manner. MSM seemed to be slightly more efficient in the spleen compared with the liver, owing to a lower ED_{50} dose in splenic tissue (17).

The acute, approximated LD_{50} after an intravenous bolus injection of MSM to mice was in the range of 150 to 200 mg Fe per kilogram (12). The safety index (LD_{50}/ED_{50}) of MSM in rodents was consequently above 100.

The biodistribution and biotransformation of MSM were studied in rats using MSM containing radiolabeled iron oxide (18). Initially, a selective uptake of MSM in the major reticuloendothelial organs was observed. The liver accumulated 85 ± 5 percent of the dose, while 7 ± 1 percent of the dose was located in the spleen 1h after injection.

With increases in time, the radioiron content in liver and spleen decreased in parallel with an increase of radioiron in the blood. One week after injection of radiolabeled MSM, 28 ± 4 percent and 4 ± 1 percent of the dose were detected in the liver and the spleen, respectively. Fifty ± 5 percent of the dose was located in the blood compartment, and all radioactivity was associated with the red blood cells. Neither renal nor fecal excretion of MSM or radiolabeled degradation products was detected in this period. The radioiron content of red blood cells increased until 6 weeks after injection and then reached a maximum level of 72 ± 7 percent of the dose.

The initially strong T2 effect of MSM was gradually reduced in the liver and spleen (Fig. 48-3). Within 2 to 5 days after injection, the contrast effect of MSM was halved, and the result matched the half-life of radioiron in liver, which was calculated to be of 4 to 5 days. No T2 change of whole blood was observed during the test period.

According to these results, the superparamagnetic iron oxide in MSM was metabolized to nonmagnetic metabolites that were redistributed from the target organs to the blood compartment.

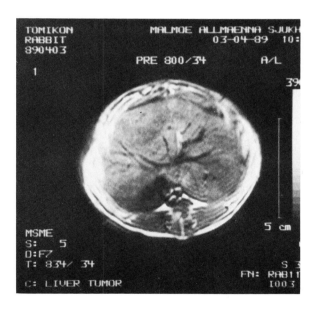
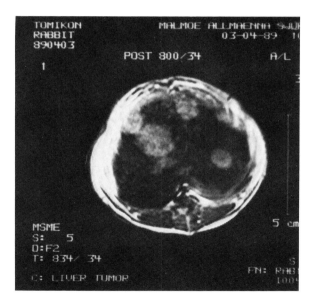

FIGURE 48-2

Images before and after intravenous injection of MSM (0.75 mg Fe/kg) to a rabbit with implanted VX2 adenocarcinoma (2.4 Tesla, TR = 800 ms, TE = 34 ms). In tumor tissue, the number and activity of macrophages are reduced and MSM is excluded from these regions. Data from Leander and Golman, Amsterdam, Society of Magnetic Resonance in Medicine 1989; 1156, abstract.

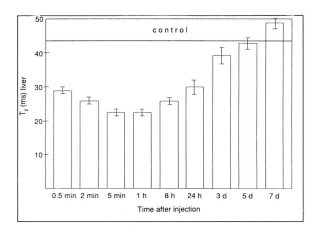

FIGURE 48-3
T2 relaxation time of mouse liver tissue at increasing time after intravenous injection of MSM (0.75 mg Fe/kg) (0.24 Tesla, 37°C). Mean values ± SD of 3 to 5 mice are plotted. (From Fahlvik AK, Holtz E, Leander P, et al: Magnetic starch microspheres: Efficacy and elimination. Invest Radiol 25:113, 1990. Reprinted by permission.)

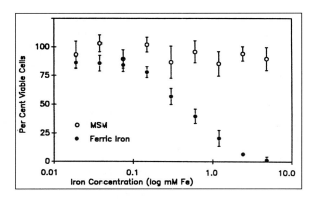

FIGURE 48-4
Macrophage toxicity of MSM and ionic iron. The cells were incubated with the test substances for 24 h, rinsed, and further cultivated for 72 h before measurement of macrophage viability. Mean values ± SD of 6 to 8 experiments are plotted. (From Fahlvik AK, Artursson P, Edman P: Magnetic starch microspheres: Interactions of a microsphere MR contrast medium with macrophages in vitro. Int J Pharmaceutics (in press). Reprinted by permission.)

The reticuloendothelial organs are important participants in the internal iron exchange and are involved in both circulation and storage of iron. Most likely, the iron oxide of MSM was solubilized, and mobilized iron entered the normal body iron pathway and was incorporated into circulating red blood cells. A similar iron-distribution profile also was observed after administration of other superparamagnetic particles (19).

After intravenous injection of MSM, microscopic examinations showed that MSM was selectively phagocytozed by macrophages in liver and spleen and subcellularly accumulated in lysosomal organelles. The iron oxide component of MSM was eliminated from the lysosomes within 3 to 7 days after injection without any morphological alterations of macrophages or other cells of the affected organs.

To study the interactions of MSM with hepatic and splenic target cells, macrophages were incubated with MSM in culture (20). No in vitro cytotoxicity of MSM, or of pure iron oxide crystals and starch as components of MSM, was detected after cellular uptake of amounts more than 80 times the ED_{50} doses for up to 4 days of incubation. However, an iron salt administered directly to the macrophages showed high cellular toxicity (Fig. 48-4). The iron oxide of MSM is rather slowly solubilized and intracellularly presented as a sustained-release preparation of ionic iron. The concentration of ionic iron is then kept below the toxic level, and the cellular mechanisms of iron handling have sufficient capacity to eliminate ionic iron as metabolite of MSM.

SUMMARY

Magnetic starch microspheres (MSM) proved to be a potent relaxation agent in vitro, as well as an efficient and safe contrast enhancer of liver and spleen in various experimental studies. Compared with most contrast media, MSM has an unusual pharmacokinetic profile. MSM has an organ-specific distribution and is highly selectively accumulated in the macrophage cells of the liver and spleen. The magnetically active iron oxide crystals of MSM are solubilized within the macrophage lysosomes, and the dissolved iron is directly incorporated into the normal body metabolism. The time-dependent biodegradation of MSM is demonstrated by relaxation analysis, MRI, histologic techniques, and pharmacokinetic

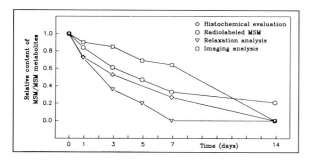

FIGURE 48-5
Relative content of MSM and iron metabolites, quantitated by different methods, in rodent liver at increase of time after intravenous injection of MSM (1 mg Fe/kg).

investigations using radiolabeled substance (Fig. 48-5). High doses of MSM, components, and metabolites of MSM are nontoxic to macrophages in vitro in the applied cytotoxicity assay.

REFERENCES

1. Freeman LM, Lan JA: Radiopharmaceutical evaluation of the hepatobiliary pathway. Nucl Med Biol 17:129, 1990.
2. Billinghurst MV: Radiopharmaceuticals for imaging the reticuloendothelial system, in Fritzberg AR (ed): Radiopharmaceuticals: Progress and Clinical Perspectives. Boca Raton, Fla., CRC Press, 1986.
3. Kudo M, Todo A, Ikekubo K, et al: Estimation of hepatic functional preserve by asialoglycoprotein receptor-binding radiolabeled synthetic ligand technetium-99m galactosylneoglycoalbumin: Preclinical and clinical studies. Jpn J Nucl Med 24:1653, 1987.
4. Peng CT: Radiopaques, in Wolff ME (ed): Burger's Medicinal Chemistry, 4th ed. New York, Wiley, 1981.
5. Foley WD: Agents in computed tomography, in Skucas J (ed): Radiographic Contrast Agents, 2d ed. Rockville, Md, Aspen, 1989.
6. Stark DD: Liver, in Stark DD, Bradley WG (eds): Magnetic Resonance Imaging. St. Louis, Mosby, 1988.
7. Lauffer RB: Hepatobiliary agents, in Runge VM (ed): Enhanced Magnetic Resonance Imaging. St. Louis, Mosby, 1989.
8. Klaveness J: Particulate agents, in Runge VM (ed): Enhanced Magnetic Resonance Imaging. St. Louis, Mosby, 1989.
9. Josephson L, Groman EV, Lewis JM, et al: A Hepatic Specific Superparamagnetic Iron Oxide Liver Imaging. Presented at Current Trends in MRI, CT and US, International Symposium, Boston 1990.
10. Stark DD, Weissleder R, Elizondo G, et al: Superparamagnetic iron oxide: Clinical application as a contrast agent for MR imaging of the liver. Radiology 168:297, 1988.
11. Wolf GL: Current status of MR contrast agents: Special report. Radiology 172:709, 1989.
12. Fahlvik AK, Holtz E, Leander P, et al: Magnetic starch microspheres: Efficacy and elimination. Invest Radiol 25:113, 1990.
13. Mosmann T: Rapid colorimetric assay for cellular growth and survival: Application to proliferation and cytotoxicity assays. J Immunol Methods 65:55, 1983.
14. Gillis P, Koenig S: Transverse relaxation of solvent protones induced by magnetized spheres: Application to ferritin, erythrocytes and magnetite. Magn Reson Med 5:323, 1987.
15. Josephson L, Lewis P, Hahn PF, Stark DD: The effect of iron oxides on proton relaxivity. Magn Reson Imaging 6:647, 1988.
16. Majumdar S, Zoghbi S, Pope CF, Gore JC: A quantitative study of relaxation rate enhancement produced by iron oxide particles in polyacrylamide gels and tissue. Magn Reson Med 9:185, 1989.
17. Fahlvik AK, Holtz E, Klaveness J: Relaxation efficacy of paramagnetic and superparamagnetic microspheres in liver and spleen. Magn Reson Imaging 8:363, 1990.
18. Fahlvik AK, Holtz E, Schrøder U, Klaveness J: Magnetic starch microspheres: Biodistribution and biotransformation. Invest Radiol 25:793, 1990.
19. Weissleder R, Stark DD, Engelstad BL, et al: Superparamagnetic iron oxide; Pharmacokinetics and toxicity. AJR 152:167, 1989.
20. Fahlvik AK, Artursson P, Edman P: Magnetic starch microspheres: Interactions of a microsphere MR contrast medium with macrophages in vitro. Int J Pharmaceutics (in press).

Index

Abdomen
  bolus-enhanced dynamic CT survey, 30–31, 36–37
  fast-scan MRI of, 106–107, 109, 112–113
  FLASH MR scan of, 106–111
  low-field MRI of, 59–62
  manganese dipyridoxyl diphosphate (Mn-DPDP), 374
Adenocarcinoma, 20, 54, 232, 427
Adenoma
  angiography of, 146
  bile duct, 187–188, 219
  biliary cystadenoma, 185, 187–188
  CT findings, 146
  cystadenoma, 220
  hemangiomas and, 139
  hepatoadenoma, 220
  hepatocellular, 142–145, 184–186
  mixed. *See* Focal nodular hyperplasia
  MRI, 147
  scintigraphy-angiographic correlation, 145
  three-dimensional T1-weighted MP-RAGE imaging of, 134
Adrenal infarction, 287
Adrenal metastasis
  CT of, 74
  MRI of, 74
Angiography. *See also* Computed tomography angiography (CT-A) and Magnetic resonance angiography (MRA)
  adenoma, 146
  Budd-Chiari syndrome, 265–266
  CT-A and, 32–34
  delayed iodine screening (DIS) and, 34–36, 241–243
  focal nodular hyperplasia, 143, 179–189
  hepatocellular adenoma, 150, 184
  liver, 7, 31–37, 139
  scintigraphic correlation of adenomas, 145

Bile Duct
  adenoma, characteristics, 187–188, 219
  anatomy, 251
  biloma, 287
  carcinoma, 281
  leak at anastomosis, 285
  liver transplantation and, 284
  necrosis, 286
Biliary cystadenoma
  characteristics of, 187
  detection of by CT and sonography, 187–188
  incidence of, 185, 187
Bolus-enhanced dynamic CT (BDCT)
  abdominal survey, 30–31, 36–37
  breast carcinoma, 45, 94, 360, 420–421, 423
  cavernous hemangioma, 191–195
  colonic carcinoma and, 6, 31–33, 174
  compared to high-field MRI, 45–47
  fatty liver, 103
  lesion detection, 31, 35–37, 76
  metastatic neoplasm, 31
  primary neoplasm, 31
Breast carcinoma
  low-field MRI, 60
  metastatic (MRI and dynamic bolus-enhanced CT), 45, 94, 360, 420–421, 423
  midfield MRI, 60
  STIR imaging of, 88
Budd-Chiari syndrome
  angiography, 265–266
  clinical features, 260–261
  color flow Doppler, 261–262
  computed tomography (CT), 262–263
  dynamic CT, 263
  hepatic venocclusive disease, 260
  hepatic venogram, 266
  IVC obstruction and, 260–261
  mesoatrial shunt MRI, 266
  MRI, 264–265
  pulsed Doppler, 262
  ^{99m}Tc-scintigraphy, 263
  therapy, use of imaging techniques, 265–267
  ultrasound, 261

431

Carcinomas
  bile duct, 281
  breast, 45, 60, 88, 94, 360, 420–421, 423
  cholangiocarcinoma, 170–173, 221
  colonic metastases, 6, 9, 42, 68, 89, 252, 254, 311, 341, 361, 408
  cystadenocarcinoma, 221
  fibrolamellar, 148–151
  gallbladder, 173
  hepatocellular. See Hepatocellular carcinoma
  liver, 196–197
  lung, metastases to liver, 61
  pancreas, 116
  renal cell, 409
  Walker's, 391
Cavernous hemangioma. See Hemangiomas
  CT-enhanced imaging of, 192
Chemical shift imaging
  CT lesion detection and, 19–27, 92, 94
  fatty infiltration of, versus spin-echo (SE) and inversion-recovery (IR) techniques, 91
  limitations, 95
  neoplasms, 92–94
  proton-spectroscopic imaging, 91–92
  superparamagnetic perfusion, 336–337
  Ultrafast MRI and, 115
Cholangioadenoma. See Bile duct adenoma
Cholangiocarcinoma, 170–171, 173, 221
Cholangioma, benign. See Bile duct adenoma
Cirrhosis
  characteristics, 172, 308–309
  CT detection and, 172, 308–312
  detection by CT during hepatic arteriography (CT-HA), 240
  Doppler ultrasound (US), 271, 272
  hepatocellular carcinoma and, 172
  MRI detection and, 309–312
  ^{31}P MRS of, 300–301
  regenerating nodules, 308–311
  superparamagnetic iron oxide (SPIO)–enhanced MRI, 412–414
  ultrasound detection and, 309–312
Colon
  adenocarcinoma, 20, 54, 232, 427
  carcinoma of
    bolus CT and, 6, 31–33, 174
    colorectal, 1–2, 5, 68,
    metastases, 6, 31–34, 42, 68, 89, 170–171, 174, 175, 252, 254, 311, 361, 341, 408
Color Doppler flow mapping
  Budd-Chiari syndrome, 261–262
  cavernous hemangioma, 191
  cirrhosis, 271, 272
  focal liver lesions
    conventional identification, 209
    Doppler ultrasonographic features, 210–211
    principles of tissue characterization, 209–210
  hepatic veins, 262, 271
  hepatitis. See Hepatitis
  liver transplantation and, 283–285, 286

portal hypertension
  characteristics of blood flow and its disturbances, 271–272
  collateral pathways, 271
  hemodynamic data, 269
  portosystemic surgical shunts, 273–274
  quantitative measurement of blood flow, 272–273
  reversal of flow in the portal venous system, 270
  thrombosis of the portal venous system, 269–270
Computed tomography (CT). See also Bolus-enhanced dynamic CT, Computed tomography angiography, Computed tomography during arterial portography, Delayed iodine scanning, Delayed scanning CT, Rapid dynamic nonincremental CT
  adenoma, 146
  adrenal metastases, 74
  biliary cystadenoma, 187–188
  body iron stores and, 317, 320–321
  Budd-Chiari syndrome, 262–263
  cavernous hemangiomas, 191
  cirrhosis detection, 172, 240, 308–312
  compared to conventional sonography, 6
  compared to CTAP, 8
  compared to MRI techniques, 6, 7, 8–13, 43–45, 55–56, 65–71, 74–80
  delayed CT (DCT), 54, 64–71
  delayed iodine screening (DIS) applications, 30, 32, 34, 36
  dynamic incremental bolus techniques, 6, 7, 54
  EOE-CT, 64, 65–71
  HCC. See Hepatocellular carcinoma
  hemangiomas. See Hemangiomas
  hepatocellular adenoma. See Hepatocellular adenoma
  Hodgkin's lymphoma, 117
  limitations, 53–54
  liver transplantation. See Transplantation of the liver
  Noncontrast CT (NCT), 64–71
  particulate biodegradable contrast medium for, 395–397
  volumetrics. See Volumetrics, hepatic lesions
  water-soluble contrast material–enhanced CT (WS-CT), 64–65
Computed tomography angiography (CT-A)
  fatty liver detection, 306–308
  fibrolamellar carcinoma, 150–151
  subsecond dynamic, 170–176
    cholangiocarcinoma, 170–171, 173, 221
    FNH. See Focal nodular hyperplasia
    gallbladder carcinoma, 170–171, 173
    HCC. See Hepatocellular carcinoma
    hepatic angiography, 32–36
    hepatic tumors, 238, 242
    metastases, 36, 170–171, 174, 175
Computed tomography during arterial portography (CTAP or AP-CT)
  colon metastases and, 7–8, 32–33
  compared to CT, 8

compared to MRI, 6, 67–71
hepatic angiography, 32–37, 241
lesion detection versus MRI, 80
liver metastases and, 8
resections and, 237–244
Contrast agents
    clinical applications
        particles, 334
        soluble complexes, 333
    design principles
        diamagnetic materials, 326–327
        ferromagnetic particles, 327–328
        paramagnetism, 327
        superparamagnetic materials, 327
    distribution in the liver, 330
    gastrointestinal contrast agents, 335–337
    pharmacokinetics and biodistribution, 329
        antibody targeting, 331
        phagocytosis, 333
        receptor targeting, 331–333
        vascular contrast agents, 329
    particulate biodegradable contrast medium for CT, 395–397
    proton relaxation enhancement
        particulate agents, 328–329
        soluble agents, 328
    reticuloendothelial, 47
    toxicity of IV MRI contrast media, 334–335
Conventional sonography, 6, 209
Cystadenocarcinoma, 221
Cystadenoma, 220

Delayed iodine scanning (DIS)
    colonic metastases, 32, 36–37
    compared to MRI, 30, 32, 34, 36
    hepatic angiography, 34–36, 241, 242
    lesion detection, 76
    tumor nodule detection versus BDCT, 36
Delayed scanning CT (DS-CT), compared to MRI, 64–71

EOE-CT, 64, 65–71
Ernst angle, 43

Fast-scan MRI
    central nervous system and abdomen, 105–113
        CE-FAST sequence, 106
        compared to high-field MRI, 43–45
        comparison of techniques, 106, 108
        FLASH, 106–111
        plausability of high-speed MRI of the abdomen, 112–113
        single-breath-hold FLASH, 107–108, 110, 111
        strategies for abdominal imaging, 110–112
Fatty liver
    anatomic distribution of fat, 306–308
    CT detection and, 306–308
    chemical-shift imaging, 91
    dynamic bolus tracking, 103
    lobular infiltration, 93–94

MRI detection and, 306–308
normal versus, 93
ultrasound, 306–308
Ferrite particles (midfield MRI)
    clinical results, 408–410
    effects at MRI, 407–408
    human toxicity, 406–407
    superparamagnetic iron oxide
        physical properties, 403–404
        physiologic considerations, 404–406
Fibrolamellar carcinoma (FLC), 148–151
    characteristics, 148–150
    detection of, MRI and CT, 150–151
    incidence, 148
FLASH MRI. *See* Fast-scan MRI
Fluoroscopic MRI, 119–127
    continuous MRI fluoroscopy, 123, 124
    continuous snapshot MRI, 126
    data acquisition, 119–121
    echo-planar imaging, 119–120
    first-in, first-out (FIFO) memory, 121
    modifications for interactive MRI, 123
    reconstruction, 121–123
    snapshot MRI, 123–126
    spleen, 125
Focal cirrhosis. *See* Cirrhosis and Focal nodular hyperplasia
Focal fat
    breast, 4
    liver, 308
Focal lesion detection
    CT compared to MRI, 73–80,
    CT compared to proton spectroscopic imaging, 92, 94
Focal nodular hyperplasia
    angiography of, 143, 179–189
    color Doppler imaging, 209–211
    detection of, MRI and CT, 139–144, 180
    dynamic CT of, 180
    hepatocellular adenoma (HA or HCA), 142–145, 181–185
    incidence, 138, 177–179, 220
    MRI detection of, 180–182
    pathologic imaging, 141, 144
    scintigraphy, 180, 181
    surgery, 220
    volumetrics and, 257–258

Gadolinium-DTPA (Gd-DTPA)–enhanced MRI
    cavernous hemangiomas and, 12–13, 167, 191, 197–198, 199
    cerebral MRI, 45
    conventional lesion characterization, 341–342, 343
    conventional lesion detection, 340–341
    current clinical role, 346–347
    dynamic MP-RAGE imaging of the liver and, 131–134
    fast-imaging of lesions, 342–346
    focal lesions MRI, 45
    future prospects, 347

Gadolinium-DTPA (Gd-DTPA)–enhanced MRI
    (continued)
    HCC. *See* Hepatocellular carcinoma
    hepatic tumor detection and, 159–160
    hepatitis. *See* Hepatitis
    rapid-acquisition spin-echo (RASE) technique
        clinical application, 362–363
        limitations and refinements, 362
        motion suppression: prior techniques, 358–359
        principles, 359–362
        results, 363
Gallbladder
    anatomy, 251
    carcinoma of, 173
    CT angiography (CT-A) of, 170–171
Gaussian curves, 256–257
Gd-BOPTA. *See* Hepatobiliary agents for MRI
Gd-DOTA meglumine
    characteristics of
        pharmacokinetic properties, 350
        physiochemical properties, 349–350
    clinical experience with
        biological safety of, 350
        diagnostic efficacy, 351
        overall safety of, 351
    MRI examinations of the liver
        diagnostic potential of Gd-DOTA, 352–353
        parameters, 352
    results and discussion
        diagnostic contribution of Gd-DOTA, 353–355
        fast versus conventional imaging sequences, 353
        role of administered dose, 353
Gradient-moment nulling, 40–42
GRASS techniques. *See* Fast-scan MRI

Hemangiomas
    adenomas and, 146
    benign
        characteristics of, 138, 213–216
        contrast-enhanced CT of, 117
        CT versus MRI, 137–146
        MRI of, 99, 100, 202, 343–345
        single-photon-emission CT (SPECT) imaging of, 205
        T1- and T2-weighted MP-RAGE images, 133
        ultrafast MRI, 117
    cavernous
        Bolus infusion CT and, 191–195
        color flow Doppler sonography, 191
        CT and, 11–12, 191, 192
        CT compared to MRI, 198–200
        diagnosis by rapid dynamic nonincremental CT. *See* Rapid dynamic nonincremental CT
        Gd-DTPA–enhanced MRI, 12, 167, 191, 197–199
        hemangiomasarcoma, 203
        hepatic abcess, 254
        incidence of, 2, 190
        liver, 2
        lungs, 3
        MRI and, 2, 3, 12–13, 194–198, 204–206
        pathology of, 2, 3, 190–191, 220
        snap-shot ultrafast MRI, 16

differentiation of, from metastases and cysts, 153–158
    malignant
        fibrolamellar carcinoma, 148–151
        hepatocellular carcinoma (HCC). *See* Hepatocellular carcinoma
        retroperitoneal metastases by MRI, 12
    surgery and, 220
    versus metastases, 193
Hepatic artery, 284
Hepatic encephalopathy
    MRI, 303, 304
    ^{31}P spectroscopic imaging, 303
Hepatic hamartoma. *See* Focal nodular hyperplasia
Hepatic metastases, 41, 46, 116, 132, 133, 135
    amorphous sign, 155
    changed morphology sign, 157
    doughnut sign, 154
    halo sign, 155
    hemochromatosis, 416
    lightbulb sign, 156
    splenic tumor nodules, 411
    superparamagnetic iron oxide (SPIO) and, 410
    target sign, 154
Hepatic resections, 234–235
    anatomy of portal and hepatic veins, 224–230
    cross-sectional imaging with US, MRI, and CT, 223–224, 232–233
    resectability of lesions, 233–234
    surgical techniques, 223, 230–232
Hepatic surgery
    anatomy, 218
    biopsy examination, 219
    cholangioadenomas, 219–220
    cholangiocarcinoma, 221
    cystadenocarcinoma, 221
    cystadenoma, 220
    diagnostic imaging, 219
    exposure for, 219
    focal nodular hyperplasia, 220
    hemangiomas, 220
    hepatoadenoma, 220
    hepatocellular carcinoma, 220–221
    issues of, 218
    metastases, 221–222
    nomenclature, 218–219
    sarcoma, 221
Hepatic veins
    anatomy, 224–230, 256
    Doppler ultrasound, 262, 271
Hepatic venocclusive disease, 260
Hepatic venogram, 266
Hepatitis
    CT detection and, 306, 307
    Doppler ultrasound, 271–272
    Gd-DTPA, 307
    MRI detection and, 306, 307
    superparamagnetic iron oxide (SPIO)–enhanced MRI detection of, 412–414
Hepatoadenoma, 220
Hepatobiliary agents for MRI
    compared with established media, 366–367, 384

comparison with other agents, 370–372
design criteria, 385
diagnostic medicine and, 366
Gd-BOPTA/Dimeg
  in vivo relaxation times and relaxivities, 389–390
  liver/tumor CNR and relaxation-rate
    enhancement, 389, 390
  MRI signal-intensity enhancement kinetics,
    388–389
  pharmacokinetics, 387–388
  physicochemical properties, 386–387
  pulse sequence influence, 390–392
iron-EHPG–enhanced MRI of liver metastases,
  368–369, 370, 371
iron-EHPG, the prototype, 367–368
manganese dipyridoxyl diphosphate (Mn-DPDP),
    development
  conclusions, 379–382
  efficacy results, 379, 380, 381
  materials and methods, 378
  Mn-DPDP, 375
  preclinical evaluation, 375–377
  safety results, 378–379
  upper abdomen and, 374
other candidates for, 369–370
potential liver MRI contrast agents, 365–366
prototype agents in development, 385–386
Hepatocellular adenoma, 142–145, 181–185
  angiography of, 150, 184
  characteristics of, 183–184, 220–221
  detection of, by CT and MRI, 142–145, 184–185, 186
  dynamic CT scan, 184–185
  focal nodular hyperplasia (FNH) and, 142–145,
    184–185
  incidence, 142, 181
Hepatocellular carcinoma (HCC), 1–2, 146–151
  characteristics of, 13, 146–147
  cirrhosis, 172
  Color Doppler flow mapping, 210–211
  colorectal liver metastases and, 1–2, 5
  CT angiography (CT-A) scan and, 34, 170–173
  CT detection and, 13, 147, 149, 150
  dynamic study, CT and MRI, 166–168
  Gd-DTPA, 346
  macroscopic classification, MRI and CT, 162–163
  microscopic classification, MRI and CT, 163
  MRI detection and, 13, 15, 146–148, 199, 265, 346
  nodular, 150
  secondary changes, and MRI, 163–166
  surgery, 220–221
  ^{99m}Tc-labeled RBC-SPECT imaging, 202–203
  tumor-like conditions, 168–169
  ultralow-field MRI, 59
Hepatomas
  diffuse hepatoma, 162
  hyperdense, 166
  massive, 163
  nodular, 164, 165–166
  pseudoglandular, 165, 167–168
High-field MRI
  adrenal mass characterization, 47
  compared to CT techniques, 45–47

compared to midfield MRI, 45
fast-scan techniques, 43–45
gradient-moment nulling (GMN), 40, 41, 42
iron oxide and
  detection of liver metastases, 418–423
  imaging parameters and timing at 1.5 Tesla,
    417–418
  pharmacology of ferrites, 415–416
lesion characterization, 39–41
respiratory-sorted phase encoding, 40, 41
reticuloendothelial contrast agents, 47
signal-to-noise ratio (SNR), 39, 45
short TI inversion recovery (STIR), 43
Hodgkin's lymphoma
  CT scan, 117
  ultrafast MRI, 117

Inferior vena cava (IVC)
  liver transplantation and, 284
  metastases and, 5–6
Intraoperative
  sonography (IOS), 6, 7, 8, 9, 187–188
  ultrasonography, 247, 250–254
    anatomy, 249–250, 251–253
    equipment, 247–248
    technical considerations, 248–249
Inversion recovery (IR) 43
  compared to midfield MRI, 50–51
  compared to STIR, 82–83
  techniques, 83
Iron-EHPG–enhanced MRI. *See* Hepatobiliary agents
    for MRI
Iron storage diseases
  detection of iron overload, 314–315
  direct measures of body iron stores
    bone marrow biopsy, 317
    liver biopsy, 316
    quantitative phlebotomy, 317
  hereditary (genetic) hemochromatosis, 313–314
  indirect measures of body iron stores
    chelator-induced urinary iron excretion, 316
    intestinal iron absorption, 316
    serum ferritin, 315
    transferrin saturation, 315
  physical methods
    CT, 317, 320–321
    dual-energy technique, 317
    IVC obstruction and, 260–261
    magnetic susceptibility measurements (by
      SQUID), 317–318
    MRI, 318–320
    MRS, 318
    nuclear resonant scattering (NRS), of gamma
      rays, 317
    secondary (acquired) hemochromatosis, 314
    single-energy technique, 317
    treatment and prognosis of iron storage diseases,
      321–323

Lesions of the liver
  arterial portography CT (AP-CT) versus MRI
    detection of, 8, 67–71

Lesions of the liver (continued)
bolus-enhanced dynamic CT (BDCT) detection of, 31, 35–37, 76, 78
color Doppler flow mapping of. See Color Doppler flow mapping
CT-A detection of, 80, 239, 244
CT detection of, 19–27, 92, 94
delayed iodine screening (DIS-CT), 76
DS-CT versus MRI detection of, 67–71
EOE-CT versus MRI detection of, 64–71
Gd-DTPA, 340–347
metastatic renal cell carcinoma, 409
midfield MRI, 49–50, 54
MRI detection of, 10, 19–27, 64–71, 76, 78, 80
MRS, 298–305
resectability, 233–234
ultralow-field MRI, 59–61
volumetrics, 256–259

Liver
angiography of, 7, 32–37, 139
BDCT. See Bolus-enhanced dynamic CT
benign tumors of, 177–189
biliary cystadenoma. See Biliary cystadenoma
carcinoma, 196–197
cirrhosis. See Cirrhosis
color Doppler flow mapping of lesions. See Color Doppler flow mapping
contrast agents. See Contrast agents
CT angiography (CT-A), 29–30, 34, 170–175, 238–242
CT appearance of, 2, 4, 8–9
CT compared to MRI of metastases, 78–79, 86, 88, 89, 153–160
CT during arterial portography (CTAP) of, 6–8, 29–30, 32, 37, 80, 238–239, 241
delayed iodine screening (DIS), 29, 32, 34–36, 76, 241, 242
fatty. See Fatty liver
FNH. See Focal nodular hyperplasia
focal fat, 308
focal lesion detection, 73–80, 92, 94. See also Lesions of the liver
Gd-DPTA. See Gadolinium-DPTA–enhanced MRI
high-field MRI and, 39–48, 415–423
intraoperative sonography (IOS), 6–9, 187–188
lesions. See Lesions of the liver
midfield MRI of, 49–57
MP-RAGE imaging of, 128–136
MRI appearance of, 3, 7
MRI compared to EOE-CT, 64–71
MRS. See Magnetic resonance spectroscopy
paraumbilical vein, 311
^{31}P spectroscopic image, 293
scintigraphy of, 7, 14–15
surgery of. See Hepatic surgery
surgical anatomy of, 5, 6
surgical versus medical metastatic disease, 7
tasks of imaging, 3, 5
tissue characterization, 14
transplantation. See Transplantation of the liver
tumors of, 75, 252, 253, 279
tumor volumetrics. See Volumetrics, hepatic lesions

Magnetic resonance angiography (MRA) of hepatic vein and portal system
case reports, 280–281, 282
discussion, 281–282
materials and methods, 277, 278
results, 277–280

Magnetic resonance imaging (MRI). See also Fluoroscopic MRI, Gadolinium-DTPA–enhanced MRI, High-field MRI, Magnetic resonance angiography, Magnetic resonance spectroscopy, Magnetization-prepared rapid gradient-echo MRI, Midfield MRI, Short TI inversion recovery MRI, Steady-state MRI, Ultrafast MRI, Ultralow-field MRI
adenomas, 147
adrenal metastases, 74
artifacts, 21, 22, 24, 25
body iron stores, 318–320
breast carcinoma detection, 45, 94, 360, 420–421, 423
Budd-Chiari syndrome, 264–265
chemical shift imaging. See Chemical shift imaging
cirrhosis, 308–312
compared to conventional sonography, 6
compared to CT, 6–7, 8–13, 65–71, 74–80
compared to CTAP, 8–9, 67–71
differentiation of hemangiomas and metastases, 13
fatty liver, 306–308
fibrolamellar carcinoma, 150–151
FNH. See Focal nodular hyperplasia
gadolinium and, 12, 13
hemangiomas. See Hemangiomas
hepatic echo-planar MRI, 115–117
hepatic encephalopathy, 303–304
hepatitis. See Hepatitis
hepatobiliary agents for. See Hepatobiliary agents for MRI
iron-EHPG–enhanced MRI. See Hepatobiliary agents for MRI
liver, appearance of, 3, 6, 7
liver transplantation and, 84, 86
mesoatrial shunts, 266
modified echo-planar technique, 16
noise, 20–22
paraumbilical vein, 311
real-time MRI image reconstruction, 122
regenerating nodules, 310, 311
reticuloendothelial MRI contrast agent, 406–407, 425–429
retroperitoneal metastases, 12
signal-to-noise ratio, 20
^{99m}Tc-labeled RBC-SPECT, 206–208
volumetrics and, 258–259

Magnetic resonance spectroscopy (MRS)
body iron stores, 318
hepatic encephalopathy, 298–305
control of intrahepatic [ATP], 302–303
diagnostic precision of ^{31}P MRS of the liver, 300, 301, 302
energy metabolism, 304
failure of urea synthesis, 301–302
"free" intrahepatic ADP concentration, 300

MRI techniques in, 304
neurotransmitter function, 304–305
normal ^{31}P MRS of human liver, 299–300
pathology, 300
phospholipid composition, 304
^{31}P MRS of cirrhosis, 300–301
quantification and pH determination, 298–299
RF-spoiling and, 101
of the liver, 289–295
alcoholic disease, 292–294
localized, 290
magnetic resonance spectroscopic imaging (MRSI or SI), 290–291
metabolic pathways, 290
metastases, 294–295
normal liver, 292
previous clinical studies, 291
quantitative clinical ^{31}P MRS, 291–292
viral hepatitis B, 294
Magnetization-prepared rapid gradient-echo (MP-RAGE) MRI, 128–136
dynamic MP-RAGE imaging of the liver, 131
gadolinium-DTPA and, 131–134
hemangiomas, 133
pulse sequences, 128–130
three-dimensional MP-RAGE imaging of the liver, 134–135
two-dimensional MP-RAGE imaging of the liver, 130–131, 132, 133
Metastases
differentiation of, from hemangiomas and cysts
combined T1- and T2-weighted pulse sequences, 155–157
morphologic criteria, 153–154, 221–222
quantitative criteria, 157–158
T1-weighted pulse sequence, 154
T2-weighted pulse sequence, 154–155
differentiation of, from primary hepatic tumors
morphologic criteria, 158–159
quantitative criteria, 159
intravenous contrast enhancement, 159–160
melanoma, 159
neoplasms, 31
splenic, 86–87, 410
surgery, 221–222
surgical versus medical disease, 5–6, 7
ultralow-field MRI, 59
vascular, 100
Midfield MRI
breast carcinoma, 60
compared to high-field MRI, 45
contrast-to-noise ratio (CNR), 49, 51, 53
CT compared to, 55–56
ferrite particles. *See* Ferrite particles
gradient-echo imaging, 52
inversion recovery (IR) compared to short TR/short TE-spin echo sequence, 50–51
lesion detection, 49–50, 54
phase-contrast imaging, 52–53
timing parameters, 51–52
tissue contrast, 49–50

Mn-DPDP. *See* Hepatobiliary agents for MRI

Neoplasms, 31
Nodular regenerative hyperplasia (NRH) or nodular transformation, 145–146
detection, 146, 148
incidence of, 145
Noise, 21–22, 50–51
contrast-to-noise ratio (CNR), 50–51, 53
ferrite-enhancement, 418
flip-angle, 101
signal-to-noise ratio (SNR), 39, 45, 54, 101
Noncontrast CT (NCT), compared to MRI, 64–71

Pancreas, carcinoma of, 116
Particulate biodegradable contrast medium for CT of the liver
materials and methods, 395–397
results, 397–401
Paraumbilical vein, 311
Portal vein,
anatomy, 224–230, 250
aneurysm, 282
CT during hepatic arteriography (CT-HA), 239
Doppler ultrasound (US), 271–273
hypertension. *See* Color Doppler flow mapping
metastases and, 5–6
magnetic resonance angiography (MRA) of, 277–282
MRI fluoroscopy, 124
thrombosis of, 285
transplantation of the liver and, 284
Proton spectroscopic imaging
chemical-shift imaging, 91–92
focal lesion detection and, 92, 94
^{31}P spectroscopic imaging
cirrhosis, 300–301
hepatic encephalopathy, 303
normal liver, 299–300
of the liver, 393
precision, 300–302

Rapid dynamic nonincremental CT
cavernous hemangiomas
incidence, 212–213
results, 213–216
RASE technique. *See* Gadolinium-DTPA–enhanced MRI
Regenerating nodules
cirrhosis and, 308–311
CT, 309
gradient-echo FLASH, 309
MRI, 310, 311
Renal cell carcinoma, 409
Resections
determining by CT-angiography, CT-HA or CT-AP
comparison of other imaging modalities, 239–243
incidence, 237–238
pitfalls, 244–245

Resections (*continued*)
   segmental localization, 243–244
   technique, 238–239
Reticuloendothelial MRI contrast agent
   superparamagnetic iron oxide (SPIO) particles
      cirrhosis detection, 412–414
      effects, 407
      enhanced MRI and, 410–412
      hepatic metastases, 410
      liver tissue, 406
      splenic tissue, 411
   superparamagnetic starch microspheres
      materials and methods, 425–426
      results and discussion, 426–428
      summary, 428–429

Sarcoma, 221
Scintigraphy
   angiographic correlation of adenomas, 145
   focal nodular hyperplasia, 180, 181
   of the liver, 7, 14–15
Serial carcinoembryonic antigen assays, 2
Short TI inversion recovery MRI (STIR)
   breast carcinomas, 88
   clinical use, 89–90
   compared to traditional inversion recovery, 82
   high-field MRI, 43
   limitations, 89
   physics, 82
   sensitivity and lesion conspicuity, 52, 85–88
   technique, 83–85
   volume of abnormality, 88–89
Shunts
   mesoatrial by MRI, 266
   portosystemic, 273–274
Sonography
   biliary cystadenoma, 187–188
Spleen
   conventional detection of, 410
   fluoroscopic imaging, 125
   imaging enhanced by SPIO, 411
   malignant splenomegaly, 412
   metastases, 86–87, 410
   superparamagnetic iron oxide (SPIO)–enhanced MRI, 410–412
Steady-state MRI
   artifacts, 98
   contrast, 98–102
   dynamic bolus tracking and, 101, 103
   FISP, 97
   FLASH and Turbo FLASH sequence, 97–98
   GRASS and Turbo GRASS sequence, 96–98
   vein thrombosis MRI, 102
Superparamagnetic iron oxide (SPIO) particles. *See* Reticuloendothelial MRI contrast agent

^{99m}Tc-labeled RBC-SPECT imaging of hemangiomas
   comparison of MRI SE sequences and, 206–208
   hemangiosarcomas, 203
   hepatocellular carcinoma, 202–203
   labeled RBC SPECT imaging, 202–204
   paraumbilical vein, 311
   single-photon-emission CT (SPECT) technique, 201–202
Transplantation of the liver
   color and pulsed Doppler imaging, 283, 285, 286
   complications
      biliary complications, 284–285, 286
      fluid collections, 285–286
      hepatic artery thrombosis, 285
      interventional radiology, 287
      miscellaneous vascular complications, 285
      other complications, 286–287
      portal vein thrombosis, 285
      rejection, 286
      vascular complications, 285
   CT imaging and, 283, 285, 286
   MRI, T1- and T2-weighted imaging, 84, 86
   postoperative considerations, 284
      anatomy, 284
      bile duct, 284
      hepatic artery, 284
      inferior vena cava, 284
      portal vein, 284
   preoperative evaluation, 283–284

Ultrafast MRI, 114–118
   chemical shift, 115
   hepatic echo-planar MRI, 115–117
   Hodgkin's lymphoma, 117
   spatial resolution, 114–115
   three-dimensional imaging, 115
   tissue contrast, compared to spin-echo (SE), gradient-echo (GE), and inversion-recovery (IR), 115
Ultralow-field MRI
   breast carcinoma, 60
   clinical applications in the abdomen and liver, 59–62
   hemangiomas, 117
   hepatocellular carcinomas, 59
   lesions, 59–61
   metastases, 59
   technical and logistical considerations, 58–59
Ultrasound
   Budd-Chiari syndrome, 261
   cirrhosis, 308–312
   fatty liver, 306–308
   intraoperative, 247, 250–251

Volumetrics, hepatic lesions
   three-dimensional reconstructions, 256–258
      focal nodular hyperplasia, 257–258
      Gaussian curves, 256–257
      materials and methods, 256–257
      MRI data and, 258–259
      results and discussion, 257–259

Walker carcinoma, 391
Water-soluble contrast material-enhanced CT, 64, 65